DRGs diagnosis-related groups
DSM-IV-TR *Diagnostic and Statistical Manual of Mental Disorders, Fourth Revision, Text Revision*
DICOM Digital Imaging and Communication in Medicine
DM disease management
EDI electronic data interchange
EDMS electronic data management system
ED/CM electronic document/content management
EHR electronic health record
EMR electronic medical record
EMAR electronic medication administration record
e-Rx electronic prescribing
ERA electronic remittance advice
ESA electronic signature authentication
EMIC Emergency Maternal and Infant Care Program
EOC episode-of-care reimbursement
EPA Equal Pay Act of 1963
EMDS Essential Medical Data Set
EPO exclusive provider organization
EIS executive information system
EOB Explanation of Benefits
XML extensible markup language
FLSA Fair Labor Standards Act of 1938
FECA Federal Employees' Compensation Act
FI fiscal intermediary
FDA Food and Drug Administration
GPCI geographic practice cost index
GUI graphical user interface
GPWW group practice without walls
HCQIP Health Care Quality Improvement Program
HIE health information exchange
HIM health information management
HIT health information technology
HIPAA Health Insurance Portability and Accountability Act of 1996
HL7 Health Level Seven
HMO health maintenance organization
HEDIS Health Plan Employer Data and Information Set

HSAs health savings accounts
HAS health systems agency
HCPCS Healthcare Common Procedure Coding System
HPD healthcare provider dimension
HAVEN Home Assessment Validation and Entry
HHA home health agency
HH PPS home health prospective payment system
HHRG home health resource group
HIS hospital information system
IPA independent practice association
IHS Indian Health Service
IS information system
IT information technology
IPF inpatient psychiatric facility
IRF inpatient rehabilitation facility
IRVEN Inpatient Rehabilitation Validation and Entry
IEEE Institute of Electrical and Electronics Engineers
IOM Institute of Medicine
IDN integrated delivery network
IDS integrated delivery system
IPO integrated provider organization
ICD-O-3 *International Classification of Diseases for Oncology, Third Edition*
ICD-9-CM *International Classification of Diseases, Ninth Revision, Clinical Modification*
ICD-10-CM *International Classification of Diseases, Tenth Revision, Clinical Modification*
ICD-10-PCS *International Classification of Diseases, Tenth Revision, Procedure Coding System*
IP internet protocol
JCAHO Joint Commission on Accreditation of Healthcare Organizations
KMS knowledge management system
LOS length of stay
LAN local area network
LTCH long-term care hospital
LUPA low-utilization payment adjustment

Health Information Management Technology

An Applied Approach

Second Edition

Merida L. Johns, PhD, RHIA

Editor

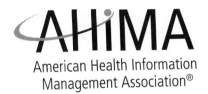

AHIMA
American Health Information
Management Association®

The Web sites listed in this book were current and valid as of the date of publication. However, Web page addresses and the information on them may change or disappear at any time and for any number of reasons. The user is encouraged to perform his or her own general Web searches to locate any site addresses listed here that are no longer valid. Web sites listed in this book are assumed to be preceded by http://www.

Please note: The Joint Commission on Accreditation of Healthcare Organizations (JCAHO) recently launched a new brand identity and is now officially called The Joint Commission. References to JCAHO remain in this edition.

ISBN 1-58426-141-2
AHIMA Product Number AB103106

AHIMA Staff:
    Claire Blondeau, MBA, Project Editor
    June E. Bronnert, RHIA, CCS, CCS-P
    Jill Burrington-Brown, MS, RHIA, FAHIMA
    Melanie A. Endicott, MBA/HCM, RHIA, CCS
    Beth Hjort, RHIA, CHPS
    Susan Hull, MPH, RHIA, CCS, CCS-P
    Karen Kostick, RHIT, CCS, CCS-P
    Elizabeth Lund, Assistant Editor
    Carol Ann Quinsey, RHIA, CHPS
    Rita A. Scichilone, MHSA, RHIA, CCS, CCS-P, CHC
    Mary H. Stanfill, RHIA, CCS, CCS-P
    Melissa Ulbricht, Editorial/Production Coordinator
    Ann Zeisset, RHIT, CCS-P, CCS
    Ken Zielske, Director of Publications

        6   7   8   9   10

American Health Information Management Association
233 North Michigan Avenue, Suite 2150
Chicago, Illinois 60601-5800

ahima.org

Contents

About the Editor and Authors

Merida L. Johns, PhD, RHIA, is president of Holistic Training Solutions, a management and education consulting firm, and is a visiting professor at The College of St. Scholastica. She received undergraduate degrees from Seattle University and graduate degrees from Alfred University and The Ohio State University. Johns was founding director of the HIT program at San Diego Mesa College and later served as director of the HIT program at Alfred State College. She also was a faculty member in the HIM program at The Ohio State University and served as program director for the nontraditional HIT–HIM progression program. In addition, she was founding director of the master's program in health informatics at the University of Alabama at Birmingham and director of the master's in information management program at Loyola University, Chicago. Johns has held numerous local, state, and national professional appointments and offices. In 1990, she received the American Health Information Management Association (AHIMA) Professional Achievement Award. Finally, she served as president of AHIMA in 1997, as a member of the AHIMA Board of Directors from 1996 to 1999, and as vice-president for education and accreditation for AHIMA until 2000.

Margret K. Amatayakul, MBA, RHIA, CHPS, CPHIT, CPEHR, FHIMSS, is president of Margret\A Consulting, LLC, located in Schaumburg, Illinois, a consulting firm specializing in computer-based patient records and associated HIM standards and regulations, such as HIPAA. She has more than thirty years of experience in national and international HIM. She is a leading authority on electronic health record (EHR) strategies for healthcare organizations and has extensive experience in EHR selection and project management. Previously, she formed and served as executive director of the Computer-based Patient Record Institute (CPRI). Other positions held include associate executive director of AHIMA, associate professor at the University of Illinois, and director of medical record services at the Illinois Eye and Ear Infirmary. She is a much-sought-after speaker, has published extensively, and has earned several professional service awards. Amatayakul also serves as an adjunct faculty member of the College of St. Scholastica and the University of Illinois at Chicago.

Elizabeth D. Bowman, MPA, RHIA, is a professor in the HIM program at the University of Tennessee Health Science Center in Memphis. She has been an HIM educator for more than twenty-five years, having received a bachelor's degree from Millsaps College and a master's degree in public administration with a concentration in healthcare administration from the University of Memphis. Bowman has chaired the AHIMA Assembly on Education and received the AHIMA Educator Award in 1999. In addition, she was awarded the Tennessee Health Information Management Association's Distinguished Member Award in 1998.

Bonnie S. Cassidy, MPA, RHIA, FAHIMA, FHIMSS, CPHQ, is president of Cassidy & Associates Consulting. She received a BS degree in medical record administration from Daemen College in Amherst, New York, and a master's degree from Cleveland State University. She is a member of the AHIMA Board of Directors and recently chaired the AHIMA Fellowship Review Committee. In 2005, she was appointed to the Certification Commission for Health Information Technology (CCHIT) Work Group on the Certification Process and in 2006 was selected to serve as a CCHIT Juror. She has held numerous elected and appointed professional positions on local, state, and national levels throughout her career. Her awards include the AHIMA 2000 Legacy Award, AHIMA's 1995 Professional Achievement Award, and the Distinguished Member Award from the Ohio Health Information Management Association (OHIMA), of which she is a past president. Her career has included working as a practitioner for two major teaching hospitals, as a consultant for three professional service companies, as adjunct faculty for two HIT programs, and as vice-president of business development for an HIM-focused consulting company.

Sandra R. Fuller, MA, RHIA, is executive vice-president and chief operating officer at AHIMA. Fuller received a bachelor's degree in health information management and a master's degree in management from the College of St. Scholastica. Formerly director of patient data services at the University of Washington Medical Center in Seattle, she completed her term as a member of AHIMA's Board of Directors at the end of 1996. She also has served on AHIMA's Council on Education and its Alliance and Program committees, and is a past president of the Washington State Health Information Management Association.

Laurinda B. Harman, PhD, RHIA, is an associate professor and chair of the department of health information management at the College of Allied Health Professions at Temple University in Philadelphia. She has been an HIM professional and educator for more than thirty years and has directed HIM baccalaureate programs at George Washington University in Washington, D.C., and The Ohio State University in Columbus. She also has served as director of education and human resource development at George Washington University and as a faculty member in the health information technology program at Northern Virginia Community College. Recently, she was editor of *Ethical Challenges in the Management of Health Information* and received the AHIMA 2001 Triumph Legacy Award for this important health information resource.

Anita C. Hazelwood, MLS, RHIA, FAHIMA, is a professor in the HIM department at the University of Louisiana at Lafayette and has been an HIM professional for nearly thirty years. She is actively involved with AHIMA's Assembly on Education (AOE) and has served on several other AHIMA committees. Hazelwood has held numerous positions with the Louisiana Health Information Management Association, including past president and delegate, and was selected as its 1997 Distinguished Member. She consults in many types of healthcare facilities and educational institutions, and conducts coding workshops for hospitals and physician offices. She has written, coauthored, and edited numerous publications, including *Basic ICD-9-CM for Physician Office Coding* and *ICD-10-CM Preview,* for which she won AHIMA's Legacy Award in 2003. She frequently serves as a reviewer for publishers of HIM-related textbooks and electronic materials.

Cheryl V. Homan, MBA, RHIA, is administrative director of information systems for the Lima Memorial Health System, located in Lima, Ohio. She received her master of business administration from Ashland University in Ashland, Ohio, and her bachelor of science in allied health professions from The Ohio State University. She has been an HIM professional for more than 20 years, served on AHIMA's Board of Directors from 1997 to 1999, and is a former president of the Ohio Health Information Management Association.

Kathleen M. LaTour, MA, RHIA, FAHIMA, is an assistant professor and chair of the department of healthcare informatics and information management (HIIM) at the College of St. Scholastica in Duluth, Minnesota. She is an active member of the Minnesota Health Information Management Association, where she was selected as the Distinguished Member in 1992. She has served as chair and member of many AHIMA councils and as a member of AHIMA's Board of Directors from 1993 to 1997. She participated in the development of the AHIMA Model Curricula for both bachelor's- and master's-level programs. LaTour has authored several articles and is the co-editor of the bachelor's-level textbook *Health Information Management: Concepts, Principles, and Practice,* second edition, a textbook published by AHIMA in 2006. She was awarded fellowship in AHIMA in recognition of sustained contributions to the field of HIM and was corecipient of AHIMA's Legacy Award in 2004.

Frances Wickham Lee, RHIA, DBA, is an associate professor in the department of health administration and policy at the Medical University of South Carolina. She received a master of business administration degree from Western Carolina University and a doctorate in business administration from the University of Sarasota. An active member of AHIMA, she received the Distinguished Member Award from the Mental Health Section of AHIMA in 1995. Lee has authored and coauthored numerous professional articles and publications, and is the coauthor of *Managing Healthcare Information Systems: A Practical Approach for Healthcare Executives.*

Carol E. Osborn, PhD, RHIA, is associate director of coding and compliance at The Ohio State University Medical Center in Columbus. An HIM professional for more than 30 years, she is a former faculty member at both the University of Illinois at Chicago and The Ohio State University. Osborn has served AHIMA at both the state and national levels, participating as state president of AHIMA's Illinois education task force and as a member of both the AHIMA Council on Education and the Item Writing Committee. She is author of *Statistical Applications for Health Information Management* and has written many articles that have appeared in the *Journal of AHIMA* and *Topics in Health Information Management.* She is a former president of the AHIMA Assembly on Education.

Bonnie J. Petterson, PhD, RHIA, is chair of the Health Information Management Department for Phoenix College in Phoenix, Arizona. She holds a PhD in educational leadership and policy studies from Arizona State University, an MS in educational psychology from the University of Wisconsin-Milwaukee, and a BS in health information administration from the University of Wisconsin-Milwaukee. She has been an educator for more than 20 years, serving both the health information administration program at the University of Wisconsin-Milwaukee and the health information technology program at Phoenix College. Previously, she worked in health information management in psychiatric, home health, and acute care hospital settings. Her AHIMA activities include past chair of the Research and AOE Program committees and service on the Educational Strategy, Workforce Research Advisory, and Awards committees. She has served in a variety of roles in state health information associations, including as AHIMA delegate from both Wisconsin and Arizona. Petterson received the mentor award from the state of Arizona.

Laurie A. Rinehart-Thompson, JD, RHIA, CHP, is an assistant professor of clinical allied medicine, Health Information Management and Systems Division, School of Allied Medical Professions, College of Medicine and Public Health at The Ohio State University. She holds a BS in medical record administration and a JD from The Ohio State University. Rinehart-Thompson has served in a variety of roles for AHIMA, including on the CHP Exam Construction (2004–2006) and Advocacy and Policy committees (2004–2005) and as a contributing author to *Ethical Challenges in the Management of Health Information.* She also served on the Ohio Health Information Management Association Board of Directors (2003–2005) and has made multiple presentations on the HIPAA Privacy Rule to HIM and other allied health professionals.

Jane Roberts, MS, RHIA, is an associate professor in health information management technology at Columbus State Community College, in Columbus, Ohio. She received a BS degree from The Ohio State University in 1988 and an MS degree in 2004. Her prior work experience includes director of medical records in acute care facilities, supervisor of medical records in a long-term care facility, and office manager in a physician office setting.

Karen S. Scott, MEd, RHIA, CCS-P, CPC, has twenty years of experience in the healthcare field. Owner of Karen Scott Seminars and Consulting, she has been an educator for many years and has taught in HIM programs at the University of Tennessee Health Science Center and Arkansas Tech University. She holds a BS in health information management and an MEd in instructional technology from Arkansas Tech University in Russellville. Scott is past president of both the Tennessee and Arkansas HIM associations and past chair of the AHIMA Council on Certification. In 2005, she was awarded the Distinguished Member Award from The Tennessee Health Information Management Association (THIMA). She teaches seminars on coding, reimbursement, medical terminology, and management throughout the country. In addition, she has published numerous articles on various healthcare topics and has written several chapters in other HIM and coding textbooks.

Carol A. Venable, MPH, RHIA, FAHIMA, is a professor and department head of health information management at the University of Louisiana at Lafayette and has been an HIM professional for nearly thirty years. She is actively involved with AHIMA's Assembly on Education (AOE), Panel of Accreditation Surveyors, and several other committees, as well as the Louisiana Health Information Management Association, where she has held many leadership positions and was selected as Distinguished Member in 1991. Previously, she was director of medical records at Lafayette General Medical Center. She has consulted in a variety of healthcare facilities and educational institutions, and conducts coding workshops for hospitals and physician offices. Venable has written, coauthored, and edited numerous publications, including *ICD-9-CM Diagnostic Coding and Reimbursement for Physician Services* and *ICD-10-CM Preview,* for which she won AHIMA's Legacy Award in 2003. She frequently serves as a reviewer for publishers of HIM-related textbooks, certification exams, and electronic materials.

Karen A. Wager, DBA, RHIA, is an associate professor in the department of health administration and policy at the Medical University of South Carolina in Charleston, where she received a master's degree in health information administration and finance. In 1998, she received a doctorate of business administration from the University of Sarasota. Wager is a member of AHIMA and has served on various association committees. She was president of the South Carolina Health Information Management Association (SCHIMA) from 1991 to 1992. Wager has authored, coauthored, and edited numerous publications and is coauthor of *Managing Healthcare Information Systems: A Practical Approach for Healthcare Executives.*

Andrea Weatherby White, PhD, RHIA, is an associate professor and program director of the master's-level program in health administration in the department of health information administration and policy at the Medical University of South Carolina. She earned her PhD in higher education administration from the University of South Carolina in 1998. She was named Teacher of the Year in 1995 and won the Excellence in Service Award in 2000. She is an active member of AHIMA. She has served as an accreditation site visitor for both health information management and health information administration educational programs.

Sue Willner, RHIA, is department chair of Santa Barbara City College's online health information technology, coding, and cancer information management programs. In her more than twenty-three years in health information management, Willner has specialized in coding and reimbursement, regulatory compliance, and data quality. She has held management positions in the hospital, managed care, and peer review organization settings and has been active as an HIM educator, speaker, and writer. Moreover, she has served in numerous volunteer roles with AHIMA and the California Health Information Association throughout her career.

Preface

Health information management (HIM) professionals are an integral part of the healthcare team. They serve the healthcare industry and the public by managing, analyzing, and utilizing the data vital for patient care and making the data accessible to healthcare providers. Whether stored on paper or in electronic files, reliable health information is critical to high-quality healthcare. Enhancing individual patient care through timely and relevant information is one of the primary goals for the HIM profession.

The American Health Information Management Association (AHIMA) represents more than 50,000 specially educated HIM professionals who work throughout the healthcare industry. AHIMA has a long history of commitment to HIM education. Among other contributions, AHIMA has developed and maintained a rigorous accreditation process for academic programs, continuously developed up-to-date curriculum models, supported faculty development, and continued to research and study the needs and future directions of HIM education.

This text, specifically developed for associate degree programs in health information technology (HIT), is an outgrowth of AHIMA's ongoing effort to provide rich resources for the education and training of new HIM professionals. In addition, it offers a ready resource for current practitioners. Its subject matter is based on AHIMA's HIM Associate Degree Entry-Level Competencies and Knowledge Clusters for 2006 and Beyond. The arrangement of information in the text provides a logical flow for skill and knowledge building among new HIT professionals. Following the prescribed curricular content found in the HIM Associate Degree Entry-Level Competencies, the text ensures coverage of information and topics considered essential for every entry-level HIT practitioner. Although the text is directed primarily at students enrolled in two-year HIT programs, students in other HIM disciplines and allied health programs also will find its content highly useful.

The fundamental organization of the text is built on the curricular content of the HIM Associate Degree Entry-Level Competencies and Knowledge Clusters. Each of the content areas is represented in the book except those relating to the biomedical sciences and to technical aspects of classification systems such as ICD. Because this is a technical-level textbook, it is designed to proceed from the specific to the global as an instructional design delivery method. This strategy is used because the book's intended audience will likely not have a previous background in healthcare delivery or, specifically, in health information management.

The book's underlying metaphor is translating basic theory into practice. A review of the cognitive and competency levels of the Entry Level Competencies reveals that HIT programs are applied in nature. Outcome expectations are that students understand theory at a basic level with a major emphasis on skill building to perform day-to-day operational tasks in health information management.

Therefore, the features used throughout the book focus on translating basic theory into practice. To accomplish this, each chapter contains the following sections:

- **Theory Into Practice:** Located at the beginning of each chapter, this section presents a case study that serves as an organizing framework for the theory presented in the chapter. This instructional design strategy "sets the stage" and "gains the learner's attention," two of the first and most basic steps in instructional design.

- **Check Your Understanding:** These sections are content review exercises. These exercises are positioned throughout each chapter so that students can reinforce their understanding of the concepts they have just read before going on to the following concepts. Multiple-choice, matching, and true-and-false formats are used.

- **Real-World Case:** Located near the end of each chapter, this section presents an actual situation faced by healthcare enterprises as reported in current literature and periodicals. The case supports the preceding instruction and moves toward selective perception.

Features in the new accompanying workbook include:

- **Real-World Case Discussion Questions:** The questions in this section are designed to initiate discussion of and elaboration on the concepts presented in the real-world case.

- **Application Exercises:** The purpose of these exercises is to give students the opportunity to put theory into practice. Because skill building is an important part of the expected outcomes for HIT students, these exercises will bring the real world into their sphere.

- **Review Quizzes:** The review quizzes are in multiple-choice format and test chapter content knowledge.

The text is segmented into five parts. **Part I, Health Data Management,** concentrates on the roles of the health information manager; the content, function, structure, and uses of health information; and how health information is managed. Chapter 1 introduces the concept of health information management. The discussion focuses on the history of the HIM profession and the evolution of the roles and functions of HIM professionals over the years. Particular emphasis is placed on HIM future roles and their relationship to the movement toward an electronic health record (EHR). Chapters 2, Functions of the Health Record, and 3, Content and Structure of the Health Record, discuss the generic components of the content, use, and structure of healthcare data. Content of the health record and documentation requirements are covered. The formats of paper and electronic record systems are investigated in chapter 3. Chapter 4, Electronic Health Records, includes a comprehensive treatment of the hybrid health record, electronic document management systems, and the transition to an EHR. Chapter 5, Healthcare Data Sets, builds on the basic knowledge presented in the previous chapters and discusses prominent healthcare data sets and their purposes and uses. Chapter 6, Clinical Vocabularies and Classification Systems, provides an introduction to clinical vocabularies and classification systems. Its purpose is to introduce the characteristics of prominent systems and help students understand how they are used throughout the healthcare system. Chapter 7, Reimbursement Methodologies, is an introduction to the uses of coded data and healthcare payment systems. It is meant to help students understand the process of reimbursement, billing procedures, use of chargemasters, and auditing. Part I concludes with Chapter 8, Health Information Technology Functions, which explains the typical functions associated with managing paper-based, hybrid, and EHR systems.

Part II, Health Statistics, Biomedical Research, and Quality Management, introduces the timely topics of healthcare service evaluation. Consisting of four chapters, part II looks at the effective use, collection, arrangement, presentation, and verification of healthcare data. Chapter 9, Secondary Data Sources, reviews various types of secondary data sources, such as registries and indexes, that are used in healthcare service evaluation. Chapter 10, Healthcare Statistics and Research, presents fundamental concepts of descriptive, vital, and facility statistics. It also talks about external and internal uses of statistics and patient data for research and the protection of patients and patient data in research. Chapter 11, Clinical Quality Management, discusses quality assessment, risk management, utilization management, and performance principles; and chapter 12, Performance Improvement, describes how the specifics of those methods are applied to clinical quality assessment.

Part III, Health Services Organization and Delivery, looks at the environment in which HIT professionals work, essentially, the U.S. healthcare delivery system. It further demonstrates the complexity of the current delivery mechanisms, systems, and regulations involving healthcare. Chapter 13 introduces the history, organization, financing, and delivery of health services in the United States. Chapter 14 discusses the ethical issues associated with health information management and presents the concepts of stewardship. Chapter 15 covers concepts basic to the U.S. legal system as they relate to the work of the HIT professional, with a focus on federal privacy and confidentiality rules and regulations applied to health information.

Part IV, Information Technology and Systems, introduces information technology (IT) concepts and provides a broad view of how IT supports the functions of healthcare delivery. Chapter 16 discusses information system concepts, components, and resources such as hardware, software, data, and network resources. The chapter helps students to conceptualize the various components necessary for development of a total health information system. Chapter 17 builds on the previous chapter and provides an overview of the application of technology to healthcare information systems and the EHR and ancillary feeder systems. Chapters 18 and 19 round out the IT section with a review of the concepts and applications of systems for decision support and with a thorough discussion of information security program development and implementation.

Finally, **Part V, Organizational Resources,** consists of one chapter, chapter 20, which introduces concepts and principles of organization and supervision. Emphasis in this final chapter is on practices associated with organizational and supervisory functions, such as budgeting, human resource supervision, and best practices in managing health information at the HIT level.

A complete glossary of HIM terms is provided at the end of the book. **Boldface** type is used in the text chapters to indicate the first substantial reference to each glossary term.

Appendices and a detailed content index complete the book.

Instructor materials for this book include lesson plans, lesson slides, and other useful resources. These resources are available to instructors in online format from the individual book page in the AHIMA Bookstore (imis.ahima.org/orders) and also are posted on the AHIMA Assembly on Education Community of Practice (AOE CoP) Web site. Instructors who are AHIMA members can sign up for this private community by clicking on the help icon within the CoP home page and requesting additional information on becoming an AOE CoP member. An instructor who is not an AHIMA member or a member who is not an instructor may contact the publisher at publications@ahima.org.

Acknowledgments

Many individuals contributed to the development of the second edition of this landmark textbook. First, the editor and AHIMA publications staff extend their sincere thanks to all the chapter authors for sharing their expertise with new entrants into the HIM profession. Developing the rich content of this text along with searching for the best examples and resources was a time-consuming process for these very busy professionals.

Second, no text is ever complete without the diligent work of the content reviewers. Their careful review and insightful suggestions ensure the essential quality of any effort of this kind. We also would like to thank the following reviewers who lent a critical eye to this endeavor:

June E. Bronnert, RHIA, CCS, CCS-P

Jill Burrington-Brown, MS, RHIA, FAHIMA

Melanie A. Endicott, MBA/HCM, RHIA, CCS

Beth Hjort, RHIA, CHPS

Susan Hull, MPH, RHIA, CCS, CCS-P

Karen Kostick, RHIT, CCS, CCS-P

Carol Ann Quinsey, RHIA, CHPS

Susan A. Schehr, RHIA

Rita A. Scichilone, MHSA, RHIA, CCS, CCS-P, CHC

Patricia L. Shaw, MEd, RHIA

Mary H. Stanfill, RHIA, CCS, CCS-P

Lydia M. Washington, MS, RHIA, CPHIMS

Ann Zeisset, RHIT, CCS-P, CCS

Additionally, the editor would like to acknowledge authors who contributed chapters to the first edition of this book. Their work served as the basis for several chapters that were revised by new authors:

Sandra Bailey, RHIA

Cathleen A. Barnes, RHIA, CCS

Mary Jo Bowie, MS, RHIA

Michelle L. Dougherty, RHIA, CHP

Michelle A. Green, MPS, RHIA, CMA, CHP

Terrell Herzig, MSHI

Joan C. Hicks, MS, RHIA

Beth M. Hjort, RHIA, CHPS

Joan Ludwig, RHIA

Keith Morneau, MS

Harry B. Rhodes, MBA, RHIA, CHPS

Foreword

To Tomorrow's Health Information Management Professionals

Health information management (HIM) is the profession dedicated to the effective management of patient information and healthcare data needed to deliver high-quality treatment and care to the public. HIM professionals who perfect their technical skills become experts in health data collection, data abstraction, enhanced coding, and monitoring, maintenance, and reporting activities while maintaining the highest standards of data integrity, confidentiality, and security. These functions encompass, among other areas, processing and using health data for treatment, billing, compliance, and surveillance. As healthcare adapts to the electronic health record (EHR) environment, the HIM professional role is critical to ensure that providers, healthcare organizations, and patients alike have access to the right healthcare information when and where it is needed.

The EHR will become a reality for nearly every healthcare organization, decision support will guide caregivers, and citizens will become knowledgeable partners in their health and wellness. Digital data and images will be accessible to support patient care. Public health and public policy will be based on accurate and timely information. The results of clinical research will be available to aid sound clinical decision making. HIM professionals will be on the front lines in delivering the benefits of electronic records and health information computing to patients, to purchasers, and to society at large.

This textbook is your guide to the complexities of knowledge and the competencies required of HIM professionals to meet the expanding roles and growing demand for highly skilled technical experts. AHIMA's 2004 Workforce Study Report emphasized that HIM professionals will be in high demand now and in the future due to the escalating speed of transition from paper and manual data entry to EHRs and that HIM practice will demand greater efficiencies, improved data quality to support evidence-based medicine, and an increased demand for information available to patients. Research shows that HIM professionals practice in more than forty work settings with more than a hundred job titles.

Health Information Management Technology: An Applied Approach, Second Edition, is written following the 2006 and Beyond Competencies and Knowledge Clusters that serve as the foundation for curricula in accredited academic programs in health information management at the associate degree level. HIM practice in a rapidly changing healthcare environment must be based on sound data and information management principles adaptable to any media and work-flow pattern. By building on the core principles outlined by editor Merida L. Johns, PhD, RHIA, and the fine array of chapter authors, you will be well prepared to take on the challenges of HIM practice in what we term an e-HIM™ or electronic HIM workplace environment.

You are tomorrow's HIM technical experts. Your efforts will ensure that health information is used fully and effectively. In addition, your efforts will ensure that health information is maintained safely and yet is accessible to the providers and patients who depend on it for high-quality service at all levels of the continuum of care. As you learn the concepts, skills, and resources to work within this environment of health information transformation, you will be fulfilling the dream of our profession's leaders: high-quality healthcare through high-quality information.

Claire Dixon-Lee, PhD, RHIA, FAHIMA
Vice President for Education and Accreditation
American Health Information Management Association

Part I
Health Data Management

Chapter 1
Introduction

Merida L. Johns, PhD, RHIA

Learning Objectives

- To understand the development of the health information management profession from its beginnings in 1928 until the present

- To understand how professional practice must evolve to accommodate changes in the healthcare environment

- To understand the responsibilities of healthcare professionals

- To become familiar with the purpose and structure of the American Health Information Management Association

- To understand the certification processes of the American Health Information Management Association

Key Terms

Accreditation

American Association of Medial Record Librarians (AAMRL)

American College of Surgeons (ACS)

American Health Information Management Association (AHIMA)

American Medical Record Association (AMRA)

Association of Record Librarians of North America (ARLNA)

Certification

Commission on Accreditation for Healthcare Informatics and Information Management Education (CAHIIM)

Communities of Practice (CoP)

Council on Certification

Credentialing

Curriculum

Health information management (HIM)

Hospital Standardization Program

House of Delegates

Registration

Introduction

Health information management (HIM) has been recognized as an allied health profession since 1928. The **Association of Record Librarians of North America** (ARLNA) was formed only 10 years after the beginning of the hospital standardization movement. The association's original objective was to elevate the standards of clinical record keeping in hospitals, dispensaries, and other healthcare facilities.

The first annual meeting of the professional organization was held in Chicago in 1929. Since then, the organization and the professionals affiliated with it have been advocates for the effective management of clinical records.

The name of the organization has changed several times throughout the years to reflect the changing healthcare environment. Today, the association is known as the **American Health Information Management Association** (AHIMA). Still, the association's underlying purpose remains the same: to ensure the accuracy, confidentiality, and accessibility of health records in every healthcare setting.

This chapter provides an introduction to the history of the HIM profession. The chapter offers insights into the current and future roles and functions of health information managers. The mission of the original organization is no less important today than it was in 1928. In fact, the role of HIM professionals is even more important in today's information- and technology-driven healthcare environment.

Those entering the HIM profession benefit from the commitment and hard work of previous visionaries in the field, who understood what it takes to develop and maintain a profession. Thus, to carry on with this legacy, today's HIM professionals must be equally committed to the original goal of "elevating standards for clinical records" as well as fulfilling the obligations of healthcare professionals.

Theory into Practice

How can healthcare organizations effectively use the Internet to support the delivery of services? What can HIM professionals do to help? In a recent article published in the *Journal of the American Health Information Management Association,* Julia Holland (2000, 50–53) describes effective strategies for using the Internet in healthcare. She begins by saying:

> Make no mistake, the Internet is keeping us all racing to stay up to date with new technologies, regulations, advances, and opportunities. But after all of the excitement has died down, the questions for healthcare remains: how can we use the power of the Internet to reengineer and support care delivery? And how does health information play a role in this process?

The healthcare industry will be working to answer these questions in the coming years, and HIM professionals are ideally positioned to lead the charge. HIM professionals have been designing and redesigning processes for decades. They are the logical and most appropriate choice to help determine how, when, and what health information will be used in the electronic healthcare world. This chapter explores what some organizations are already doing along these lines and how HIM professionals can get involved.

What is health information anyway? The answer depends on who is answering the question:

- For HIM professionals, health information is information that has traditionally been stored in a paper chart, whether it is housed in a hospital, physician's office, clinic, health department, or any other facility that provides patient care.

- For healthcare consumers, who take a broader view, health information is anything related to any healthcare encounter they have experienced in their lives, including insurance payments, physician's office visits, and prescription records.

- For insurance companies and other organizations that pay for healthcare services, health information is the coded data submitted to support billing, plus any miscellaneous information required to further explain diagnoses and treatments.

The list goes on and on. Sooner or later, someone will need all the information accumulated along the entire continuum of patient care. The trick has always been to determine *who* should access *what* information and *how* to make it appropriately available in a cost-effective manner.

Vendors have touted the electronic medical record for years, but many organizations are still seeking a fully functional product that meets their information demands, not to mention the need to become more efficient and economical. Although traditional vendors understand the many relationships that complicate the healthcare information environment, their advances in technology are falling behind the lightning-fast pace of the demands that HIM professionals face.

Why use the Internet? The pros and cons of this question are still being debated. From a technology and traffic standpoint, the Internet is the only single medium available capable of handling the estimated 30 billion transactions per year healthcare generates (Gardner 2000, 67). These transactions include payments, treatment approvals, prescriptions, laboratory orders, and reports of test results. In addition, an increasing number of people are using the Internet either daily or intermittently to become familiar with navigating and gathering information. Add the ease with which a person can potentially access his or her own or family health information without having to make an appointment, take off from work, get in the car, fight traffic, and wait to see the doctor, and the Internet appears to be the perfect solution. But is it?

For the HIM professional, the Internet presents exciting opportunities for process reengineering in support of care delivery. Think about all the information that is manually passed through an HIM department on a daily basis, and then consider the effect of automating that information. With all these issues covered, the HIM department's cost to the organization would decrease significantly, and service and customer satisfaction would increase.

For example:

- Maintaining a large staff of file clerks would no longer be necessary because all the information would be generated and stored electronically.

- Most traditional release of information processes would be transformed. Most insurers would likely use the Internet to request and receive the information needed to support rapid and accurate billing and reimbursement if they were confident that the information was secure.

- Multifacility organizations and off-campus offices would no longer present the problems associated with chart tracking and chart transportation. These problems have plagued the HIM profession for decades and limited the ability of health-care organizations to operate efficiently and provide high-quality services.

- Electronic authentication would shorten chart completion turnaround time, thereby lowering the number of delinquent records, which is frequently an issue for accreditation.

The HIM professional must become an ally to the leaders making Internet and technology decisions. The potential opportunities are endless. For instance, HIM professionals can address issues of data quality such as legibility, completeness, timeliness, and accuracy, to name a few. They can contribute to the success of many consumer-related endeavors such as personal health records. And HIM professionals' skills will continue to be in demand in areas such as developing organizational health information policies and interpreting regulations and accreditation standards.

Early History of Health Information Management

Today's HIM professionals are the benefactors of the wisdom, insight, and fortitude of pioneers whose untiring commitment is reflected in today's dynamic profession. The history of the HIM profession is witness to how a small group of dedicated individuals can come together and make a difference for decades to come.

The early history of the health information profession was summarized by Edna K. Huffman in an article appearing in the March 1941 issue of the *Bulletin of the American Association of Medical Record Librarians* (Huffman 1941). Three distinct steps influenced development of the profession. These included the hospital standardization movement, the organization of records librarians, and the approval of formal educational processes and a curriculum for medical record librarians.

Hospital Standardization

Before 1918, the creation and management of hospital medical records were the sole responsibility of the attending physician. Physicians in the early twentieth century, like many physicians today, often disliked doing paperwork. Unless the physician was interested in medical research, the medical records in the early twentieth century were "practically worthless and consisted principally of nurses notes" (Huffman 1941, 101).

Medical records of that time did not contain graphical records or laboratory reports. Because there was no general management of medical record processes, the incomplete records were often filed as received on discharge of the patient. Hospitals made no effort to ensure that the deficient portions were completed. Furthermore, no standardized vocabulary was used to document why the patient was admitted to the hospital or what the final diagnosis upon discharge was.

In 1918, the hospital standardization movement was inaugurated by the **American College of Surgeons** (ACS). The purpose of the **Hospital Standardization Program** was to raise the standards of surgery by establishing minimum quality standards for hospitals. The ACS realized that one of the most important items in the care of any patient was a complete and accurate report of the care and treatment provided during hospitalization. Specifically, the standard required the following (Huffman 1941, 101):

> Accurate and complete medical records [must] be written for all patients and filed in an accessible manner in the hospital, a complete medical record being one which includes identification data; complaint; personal and family history; history of the present illness; physical examination; special examinations such as consultations, clinical laboratory, x-ray and other examinations; provisional or working diagnosis; medical or surgical treatment; gross or microscopical pathological findings; progress notes; final diagnosis; condition on discharge; follow-up; and, in case of death, autopsy findings.

It was not long before hospitals realized that to comply with the hospital standards, new medical record processes had to be implemented. In addition, new staff had to be hired to ensure that the new processes were appropriately carried out. Furthermore, hospitals recognized that medical records must be maintained and filed in an orderly manner and that cross-indexes of disease, operations, and physicians must be compiled. Thus, the job position of medical record clerk was established.

Organization of the Association of Records Librarians

A nucleus of 35 members of the Club of Record Clerks met at the Hospital Standardization Conference in Boston in 1928. Near the close of the meeting, the Association of Record Librarians of North America (ARLNA) was formed. During its first year, the association had a charter membership of 58 individuals. Members were admitted from 25 of the 48 states, the District of Columbia, and Canada (Huffman 1985). The ARLNA was the predecessor of the American Health Information Management Association (AHIMA).

Approval of Formal Education and Certification Programs

Early HIM professionals understood that for an occupation to be recognized as a profession, there must be preliminary training. They also understood that such training needed to be distinguished from mere skill. That is, it needed to be intellectual in character, involving knowledge and, to some extent, learning. Therefore, work began on the formulation of a prescribed course of study as early as 1929. In 1932, the association adopted a formal **curriculum.**

The first schools for medical record librarians were surveyed and approved by the ARLNA in 1934. By 1941, 10 schools had been approved to provide training for medical record librarians. This formal **accreditation** process of academic programs was the precursor to the current accreditation program still sponsored by AHIMA today under the auspices of the **Commission on Accreditation for Health Informatics and Information Management Education** (CAHIIM).

The Board of Registration was instituted in 1933. The founders of the profession recognized that the existence of unqualified workers in the field lowered the standards of their profession. Therefore, they organized a **certification** board so that there would be a baseline by which to measure qualified medical record librarians. The Board of Registration established criteria for eligibility for **registration.** The board also developed and administered the qualifying examination. Today, the role of the Board of Registration is played by AHIMA's **Council on Certification** (COC).

Development of the HIM profession coincided with the professionalization of other healthcare disciplines such nursing, x-ray technology, and laboratory technology. All these disciplines established registration and/or training programs around the same time.

The professional membership of the association of HIM professionals grew steadily over the subsequent decades. Although the names of the association and the credentials have changed several times during the past decades, the fundamental elements of the profession— formal training requirements and certification by examination—have remained the same.

Evolution of Practice

The various names given to the medical record association and its associated credentials reveal a lot about the evolution of the profession and its practice. In 1928, the organization's name was the Association of Record Librarians of North America (ARLNA). In 1944, Canadian members formed their own organization, and the name of the organization was changed to the **American Association of Medical Record Librarians** (AAMRL). In 1970, the organization changed its name again to eliminate the term *librarian.* The organization's name became the **American Medical Record Association** (AMRA). The organization underwent another name change in 1991 to become the American Health Information Management Association (AHIMA).

The organization's title changes in 1970 and 1991 reflected the changing nature of the roles and functions of the association's professional membership. In 1970, the term *administrator* mirrored the work performed by members more accurately than the term *librarian.* Similarly, in 1991, association leaders believed that the management of information, rather than the management of records, would be the primary function of the profession in the future.

The names of the credentials conferred by the organization changed as the association's name changed. In 1999, the AHIMA **House of Delegates** approved a credential name change. Registered record administrator (RRA) became registered health information administrator (RHIA), and accredited record technician (ART) became registered health information technician (RHIT).

What does the changing of the organization and credential names say about the profession? Probably one of the most significant things that it indicates is a major shift in what professionals do and how they fit within their environment. The combined forces of new information technologies and the demands for increased, better, and more timely information require the profession to change radically.

Traditional Practice

The original practice of health information management was based on the Hospital Standardization Program, initiated in 1918. The program emphasized the need to ensure that complete and accurate medical records were compiled and maintained for every patient. Accurate records were needed to support the care and treatment provided to the patient as well as to conduct various types of clinical research. This emphasis remained fundamental to the profession through 1990. For example, a review of the professional practice standards published by AMRA in 1984 and updated in 1990 shows a model of practice that was highly quantitative and department based (Johns 1991, 57).

Further evaluation of the 1990 professional practice standards discloses that the tasks of medical record practitioners at that time involved planning, developing, and implementing systems designed to control, monitor, and track the quantity of record content and the flow, storage, and retrieval of medical records. In other words, activities primarily centered on the medical record or reports within the record as a physical unit rather than on the data elements that make up the information within the medical record.

At that time, very few standards "addressed issues relating to determination of the completion, significance, organization, timeliness, or accuracy of information contained in the medical record or its usefulness to decision support" (Johns 1991, 57). Figure 1.1 illustrates how traditional practice focused on the management of medical records as objects.

Information-Oriented Management Practice

The traditional model of practice shown in figure 1.1 would not be appropriate for today's information-intensive and automated healthcare environment. The traditional model of practice is department focused. Tasks are devoted primarily to processing and tracking records rather than processing and tracking information.

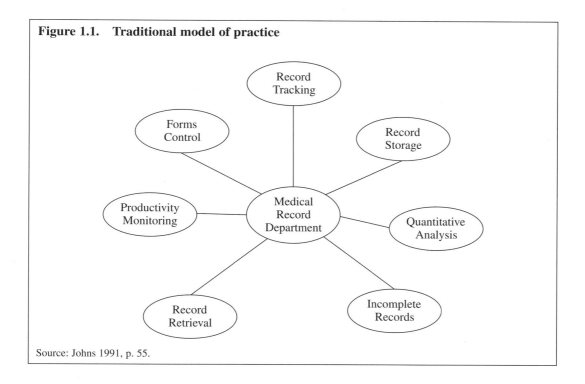

Figure 1.1.   Traditional model of practice

Source: Johns 1991, p. 55.

Studies have consistently shown that 25 to 40 percent of a hospital's operating costs are devoted to information handling. Obviously, information management has become a top priority for healthcare institutions (Blum 1986; Protti 1984). In today's information age, information crosses departmental boundaries and is broadly disseminated throughout the organization. In fact, information grows out of data manipulation from a variety of shared data sources. An information-oriented management model includes tasks associated with a broad range of information services. Therefore, the tasks performed as a health information manager—in contrast to tasks performed as a medical record manager—are information based, "emphasizing data manipulation and information management tasks and focusing on the provision of an extensive range of information services" (Johns 1991, 59).

Vision 2006

What new information services and functions are being performed by health information managers? In 1996, AHIMA developed a vision of the future for health information managers. The initiative was called Vision 2006. Vision 2006 identified many new roles that information managers would likely assume in the upcoming information-focused decades. Moreover, it demonstrated the difference between traditional practice and information-oriented practice. Table 1.1 shows the differences between tasks in traditional and information-focused practice (as envisioned through AHIMA's Vision 2006 initiative).

As table 1.1 shows, the traditional model of practice is department based and the health information manager's activities are usually performed in the medical record department. In the new model, tasks are information based and many of the health information manager's activities are performed outside the HIM department. Indeed, many health information managers work entirely in other areas of the facility and in other set-

Table 1.1.   Comparison of traditional HIM and Vision 2006 roles

Traditional HIM	Vision 2006
Department based	Information based
Physical records	Data item definition Data modeling Data administration Data auditing
Aggregation and display of data	Electronic searches Shared knowledge sources Statistical and modeling techniques
Forms and records design	Logical data views Data flow and reengineering Application development Application support
Confidentiality and release of information	Security, audit, and control programs Risk assessment and analysis Prevention and control measures

tings. They work in a variety of functional areas, such as quality improvement, decision support, information systems, utilization management, data privacy, data security, and so on. Instead of working primarily in hospitals, many work in ambulatory care facilities and other nontraditional settings.

A second important difference is that the traditional model of practice is based on creating, tracking, and storing physical records. In today's information-intense environment, the physical (paper-based) health record is being replaced by the computer-based health record. The information in computer-based records is created, compiled, and stored in many different areas within the enterprise and is brought together electronically only when needed. The tasks performed by a health information manager focus on such activities as maintaining data dictionaries, developing data models, performing data administration tasks, and ensuring data quality through a variety of auditing tasks.

Another difference between the two models of practice centers on tasks associated with data analysis and interpretation. In the traditional model of practice, the tasks involve the aggregation and display of data. However, today's information world is much more complicated than it was two or three decades ago and contains more enabling technologies to search and analyze data. Thus, the health information manager who works in decision support or quality improvement today must use sophisticated computer-based tools to analyze data from a variety of data sources.

With more emphasis being placed on the development of an electronic record, health information managers will find that the tasks they perform are less concerned with paper forms design. Instead, the tasks will focus more on developing good user interfaces for electronic medical records.

Finally, health information practitioners have always been concerned with the privacy and confidentiality of data. The tasks in the traditional model of practice were confined principally to issues involving release of information. However, in a more technologically sophisticated world, these tasks are shifting to include enterprise-wide responsibilities for computer data security programs as well as organization-wide privacy programs.

AHIMA's e-HIM Task Force in 2003 confirmed the information-handling focus of HIM practice where the state of health information is described as electronic, patient centered, comprehensive, longitudinal, accessible, and credible (AHIMA 2003).

Workforce 2004

In 2004, AHIMA completed an extensive study called "Data for Decisions: The HIM Workforce and Workplace," commonly referred to as Workforce 2004 (AHIMA 2004). The purpose of the study was to understand the status of AHIMA members, education programs accredited by AHIMA, and employers of HIM professionals. The study results help to assess the future direction of the work of HIM professionals.

Many challenges face HIM professionals as a shift occurs from a paper-based to an electronic medical record. The shift to an electronic medical record will not be instantaneous. This means that HIM professionals are likely to be responsible for hybrid patient records, records that are partly in paper format and partly electronic. Thus, HIM professionals will be working with information that may or may not be integrated and may or may not be stored in common repositories.

Like Vision 2006, Workforce 2004 predicts that HIM professionals will be working in a broader set of roles as the electronic record expands. HIM professionals will:

- Work in oversight and accreditation to ensure that established standards are met
- Educate patients, providers, and administrators about privacy, content, access, and interpretation of the patient record
- Work with patients to help them access and understand information in their health records
- Work as data experts extracting and abstracting patient records
- Function as guardians of the record and manage access to its content
- Monitor compliance with information standards and regulatory requirements
- Work as data analysts supporting clinical researchers and business analysts

The study also concludes that there is a need for health information technician (HIT) roles to adjust from supervisory functions to a more technical workforce with critical and analytical thinking skills. The emphasis in the future for HITs will be in the areas of coding, data management, and data-abstracting skills.

From Traditional Roles to Future Opportunities

In the Vision 2006 initiative, AHIMA identified several new roles as opportunities for health information managers in 2006 and beyond. These new roles are based on the information model of practice and include the following (AHIMA 1999b):

- The health information manager for integrated systems is responsible for the organization-wide direction of health information functions.
- The clinical data specialist is responsible for data management functions, including clinical coding, outcomes management, and maintenance of specialty registries and research databases.
- The patient information coordinator assists consumers in managing their personal health information, including personal health histories and release of information.
- The data quality manager is responsible for data management functions that involve formalized continuous quality improvement activities for data integrity throughout the organization, such as data dictionary and policy development and data quality monitoring and audits.
- The information security manager is responsible for managing the security of electronically maintained information, including the promotion of security requirements, policies, and privilege systems and performance auditing.
- The data resource administrator manages the data resources of the organization, such as data repositories and data warehouses.
- The research and decision support specialist provides senior managers with information for decision making and strategy development.

Figure 1.2 illustrates the interrelationships among these roles with the patient as the center and primary focus of all information management tasks.

In 2003, the roles and competencies required of HIM professionals were defined by the e-HIM Task Force and incorporated into a Vision Statement of HIM Practice in 2010. Vision 2010 defines HIM as "the body of knowledge and practice that ensures the availability of health information to facilitate real-time healthcare delivery and critical health related decision-making for multiple purposes across diverse organizations, settings, and disciplines." Because of the expanded role of technology, HIM professionals will need to work closely with information technology professionals. Importantly, the task force confirms that HIM professionals will work as information brokers by ensuring timely and accurate sharing, transferring, and interpreting of health information.

Vision 2006 and Vision 2010 are essentially a strategic blueprint of the changes that the HIM profession will likely undergo over the next decade and beyond. It is important to remember, however, that the healthcare environment is constantly changing. Therefore, the roles of HIM professionals will continue to evolve to meet the needs of the healthcare delivery system. The future of the HIM profession is positive. However, for individual members of the profession to be successful, each must engage in a program of lifelong learning. This means that change today is an everyday occurrence. Health information professionals must commit themselves to continually upgrade their skills so that they can be ready to step into new job opportunities.

Figure 1.2.   Vision 2006 roles

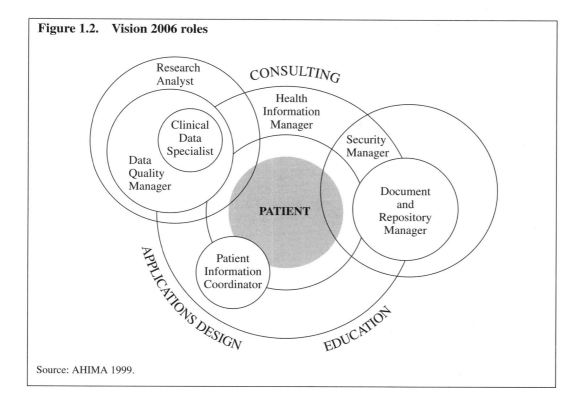

Source: AHIMA 1999.

Check Your Understanding 1.1

Instructions: Choose the word, term, or phase that completes each of the following sentences.

1. _____ HIM has been recognized as an allied health profession since _____.
   a. 1910
   b. 1918
   c. 1928
   d. 2006

2. _____ The hospital standardization movement was inaugurated by the _____.
   a. American Health Information Management Association
   b. American College of Surgeons
   c. Record Librarians of North America
   d. American College of Physicians

3. _____ Throughout the years, HIM roles have _____.
   a. Remained the same
   b. Broadened in scope
   c. Become more focused
   d. Diminished

4. _____ The traditional model of HIM practice was _____.
   a. Department based
   b. Information based
   c. Electronically based
   d. Analytically based

5. _____ The new model of HIM practice is _____.
   a. Information focused
   b. Record focused
   c. Department focused
   d. Traditionally focused

Today's Professional Organization

The health information management profession began with establishment of the ARLNA in 1928. As previously described, the organization's name has changed several times. The last name change occurred in 1991, when the professional organization assumed the name of AHIMA. The most recent name change reflects the requirements of the information age and, subsequently, the needs of the healthcare delivery system and the new roles of health information managers.

Mission

Before studying AHIMA's structure, it is important to understand why the organization exists and what contributions it makes to both its members and the healthcare system in general. The mission of an organization explains what the organization is and what it does. In other words, it describes the organization's distinctive purpose. Figure 1.3 shows AHIMA's current mission statement.

AHIMA is a membership organization. The majority of its members are credentialed HIM professionals who work throughout the healthcare industry. These professionals serve the healthcare industry and the public by managing, analyzing, and utilizing information

---

Figure 1.3.   American Health Information Management Mission Statement, 2001

The American Health Information Management Association is the community of professionals engaged in health information management, providing support to members and strengthening the industry and profession.

AHIMA:
- Provides career, professional development, and practice resources
- Sets standards for education and certification
- Advocates public policy that advances HIM practice
- Facilitates member communication
- Promotes the contributions of its members

AHIMA values:
- A code of ethical health information management practices
- The public's right to private and high-quality health information
- The celebration and promotion of diversity

---

vital for patient care and making it accessible to healthcare providers when and where it is needed.

The primary focus of the organization is to foster the professional development of its members through education, certification, and lifelong learning. By doing this, AHIMA promotes the development of high-quality information that benefits the public, the healthcare consumer, healthcare providers, and other users of clinical data. The organization has certification programs that set high standards to ensure the qualifications of the individuals who practice as health information managers and technicians. In addition, it supports numerous continuing education (CE) programs to help its credentialed members and others maintain their knowledge base and skills.

To accomplish its mission, AHIMA expects that all its members will follow a Code of Professional Ethics. (A complete discussion of ethical principles and the AHIMA Code of Ethics is provided in chapter 14.) As the Code of Ethics (p. 663) demonstrates, all members of AHIMA are expected to act in an ethical manner and comply with all laws, regulations, and standards governing the practice of health information management. As professionals, members are expected to continually update their knowledge base and skills through CE and lifelong learning. HITs and managers are expected to promote high standards of HIM practice, education, and research. Additionally, they are expected to promote and protect the confidentiality and security of health records and health information.

Membership

Today, AHIMA has more than 50,000 members. To accommodate the diversity in membership, the organization has several membership categories.

Active members are those who hold an AHIMA credential and are entitled to all membership privileges, including the right to vote and to serve in the House of Delegates. Active membership provides HIM professionals the best opportunity to participate in the organization and to offer input to the current and future practices of the profession.

Associate members also include individuals interested in the purposes of AHIMA, but who do not hold a professional AHIMA credential. Associate members have all the rights and privileges of membership, including the right to serve on committees and subcommittees with voice and vote. They are not, however, entitled to other voting privileges and may not hold office or serve as delegates.

Student members include any students formally enrolled in AHIMA-accredited college programs in health information management. The student membership category gives entry-level professionals an opportunity to participate on a national level in promoting sound HIM practices. Student members have all the rights and privileges of membership, including the right to serve on committees and subcommittees in designated student positions with voice, but no vote.

The other membership category includes honorary members. Honorary memberships are conferred by the organization on individuals who have made a significant contribution to health information management or rendered distinguished service in the HIM profession or its related fields. Honorary membership is awarded by the Board of Directors or by a simple majority vote of the House of Delegates.

Structure and Operation

Every organization needs a management structure in order to operate effectively and efficiently. AHIMA is made up of two components: a volunteer component and a staff component. The volunteer structure establishes the organization's mission and goals, develops policy, and provides oversight for the organization's operations. The staff component of the organization carries out the operational tasks necessary to support the organization's mission and goals. The staff works within the policies established by the volunteer component.

Association Leadership

As a nonprofit membership association, AHIMA depends on the participation and direction of volunteer leaders from the HIM community. AHIMA's members elect the delegates who serve in the governing bodies of the organization. Members of AHIMA's Board of Directors as well as members of the COC and representatives on the CAHIIM Board of Commissioners are elected by the membership.

AHIMA's Board heads up the volunteer structure. It also has responsibility for managing the property, affairs, and operations of AHIMA.

As the preceding list demonstrates, the Board of Directors is charged with tremendous responsibility. Its members include the president, the president-elect, the past president, nine elected directors, and the executive director of the organization. Except for the executive director, all members of the Board are elected by the membership and serve three-year terms of office. Members of the Board must be active members of the association.

In addition to the Board of Directors, two other groups are elected directly by the overall membership: the COC and the CAHIIM. The COC is responsible for overseeing AHIMA's certification process and for setting policies and procedures. Similarly, CAHIIM is responsible for overseeing AHIMA's accreditation of college programs in health information technology and health information administration.

Communities of Practice

The **Communities of Practice** (CoP) make up a virtual network of AHIMA members who communicate via a Web-based program managed by AHIMA. The CoP provides the following benefits to members only:

- CoP makes it possible for members to contact other members for quick problem-solving, support, advice, and career-building tips and opportunities. It also makes it possible to share best practices.

- CoP makes it possible for members to search for other members with similar interests and backgrounds.

- CoP provides links to other sites that provide specialized HIM information.

- CoP includes a professional library of HIM standards, guidelines, practice briefs, and other resources.

National Committees

AHIMA's president appoints the members of the association's national committees. These committees support the mission of the organization and work on specific projects as designated by the president and the Board of Directors. Examples of the national committees include the Awards Committee, the Bylaws Committee, the Coding Policy and Strategy Committee, and the Fellowship Review Committee.

House of Delegates

The House of Delegates is an extremely important component of the volunteer structure. It conducts the official business of the organization and functions as AHIMA's legislative body. The House of Delegates meets annually, usually in conjunction with the national meeting. Each state HIM association elects representatives to the House of Delegates to serve for a specified term of office. For that reason, the House of Delegates is similar to the legislative branch of the U.S. government. Its specific powers include the following:

- Approving the standards that govern the profession, including:

  —The AHIMA Code of Ethics

  —The guide to the interpretation of the Code of Ethics

  —The grounds for disciplinary action (minimum standards)

  —The standards for initial certification

  —The standards for maintenance of certification

  —The standards for HIM associate and baccalaureate degrees

- Electing the members of the AHIMA Nominating Committee, except the chairman and appointed members

- Advising the Board of Directors in the development and modification of the association's plans

- Approving dues for all membership categories except corporate

- Levying special assessments

- Approving members' continuing education fee

- Approving amendments to AHIMA's bylaws

- Approving the standing rules of the House of Delegates

- Approving resolutions

State and Local Associations

In addition to its national volunteer organization, AHIMA supports a system of component organizations in every state, plus Washington, D.C., and Puerto Rico. Component state associations (CSAs) provide their members with local access to professional education, networking, and representation. CSAs also serve as an important forum for communicating information relevant to national issues and keeping members informed of regional affairs that affect health information management.

Many states also have local or regional organizations. For newly credentialed professionals, the state and local organizations are ideal avenues for becoming involved with volunteer work within the professional organization. Most HIM professionals who serve in the House of Delegates or serve on AHIMA's Board of Directors got their start in volunteer services with local, regional, and state associations.

Staff Structure

AHIMA's headquarters are located in Chicago. The staff required to run the day-to-day operations of the organization is organized into a number of divisions. The executive director is the individual responsible for overseeing day-to-day operations. A team of executives, managers, and staff support the executive director. Examples of the staff departments include, among others, member services, certification, accreditation and education, professional practice services, publications, marketing, and policy and government relations.

Accreditation of Educational Programs

AHIMA has a long tradition of commitment to HIM education. As discussed previously, the first prescribed curriculum for the training of medical record professionals was proposed in 1929. The first educational programs were accredited in 1934. Since that time, the association has developed and maintained a rigorous accreditation process for academic programs, continuously developed up-to-date curriculum models, and supported educational programs in a variety of ways.

The House of Delegates is responsible for approving standards for the accreditation of educational programs in health information management at the associate and baccalaureate levels. CAHIIM is the accrediting agency for degree-granting programs in health informatics and information management. CAHIIM serves the public interest by establishing quality standards for the educational preparation of future HIM professionals. When a program is accredited by CAHIIM, it means that it has voluntarily undergone a rigorous review process and has been determined to meet or exceed the standards mutually established by the CAHIIM and AHIMA. CAHIIM accreditation is a way to recognize and publicize best practices for HIM education programs.

CAHIIM reviews formal applications from college programs that apply for Candidacy status. After a successful review of the application documentation, a program may be deemed a Candidate for Accreditation for up to two years. Students enrolled in programs that are placed in Candidacy status are eligible to join AHIMA as student members. Within an agreed upon timeframe, the college program prepares a self-assessment document and a campus site visit occurs. A report of site visit is reviewed by the CAHIIM Board of Commissioners and a final determination is made as to the ability of the college program to meet the accreditation Standards for curriculum, facility, resources, and other requirements. The accreditation of educational programs is important because only those individuals who graduate from an approved program may sit for the national **credentialing** examinations for registered health information technician (RHIT) or registered health information administrator (RHIA).

Certification and Registration Program

The founding members of the organization recognized early on the necessity of setting standards for medical record practitioners. In 1933, the association organized a certifying board known as the Board of Registration. This board was developed "so that there might be a yard-stick by which qualified medical record librarians could be determined" (Huffman 1941, 101). To become a registered record librarian (RRL) in 1940, a candidate needed to:

- Be at least 21 years of age
- Be a graduate of a school for record librarians approved by AAMRL
- Be currently employed in medical records work
- Pass a qualifying credentialing examination

As the field of health information management became more complex, the association recognized the need to expand its credentialing program. Today, the AHIMA certification program encompasses several different types of credentials, including:

- Registered health information technician (RHIT)
- Registered health information administrator (RHIA)
- Certified coding associate (CCA)
- Certified coding specialist (CCS)
- Certified coding specialist—physician based (CCS-P)
- Certified in healthcare privacy (CHP)
- Certified in healthcare privacy and security (CHPS)
- Certified in healthcare security (CHS)

Each of these credentials has specific eligibility requirements and a certification examination. To achieve certification from AHIMA, individuals must meet the eligibility requirements for certification and successfully complete the certification examination.

Because the HIM profession is constantly changing, certified individuals must demonstrate that they are continuing to maintain their knowledge and skill base. Therefore, to maintain their certification, individuals who hold any of AHIMA's credentials must complete a designated set of CE credits. Activities that qualify for CE credits include such things as attending workshops and seminars, taking college courses, participating in independent study activities, and engaging in self-assessment activities. AHIMA's Web site provides information on the most recent requirements for maintenance of certification.

Foundation of Research and Education in Health Information Management

The Foundation of Research and Education in Health Information Management (FORE) actively promotes education and research in the HIM field. Founded in 1962, FORE is a separately incorporated affiliate organization created and managed by AHIMA.

The HIM industry is based on the belief that high-quality healthcare requires high-quality information. FORE has provided the knowledge, research, and education infrastructure for this industry. Its role is to envision the future direction and needs of the field and to respond with strategies, information, planning, and programs that will keep the HIM profession on the cutting edge.

Some of the initiatives that have been spearheaded by FORE include the Leadership Recognition Program, the benchmarking and best practices research initiative, the legal and regulatory clearinghouse and curriculum, and various faculty support initiatives. In addition, the foundation administers a number of programs, including the scholarship, student loan, and research programs.

Check Your Understanding 1.2

Instructions: Choose the word, term, or phrase that completes each of the following sentences.

1. _____ The primary focus of AHIMA is to _____.
   a. Ensure that medical records are complete
   b. Implement an electronic record in hospitals
   c. Foster professional development of its members
   d. Set and implement standards

2. _____ Every member of AHIMA is expected to _____.
   a. Follow the AHIMA Code of Ethics
   b. Continually update his or her knowledge base
   c. Promote high standards of practice
   d. All of the above

3. _____ Active members of AHIMA include those who _____.
   a. Hold an AHIMA credential
   b. Do not hold an AHIMA credential
   c. Are students in HIM programs
   d. Have made a significant contribution to HIM but have no credential

4. _____ The membership of AHIMA elects members of _____.
   a. The AHIMA Board of Directors
   b. The Council on Certification
   c. The Commission on Accreditation for Healthcare Informatics and Information Management
   d. All of the above

5. _____ The _____ functions as the legislative body of AHIMA.
   a. Board of Directors
   b. House of Delegates
   c. COC
   d. CAHIIM

Summary

The health information management profession has a rich history. It continues to prosper today as it takes advantage of new opportunities and accommodates the changes ushered in by the information age. At the beginning of the organization's inception in 1928, founding members realized the need to direct the field of medical records toward professional standing. This required the development of a formal organization devoted to establishing standards and best practices for the discipline, including the creation of a prescribed training curriculum and the launch of a formal certification program. Amazingly, all this was accomplished in only six short years from the formation of the organization in 1928, to the establishment of a credentialing program in 1933, to the first accreditation of academic programs in 1934.

The professional association, beginning first as the Association of Record Librarians of North America and continuing today as the American Health Information Management Association, has demonstrated remarkable resilience in an ever-changing healthcare delivery system. Thanks to the foresight and insight of health information professionals through the decades, the organizational structure of the association has adapted to the membership's changing needs:

- Credentialing programs have been expanded to represent the diversity of work tasks in the discipline.

- Accreditation standards for academic programs have continued to become more rigorous, reflecting program outcomes and the growing need for better-trained and qualified graduates.

- Advocacy for confidentiality and patients' rights continues to be a fundamental objective as AHIMA's expertise and input are sought in the development of federal policy.

- The role and definition of professional practice have been studied and changed to meet new demands.

The new generation of HIM professionals has inherited a powerful legacy from HIM pioneers. The growth and viability of the profession in years to come will depend on the dedication of current professionals to actively participate in the professional organization at the local, state, and national levels and to commit to continually updating their knowledge base and skills through lifelong learning.

References

American Health Information Management Association. 2004. *Data for Decisions: The HIM Workforce and Workplace.* Chicago: AHIMA.

American Health Information Management Association. 2003. *A Vision of the e-HIM Future: A Report from the AHIMA e-HIM Task Force.* Chicago: AHIMA.

American Health Information Management Association. 1999b. Vision 2006. Updated and adapted from an article originally published in *AHIMA Advantage* 2:1 (January 1998).

American Medical Record Association. 1990. *Professional Practice Standards.* Chicago: AMRA.

American Medical Record Association. 1984. *Professional Practice Standards.* Chicago: AMRA.

Blum, B. I. 1986. *Clinical Information Systems.* New York: Springer-Verlag.

Commission on Accreditation for Health Informatics and Information Management Education, *Accreditation Standards for Health Information Management at the Associate Degree Level,* 2005.

Gardner, Elizabeth. 2000. Healing the health care business. *Internet World* 6(10):67.

Holland, Julia. 2000. Worlds collide: Health information meets the Internet. *Journal of American Health Information Management Association* 71(10):50–53.

Huffman, Edna K. 1941 (March). Requirements and advantages of registration for medical record librarians. *Bulletin of the American Association of Medical Record Librarians.*

Huffman, Edna K. 1985. *Medical Record Management,* 8th ed. Berwyn, IL: Physicians' Record Company.

Johns, Merida L. 1991. Information management: A shifting paradigm for medical record professionals? *Journal of the American Medical Record Association* 62(8).

Protti, D. J. 1984. Knowledge and skills expected of health information scientists: A sample survey of prospective employers. *Methods of Information in Medicine* 23:204–8.

Chapter 2
Functions of the Health Record

Cheryl Homan, MBA, RHIA

Learning Objectives

- To define the term *health record*
- To understand the various uses of the health record
- To identify the different users of the health record and its importance to each user
- To describe the functions of the health record
- To describe the components of health record data quality
- To understand the patient's right to privacy and the requirements for maintaining the confidentiality of patient-identifiable health information
- To recognize the importance of information security
- To identify the roles and responsibilities of health information management professionals in the development and maintenance of health record systems

Key Terms

Accreditation organizations

Aggregate data

Allied health professionals

Centers for Medicare and Medicaid Services (CMS)

Coding specialist

Confidentiality

Data

Data accessibility

Data accuracy

Data comprehensiveness

Data consistency

Data currency

Data definition

Data granularity

Data precision

Data quality management

Data relevancy

Data timeliness

Diagnostic codes

Electronic health record (EHR)

Health record

Information

Integrated health record format

Privacy

Problem-oriented health record format

Procedural codes

Quality improvement organizations (QIOs)

Reimbursement

Source-oriented health record format

Third-party payers

Transcriptionists

Utilization management organization

Introduction

The **health record** is the principal repository (storage place) for **data** and **information** about the healthcare services provided to an individual patient. It documents the who, what, when, where, why, and how of patient care.

Healthcare providers have created and maintained records of the medical care provided to individual patients for centuries. However, modern documentation standards for the health record did not begin to appear until the early twentieth century.

Today, almost every person in the United States has at least one health record with his or her identification on it. Moreover, every time a person consults a new healthcare provider, another health record is created. Thus, it is very likely that any given patient may have multiple health records.

The health record is known by different names in different healthcare settings. The records of acute care patients who receive services as hospital inpatients are often called *patient records*. Physicians and physicians' office personnel typically use the term *medical record*. The records of patients in long-term care facilities are often called *resident records*. Facilities that provide ambulatory behavioral health services sometimes refer to *client records*. Paper-based health records are also sometimes called charts, especially in hospital settings. No matter what term is used, however, the primary function of the health record is to document and support patient care services.

Although sometimes used interchangeably, the terms *data* and *information* do not mean the same thing. *Data* represent the basic facts about people, processes, measurements, conditions, and so on. They can be collected in the form of dates, numerical measurements and statistics, textual descriptions, checklists, images, and symbols. After data have been collected and analyzed, they are converted into a form that can be used for a specific purpose. This useful form is called *information*. In other words, data represent facts and information represents meaning.

Today, the management of health record systems and services is the primary responsibility of health information management (HIM) professionals. As discussed in chapter 1, the HIM profession has evolved as healthcare delivery has changed since individual patient records were first created almost a hundred years ago. The ongoing development of computerized healthcare applications and standards continues to bring change to the profession.

The traditional practice of health record management was based on the collection of data on paper forms stored in paper file folders. Paper-based documentation systems are gradually being replaced with electronic systems. Today's HIM professionals are challenged with managing hybrid record environments that are partially electronic and partially paper based. Future professional practice will be based on the electronic collection, storage, and analysis of healthcare information created and maintained in interactive **electronic health record** (EHR) systems.

Theory into Practice

Until recently, most healthcare providers documented their services directly in the paper-based records of their patients. That is, they handwrote or dictated their clinical notes and orders and filled out paper data-collection forms. Dictated reports were typewritten by **transcriptionists** and then checked by clinicians for accuracy. All these paper-based materials were then filed in paper folders or clipped together in paper charts.

Today, information technology is revolutionizing the way healthcare data and information are created, collected, and stored. Virtually every healthcare organization uses computer technology to collect, store, or retrieve some portion of a patient's healthcare data. For example, the results of laboratory tests have been routinely reported via computer printouts for some time. In many environments, healthcare providers can also access these results via computer workstations and other computerized output devices.

Movement toward EHRs has become part of the national agenda in the United States. Eventually, every healthcare organization will need to adopt a "paperless" health record system. In 2001, the National Committee on Vital and Health Statistics (NCVHS) issued a report and recommendations detailing how to build a national health information infrastructure (NCVHS 2001). Based on these recommendations and in an effort to reduce healthcare costs, improve care, and avoid medical errors, President George W. Bush has outlined a plan to achieve EHRs for most Americans by 2014. The Office of the National Coordinator for Health Information Technology (ONC), a sub-Cabinet-level post at the Department of Health and Human Services (HHS), is coordinating this national effort.

While a national infrastructure for EHRs is being created, individual healthcare providers are learning how to use computers and digital devices that will soon replace paper-based health records. A significant challenge for healthcare organizations is the development of effective documentation procedures and screens (the electronic data collection formats that will replace paper forms) that save personnel time. In addition, EHR technologies and systems must be designed and implemented so as not to intrude on the human relationship between provider and patient. To make EHRs a reality, physicians, nurses, and other clinicians need to be comfortable with using devices such as personal data assistants (PDAs) and computer keyboards in place of paper and pen.

Purposes of the Health Record

Health records are used for a number of purposes related to patient care. The primary purposes of the health record are associated directly with the provision of patient care services. The secondary purposes of the health record are related to the environment in which healthcare services are provided. The secondary purposes are not related directly to specific patient care encounters (Dick, Steen, and Detmer 1997, 77–79).

Primary Purposes

According to the Institute of Medicine (Dick, Steen, and Detmer 1997, 77–78), the primary purposes of the health record can be classified into the following categories:

- *Patient care delivery:* The health record documents the services provided by clinical professionals and **allied health professionals** working in a variety of settings. Health record documentation helps physicians, nurses, and other clinical care professionals make informed decisions about diagnoses and treatments. The health record is also a tool for communication among the individual patient's different caregivers. Effective communication ensures the continuity of patient services. Moreover, the detailed information stored in health records allows healthcare providers to assess and manage risk. Finally, the health record represents legal evidence of the services received by the individual patient.

- *Patient care management:* Patient care management refers to all the activities related to managing the healthcare services provided to patients. The health record assists providers in analyzing various illnesses, formulating practice guidelines, and evaluating the quality of care.

- *Patient care support processes:* Patient care support encompasses the activities related to the handling of the healthcare organization's resources, the analysis of trends, and the communication of information among different clinical departments.

- *Financial and other administrative processes:* Because the health record documents the patient's course of illness and treatment, the information in it determines the payment the provider will receive in every type of reimbursement system. Health record data elements are trended to assist in managing and reporting costs.

- *Patient self-management:* Individuals are becoming more actively involved in managing their own health and healthcare and are therefore becoming a primary user of the health record (IOM 2003, 5).

Figure 2.1 (p. 28) lists examples of the primary uses of the health record.

Secondary Purposes

The secondary purposes of the health record are not associated with specific encounters between patient and healthcare professional. Rather, they are related to the environment in which patient care is provided. According to the Institute of Medicine (IOM), education, research, regulation, and policy making are all considered secondary purposes of the health record (Dick, Steen, and Detmer 1997, 76–77). Figure 2.2 (p. 29) lists some examples of the secondary purposes of the health record. In 2003, public health and homeland security were added to the list of secondary purposes (IOM 2003, 5).

Check Your Understanding 2.1

Instructions: Indicate whether the following statements are true or false (T or F).

1. _____ The health record is the principal repository (storage place) for data and information about the healthcare services provided to individual patients.

2. _____ The lab test result "hemoglobin: 14.6 gm/110 ml" is considered information.

3. _____ All the primary purposes of the health record are associated directly with the provision of patient care services.

4. _____ Review of the health record by the physician to determine how to treat the patient is considered one of its primary purposes.

5. _____ The secondary purposes of the health record are related to the environment in which healthcare services are provided but are not related directly to specific patient care encounters.

6. _____ Submitting health record documentation to a third-party payer for the purpose of substantiating a patient bill is considered a secondary purpose of the health record.

7. _____ Use of the health record to study the effectiveness of a given drug is considered a primary use of the health record.

8. _____ Use of healthcare information by a state government agency to establish funding for smoking cessation programs is considered a secondary use of the health record.

9. _____ Use of health information by a respiratory therapy student to write a report as part of a requirement for a course he is taking is considered a primary use of the health record.

10. _____ The terms *data* and *information* mean the same thing.

Figure 2.1.   Primary purposes of the health record

Patient Care Delivery (Patient)
- To document services received
- To constitute proof of identity
- To self-manage care
- To verify billing

Patient Care Delivery (Provider)
- To foster continuity of care (that is, to serve as a communication tool)
- To describe diseases and causes (that is, to support diagnostic work)
- To support decision making about diagnosis and treatment of patients
- To assess and manage risk for individual patients
- To facilitate care in accordance with clinical practice guidelines
- To document patient risk factors
- To assess and document patient expectations and patient satisfaction
- To generate care plans
- To determine preventive advice or health maintenance information
- To provide reminders to clinicians
- To support nursing care
- To document services provided

Patient Care Management
- To document case mix in institutions and practices
- To analyze severity of illness
- To formulate practice guidelines
- To manage risk
- To characterize the use of services
- To provide the basis for utilization review
- To perform quality assurance

Patient Care Support
- To allocate resources
- To analyze trends and develop forecasts
- To assess workload
- To communicate information among departments

Financial and Other Administrative Processes
- To document services for payments
- To bill for services
- To submit insurance claims
- To adjudicate insurance claims
- To determine disabilities (for example, workmen's compensation)
- To manage costs
- To report costs
- To perform actuarial analysis

Source: Adapted from Dick, Steen, and Detmer 1997, 78, and IOM 2003, 5.

Figure 2.2. Secondary purposes of the health record

Education
- To document the experience of healthcare professionals
- To prepare conferences and presentations
- To teach healthcare students

Regulation
- To serve as evidence in litigation
- To foster postmarketing surveillance
- To assess compliance with standards of care
- To accredit professionals and hospitals
- To compare healthcare organizations

Research
- To develop new products
- To conduct clinical research
- To assess technology
- To study patient outcomes
- To study effectiveness and cost-effectiveness of patient care
- To identify populations at risk
- To develop registries and databases
- To assess the cost-effectiveness of record systems

Public Health and Homeland Security
- To monitor public health
- To monitor bioterrorism activity

Policy Making and Support
- To allocate resources
- To conduct strategic planning

Industry
- To conduct research and development
- To plan marketing strategy

Source: Adapted from Dick, Steen, and Detmer 1997, 79, and IOM 2003, 5.

Users of the Health Record

The primary users of health records are patient care providers. However, many other individuals and organizations also use the information in health records. Managed care organizations, integrated healthcare delivery systems, regulatory and **accreditation organizations,** licensing bodies, educational organizations, **third-party payers,** and research facilities all use information that was originally collected to document patient care.

The IOM broadly defines the users of health records as "those individuals who enter, verify, correct, analyze, or obtain information from the record, either directly or indirectly through an intermediary" (Dick, Steen, and Detmer 1997, 75). All the users of health records influence clinical care in some way, but they use the information from health records for various reasons and in different ways. Some users (for example, nurses, physicians, and **coding specialists**) refer to the health records of specific patients as a part of their daily work. Many other users, however, never have direct access to the records of individual patients.

Instead, they use clinical and demographic information collected from the records. Figures 2.3 and 2.4 list examples of the individual and institutional users of health records (Dick, Steen, and Detmer 1997,76–77).

Individual Users

As already noted, many individuals depend on the information in health records to perform their jobs. Some of these individual users are identified in the following paragraphs.

Patient Care Providers

The individuals who provide direct patient care services include physicians, nurses, nurse practitioners, allied health professionals, and other clinical personnel. Allied health professionals include physician assistants, physical therapists, respiratory therapists, occupational therapists, radiology technicians, and medical laboratory technicians. Other medical professionals also provide clinical services. These individuals include pharmacists, social workers, dietitians, psychologists, podiatrists, and chiropractors.

Direct patient care providers document their services directly in their patients' health records. Other service providers (for example, medical laboratory technicians) submit separate written reports that become part of individual health records.

Healthcare providers offer services to a number of patients during any given period of time. For providers, the health record serves as a device for communicating vital information among departments and across disciplines and settings.

Figure 2.3.   Representative individual users of health records

Patient Care Delivery (Providers)
- Chaplains
- Dental hygienists
- Dentists
- Dietitians
- Laboratory technologists
- Nurses
- Occupational therapists
- Optometrists
- Pharmacists
- Physical therapists
- Physicians
- Physician assistants
- Podiatrists
- Psychologists
- Radiology technologists
- Respiratory therapists
- Social workers

Patient Care Delivery (Consumers)
- Patients
- Families

Patient Care Management and Support
- Administrators
- Financial managers and accountants
- Quality managers
- Records professionals
- Risk managers
- Unit clerks
- Utilization review managers

Patient Care Reimbursement
- Benefit managers
- Insurers (federal, state, and private)

Other
- Accreditors
- Government policy makers and legislators
- Lawyers
- Healthcare researchers and clinical investigators
- Health sciences journalists and editors

Source: Adapted from Dick, Steen, and Detmer 1997, 76.

Figure 2.4.   Representative institutional users of health records

Healthcare Delivery (Inpatient and Outpatient)
- Alliances, associations, networks, and systems of providers
- Ambulatory surgery centers
- Donor banks (blood, tissue, organs)
- Health maintenance organizations
- Home care agencies
- Hospices
- Hospitals (general and specialty)
- Nursing homes
- Preferred provider organizations
- Physician offices (large and small group practices, individual practitioners)
- Psychiatric facilities
- Public health departments
- Substance abuse programs

Management and Review of Care
- Medicare peer review organizations
- Quality management companies
- Risk management companies
- Utilization review and utilization management companies

Reimbursement of Care
- Business healthcare coalitions
- Employers
- Insurers (federal, state, and private)

Research
- Disease registries
- Health data organizations
- Healthcare technology developers and manufacturers (equipment and device firms, pharmaceutical firms, and computer hardware and software vendors for patient record systems)
- Research centers

Education
- Allied health professional schools and programs
- Schools of medicine
- Schools of nursing
- Schools of public health

Accreditation
- Accreditation organizations
- Institutional licensure agencies
- Professional licensure agencies

Policy Making
- Federal government agencies
- Local government agencies
- State government agencies

Source: Adapted from Dick, Steen, and Detmer 1997, 77.

Patient Care Managers and Support Staff

Patient care managers and support staff oversee the services provided to patients within their organization. The health record provides the data they need to evaluate the performance of individual patient care providers and to determine the effectiveness of the services provided. The patient care manager refers to the documentation in the health record when questions arise about a specific patient's course of treatment or about the services the patient received.

Patient care managers also are responsible for the overall evaluation of services rendered for their particular area of responsibility. To identify patterns and trends, they take details from individual health records and then put all the information together in one place. On the basis of these combined **aggregate data,** the managers recommend changes to patient care processes, equipment, and services. The goal of the changes is to improve the future outcomes of patient care.

Coding and Billing Staff

Healthcare **reimbursement** is based on the documentation contained in the health record. By referring to the records of individual patients, coding specialists identify the patients' diagnoses as well as the therapeutic procedures they underwent and the services they received. Using this information, coding specialists assign appropriate **diagnostic** and **procedural codes.** The coded information is then used to generate a patient bill and/or a claim for reimbursement to a third-party payer, such as a commercial health insurance company or government-sponsored health program such as Medicare.

Some third-party payers require billers to submit copies of portions of the health record along with the claims. The health record documentation substantiates the need for services and the fact that such services were provided.

Other Individual Users

Many other individuals may use the health record as a source of information.

Patients
Today, patients are taking an active interest in their own health and in the preventive and therapeutic healthcare they receive. Recent federal legislation—the Health Insurance Portability and Accountability Act (HIPAA) of 1996—includes health record security and privacy provisions. HIPAA grants most patients the right to see their health records. In addition, they have the right to correct the information in their records and to add missing information. They also can verify billed services.

Employers
Employers use information based on the health records of their employees to determine the extent and effects of occupational hazards. They also use health record information to manage healthcare and disability insurance benefits for their employees. Moreover, individual employees' disability claims must be supported by the information in their health records.

Lawyers
The health record is considered legal documentation of the healthcare services provided to patients. Attorneys for healthcare organizations use it as a tool to protect the legal interests of the facility and its patient care providers. The legal representatives of physicians and their malpractice insurance carriers also depend on the documentation in the health record. Attorneys for patients who bring civil suits use health records to support claims for com-

pensation of medical malpractice. Attorneys also use information from the health record to determine the mental competency of individuals.

Law Enforcement Officials

Law enforcement officials, such as police officers, agents of the Federal Bureau of Investigation (FBI), sheriffs, and marshals, also may use the health record in limited situations. For example, health records are used in the investigation of gunshot injuries, child abuse and neglect, domestic violence, and other crimes. Law enforcement officials also use information contained in health records to identify and locate suspects, fugitives, material witnesses, and missing persons.

Healthcare Researchers and Clinical Investigators

Clinical research is the process by which the effectiveness of treatment methods is evaluated and improved methods for future care are developed. Researchers review health records for the particular population being studied and extract data. The data help them to evaluate and make decisions about disease processes and treatments. Healthcare researchers and clinical investigators also use aggregate health record data.

Health Science Publishers and Journalists

Healthcare consumers continue to seek more and more information about developments in clinical research, alternative medicine, preventive medicine, and public health. The Internet offers extensive healthcare information to Americans. Radio, television, and print journalists also look for legitimate sources of information on healthcare topics.

Government Policy Makers

Local, state, and federal government policy makers are responsible for evaluating the overall health and well-being of the populations they serve. Government agencies establish the requirements for reporting cases of certain communicable diseases. They also require the reporting of information relevant to health-related social issues such as gunshot wounds, teenage pregnancies, and drug abuse. The health record is the source for the information needed to meet such reporting requirements. Policy makers develop aggregate information, which serves as the basis for investigations of the health patterns and trends in a given population. Using this information, policy makers can develop and fund community programs.

Institutional Users

A number of organizations depend on access to healthcare-related information. The health record is the most reliable source of such information.

Healthcare Delivery Organizations

Healthcare delivery organizations include physicians' practices, ambulatory clinics, blood and tissue donor banks, home care agencies, hospices, acute care hospitals, rehabilitation hospitals, psychiatric hospitals, long-term care facilities, and public health departments and clinics. Such organizations use data from health records in providing services, evaluating and monitoring the use of resources, seeking reimbursement for the services provided, and planning and marketing services.

Third-Party Payers

Third-party payers are organizations responsible for the reimbursement of healthcare services covered by some kind of insurance program. Third-party payers include commercial health insurance companies, managed care organizations, self-insured employers, and the fiscal (or financial) intermediaries representing Medicare and Medicaid. Third-party payers review individual health records to determine whether the documentation supports the provider's claim for reimbursement. Claims that are not supported by adequate health record documentation are often denied. Many third-party payers enter into contractual arrangements with medical review organizations to perform the actual review of health records.

Medical Review Organizations

Quality improvement organizations and **utilization management organizations** evaluate the adequacy and appropriateness of the care provided by healthcare organizations. Medical review organizations work under contract with the federal government. These organizations examine the individual health records for specific episodes of care to determine whether the services were medically necessary. Depending on the organization, this process may take place on a concurrent basis while the patient is still under treatment or on a retrospective basis after the patient has received services. The results of the medical reviews are usually linked directly to the level of reimbursement paid to the provider.

Research Organizations

Organizations performing healthcare-related research study the current healthcare environment to prove or disprove hypotheses related to disease processes and treatments. Research organizations include disease registries, research centers, and health data companies. In some instances, the law may require healthcare providers to provide aggregate data from health records on specific disease processes. In other instances, participation is voluntary. Healthcare providers committed to health education and research work closely with research organizations to develop and test experimental patient care protocols and to provide the relevant data from the health record.

Educational Organizations

Healthcare professionals undergo rigorous professional education based on classroom and hands-on training. Medical schools, dental schools, nursing schools, and allied health training programs frequently use health records as sources of case study information.

Accreditation Organizations

The mission of every accreditation organization is to improve the quality of services offered in healthcare facilities. Participation in accreditation programs is voluntary. Accreditation organizations include the Joint Commission on Accreditation of Healthcare Organizations, the American Osteopathic Association, the Commission on Accreditation of Rehabilitation Facilities, and the Accreditation Association for Ambulatory Health Care.

Every participating healthcare organization is subject to a periodic accreditation survey. Surveyors visit each facility and compare its programs, policies, and procedures to a pre-published set of performance standards. A key component of every accreditation survey is a review of the facility's health records. Surveyors review the documentation of patient care services to determine whether the standards for care are being met. They then use the results of the review to make the overall accreditation decision. The surveys usually involve the direct review of a sample of health records from recent and current patients along with a review of aggregate statistics related to expected patient outcomes.

Government Licensing Agencies

The goal of local, state, and federal licensing agencies is to make sure that the healthcare facilities in their areas provide effective and appropriate care to healthcare consumers. Licensing agencies include state licensing bureaus and federal and state departments responsible for certifying facilities that receive funding from the federal, state, and local governments. As part of the licensing process, health records are reviewed to determine whether the facility is complying with the licensing regulations in that geographic area.

Policy-Making Bodies

The **Centers for Medicare and Medicaid Services** (CMS) is a division of the U.S. Department of Health and Human Services. (Until 2001, it was known as the Health Care Financing Administration, or HCFA.) CMS is responsible for administering the federal Medicare program and the federal portion of the Medicaid program.

Data taken from health records and supplied by healthcare organizations as part of the Medicare billing and reimbursement process are kept in a national database. The database is used to make decisions related to healthcare reimbursement mechanisms, the effectiveness of healthcare services, and the general health of the Medicare population. Although the content and sources of data differ, similar information databases are maintained at the state level.

In addition to the information kept in federal and state databases, policy-making bodies rely on the support of various health-related organizations that have been created to support high standards of healthcare in the United States. Although their overall mission varies, organizations such as the American Medical Association, the American Psychiatric Association, the American Hospital Association, the American Health Information Management Association, the American College of Surgeons, and the American College of Physicians all develop healthcare standards. They also make recommendations to the federal and state governments on healthcare policy issues.

Check Your Understanding 2.2

Instructions: Indicate whether the following statements are true or false (T or F).

1. _____ A physical therapist documenting in the health record is an institutional health record user.

2. _____ A surveyor from the American College of Surgeons reviewing a health record to determine compliance with the Commission on Cancer standards is an institutional health record user.

3. _____ An HIM professional extracting data from a paper-based record for an analysis of infection rates requested by hospital administration is an individual health record user.

4. _____ A patient requesting a copy of her health record is an individual health record user.

5. _____ An auditor employed by Medicare that is reviewing health records for a mortality study is an individual health record user.

6. _____ A physician who has a contract with the state department of health to analyze the factors associated with an influenza outbreak in the state is an institutional health record user.

7. _____ Epidemiologists from the U.S. Department of Homeland Security studying the incidence of life-threatening organisms are individual health record users.

8. _____ A physician reviewing a health record of his patient to determine a diagnosis is an individual health record user.

9. _____ A police officer investigating a missing person report is an institutional health record user.

10. _____ An attorney defending a healthcare organization in a civil complaint from a patient is an individual health record user.

Functions of the Health Record

The primary function of the health record is to store patient care documentation. A number of systems, policies, and processes make it possible to collect patient care documentation efficiently and to store it in easily accessible and secure formats of high quality.

Besides storage of patient care documentation, the health record has other equally important functions. These include helping physicians, nurses, and other caregivers make diagnoses and choose treatment options. Paper-based health record formats limit these types of clinical decision making functions. With the implementation of EHR systems, the function of the health record as an interactive tool for clinical problem solving and decision making will increase.

Storage of Information

As noted earlier, the main function of the health record is to store patient care data and information. According to the IOM (Dick, Steen, and Detmer 1997, 81–93), the attributes associated with the storage function are accessibility, quality, security, flexibility, connectivity, and efficiency.

Accessibility

Authorized users of the health record must be able to access information easily when and where they need it. Every health record system should allow record access 24 hours a day.

Any organization that maintains health records for individual patients must have systems in place that identify each patient and support efficient access to information on each patient. The systems must be able to do this regardless of the format in which the record is stored.

Quality

Clinicians, patients, administrators, researchers, and many other individuals and organizations rely on the quality of the information in the health record. In large part, the quality of such information depends on the design of the organization's systems and processes for collecting the original information.

Health record information is collected in different ways and from numerous sources. Patients and their families provide information to healthcare providers. Healthcare providers retrieve information from the documentation of previous patient encounters. Physicians and other providers make direct observations about the patient, assess clinical problems, provide diagnostic and therapeutic services, and evaluate the results of therapy. The data generated by electronic diagnostic and monitoring equipment such as laboratory results and tracings from heart monitors are also included in the health record. All this information is recorded on paper forms or in computer formats to become part of the health record.

Data Quality Management
To accomplish the primary and secondary purposes of the health record, the data in it must be of the highest quality. Incomplete or missing data (for example, unrecorded lab results) could compromise patient care. Likewise, they may contribute to incorrect assumptions made by policy makers. Further, incomplete or missing data could result in inaccurate research findings. One of the HIM professional's most important roles is to ensure that the health record contains the highest-quality data possible.

In 1998, the American Health Information Management Association (AHIMA) developed a **data quality management** model, which is based on four domains (Cassidy et al. 1998):

- *Data applications:* The purposes for which data are collected
- *Data collection:* The processes by which data are collected
- *Data warehousing:* The processes and systems by which data are archived (saved for future use)
- *Data analysis:* The processes by which data are translated into information that can be used for designated application

The data quality management model applies the following quality characteristics to the four quality management domains:

- Accuracy
- Accessibility
- Comprehensiveness
- Consistency
- Currency
- Definition
- Granularity
- Precision
- Relevancy
- Timeliness

Data accuracy means that data are correct. The data should represent what was intended or defined by the original source of the data. For example, the patient's emergency contact information recorded in a paper record or a database should be the same as what the patient said it was. Results of laboratory testing for a particular patient should reflect the results generated by the laboratory equipment. Data related to the medication provided to a particular patient should reflect the actual date, time, and medication administered. The accuracy of the data placed in the health record depends on a number of factors, including:

- The patient's physical health and emotional state at the time the data were collected
- The provider's interviewing skills
- The provider's recording skills
- The availability of the patient's clinical history
- The dependability of the automated equipment
- The reliability of the electronic communications media

Data accessibility means that the data are easily obtainable. The following factors affect the accessibility of health record data and information:

- Whether previous health records are available when and where they are needed
- Whether dictation equipment is accessible and working properly
- Whether transcription of dictation is accurate, timely, and readily available to healthcare providers
- Whether computer data-entry devices are working properly and are readily available to healthcare providers

Data comprehensiveness means that all the required data elements are included in the health record. In essence, comprehensiveness means that the record is complete. In both paper-based and computer-based systems, having a complete health record is critical to the organization's ability to provide excellent patient care and to meet all regulatory, legal, and reimbursement requirements. In general, the health record must include the following data elements:

- Patient identification
- Consents for treatment
- Advance directives
- Problem list
- Diagnoses
- Clinical history
- Diagnostic test results
- Treatments and outcomes
- Conclusions and follow-up requirements

Data consistency means that the data are reliable. Reliable data do not change no matter how many times or in how many ways they are stored, processed, or displayed. Data values are consistent when the value of any given data element is the same across applications and systems. Related data items also should be reliable. For example, the clinical history for a male patient would never include a hysterectomy as a past surgical procedure.

Legitimate documentation inconsistencies do occur in health records. Any given health record may contain numerous references to the patient's diagnosis in terms of:

- The admitting diagnosis
- The diagnostic impression upon physical examination
- The postoperative diagnosis
- The pathology diagnosis
- The discharge diagnosis

Any inconsistencies among the various types of diagnoses would be legitimate. The different diagnoses incorporate the results of tests and findings not available at the time the previous documentation took place.

In other instances, however, data inconsistencies in the health record are not acceptable. For example, a nursing assessment might indicate that the patient is deaf when there is no documentation by the physician that the patient's hearing is compromised. Another unacceptable inconsistency occurs when different healthcare providers use different terminology. For example, different providers might use the words *cyst, lesion,* and *abscess* interchangeably in documenting a skin condition for the same patient. Such inconsistencies create difficulties for other caregivers and can be very confusing to external users of the health record.

Data currency and **data timeliness** mean that healthcare data should be up-to-date and recorded at or near the time of the event or observation. Because care and treatment rely on accurate and current data, an essential characteristic of data quality is the timeliness of the documentation or data entry.

Data definition means that the data and information documented in the health record are defined. For information to be meaningful, it must be pertinent. Users of the data must understand what the data mean and represent. Every data element should have a clear definition and a range of acceptable values.

Data granularity requires that the attributes and values of data be defined at the correct level of detail. For example, numerical values for laboratory results should be recorded to the appropriate decimal place as required for the meaningful interpretation of test results.

Data precision is the term used to describe expected data values. As part of data definition, the acceptable values or value ranges for each data element must be defined. For example, a precise data definition related to gender would include three values: male, female, and unknown. Precise data definition yields accurate data collection. In paper-based health records, much of the documentation and data is collected in narrative format and it is difficult to apply the concept of data precision to narrative text. The movement toward computerized patient records provides the perfect opportunity to improve data precision in health records.

Data relevancy means that the data in the health record are useful. The reason for collecting the data element must be clear to ensure the relevancy of the data collected. In paper-based health records, the volume of detail provided often limits the usefulness of the data and information (Abdelhak 2001). For example, nursing documentation is often lengthy and physicians and other caregivers may not have sufficient time to review it.

Security

Healthcare organizations and the clinical professionals who provide patient care services depend on the accuracy and accessibility of the information collected and stored in the health record. In addition, healthcare administrators, third-party payers, government agencies, accreditation organizations, and medical researchers all must have access to detailed healthcare information in order to fulfill their functions. However, these legitimate needs for access to information must be balanced against the public's expectation that healthcare providers will respect and protect the **privacy** of their patients.

Privacy, **confidentiality,** and security are related, but distinct, concepts. In the context of healthcare, *privacy* can be defined as the right of individuals to control access to their personal health information. *Confidentiality* refers to the expectation that the personal information shared by an individual with a healthcare provider during the course of care will be used only for its intended purpose. *Security* is the protection of the privacy of individuals and the confidentiality of health records. In other words, security allows only authorized users to access health records. In the broader sense, security also includes the protection of healthcare information from damage, loss, and unauthorized alteration. (Privacy, confidentiality, and security are discussed in more detail in chapters 14, 15, and 19.)

Requirements for Access, Flexibility, Connectivity, and Efficiency

For the health record to fulfill its intended purposes, several conditions must be met. Essentially, these involve how the health record is made available to legitimate users and how it is stored and maintained.

Access

To be useful, the health record must be made available to legitimate users. As mentioned earlier, protecting the confidential nature of the health record is extremely important and is one of the HIM professional's primary responsibilities.

In paper-based health record systems, access control is relatively straightforward. The records are stored in locked storage areas that are accessible only to authorized HIM staff. When needed for patient care purposes, the health record is retrieved from the file and forwarded to the appropriate service area. The record is then logged out according to a prescribed procedure. In this way, the HIM staff knows where to find the record in the event it is needed by another department or provider.

EHR systems have the same access control requirements that paper-based systems do. However, the mechanisms for controlling access to confidential information are different. Access control mechanisms are built in to EHRs. Technology-based access control mechanisms include the use of passwords, access cards or tokens, biometric devices, workstation restrictions, and role-based restrictions. (See chapter 19 for additional information on access control.)

Flexibility

Health record data should be flexible enough to meet the needs of all the record's different users. In paper-based health record systems, this characteristic cannot be fully realized. Standardized forms are designed to make data readily available and meaningful to those caring for the patient. However, these forms may not support the needs of everyone who uses the health record. For example, individual physicians may wish to view laboratory results in ways that a single standard display does not permit.

When designed appropriately, EHR systems can be extremely flexible in the way they display and present information. Authorized caregivers and other legitimate health record users display the information they need in the formats they prefer. For example, caregivers may wish to see views of the data by source, encounter, problem, date, or any number of other variables. Further, they may need data in detail or in summary form. Some users may only need to know the presence or absence of certain data, not necessarily the nature of the data. In these instances, the EHR has the potential to accommodate these needs and enhance the confidentiality of patient-identifiable health information.

Connectivity

Connectivity refers to the capacity of health record systems to provide communication linkages and allow the exchange of health record data among information systems. Communications technology can be used within individual organizations to connect the various information systems that contain electronic components of the health record. Health record information that is not stored in an electronic format, however, must be transferred from place to place within the organization in a paper-based format. The complete implementation of EHR systems will make full use of the technologies available.

Efficiency

Efficiency is another component of health record storage that will be improved in computer-based systems. As noted earlier, providing access to paper-based health records is an inefficient process, especially when information must be transferred between providers and facilities. Even internal transfers of health records can be troublesome because paper records may be needed in more than one place at a time. Moreover, paper records can be easily misplaced by users or misfiled by staff.

Another factor related to efficiency is the structure of the data. Today, much of the data entered into a computer-based system for storage has been scanned in from paper forms. Thus, most of the data are unstructured and cannot be used to make meaningful comparisons. For example, transcribed reports and data obtained from document imaging systems provide electronically stored text, but the information cannot be analyzed efficiently. In fully functional EHR systems, structured data capture processes will use controlled vocabularies and code sets. Data collected in standard forms can be analyzed efficiently and compared through computer software applications.

Guidance in Clinical Problem Solving

Physicians, nurses, and other caregivers use the information in individual health records as the basis for making diagnoses and choosing treatment options. A properly formatted health record can guide clinicians through the process of solving clinical problems. *Health record format* refers to the organization of electronic information or paper forms within the individual record.

Three types of formats are commonly used in paper-based record systems: source-oriented, problem-oriented, and integrated. The **source-oriented health record format** organizes the information according to the patient care department that provided the care. This format is used by most acute care hospitals. The **problem-oriented health record format** is a documentation approach in which the physician defines each clinical problem individually. Information about the problems is organized into four components: the database, the problem list, initial plans, and progress notes. The **integrated health record format** organizes all the paper forms in strict chronological order and mixes the forms created by different departments. (Chapter 3 discusses health record formats in more detail.)

Over the years, there has been a lot of debate about which record format is most useful for clinical problem solving. In 1991, the IOM's Committee on Improving the Patient Record studied various formats. The committee could not agree on which format would be the most useful in improving patient care. It felt that a mere translation of current record formats from paper media to computer media would not result in meaningful improvements.

The report of the study (Dick, Steen, and Detmer 1997) noted that current record systems are based on clinician behaviors and record forms that produce substantial waste, imprecision, and complexity. It concluded that the movement toward EHR systems will give healthcare organizations and providers the opportunity to study and improve clinical approaches. Improvements in clinical care then will be reflected in the health record format (Dick, Steen, and Detmer 1997).

Today, developing EHR systems are introducing new formats and functionality. Results management, order entry, and order management were added to the EHR functional model by the IOM in 2003 (IOM 2003, 7–8).

Results Management

Having ready access to all types of results, including laboratory results, radiology results, and other test results, over a period of time helps providers make informed choices for diagnoses and treatment and increases quality of care. With EHRs, both current and previous computerized results can be displayed automatically for care providers to improve effectiveness and efficiency of treatment while reducing the cost of care by eliminating duplicate testing. EHR formats for trending and comparing results over time are not available in paper-based systems.

Order-Entry/Order Management

Computerized physician/provider order-entry (CPOE) systems have been developed to improve quality of care (Amatayakul 2004, 10). Whereas paper-based health records capture handwritten orders, CPOE provides physicians and other providers the ability to place orders via the computer from any number of locations and adds decision support capability to enhance patient safety. Early adopters of this technology have been able to eliminate lost orders, eliminate issues with illegible handwriting, eliminate duplicate orders, reduce medication errors, and reduce the time to fill orders (IOM 2003, 8). CPOE presents another new format and provides a health record functionality that is unique to the EHR.

As the EHR evolves, new formats will continue to be developed. Some will be more effective than others in encouraging the use of efficient, scientific problem-solving methods in the clinical process.

Clinical Decision Support

Effective and efficient patient care requires a great deal of complex information. To be an effective tool in clinical decision support, the health record needs to be more than a simple repository of patient care data (Dick, Steen, and Detmer 1997). Fully functional EHR systems will provide a number of decision-making tools that are not currently available in health record systems.

Clinical decision support tools can review structured electronic data and alert practitioners to out-of-range laboratory values or dangerous trends before problems become evident. The tools can recall relevant diagnostic criteria and treatment options on the basis of the data in the record. This will support the physician as he or she considers various diagnostic and treatment alternatives. Because the human memory is imperfect, such tools can provide a consistent supplementary knowledge base grounded in the latest clinical research.

In addition, computer-based clinical decision support tools can give clinicians instant access to pharmaceutical formularies, referral databases, and reference literature. This type of ready access provides clinicians with updates to information that they may use infrequently. Further, these applications can help healthcare professionals learn about new developments because the bibliographic information in the decision support databases is always up-to-date.

Standard commercial software packages also can be included in health information systems so that descriptive, graphical, and statistical analyses of clinical data can be carried out. Such analyses may be limited to a specific case or performed on aggregate data to identify trends in a larger patient population. This functionality cannot be readily accomplished in paper-based record systems without a significant investment in staff time.

Check Your Understanding 2.3

Instructions: Match the following terms with the correct definitions.

1. ____ Electronic health record
2. ____ Confidentiality
3. ____ Data consistency
4. ____ Data comprehensiveness
5. ____ Data granularity
6. ____ Health record
7. ____ Privacy
8. ____ Security

a. A characteristic of data that is reliable
b. A characteristic of data whose values are defined at the appropriate level of detail
c. Documentation of the services provided to patients by clinicians
d. An interactive health record that has functions beyond storage
e. A program designed to protect patient privacy and to prevent unauthorized access, alteration, or destruction of health records
f. A comparison of actual system activity with expected activity
g. An individual's right to control access to his or her personal information
h. The expectation that the personal information shared by an individual with a healthcare provider during the course of care will be used only for its intended purpose
i. A characteristic of data that includes every required data element

---

Real-World Case #1

The following case study is adapted from a publication by Susan Helbig in the October 2004 IFHRO Congress and AHIMA Convention Proceedings.

The Department of Veterans Affairs (VA) has been implementing components of the electronic health record since the late 1990s. The system is designed to provide for reuse of the information previously documented on a given patient with copy/paste functionality. However, HIM professionals in many VA facilities began to experience health record integrity concerns as a result of this functionality. Busy clinicians were using the copy/paste function to take information from one document in the health record to another document to speed up the documentation process. According to Helbig, discharge summaries and progress notes were becoming extremely long because of all the copying of information from other portions of the record and because the information copied did not always reference the initial author. Coders were having difficulty determining what was actually done during a particular encounter as a result of the copy/paste practice.

In 2002, a study was initiated at VA Puget Sound Health Care System in Washington State to quantify the extent and effect of the concern. The health records of 243 patients with 29,386 notes and 6,322 copy events were reviewed as part of the study. The study found a relatively low rate of high-risk copying, but at least one high-risk event for every 10 patients reviewed.

Real-World Case #2

The following case study is adapted from a published proceeding by Liu Aimin for the October 2004 IFHRO Congress and AHIMA Convention.

In November 2002, the first case of SARS (severe acute respiratory syndrome) was found in China. By June 2003, there were more than 5,000 diagnosed cases and more than 300 deaths due to SARS in China alone. SARS was not officially announced as an infectious disease by the Chinese Disease Control. Therefore, multiple entities, including the government, health authority, and health bureau, were all trying to gather information on SARS in different formats and on different forms. According to Aimin (2004, 2), "In Spring 2003, SARS was out of control due to incorrect information."

When the HIM departments of facilities received SARS paper-based health records, the records had to be pasteurized to prevent spread of the SARS infection. Department staff were unable to complete discharge record processing until pasteurization was complete.

To study SARS and develop an information system, the Chinese Health Ministry commissioned a SARS research project to collect SARS records from severely affected areas, compare forms, and abstract key data elements. This project is being conducted by the Chinese Medical Record Association, which is affiliated with the Chinese Hospital Association.

Summary

The health record is the principal repository of data and information about the healthcare services provided to patients. A number of individuals and institutions use it as a source of information, but the primary users are the clinical professionals who provide direct patient care. Secondary users include healthcare managers and administrators, government agencies and policy makers, third-party payers, researchers, educators, and accreditation organizations.

The primary function of the health record is the storage of patient care information. The most important attributes of record storage include accessibility, quality, security, flexibility, connectivity, and efficiency. The full implementation of interactive electronic health record systems will add more functionality to the health record that traditional paper-based records cannot provide. In addition to storing health information, EHRs will provide knowledge resources to help clinicians solve diagnostic problems, support clinical decision making and administrative processes, and provide support for electronic reporting for population health management.

The concepts of privacy, confidentiality, and security are central to health information management. Patients have the right to expect that healthcare providers will respect their privacy and guard their healthcare information against unauthorized access. Confidentiality forms the basis of meaningful patient–provider relationships. Without the protection of confidentiality, patients would be reluctant to be honest and open about issues related to their health. Security ensures that the information stored in a health record is protected from unauthorized alteration, damage, and loss.

References

Abdelhak, Mervat, et al. 2001. *Health Information: Management of a Strategic Resource,* 2nd ed. Philadelphia: W.B. Saunders Company.

Aimin, Liu. 2004 (October). The impact of SARS on the Chinese health information system. *2004 IFHRO Congress and AHIMA Convention Proceedings.* Chicago: AHIMA.

Amatayakul, Margaret K. 2004. *Electronic Health Records: A Practical Guide for Professionals and Organizations,* 2nd ed. Chicago: American Health Information Management Association.

American Health Information Management Association. 2000. *Evolving HIM Careers: Seven Roles for the Future.* Chicago: AHIMA.

Cassidy, Bonnie, et al. 1998. Practice brief: Data quality management model. *Journal of American Health Information Management Association* 69(6).

Cofer, Jennifer, editor. 1994. *Health Information Management,* 10th ed. Berwyn, IL: Physicians' Record Company.

Dick, Richard S., Elaine B. Steen, and Don E. Detmer, editors. 1997. *The Computer-Based Patient Record: An Essential Technology for Health Care,* rev. ed. Washington, DC: National Academy Press.

Drazen, Erica. 2001. Is this the year of the computer-based patient record? *Healthcare Informatics* (2):94–98.

Fernandez, Lorraine, et al. 1997. Practice brief: Master patient (person) index (MPI)—recommended core data elements. *Journal of American Health Information Management Association* 68(7).

Glondys, Barbara. 1999. *Documentation for the Acute Care Patient Record.* Chicago: AHIMA.

Hagland, Mark. 2000. Moving gradually toward a paperless world. *Journal of American Health Information Management Association* 71(8):26–31.

Helbig, Susan. 2004 (October). Copying and pasting in the EHR-S: An HIM perspective. *2004 IFHRO Congress and AHIMA Convention Proceedings.* Chicago: AHIMA.

Hjort, Beth. 2000. Practice brief: Security audits. *Journal of American Health Information Management Association* 71(8).

Institute of Medicine. 2003. *Key Capabilities of an Electronic Health Record System: Letter Report.* Available online from nap.edu.

National Committee on Vital and Health Statistics. 2001. *A Strategy for Building the Health Information Infrastructure.* U.S. Department of Health and Human Services. Washington, DC: HHS.

Skurka, Margaret A. 1998. *Health Information Management: Principles and Organization for Health Record Services,* rev. ed. Chicago: AHA Press.

Transforming Health Care: The President's Health Information Technology Plan. 2004. Available online from whitehouse.gov/infocus/technology/ economic_policy200404/chap3.html.

Welch, Julie. 2000. Practice brief: Authentication of health record entries. *Journal of American Health Information Management Association* 71(3).

Chapter 3
Content and Structure of the Health Record

Bonnie J. Petterson, PhD, RHIA

Learning Objectives

- To understand the content of health records in various healthcare settings
- To recognize the documentation requirements of accreditation organizations and state and federal government agencies
- To describe the different formats used for health records in healthcare organizations
- To understand the advantages of electronic health records over paper-based and hybrid health records

Key Terms

Accreditation

Accreditation Association for Ambulatory Health Care (AAAHC)

Advance directive

American Osteopathic Association (AOA)

Anesthesia report

Authorization to disclose information

Autopsy report

Care plan

Certification

Commission on Accreditation of Rehabilitation Facilities (CARF)

Computer-based patient record (CPR)

Conditions for Coverage

Conditions of Participation

Consent to treatment

Consultation report

Deemed status

Discharge summary

Electronic health record (EHR)

Electronic medical record (EMR)

Expressed consent

Hybrid health record

Imaging technology

Implied consent

Integrated health records

Joint Commission on Accreditation of Healthcare Organizations (JCAHO)

Licensure

Medical history

Medical staff privileges

Medicare Conditions of Participation or Conditions for Coverage

Minimum Data Set (MDS) for Long-Term Care

National Committee for Quality Assurance (NCQA)

Operative report

Outcomes and Assessment Information Set (OASIS)

Palliative care

Pathology report

Patient assessment instrument (PAI)

Patient history questionnaire

Patient Self-Determination Act (PSDA)

Patient's bill of rights

Personal health record (PHR)

Physical examination report

Physician's orders

Problem list

Problem-oriented health records

Progress notes

Recovery room report

Resident assessment instrument (RAI)

Resident assessment protocol (RAP)

Source-oriented health records

Transfer record

Introduction

As explained in chapter 2, the health record has multiple purposes. One of its primary purposes is the documentation of patient care. It represents the main communication mechanism used by healthcare providers in the delivery of patient treatment. Without it, providers would be unable to provide safe and effective care.

For more than a century, health records were created and maintained in paper-based formats. In recent years, however, many healthcare providers have implemented computer-based health records. As the demand for health information increases and as healthcare facilities adopt advanced information technology, computer-based records will eventually replace most paper-based health records. A number of different terms have been used to describe computer-based records. Today, **electronic health record** (EHR) is the term used most widely by the federal government and other entities. It refers to a health record available electronically allowing communication across providers and permitting real-time decision making. It also allows for efficient reporting mechanisms. Other terms used more commonly in the past include **electronic medical record** (EMR) and **computer-based patient record** (CPR) (Mon 2004a). When a facility is transitioning from paper to electronic systems and uses components of both, the record is referred to as a **hybrid health record.** Chapter 4 discusses the EHR in more detail.

This chapter describes the basic content of acute care health records and then provides specialized information requirements of other healthcare settings. It also introduces the documentation methods required by government and accreditation organizations. Finally, the chapter discusses the formats of paper-based, hybrid, and electronic health records and compares their strengths and weaknesses.

Theory into Practice

Major shifts in the way physicians, organizations, hospitals, and other health settings manage health records are beginning to appear throughout the United States. The following real-life case is an example of the steps an organization takes in the transition from paper-based health record formats to computer-based systems.

Mayo Clinic Hospital, a 205-bed acute care hospital located in Phoenix, Arizona, has close to 350 physicians from more than 65 medical and surgical specialties on its medical staff.

The Phoenix hospital opened in the fall of 1998 with a hybrid health record. Much of the care record is entered and accessed via vendor-purchased, site-edited software. The conditions of admission, consents and authorizations, physician progress notes, physician orders, anesthesia and sedation reports, interoperative records, emergency and ambulatory surgery records, and patient discharge instructions and referrals are paper documents. Emergency visit documents are gathered six hours after patient release and are scanned into the electronic system. All dictated physician reports (history and physicals, operative reports, consultations, and discharge summaries) are immediately available in the electronic record after transcription. Paper versions of the reports are scanned into the imaging system upon patient discharge for purposes of obtaining physicians' electronic signatures. All other documentation, including that done by nursing, therapists, and other health professionals, and diagnostic or therapeutic testing, including imaging, are recorded and reported electronically. The facility is currently investigating a computerized physician order-entry (CPOE) component and anticipates that it, along with an automated prescription pad, will be its next electronic addition.

Discharge record analysis (reviewing the record upon patient discharge for missing elements) is done by health information personnel using a computer. The system filters documents so that only those needing review are accessed. Electronic signatures are used and physicians can enter the system at any of the Arizona Mayo sites. E-mail notices to physicians on record deficiencies are generated automatically upon completion of analysis. Although the parts of the record generated on paper are stored for a very short period of time after scanning, all release of information and other processes, including coding, use the computer-based record.

About fourteen miles away, Mayo Clinic's outpatient clinic practice uses the same electronic record. Computers are located in each examination room and in stations outside the rooms. Information such as current medications and allergies can be entered directly. Progress notes from all patient visits at the clinic and from the three primary care practice sites located elsewhere in the metropolitan area are dictated immediately after each visit. Similar to hospital-dictated reports, they are transcribed and made immediately available as part of the electronic record. Paper documents in the outpatient setting include consents, insurance cards, and miscellaneous specialty-specific documentation. All paper documents are picked up hourly by health information personnel, scanned and indexed into the imaging system, and reviewed for quality. The scanned material is available in the electronic record within two to four hours of the pickup time.

Kathie Falk, supervisor of medical records at Mayo Clinic Hospital, and Yolanda Nichols, her counterpart at the clinic, note, however, that the Mayo facilities in Rochester, Minnesota, and Jacksonville, Florida, currently have site-specific electronic records. There is some sharing of information (for example, Minnesota and Arizona have the same registration/billing systems, utilize the same transcription database, and all three sites use the same radiology system). Improving interoperability across the country is a Mayo goal.

Content of the Health Record

First and foremost, the health record is a tool for documenting patient care. The information in the health record is provided directly by the healthcare professionals who participate in the patient's care. This information is used for:

- Planning and managing diagnostic, therapeutic, and nursing services
- Evaluating the adequacy and appropriateness of care
- Substantiating reimbursement claims
- Protecting the legal interests of the patient, the healthcare provider, and the healthcare organization

In addition, the health record is a tool used by the patient's caregivers to communicate with each other. Finally, information collected from health records is used for research, public health, and educational and organizational activities such as medical research, professional training, performance improvement, risk management, and strategic planning.

The health record generally contains two types of data: clinical and administrative. *Clinical data* document the patient's medical condition, diagnosis, and treatment as well as the healthcare services provided. *Administrative data* include demographic and financial information as well as various consents and authorizations related to the provision of care and the handling of confidential patient information.

The content of the health record varies, depending on the healthcare setting and the provider's medical specialty. Record content is determined primarily by practice needs and pertinent standards. Standards are statements of expected behavior or reference points against which structures, processes, or outcomes can be measured. Standards for documentation can be found in the following four main sources:

- *Facility-specific standards:* Standards might be found in facility policies and procedures and, when a facility has an organized medical staff, in the medical staff bylaws, rules, and regulations. Facility-specific guidelines govern the practice of physicians and others within a specific organization.

- *Licensure requirements:* Before they can provide services, most healthcare organizations must be licensed by government entities such as the state or county in which they are located and must maintain a license as long as care is provided.

- *Government reimbursement programs:* Standards are applied to facilities that choose to participate in federal government reimbursement programs such as Medicare and Medicaid. These standards are titled **Conditions of Participation** or **Conditions for Coverage.** Facilities are said to be certified if the standards are met.

- *Accreditation standards:* Accreditation is the end result of an intensive external review process that indicates a facility has voluntarily met the standards of the independent accrediting organization (such as the **Joint Commission on Accreditation of Healthcare Organizations** [JCAHO]).

Standards of these groups not only address content, but often also outline time limits for completion of particular portions of the health record. Healthcare data sets also help determine elements of record content. For example, the Uniform Ambulatory Care Data Set outlines what data should be documented in facilities where ambulatory care is delivered. Data sets are discussed in chapter 5.

Content of Hospital Acute Care Records

This section describes the basic content of health records maintained by acute care hospitals. (See table 3.1 for a summary of the basic components of an acute care health record.) The basic components will be found in a record whether the record is paper based, hybrid, or computer based. The health record content requirements for other healthcare settings and medical specialties are discussed in the following section.

Clinical Data

The patient's attending or primary physician usually gives the hospital some preliminary information about the patient before he or she is admitted to the hospital. (Admission is the process of formal registration for hospital services.) Such information includes an admitting or working diagnosis, sometimes also called a provisional diagnosis. The diagnosis identifies the condition or illness for which the patient needs medical care. This information is recorded on an admission or registration record, also referred to as a face sheet in paper-based systems. The admission record also includes demographic and financial data about the patient. (See the administrative data section later in this chapter.)

Table 3.1. Basic components of the acute care health record	
Component	**Function**
Registration record	Documents demographic information about the patient
Medical history	Documents the patient's current and past health status
Physical examination	Contains the provider's findings based on an examination of the patient
Clinical observations	Provide a chronological summary of the patient's illness and treatment as documented by physicians, nurses, and allied health professionals
Physician's orders	Document the physician's instructions to other parties involved in providing the patient's care, including orders for medications and diagnostic and therapeutic procedures
Reports of diagnostic and therapeutic procedures	Describes the procedures performed and gives the names of clinicians and other providers; includes the findings of x-rays, mammograms, ultrasounds, scans, laboratory tests, and other diagnostic procedures
Consultation reports	Document opinions about a patient's condition furnished by providers other than the attending physician
Discharge summary	Concisely summarizes the patient's stay in a hospital
Patient instructions	Document the instructions for follow-up care that the provider gives to the patient or the patient's caregiver
Consents, authorizations, and acknowledgments	Document the patient's agreement to undergo treatment or services, permission to release confidential information, or recognition that information has been received

The following types of clinical data are documented in the health record during the patient's hospital stay:

- Patient's **medical history** and pertinent family history
- Report of the patient's initial physical examination
- Attending physician's diagnostic and therapeutic orders
- Clinical observations of the providers who care for the patient
- Reports and results of every diagnostic and therapeutic procedure performed
- Reports of consulting physicians
- Patient's **discharge summary**
- Final instructions to the patient upon discharge

Medical History

A complete medical history documents the patient's current complaints and symptoms and lists his or her past medical, personal, and family history. In acute care, the medical history is usually the responsibility of the attending physician. Medical histories obtained by specialists such as gynecologists and cardiologists concentrate on the organ systems involved in the patient's current illness. Table 3.2 shows the information that is usually included in a medical history.

Table 3.2.   Information usually included in a complete medical history

Components of the History	Complaints and Symptoms
Chief complaint	Nature and duration of the symptoms that caused the patient to seek medical attention as stated in his or her own words
Present illness	Detailed chronological description of the development of the patient's illness, from the appearance of the first symptom to the present situation
Past medical history	Summary of childhood and adult illnesses and conditions, such as infectious diseases, pregnancies, allergies and drug sensitivities, accidents, operations, hospitalizations, and current medications
Social and personal history	Marital status; dietary, sleep, and exercise patterns; use of coffee, tobacco, alcohol, and other drugs; occupation; home environment; daily routine; and so on
Family medical history	Diseases among relatives in which heredity or contact might play a role, such as allergies, cancer, and infectious, psychiatric, metabolic, endocrine, cardiovascular, and renal diseases; health status or cause and age at death for immediate relatives
Review of systems	Systemic inventory designed to uncover current or past subjective symptoms that includes the following types of data: • *General:* Usual weight, recent weight changes, fever, weakness, fatigue • *Skin:* Rashes, eruptions, dryness, cyanosis, jaundice; changes in skin, hair, or nails • *Head:* Headache (duration, severity, character, location) • *Eyes:* Glasses or contact lenses, last eye examination, glaucoma, cataracts, eyestrain, pain, diplopia, redness, lacrimation, inflammation, blurring • *Ears:* Hearing, discharge, tinnitus, dizziness, pain • *Nose:* Head colds, epistaxis, discharges, obstruction, postnasal drip, sinus pain • *Mouth and throat:* Condition of teeth and gums, last dental examination, soreness, redness, hoarseness, difficulty in swallowing • *Respiratory system:* Chest pain, wheezing, cough, dyspnea, sputum (color and quantity), hemoptysis, asthma, bronchitis, emphysema, pneumonia, tuberculosis, pleurisy, last chest x-ray • *Neurological system:* Fainting, blackouts, seizures, paralysis, tingling, tremors, memory loss • *Musculoskeletal system:* Joint pain or stiffness, arthritis, gout, backache, muscle pain, cramps, swelling, redness, limitation in motor activity • *Cardiovascular system:* Chest pain, rheumatic fever, tachycardia, palpitation, high blood pressure, edema, vertigo, faintness, varicose veins, thrombophlebitis • *Gastrointestinal system:* Appetite, thirst, nausea, vomiting, hematemesis, rectal bleeding, change in bowel habits, diarrhea, constipation, indigestion, food intolerance, flatus, hemorrhoids, jaundice • *Urinary system:* Frequent or painful urination, nocturia, pyuria, hematuria, incontinence, urinary infections • *Genitoreproductive system:* Male—venereal disease, sores, discharge from penis, hernias, testicular pain, or masses; female—age at menarche, frequency and duration of menstruation, dysmenorrhea, menorrhagia, symptoms of menopause, contraception, pregnancies, deliveries, abortions, last Pap smear • *Endocrine system:* Thyroid disease; heat or cold intolerance; excessive sweating, thirst, hunger, or urination • *Hematologic system:* Anemia, easy bruising or bleeding, past transfusions • *Psychiatric disorders:* Insomnia, headache, nightmares, personality disorders, anxiety disorders, mood disorders

Physical Examination Report

The **physical examination report** represents the attending physician's assessment of the patient's current health status. This report should document information on all the patient's major organ systems. Table 3.3 lists the components that are usually included in this report.

Diagnostic and Therapeutic Orders

Physician's orders are the instructions the physician gives to the other healthcare professionals who actually perform diagnostic tests and treatments, administer medications, and provide specific services to a particular patient. Admission and discharge orders should be found for every patient unless the patient leaves the facility against medical advice (AMA), but other orders will vary from patient to patient. All orders must be legible and include the date and the physician's signature. In electronic systems, signatures are attached via an authentication process. See figure 3.1 for an example of a physician's orders in an electronic format.

Standing orders are orders the medical staff or an individual physician has established as routine care for a specific diagnosis or procedure. Standing orders are commonly used in hospitals, ambulatory surgery facilities, and long-term care facilities. An example is shown in figure 3.2. Usually, standing orders are preprinted on a single sheet of paper or available via a standard computer screen. Like other physicians' orders, they must be signed and dated.

Physicians may communicate orders verbally or via the telephone when the hospital's medical staff rules allow. State law and medical staff rules specify which practitioners are allowed to accept and execute verbal and telephone orders. How the orders are to be authenticated as well as the time period allowed for authentication also may be specified.

Clinical Observations

In acute care hospitals, the documentation of clinical observations is usually provided in **progress notes.** The purpose of documenting the clinical observations of physicians, nurses, and other caregivers is to create a chronological report of the patient's condition and response to treatment during his or her hospital stay. The patient's condition determines the frequency of the notes.

The rules and regulations of the hospital's medical staff specify which healthcare providers are allowed to enter progress notes in the health record. Typically, the patient's attending physician, consulting physicians who have **medical staff privileges,** house medical staff, nurses, nutritionists, social workers, and clinical therapists are authorized to enter progress notes. Depending on the record format used by the hospital, each discipline may maintain a separate section of the health record or the observations of all the providers may be combined in the same chronological or integrated health record. (Source-oriented and integrated health records are discussed later in this chapter.)

Progress notes serve to justify further acute care treatment in the facility. In addition, they document the appropriateness and coordination of the services provided.

Special types of notes are frequently found in a record. For example, prior to the administration of anything other than local anesthesia, the anesthesiologist visits the patient and documents important factors about the patient's condition that may have an impact on the anesthesia chosen or its administration. Allergies and drug reactions would

Table 3.3.   Information usually documented in the report of a physical examination

Report Components	Content
General condition	Apparent state of health, signs of distress, posture, weight, height, skin color, dress and personal hygiene, facial expression, manner, mood, state of awareness, speech
Vital signs	Pulse, respiration, blood pressure, temperature
Skin	Color, vascularity, lesions, edema, moisture, temperature, texture, thickness, mobility and turgor, nails
Head	Hair, scalp, skull, face
Eyes	Visual acuity and fields; position and alignment of the eyes, eyebrows, eyelids; lacrimal apparatus; conjunctivae; sclerae; corneas; irises; size, shape, equality, reaction to light, and accommodation of pupils; extraocular movements; ophthalmoscopic exam
Ears	Auricles, canals, tympanic membranes, hearing, discharge
Nose and sinuses	Airways, mucosa, septum, sinus tenderness, discharge, bleeding, smell
Mouth	Breath, lips, teeth, gums, tongue, salivary ducts
Throat	Tonsils, pharynx, palate, uvula, postnasal drip
Neck	Stiffness, thyroid, trachea, vessels, lymph nodes, salivary glands
Thorax, anterior and posterior	Shape, symmetry, respiration
Breasts	Masses, tenderness, discharge from nipples
Lungs	Fremitus, breath sounds, adventitious sounds, friction, spoken voice, whispered voice
Heart	Location and quality of apical impulse, trill, pulsation, rhythm, sounds, murmurs, friction rub, jugular venous pressure and pulse, carotid artery pulse
Abdomen	Contour, peristalsis, scars, rigidity, tenderness, spasm, masses, fluid, hernia, bowel sounds and bruits, palpable organs
Male genitourinary organs	Scars, lesions, discharge, penis, scrotum, epididymis, varicocele, hydrocele
Female reproductive organs	External genitalia, Skene's glands and Bartholin's glands, vagina, cervix, uterus, adnexa
Rectum	Fissure, fistula, hemorrhoids, sphincter tone, masses, prostate, seminal vesicles, feces
Musculoskeletal system	Spine and extremities, deformities, swelling, redness, tenderness, range of motion
Lymphatics	Palpable cervical, axillary, inguinal nodes; location; size; consistency; mobility and tenderness
Blood vessels	Pulses, color, temperature, vessel walls, veins
Neurological system	Cranial nerves, coordination, reflexes, biceps, triceps, patellar, Achilles, abdominal, cremasteric, Babinski, Romberg, gait, sensory, vibratory
Diagnosis(es)	

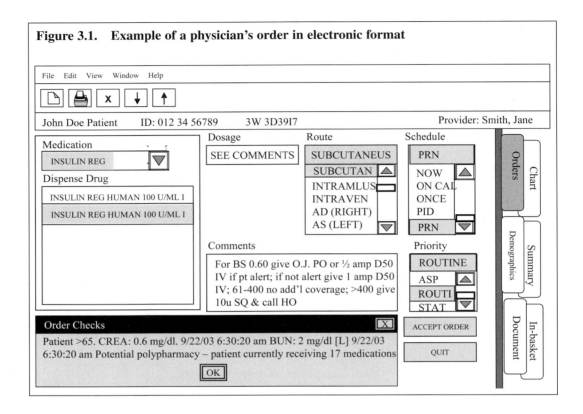

Figure 3.1.   Example of a physician's order in electronic format

be noted. A postanesthesia note also should be found describing the patient's recovery from the anesthetic. Similarly, the surgeon responsible for a major procedure must document a pre- and postsurgical patient evaluation. In addition, nurses are responsible for specific patient admission and discharge notes and, if a patient should die while hospitalized, both physician and nursing notes are important.

Just as physician documentation begins with the history and physical examination, nurses and allied health professionals may begin their care with assessments focused at understanding the patient's condition from the perspective of their specialized body of knowledge. Figure 3.3 provides an example of an admission nursing assessment. Often a **care plan** may then follow the assessment. A care plan is a summary of the patient's problems from the nurse or other professional's perspective with a detailed plan for interventions.

Nurses also maintain chronological records of the patient's vital signs (blood pressure, heart rate, respiration rate, and temperature) and separate logs that show what medications were ordered and when they were administered. Other chronological monitors also may be ordered depending on the patient's diagnosis. Sometimes these records are referred to as flow records because they show trends over time or the data may be represented in graphic form for ease in communication. (See figure 3.4 for an example of monitors in electronic format.) Special interventions such as the use of restraints also requires focused documentation.

Figure 3.2.   Example of a physician's standing order in paper format

Midwest Medical Center

HEPARIN ORDER: REGULAR UNFRACTIONATED
HEPARIN FOR ADULTS

	PATIENT LABEL

Diagnosis:_____

Allergies:_____

Total Body Weight: _____lb = _____ kg

Warning: Due to an increased risk of serious bleeding, patients should not receive both regular heparin and low-molecular-weight heparin.

Patients should also be evaluated for continuance of other medications such as aspirin, clopidogrel, and NSAID therapy.

1. Check baseline PTT, PT/INR, heme panel

2. Check the appropriate bolus regimen according to diagnosis/disease
    a. ☐ No initial bolus
    b. ☐ Acute coronary syndrome—heparin bolus 75 units/kg = _____ units IV
        (round to the nearest 1000 units—maximum bolus = 10,000 units)
    c. ☐ In combination with thrombolytic therapy for acute MI (TNKase, Retavase, TPA)
        ☐ 5000 units bolus if 65 kg or greater
        ☐ 4000 units bolus if less than 65 kg
    d. ☐ Treatment of DVT/PE—heparin bolus 80 units/kg = _____ units IV
        (round to the nearest 1000 units—maximum bolus = 10,000 units)

3. Following bolus, begin IV heparin infusion (check the appropriate regimen):
    • Premixed IV bag contains heparin 25,000 units in 250 ml of D5W (100 units/ml)
    • Maximum initial infusion rate not to exceed 2000 units/h
    ☐ All cardiology regimens: 16 units/kg/h = _____ ml/h
    ☐ Treatment of DVT or PE: 18 units/kg/h = _____ ml/h

4. Check PTT 6 hours after initiation of heparin infusion

5. Adjust heparin based on guidelines below
    (document all changes on MAR and physician's orders sheet):

PTT (seconds)	Bolus Dose	Rate Changes	Repeat PTT after Each Dosage Change
PTT <35	Bolus 4000 units	Increase rate 200 units/h	6 h
PTT 35–45	Bolus 3000 units	Increase rate 200 units/h	6 h
PTT 46–70	No bolus	No rate change	Next a.m.
PTT 71–90	No bolus	Decrease rate 100 units/h	6 h
PTT 91–100	No bolus	Hold infusion 1 h, then decrease rate by 200 units/h	6 h
PTT >100	No bolus	Hold infusion 1 h, then decrease rate by 300 units/h	6 h

6. Check PTT and heme panel every morning (while patient is on heparin protocol).

7. Check stools daily for occult blood and notify physician if positive.

8. Notify physician for bleeding, hematoma, or heart rate above 120 bpm.

Physician Signature:_____ Date/Time:_____
RN Signature:_____ Date/Time:_____

HEPARIN ORDER
000013 (11/2002)

Figure 3.3.   Example of an initial nursing assessment in paper format

Midwest Medical Center

INITIAL NURSING ASSESSMENT

PATIENT LABEL

Baseline Information

| Date: | Time: | Age: | Arrived: AMB   WC   Stretcher   EMS   Carried   Other: | Primary MD: |

Initial/Chief Complaint/History of Present Illness:

| T:
PO   R   TM | P: | R: | BP: R   L | $\oplus O_2$
Sats   % | Sex:
M   F | Height: | Weight: Actual:
Stated: |

| $\oplus$ Tetanus/Immunizations: | Pneumococcal Vaccine   ☐ No   ☐ Yes   Most Recent Date: |
| $\oplus$ Pregnant   ☐ No   ☐ Yes | LNMP: | Influenza Vaccine   ☐ No   ☐ Yes   Most Recent Date: |

Allergies: ☐ None   ☐ Medications   ☐ Latex   ☐ Food   ☐ Anesthesia   ☐ Other

List Names and Reactions:

TB Assessment (Initiate airborne isolation if 4 or more criteria are checked yes)

Persistent Cough > 2 weeks ☐ No ☐ Yes	Abnormal Chest X-Ray	☐ No ☐ Yes	Respiratory Isolation
Fever > 100.4 (night sweats) ☐ No ☐ Yes	Physician Order for AFB (smear/culture)	☐ No ☐ Yes	Ordered ☐ No ☐ Yes
Unexplained Weight Loss ☐ No ☐ Yes	Recent Exposure to Person with Suspected TB or +PPD	☐ No ☐ Yes	

RN/LPN Signature: _____

☐ See Home Medication Orders   Medication/Over the Counter/Herbal History   ☐ Investigation Drugs/Devices

Medication	Dose	Freq	Last Dose	Medication	Dose	Freq	Last Dose

Hospitalizations/Surgeries:

Medical History

Neurological	☐ No	☐ Yes		Sensory Impairment	☐ No	☐ Yes	
Cardiovascular	☐ No	☐ Yes		Endocrine	☐ No	☐ Yes	
Hypertension	☐ No	☐ Yes		Blood Disorder	☐ No	☐ Yes	
Respiratory	☐ No	☐ Yes		Cancer	☐ No	☐ Yes	
Gastrointestinal	☐ No	☐ Yes		Psychological	☐ No	☐ Yes	
Renal/Urological	☐ No	☐ Yes		Tobacco Use	☐ No	☐ Yes	
Gynecological	☐ No	☐ Yes		Alcohol/Drug Use	☐ No	☐ Yes	
Musculoskeletal	☐ No	☐ Yes		Infectious Disease	☐ No	☐ Yes	
Integumentary	☐ No	☐ Yes		Cough/Cold Past 2 Weeks	☐ No	☐ Yes	
EENT	☐ No	☐ Yes		Anesthesia	☐ No	☐ Yes	

Source of Information   ☐ Patient   ☐ Family   ☐ Unable to Obtain   ☐ Other   ☐ Medications Sent Home with Patient: _____

| Arrival Date: | Arrival Time: | T:
PO   R   TM | P: | R: | BP: R   L | O_2 Sats   %:
(If applicable) |

RN Initial: _____   RN Signature: _____   Date: _____   Time: _____   Unit: _____

RN Initial: _____   RN Signature: _____   Date: _____   Time: _____   Unit: _____

INITIAL NURSING ASSESSMENT
000039 (10/2002)

Figure 3.4. Example of special progress notes in electronic format

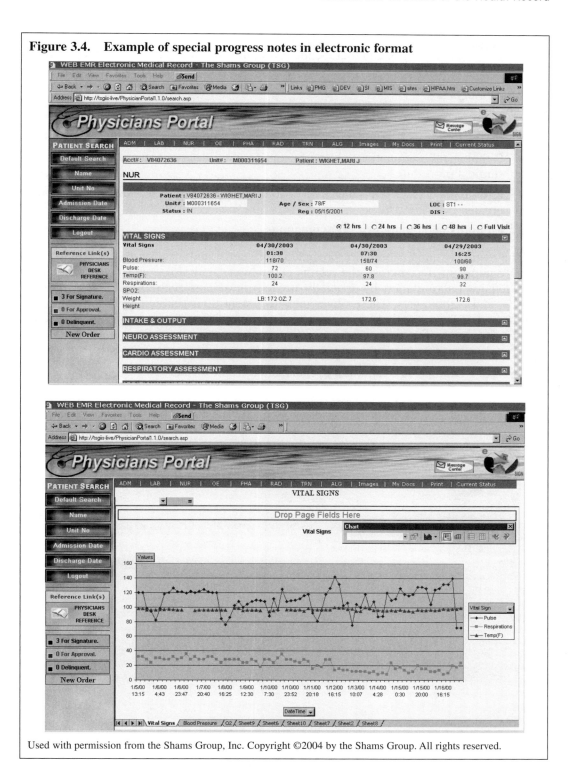

Reports of Diagnostic and Therapeutic Procedures

The results of all diagnostic and therapeutic procedures become part of the patient's health record.

Diagnostic Reports

Diagnostic procedures include the following:

- Laboratory tests performed on blood, urine, and other samples from the patient
- Pathological examinations of tissue samples and tissues or organs removed during surgical procedures
- Radiological scans and images of various parts of the patient's body and specific organs
- Monitors and tracings of body functions

The results of most laboratory procedures are generated electronically by automated testing equipment. In contrast, the results of monitors, radiology, and pathology procedures require interpretation by specially trained physicians such as cardiologists, radiologists, and pathologists. These physicians document their findings in reports that then become part of the patient's permanent record, along with copies or samples of the tracing, images, and scans. (See figures 3.5 and 3.6.)

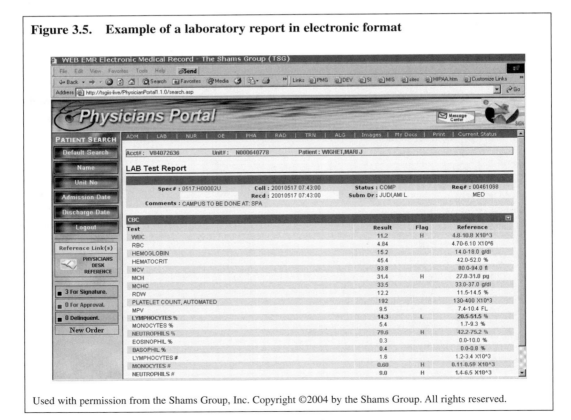

Figure 3.5.   Example of a laboratory report in electronic format

Figure 3.6.   Example of an electrocardiography report in paper format

University of Anystate Hospitals

GRAPHIC EKG REPORT

PATIENT, PETUNIA P.
000000001
DOB: 08/14/1949

NAME: Patient, Petunia

TECHNICIAN: SKH

PROCEDURE DATE/TIME: 10/11/04 9:59:02

CARDIOLOGIST: Julius W. Cardiolini, MD

SEX/RACE: Female, White

REPORT DATE: 10/08/04

REQUESTED BY: M. Gynesurg, MD

RESULTS: Normal EKG
PR   200   Normal sinus rhythm rate: 59
QRST   73
QT   407
QTc   403
Axes
P   28
QRS   36
T   35

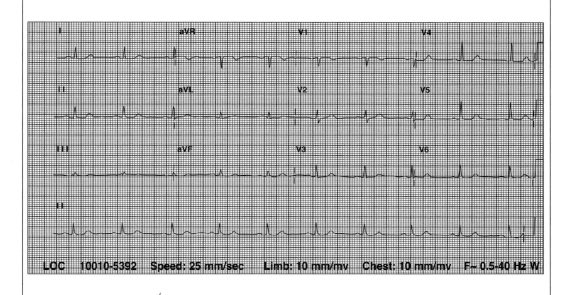

LOC   10010-5392   Speed: 25 mm/sec   Limb: 10 mm/mv   Chest: 10 mm/mv   F~ 0.5-40 Hz W

_____   10/8/04
Julius W. Cardiolini, MD   Date
Cardiologist

Operative Reports

Any major diagnostic procedure and surgical event requires special documentation. First, the patient must consent to the procedure after an explanation and an opportunity to ask questions. Often special documents or screens are designed to provide evidence of consent, including the appropriate signature. The need to obtain the patient's consent before medical and surgical procedures is based on the legal concept of battery. Battery is the unlawful touching of a person without his or her implied or expressed consent.

Implied consent is assumed when a patient voluntarily submits to treatment. The rationale behind this assumption is that one can reasonably assume that the patient understands the nature of the treatment or would not submit to it. **Expressed consent** is a consent that is either spoken or written. Although courts recognize both spoken and written consent, spoken consent is more difficult to prove.

It is primarily the physician's responsibility to make sure that the patient understands the nature of the procedure and alternative treatments as well as the procedure's risks, complications, and benefits before the procedure is performed. Medical staff rules or hospital policies usually list which types of services and procedures always require written consent from the patient. Generally, procedures that involve the use of anesthetics, the administration of experimental drugs, the surgical manipulation of organs and tissues, and significant risk of complications require written consent. In addition, some states have passed laws that require written consent forms for certain types of testing procedures (for example, HIV testing). Written consents should be witnessed by at least one individual and should be obtained prior to the service or procedure. The original copies of consent forms should always become part of the patient's health record. Figure 3.7 provides an example of an operative consent.

Preoperative notes are made by the anesthesiologist and surgeon prior to the procedure, and nurses report preoperative patient preparations. The entire procedure itself is then recorded, along with an anesthesia record, an operative report, and a postanesthesia or recovery room report. When tissue is removed for evaluation, a pathology report also must be present.

The **anesthesia report** notes any preoperative medication and response to it, the anesthesia administered with dose and method of administration, the duration of administration, the patient's vital signs while under anesthesia, and any additional products given the patient during the procedure. The anesthesiologist or nurse anesthetist is responsible for this documentation. An anesthesia record that includes the preanesthesia evaluation is shown in figure 3.8.

The **operative report** describes the surgical procedures performed on the patient. Each report usually includes the following information:

- Patient's preoperative and postoperative diagnosis
- Descriptions of the procedures performed
- Descriptions of all normal and abnormal findings
- Descriptions of any unique or unusual events during the course of the surgery
- Number of ligatures, sutures, packs, drains, and sponges used
- Descriptions of any specimens removed
- Names of the surgeons and their assistants
- Date and duration of the surgery

Figure 3.7. Example of an informed consent for operation with blood products

University of Anystate Hospitals

**INFORMED CONSENT FOR OPERATION/
PROCEDURE/ANESTHESIA INCLUDING
BLOOD AND BLOOD PRODUCTS**

PATIENT LABEL

1. I give permission to Dr.(s) _____ to perform
   the following procedure(s): _____
   _____
   _____ on _____ (patient's name).

2. I understand that during the procedure(s), new findings or conditions may appear and require an additional procedure(s) for proper care.

3. My physician has explained the following items:
   - the nature of my condition
   - the nature and purpose of the procedure(s) that I am now authorizing
   - the possible complications and side effects that may result, problems that may be experienced during recuperation, and the likelihood of success
   - the benefits to be reasonably expected from the procedure(s)
   - the likely result of no treatment
   - the available alternatives, including the risks and benefits
   - the other possible risks that accompany any surgical and diagnostic procedure (in addition to those already discussed). I acknowledge that neither my physician nor anyone else involved in my care has made any guarantees or assurances to me as to the result of the procedure(s) that I am now authorizing.

4. I know that other clinical staff may help my physician during the procedure(s).

5. I understand that the procedure(s) may require that I undergo some form of anesthesia, which may have its own risks.

6. Any tissue or specimens taken from my body as a result of the procedure(s) may be examined and disposed of, retained, preserved, or used for medical, scientific, or teaching purposes by the hospital.

7. I understand that my procedure(s) may be photographed or videotaped and that observers may be present in the room for the purpose of advancing medical care and education.

8. I understand that during or after the procedure(s) my physician may find it necessary to give me a transfusion of blood or blood products. My physician has explained the alternatives to, and possible risks of, transfusion.

9. I understand what my physician has explained to me and have had all my questions fully answered.

10. Additional comments: _____
    _____

After talking with my physician and reading this form, I give my consent to the procedure(s) described above.

Signature of Patient or
Legal Representative: _____ Date: _____ Time: _____

If Legal Representative, Relationship to Patient: _____

Witness: _____

Verbal or Telephone Consent

Name of Legal Representative: _____ Date: _____ Time: _____

Relationship to Patient: _____

Witness: _____ Witness: _____

I have explained the risks, benefits, potential complications, and alternatives of the treatment to the patient and have answered all questions to the patient's satisfaction, and he/she has granted consent to proceed.

Physician Signature: _____ Date: _____ Time: _____

INFORMED CONSENT FOR OPERATION
000015 (11/2002)

Figure 3.8.   Example of a preanesthesia and anesthesia record in a paper format

University of Anystate Hospitals

ANESTHESIA RECORD
PAGE 1 OF 2

PATIENT LABEL

Date: _____   Time: _____
Age: _____ Sex: _____ Height: _____ Weight: _____ BP: _____ P: _____ R: _____ T: _____
Lab: _____ Status: _____
Allergies: _____ Last Intake: _____
Premedication: _____

☐ **Patient reassessed immediately prior to induction. Condition satisfactory for planned anesthesia.**

Vital Signs

Time		Machine Check

(Graph grid with vital signs plotting area)

Legend (left column):
Systolic ∨
Diastolic ∧
Pulse ∧∧
Respiration ○ Spon ● Assist ⊙ Controlled
Surgery Start/End ⊗
Anesthesia Start/End ✕
Anesthesia Start _____
Anesthesia End

Scale values: 240, 220, 200, 180, 160, 140, 120, 100, 80, 60, 40, 20, 15, 10, 5

Right column labels:
Machine Check
Initials
Patient Position
☐ General
☐ Regional
☐ Local
☐ Monitored
☐ IVs (spinal/EPI needle)
Position
Prep
Site
Agent
Paresthesia
Catheter
Sensory Block TO
☐ Heat/Moisture Exchanger
☐ Warming Blanket
☐ Fluid Warmer
☐ Bair Hugger
Endotracheal Tube
Cuff Inflated
Laryngoscope Blade
Stylet
Direct Vision
Blind

Figure 3.8.   (Continued)

University of Anystate Hospitals

ANESTHESIA RECORD
PAGE 2 OF 2

PATIENT LABEL

Monitors
- ☐ NIBP   ☐ R   ☐ L
- ☐ APB   ☐ R   ☐ L
- ☐ T (site): _____
- ☐ Pulse oximeter (site): _____
- ☐ ECG (lead): _____
- ☐ Airway gas monitor
- ☐ FiO$_2$ analyzer
- ☐ Pulmonary artery
- ☐ CVP
- ☐ EEG
- ☐ Stethoscope (site): _____
- ☐ SSEP
- ☐ Peripheral nerve stimulator
- ☐ Capnography

Remarks

Fluid		Fluid		Fluid		Fluid		Fluid		Fluid	
Start	Finish	Start	Finish	Start	Finish	Start	Finish	Start	Finish	Start	Finish

Operation

Surgeon   Anesthesiologist   Date

Recovery Room   Time: _____
BP
P   T   °F   Endotracheal
Condition   SpO$_2$ %   In ☐   Out ☐

Preanesthesia Evaluation

Review of Clinical Data

- ☐ Yes   ☐ No   Patient Medical History Reviewed
- ☐ Yes   ☐ No   Current Medications Reviewed
- ☐ Yes   ☐ No   Allergies Reviewed
- ☐ Yes   ☐ No   ☐ N/A   Lab Results Reviewed
- ☐ Yes   ☐ No   ☐ N/A   CXR Results Reviewed
- ☐ Yes   ☐ No   ☐ N/A   EKG Results Reviewed

Pertinent Physical Exam

	Normal	Abnormal	Comments
EENT			
Respiratory			
Cardiac			
Mental Status			

Anesthesia History

- ☐ Yes   ☐ No   Past Hx of Anesthesia Complications
- ☐ Yes   ☐ No   Family Hx of Anesthesia Complications
- ☐ Yes   ☐ No   History of Malignant Hyperthermia

ASA Classification

1   2   3   4   5   E

Airway Evaluation

Dentures:	☐ None ☐ Upper ☐ Lower
Capped Teeth:	☐ None ☐ Yes
Condition of Teeth:	☐ Good ☐ Fair ☐ Poor

Estimated Intubation Difficulty:

☐ Normal   ☐ Moderately Difficult   ☐ Difficult

Anesthesia Plan

- ☐ General
- ☐ Spinal
- ☐ Epidural
- ☐ Regional Block
- ☐ Rapid Sequence Intubation
- ☐ MAC
- ☐ Epidural for POPM

☐ Alternatives, risks of anesthesia, and potential complications were discussed. Patient and/or guardian state understanding and acceptance of anesthesia plan.

Comments:

_____   _____
Anesthesiologist   Date

ANESTHESIA RECORD
000017 (11/2002)

(See figure 3.9.) The operative report should be written or dictated by the surgeon immediately after surgery and become part of the health record. When there is a delay in dictation or transcription, a progress note describing the surgery should be entered into the patient's record.

Immediately after the procedure, the patient is usually evaluated for a period of time in a special unit called a recovery room. Monitoring is important to make sure the patient sufficiently recovers from the anesthesia and is stable enough to be moved to another location. The **recovery room report** includes the postanesthesia note (if not found elsewhere), nurses' notes regarding the patient's condition and surgical site, vital signs, and intravenous fluids and other medical monitoring.

A **pathology report** is dictated by a pathologist after examination of tissue received for evaluation. This report usually includes descriptions of the tissue from a gross or macroscopic (with the eye) level and representative cells at the microscopic level along with interpretive findings. Sometimes an initial tissue evaluation occurs while the surgery is in progress to give the surgeon information important to the remainder of the operation. A full written report then would follow. (See figure 3.10.)

Consultation Reports

The **consultation report** documents the clinical opinion of a physician other than the primary or attending physician. The consultation is requested by the primary or attending

---

Figure 3.9.   Example of an operative report in electronic format

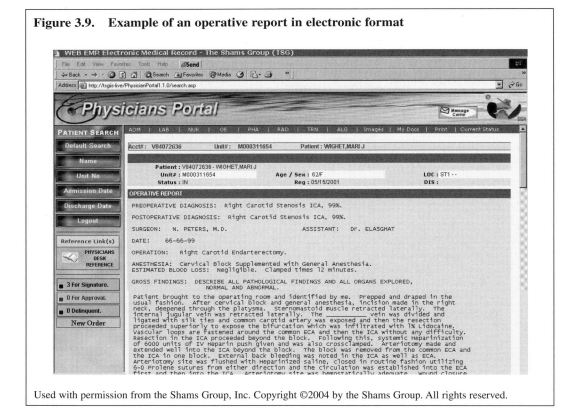

Figure 3.10. Example of a surgical pathology report in electronic format

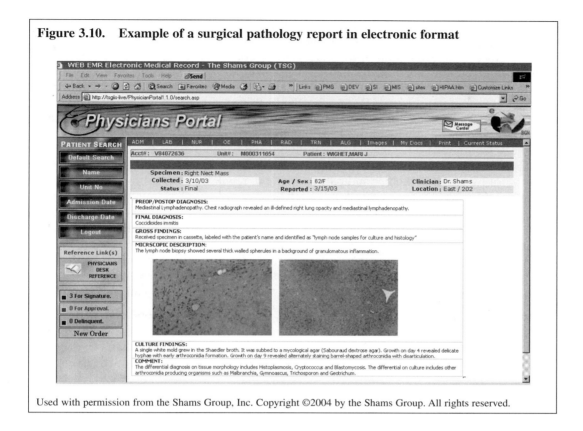

physician. The report is based on the consulting physician's examination of the patient and a review of his or her health record.

Some organizations make consultation requests by telephone and provide the consultant with selected information from the patient's record. The consultant then dictates his or her findings and returns them to the requesting physician.

Other organizations use a consultation form. The first part of the form communicates the consultation request and provides the consultant with pertinent patient history. The consultant then uses the second part to document and return his or her opinion to the requesting physician.

Deliveries and Newborns

Each individual that is admitted to a healthcare setting must have a health record. A record on a newborn is generated upon live birth. The mother's hospital obstetric record is separate from the infant's record and actually begins in her practitioner's office. In the case of a baby born deceased, however, all information about the baby and the mother is maintained in the mother's health record. (See information pertaining to obstetric/gynecologic care later in this chapter.)

Obstetric delivery records include a prenatal care summary provided by the practitioner's office, an admission evaluation by the attending physician to update the summary, and a record of labor, including information on contractions, fetal heart tones, examination of the birth canal, medications given, and vital signs. The delivery record includes type of delivery; medications administered, including anesthesia, description of the birth process and any blood loss; evaluation of the placenta and cord; and information about any other delivery interventions. Data about the baby also will be recorded in the mother's record, including sex, weight, length, Apgar scores, any abnormal findings, and any treatments given. Postpartum care records begin after the birth and contain progress notes by physicians and nurses and other care providers in addition to the results of any diagnostic tests, treatments, and medications received by the mother.

The newborn record begins with the birth history, which may be the same or similar to the mother's labor and delivery data noted above. Newborn identification generally includes bands worn by both the mother and baby, which are regularly checked for matching information, and the infant's footprints. A thorough newborn physical examination is completed shortly after the baby's birth with periodic updates throughout hospitalization. Head and chest measurements are part of an evaluation of all body systems. Nursing documentation includes information on the baby's feeding and elimination status, weight, vital signs, appearance, response to environment, sleeping patterns, and condition of the cord stump. Any special tests, treatments, and medications will also be noted. More extensive documentation will be found if a baby is born prematurely or requires intensive care services.

Discharge Summaries, Patient Instructions, and Transfer Records

The **discharge summary** is a concise account of the patient's illness, course of treatment, response to treatment, and condition at the time the patient is discharged (officially released) from the hospital. Because it provides an overview of the entire medical encounter it:

- Ensures the continuity of future care by providing information to the patient's attending physician, referring physician, and any consulting physicians

- Provides information to support the activities of the medical staff review committee

- Provides concise information that can be used to answer information requests from authorized individuals or entities

The discharge summary is the responsibility of, and must be signed by, the attending physician. A paper-based record summary is found in figure 3.11. If the patient's stay is not complicated and lasts less than 48 hours or involves an uncomplicated delivery or normal newborn, a discharge note in place of a full summary is often acceptable.

The summary also includes instructions for follow-up care to be given to the patient or his or her caregiver at the time of discharge. It is vital that the patient be given clear, concise instructions. Ideally, patient instructions are communicated both verbally and in writing. The healthcare professional who delivers the instructions to the patient or caregiver should sign the record to indicate that he or she has issued them. In addition, the person receiving the instructions should sign to verify that he or she understands them. A copy of the written instructions then becomes part of the health record. (See figure 3.12.)

When someone other than the patient assumes responsibility for the patient's aftercare, the record should indicate that the instructions were given to the responsible party. Documentation of patient education may be accomplished by using formats that prompt the person providing instruction to cover important information.

Figure 3.11.   Example of a discharge summary in paper format

Midwest Medical Center

DISCHARGE SUMMARY

> SAYLORMEN, POPEYE T.
> 333333333
> DOB: 02/09/1961

PHYSICIAN/SURGEON: Philip P. Heartstopper, MD

DATE OF DISCHARGE: 05/18/2003

PRINCIPAL OPERATION AND PROCEDURE: OPCAB × 3, left internal mammary artery of the LAD, saphenous vein graft to D-1, and saphenous vein graft to OM-1

HISTORY OF PRESENT ILLNESS: Mr. Saylormen was seen at the request of Dr. Doctor regarding surgical treatment of ischemic heart disease. He is a 42-year-old male with a family history of coronary artery disease. He smokes a pipe and had a previous myocardial infarction approximately three years ago. His current status is postangioplasty. While working on a construction project, he developed anginal-type symptoms and was seen in the emergency room and then admitted to the hospital for further evaluation.

ADMITTING DIAGNOSIS: Coronary artery disease

HOSPITAL COURSE: The patient underwent cardiac catheterization and was found to have significant three-vessel coronary artery disease. It was felt that he would benefit from undergoing an OPCAB procedure. On 05/14/03, the patient underwent OPCAB × 3 as described above. The patient tolerated the procedure well and returned to the Cardiothoracic Intensive Care Unit hemodynamically stable. On postoperative day one, he was weaned from mechanical ventilation, extubated, and transferred to the Cardiothoracic Step-Down Unit, where he continued on a progressive course of recovery. On postoperative day four, he was up and about in his room and the halls without difficulty. Upon discharge, he was tolerating his diet well. His lungs were clear. His abdomen was soft, and his incisions were unremarkable. His vital signs were stable. He was in normal sinus rhythm. His heart rate was in the 70s and 80s. Blood pressure had been running consistently in the low 110s/60s. He was afebrile. Oxygen saturations on room air were reported at 97%.

LABORATORY DATA AT DISCHARGE: BUN 14, Creatinine 0.9, H&H 8.8 and 25.4

MEDICATIONS AT DISCHARGE: Lisinopril 5 mg q.d.; Lipitor 80 mg q.d.; metoprolol 50 mg q.d.; aspirin 81 mg q.d.; Darvocet-N 100—one to two tablets every 4–6 hours as needed for pain; iron sulfate 325 mg q.d. × 30 days; and Colace 100 mg b.i.d. × 30 days

DIET: He may follow a regular diet.

FINAL DIAGNOSIS: Coronary artery disease

DISPOSITION: No lifting greater than 10 pounds. No driving for 4–6 weeks. He may shower but he should not take a tub bath. Follow up with Dr. Doctor in 1–2 weeks.

_____   5/18/03
Philip P. Heartstopper, MD   _____
                                                   Date

d: 05/18/2003
t: 05/19/2003
PPH, MD/mb

Figure 3.12.   Example of patient instructions provided at discharge

University of Anystate Hospitals

PATIENT/FAMILY INSTRUCTIONS
PAGE 1 OF 2

PATIENT LABEL

This is a guide for your care. Call your doctor for any problems or changes that concern you.

Diet

Diet: _____ If on special diet and have questions, call dietitian.

Managing Your Meds Discussed
(Place a checkmark if medication handouts given)

Medications (list all medications)

Name/Dose	How to Take	

Activities/Special Care

Activities (Check as indicated)
- ☐ Crutches/walker
- ☐ Walk with assistance
- ☐ Gradually resume normal activity
- ☐ Bedrest
- ☐ Other _____

Dressing and Wound Care
(Report increased pain, redness, swelling, drainage, or fever)
- ☐ Doctor to change dressing
- ☐ Keep dressing dry
- ☐ If no dressing, keep incision clean and dry
- ☐ Clean wound and change dressing

Additional Instructions (PEARLS)

Follow-Up (appointments/equipment/referrals)

Agency	Phone	Arrangements (instructions provided by agency)

Dr. _____ _____ Date/Time _____ ☐ Call for an appointment
Dr. _____ _____ Date/Time _____ ☐ Call for an appointment
Dr. _____ _____ Date/Time _____ ☐ Call for an appointment

I understand the above instructions and have the ability to carry these out after discharge. I am aware of the importance of medical follow-up with my doctor.

Patient/Patient Rep. Signature: _____ Date: _____

RN Signature: _____ Date: _____

Figure 3.12. (Continued)

University of Anystate Hospitals

PATIENT/FAMILY INSTRUCTIONS
PAGE 2 OF 2

PATIENT LABEL

Discharge Date: _____ Time: _____ Mode: _____

Discharged With:

☐ Family member ☐ Friend ☐ By self ☐ Other:_____

Escorted by: ☐ Hospital Attendant ☐ Ambulance Attendant

RN Discharge Assessment

_____

_____

_____

_____

_____

Continuing Care Assessment

Care Plan ☐ All goals resolved on IPOC/clinical path/plan of care. Exceptions documented.

Discharge with: ☐ Self/family care • Patient and/or family verbalized an understanding of instructions. Person (s) to assist if needed:_____

Discharge with: ☐ Support services • Patient will receive follow-up with a referral agency or extended care facility. See front of form.

Discharge to: ☐ Home ☐ Home with home health ☐ Extended care facility ☐ Other:_____

☐ Patient Expired Date: Time: Valuables Given to: ☐ Family ☐ Funeral Home ☐ Security
☐ Patient Left without Permission Date: Time:

RN Signature: _____ Date: _____

PATIENT INSTRUCTIONS
5435680 (03/2002)

When a patient is being transferred from the acute setting to another health care organization, a **transfer record** may be initiated. This record also is called a referral form. A brief review of the patient's acute stay along with current status, discharge and transfer orders, and any additional instructions will be noted. Social service and nursing personnel often complete portions of the transfer record.

Despite the best efforts of hospital caregivers and physicians, some patients die while they are hospitalized. In such cases, the attending physician should add a summary statement to the patient's health record to document the circumstances surrounding the patient's death. The statement can take the form of a final progress note or a separate report. The statement should indicate the reason for the patient's admission, his or her diagnosis and course in the hospital, and a description of the events that led to his or her death.

Autopsy Reports

An **autopsy report** is a description of the examination of a patient's body after he or she has died. Also called necropsies, autopsies are usually conducted when there is some question about the cause of death or when information is needed for educational or legal purposes. The purpose of the autopsy is to determine or confirm the cause of death or to provide more information about the course of the patient's disease.

The autopsy report is completed by a pathologist and becomes part of the patient's permanent health record. The authorization for the autopsy, signed by the patient's next of kin or by law enforcement authorities, must be obtained prior to the autopsy and also should become part of the record.

Administrative Data

As noted earlier in this section, an acute care health record contains the patient's demographic and financial information as well as a summary of the reason the patient is seeking treatment. Commonly, the administrative information is collected by hospital admitting personnel who personally ask the patient or the patient's representative for the information needed to complete the admissions form.

Today, most hospitals collect admissions information electronically. For hospitals that maintain a paper-based health record system, a printout of the admissions information is placed in the health record. In both paper-based and electronic health record systems, the admissions information then becomes a permanent part of the patient's record. The admissions information may be referred to as a face sheet, a registration form, or a registration record.

Demographic and Financial Information

Demographics is the study of the statistical characteristics of human populations. In the context of healthcare, demographic information includes the following elements:

- Patient's full name
- Patient's identification number or health record number as assigned by the healthcare facility
- Patient's address
- Patient's date of birth

- Patient's place of birth
- Patient's gender
- Patient's race or ethnic origin
- Patient's marital status
- Name and address of patient's next of kin
- Date and time of admission
- Type of admission (inpatient or outpatient)
- Hospital's name, address, and telephone number

The financial information maintained in the acute care health record is limited to the insurance information collected from the patient at the time of admission. This information includes the name of the expected payer, the name of the policy holder (or insured), the gender of the policy holder, the patient's relationship to the policy holder, the employer of the policy holder, individual and group insurance policy numbers, and the patient's Social Security number. (See figure 3.13.)

Consents, Authorizations, and Acknowledgments

Healthcare providers are required to obtain written consents or authorizations before they may provide invasive diagnostic procedures and surgical interventions or release confidential patient information.

Figure 3.13.   Example of an admission record in electronic format

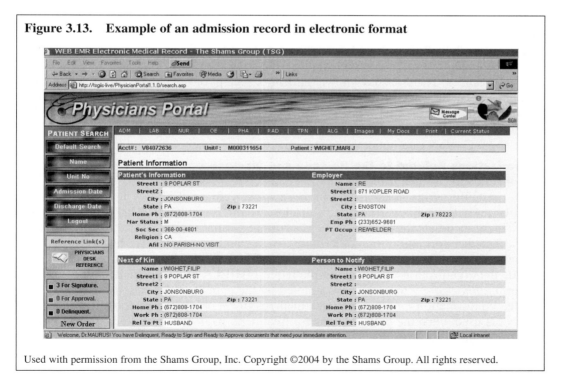

Used with permission from the Shams Group, Inc. Copyright ©2004 by the Shams Group. All rights reserved.

Consents for procedures were discussed in the operative reports section of this chapter. Acknowledgments usually apply to the patient's confirmation that he or she has received specific information from the healthcare facility.

Consent to Treatment

Many healthcare facilities obtain a **consent to treatment** from patients or their legal representatives before providing care or services except in emergency situations. This type of consent documents the patient's permission for routine services, diagnostic procedures, and medical care (Abdelhak 2001, 91). However, privacy legislation has made this step a matter of facility choice.

In 2001, the Department of Health and Human Services (HHS) published the first comprehensive set of federal rules dealing with health information privacy and security. The rules were established to implement the provisions of the Health Insurance Portability and Accountability Act (HIPAA) of 1996 and provide some uniformity to related practices across the country. (The privacy rule is discussed in detail in chapter 15; the security rule is discussed in chapter 19.)

The final privacy rule became effective October 15, 2002. It permits all covered entities (those to whom the regulations apply) to use and disclose patients' protected health information for their own treatment, payment, or healthcare operations and for treatment, payment, and certain healthcare operations of other parties without prior written permission from the patients or the patients' legal representatives. HHS stresses that covered entities may still voluntarily elect to obtain such consents. Many do because they are considered an integral part of healthcare professional ethical and practice standards. Covered entities have complete discretion in designing their consent process if they choose this alternative. When a consent is obtained, it must become part of the patient's record.

Notice of Privacy Practices

The privacy rule requires providers with a direct treatment relationship with a patient to secure the patient's written acknowledgment that he or she received the provider's notice of privacy practices. The signed acknowledgment of receipt of the notice of privacy practices should be obtained when service is first provided to a patient and should become part of the health record. When the first service is for emergency care and the patient is unable to sign, the provider is allowed to obtain the acknowledgment after the emergency treatment has been given. Content of a notice of privacy practices is further described in chapter 15.

Authorizations Related to the Release and Disclosure of Confidential Health Information

In the past, the terms *consent* and *authorization* were used almost interchangeably to describe an individual's permission to disclose health information. The terms referred to the written documentation of the patient's formal permission to release his or her confidential health information to another party. As a standard of practice, healthcare providers only obtained the individual's permission to disclose health information when parties outside the organization were making the request. HIPAA privacy legislation now applies the term *authorization* to permission granted by the patient or the patient's representative to release information for other than treatment, payment or healthcare operations. The term *consent* is used when the permission is for treatment, payment or healthcare operations.

An **authorization to disclose information** allows the healthcare facility to verbally disclose or send health information to other organizations. The patient or his or her legal representative signs the authorization. Under the HIPAA privacy rule, covered providers are required to obtain a written authorization for the use or disclosure of protected health information for purposes not related to treatment, payment, or healthcare operation. The HIPAA privacy rule establishes federal guidelines for the content and use of authorization forms. Guidelines also indicate who may provide consent and when an authorization can be revoked. (See chapter 15.) Individual states may have laws or regulations that define the content of authorizations. When such laws or regulations exist, the facility should consult the HIPAA privacy rule to determine how to apply the state requirements (Hughes 2001). Usually the most restrictive guideline is the one followed.

The HIPAA privacy rule also requires special handling when releasing some psychotherapy documentation. In addition, many states have laws and regulations that address the use and disclosure of behavioral health and psychotherapy records. A federal confidentiality rule for alcohol and drug abuse treatment records applies to the records of participants in federally assisted alcohol or drug abuse programs. Other laws may address those with the human deficiency virus (HIV) or acquired immune deficiency syndrome (AIDS) and other disorders. If these other laws and regulations more stringently protect individual health information or provide the individual greater access or control over their protected health information, they will not be preempted by HIPAA.

The HIPAA privacy rule requires most healthcare providers to obtain written authorization for specific disclosures not otherwise permitted by law. However, healthcare providers may require patients to give their permission as a condition of treatment and managed care organizations and health insurance plans may require authorization as a condition of service enrollment.

Advance Directives

An **advance directive** is a written document that names the patient's choice of legal representative for healthcare purposes. The person designated by the patient is then empowered to make healthcare decisions on behalf of the patient in the event that the patient is no longer capable of expressing his or her preferences. Living wills and durable powers of attorney for healthcare are two examples of advance directives. Physician orders for "do not resuscitate" (DNR) and "do not attempt intubation" (DNI) should be consistent with the patient's advance directives.

The federal **Patient Self-Determination Act** (PSDA) went into effect in 1991. The PSDA requires healthcare facilities to provide written information on the patient's right to execute advance directives and to accept or refuse medical treatment. Healthcare organizations that accept Medicare or Medicaid patients are required to adhere to the following provisions of the PSDA:

- Healthcare organizations must develop policies that meet the requirements of state law regarding the patient's right to accept or refuse medical treatment and to develop advance directives.

- Upon admission, healthcare organizations must provide written information to the patient that describes the treatment decisions that patients may make and the hospital's related policies.

- Healthcare organizations must document the fact that the patient has an advance directive in his or her health record. However, they are not required to make a copy of the directive a permanent part of the patient's health record.

Acknowledgments of Patient's Rights

Acknowledgment forms are used to document the fact that information about the patient's rights while under care was provided to the patient. Referred to as the **patient's bill of rights, Medicare Conditions of Participation** require hospitals to provide patients this information. The information must include the right to:

- Know who is providing treatment
- Confidentiality
- Receive information about treatment
- Refuse treatment
- Participate in care planning
- Be safe from abusive treatment

There are two common ways to document the receipt of rights' information in the health record. First, the patient or his or her legal representative can sign a document to indicate that the patient received the bill of rights. Second, the facility can have the patient sign and date the actual bill of rights and place it in the health record.

Other Administrative Information

Some healthcare facilities place property lists and birth and death certificates in health records. When a patient brings personal property and valuables to the healthcare facility, the facility may document them in the health record. Items such as eyeglasses, hearing aids, prostheses, and other special medical equipment should be documented. When items are kept in a secure location by the facility, that fact should be documented on the property/valuable list.

State governments use birth and death certificates to collect vital information and health statistics. The content requirements vary somewhat according to relevant state law. In some states, the certificates are prepared by hospitals. Copies of the certificates are often included in the patients' health records.

Check Your Understanding 3.1

Instructions: Choose the most appropriate answer for the following questions.

1. _____ Which two major types of data are contained in the health record?
   a. Nursing and physician
   b. Administrative and clinical
   c. Demographic and financial
   d. Surgical and medical

2. _____ Which of the following terms refers to state or county regulations that healthcare facilities must meet to be permitted to provide care?
   a. Accreditation
   b. Bylaws
   c. Certification
   d. Licensure

3. _____ Which of the following would not be found in a medical history?
   a. Chief complaint
   b. Vital signs
   c. Present illness
   d. Review of systems

4. _____ An attending physician requests the advice of a second physician who then reviews the health record and examines the patient. The second physician records impressions in what type of report?
   a. Consultation
   b. Progress note
   c. Operative report
   d. Discharge summary

5. _____ Which specialized type of progress note provides healthcare professionals impressions of patient problems with detailed treatment action steps?
   a. Flow records
   b. Vital signs record
   c. Care plan
   d. Surgical note

6. _____ Written or spoken permission to proceed with care is classified as _____.
   a. Expressed consent
   b. Acknowledgment
   c. Advance directives
   d. Implied consent

7. _____ Which of the following reports provides information on tissue removed during a procedure?
   a. Operative report
   b. Laboratory report
   c. Pathology report
   d. Anesthesia report

8. _____ Sleeping patterns, head and chest measurements, feeding and elimination status, weight, and Apgar scores are recorded in which of the following records?
   a. Obstetric
   b. Newborn
   c. Surgical
   d. Emergency

9. _____ Which of the following is not considered patient demographic information?
   a. Patient's date of birth
   b. Name of next of kin
   c. Type of admission
   d. Admitting diagnosis

10. _____ Which of the following administrative documents names the patient's choice of legal representative for healthcare purposes?
    a. Advance directive
    b. Patient's bill of rights
    c. Notice of privacy practices
    d. Authorization for release of information

Specialized Health Record Content

There are differences as well as similarities among the health records maintained by different healthcare facilities. The healthcare setting (acute care, ambulatory care, long-term care, and so on) is one factor. For example, the records of residents in long-term care facilities often contain immunization records and must contain documentation of communication of patient's rights. Acute care records, in contrast, do not usually contain immunization records but do contain acknowledgment of receipt of a bill of rights.

The content of the health records in various healthcare settings also depends on external factors such as which accreditation standards apply. For example, JCAHO issues specific health information standards for acute care hospitals. However, the standards of the **Commission on Accreditation of Rehabilitation Facilities** (CARF) are more frequently used by rehabilitation hospitals.

State and local laws in the facility's specific geopolitical location also may affect record content. In addition, the content of records can be affected by the rules that apply to facilities that receive funding from the federal government. For example, some federal regulations only apply to healthcare facilities that treat Medicare enrollees.

The content of health records also depends on the type of medical services the patient requires. For example, the content of the record for an obstetrics patient would be different from the content of the record for a neurosurgical patient. Content also depends in part on the duration of medical services. For example, the content of a long-term rehabilitation record would be different from the content of an emergency services record.

Health record content also may be affected by the traits of individual patients (for example, age, functional status). Finally, the complexity of the patient's medical condition is yet another factor.

Information Pertaining to Emergency Care

The delivery of emergency care services occurs primarily in hospital-based emergency departments and freestanding urgent care centers. Emergency care documentation is limited to information about the patient's presenting problem and the diagnostic and therapeutic services provided during the episode of care. The services provided in emergency situations concentrate on diagnosing the medical problem and stabilizing the patient. Although minor injuries and illnesses may require no further medical treatment, emergency patients often must be referred to ambulatory care providers for follow-up care. Seriously ill patients are admitted to a hospital for ongoing acute care treatment.

For emergency care records, documenting the instructions given to the patient, as well as the patient's presenting complaint, evaluation, and assessment, is important. Thorough documentation is needed to justify reimbursement, protect the facility or the patient in potential legal proceedings, and ensure continuity of care.

The following information must be entered into the patient's health record for each emergency care visit:

- Patient identification (or the reason it could not be obtained)
- Time and means of the patient's arrival at the facility

- Pertinent history of the illness or injury and physical findings, including the patient's vital signs
- Emergency care given to the patient prior to arrival
- Diagnostic and therapeutic orders
- Clinical observations, including the results of treatment
- Reports and results of procedures and tests
- Diagnostic impression
- Medications administered
- Conclusion at the termination of evaluation/treatment, including final disposition, the patient's condition on discharge or transfer, and any instructions given the patient, the patient's representative, or another healthcare facility for follow-up care
- Documentation of cases when the patient left the facility against medical advice

Information Pertaining to Ambulatory Care

The records of healthcare services provided in physicians' offices, group practices, clinics, and outpatient settings typically include the following materials:

- Registration forms
- Problem lists
- Medication lists
- Patient history questionnaires
- History and physicals
- Progress notes
- Results of consultations
- Diagnostic test results
- Miscellaneous flow sheets (for example, pediatric growth charts and immunization records and specialty-specific flow sheets)
- Copies of records of previous hospitalizations or treatment by other healthcare practitioners
- Correspondence
- Consents to disclose information
- Advance directives

Many of the data found in ambulatory care settings are similar to those found in acute care hospitals. The registration record used in a physician's office, for example, includes the same demographic and financial information as a hospital admissions record.

Ambulatory care records, however, do include several elements unique to the ambulatory setting. For example, ambulatory records usually contain a **problem list** whose function is to facilitate ongoing patient care management. The problem list describes any significant current and past illnesses and conditions as well as the procedures the patient has undergone. Sometimes problems are separated into acute (short term such as otitis media) and chronic (such as diabetes mellitus) categories. The problem list also may include information on the patient's previous surgeries, allergies, and drug sensitivities. Some physician practices place information on the patient's current prescription medications on the problem list. Others maintain a separate medication list. (See figure 3.14 for an example of a problem list.)

Some physician practices also use a structured format to collect past medical history information from the patient. This is called a **patient history questionnaire.**

Ambulatory care settings may earn accreditation from the **Accreditation Association for Ambulatory Health Care** (AAAHC), JCAHO, the **American Osteopathic Association** (AOA), the **National Committee for Quality Assurance** (NCQA), or other specialized groups. All have health information documentation standards. Most physician practices do not participate in voluntary accreditation programs, but some clinics, outpatient settings, and managed care organizations choose to do so.

Information Pertaining to Obstetric/Gynecologic Care

Some ambulatory care records have special requirements. According to the American College of Obstetricians and Gynecologists (ACOG), the documentation of obstetric care must include a comprehensive personal and family history, a detailed physical examination report, a treatment plan, and patient instructions (ACOG 1996). Specifically, the following kinds of information should be maintained for both obstetric and gynecologic patients:

- Medical history
  —Reason for visit
  —Health status
  —Dietary/nutritional assessment
  —Physical fitness and exercise status
  —Tobacco, alcohol, and drug usage
  —History of abuse or neglect
  —Sexual practices, including high-risk behaviors and method of contraception
- Physical examination
- Periodic laboratory testing, including Pap tests and mammography, cholesterol levels, and fecal blood test
- Additional laboratory testing needed for high-risk groups, including:
  —Hemoglobin levels
  —Bacteriuria testing
  —Fasting glucose testing
  —Testing for sexually transmitted diseases
  —HIV testing

Figure 3.14.   Example of a problem list in paper format

		PROBLEM LIST		
Identification Number				
Medical Record Number				
Last Name		First Name		Middle Initial
Date of Birth				

PROBLEM NUMBER	DATE ENTERED	LIST SIGNIFICANT ACUTE AND CHRONIC CONDITIONS INCLUDING SURGICAL PROCEDURES	PROBLEM RESOLVED	DATE RESOLVED
1				
2				
3				
4				
5				
6				
7				
8				
9				
10				
11				
12				
13				
14				
15				
16				
17				
18				
19				
20				

—Tuberculosis skin testing

—Lipid profile

—Thyroid testing

—Colonoscopy

Information Pertaining to Pediatric Care

The records of infants, children, and adolescents also require special content. These ambulatory care records should include the following:

- Past medical history
- Birth history
- Nutritional history
- Personal, social, and family history
- Growth and development record
- Review of systems

In addition, the records should include documentation of well-child visits and immunizations as well as visits for medical concerns, including any medications prescribed.

Information Pertaining to Ambulatory Surgical Care

The operating room (OR) records maintained by freestanding ambulatory surgery centers are very similar to those maintained by hospital-based surgery departments. Specifically, Medicare regulations require that ambulatory surgery records include the following information:

- Patient identification
- Significant medical history and the results of the physical examination
- Preoperative studies (studies performed before surgery)
- Findings and techniques of the operation, including the pathologist's report
- Allergies and abnormal drug reactions
- Record of anesthesia administration
- Documentation of the patient's informed consent to treatment
- Discharge diagnosis

The ambulatory surgery record should also include documentation of the patient's course in the recovery room. Many ambulatory surgery centers also telephone patients at home after their surgery as a routine follow-up procedure. The patient's record should include records of any follow-up calls. In addition to JCAHO, the American Association for Accreditation of Ambulatory Surgery Facilities has standards that apply to this type of setting.

Information Pertaining to Long-Term Care

Long-term care is provided in a variety of facilities, including the following:

- Skilled nursing facilities (SNFs)

- Subacute care facilities

- Nursing facilities (NFs) (also known as convalescent care centers)

- Intermediate care facilities (ICFs)

- ICFs for the mentally retarded (ICF-MRs)

- Assisted-living facilities

The regulations that govern long-term care facilities have established strict documentation standards. Most SNFs, NFs, and ICF-MRs are governed by both federal and state regulations, including the Medicare Conditions of Participation. Assisted-living facilities are usually governed only by state regulations. Most long-term care providers do not participate in voluntary accreditation programs, although JCAHO does have long-term care facility standards.

The health records of long-term care patients are based on ongoing assessments and reassessments of the patient's (or resident's) needs. An interdisciplinary team develops a plan of care for each patient upon admission to the facility, and the plan is updated regularly over the patient's stay. The team includes the patient's physician and representatives from nursing services, nutritional services, social services, and other specialty areas (such as physical therapy), as appropriate.

In SNFs, the care plan is based on a format required by federal regulations. The care plan format is called the **resident assessment instrument** (RAI). The RAI is based on the **Minimum Data Set** (MDS) **for Long-Term Care.** The overall RAI framework includes the MDS, triggers, utilization guidelines, and **resident assessment protocols** (RAPs). The patient is assessed and reassessed at defined intervals as well as whenever there is a significant change in his or her condition.

The RAI is a critical component of the health record. In addition to development of the care plan, Medicare uses the MDS form to determine reimbursement. Many states also use it to determine Medicaid payments, and accreditation surveyors use information from it during the survey process.

The MDS is submitted electronically to each state health department and then on to the Centers for Medicare and Medicaid Services (CMS). At CMS, demographic and quality indicator information is compiled and provided as feedback to each facility.

The physician's role in a long-term care facility is not as visible as it is in other care settings. The physician develops a plan of treatment, which includes the medications and treatments provided to the resident. He or she then visits the resident in the facility on a thirty- or sixty-day schedule unless the resident's condition requires more frequent visits. At each visit, the physician reviews the plan of care and physician's orders and makes changes as necessary. Between visits, the physicians are contacted when nursing identifies changes in the resident's condition.

Other specialized assessments and interdisciplinary progress notes are included in the long-term care health record. The following list identifies the most common components of long-term care records:

- Identification and admission information
- Personal property list, including furniture and electronics
- History and physical and hospital records
- Advance directives, bill of rights, and other legal records
- Clinical assessments
- RAI/MDS and care plan
- Physician's orders
- Physician's progress notes/consultations
- Nursing or interdisciplinary notes
- Medication and records of other monitors, including administration of restraints
- Laboratory, radiology, and special reports
- Rehabilitation therapy notes (physical therapy, occupational therapy, and speech therapy)
- Social services, nutritional services, and activities documentation
- Discharge documentation

If paper-based records are found in a long-term setting, a process called record thinning may occur at intervals during the patient's stay. Records of patients whose stay extends to months or years become cumbersome to handle. Selected material may be removed and filed elsewhere according to facility guidelines. Any material removed must remain accessible when needed for patient care and service evaluation.

Information Pertaining to Home Health Care

Home health agencies provide medical and nonmedical services in the patient's home or place of residence. Home health care has seen an increase in the volume of patients due to growth in the aged population, the desire of Americans to live at home as long as possible, and cost savings over residential settings such as long-term care facilities.

Federal regulations govern the home care agencies that accept Medicare enrollees. States also have licensure regulations for home care agencies. Organizations such as JCAHO and the Community Health Accreditation Program of the National League for Nursing also provide accreditation services for some home health agencies.

Medicare regulations and accreditation standards have established documentation requirements. They also mandate periodic assessments. For agencies that are certified for Medicare, the home health certification/plan of care is a central component of documentation. This document is a plan of treatment established by a physician. It details the patient's diagnoses, impairments, goals, rehabilitation potential, and the type and frequency of services to be provided. The physician reviews and renews the home health certification/plan of care at least once during a sixty-day episode. Between renewals, certification is updated via the physician's telephone orders. There are no requirements for physician visits in home care; patients are responsible for seeing their physicians as necessary.

Medicare-certified home health care also uses a standardized patient assessment instrument called the **Outcomes and Assessment Information Set** (OASIS). OASIS items are a component of the comprehensive assessment that is the foundation for the plan of care. OASIS is completed at the start or resumption of care, with each sixty-day episode, with a significant change in condition, and upon patient transfer or discharge. It is the basis for reimbursement under Medicare. OASIS is submitted electronically to the state health department and then to CMS. Unique to home care is a service agreement that details the type and frequency of services, the charges for the services, and the parties responsible for payment.

Other documentation in a home care record is driven by the services ordered by the physician and agreed to by the patient. Each visit to the patient is documented in his or her health record. Home health aides may assist the patient with activities of daily living such as bathing and housekeeping, which allows the patient to remain at home. Documentation of this type of intervention is also necessary.

Some parts of home care records may be kept in the patient's home to facilitate communication among multiple caregivers or services. Technology has affected home care through the use of portable computers such as laptops and personal data assistants (PDAs).

The home care record usually includes the following types of documentation:

- Initial database/demographics and service agreement

- Certification and plan of treatment

- Physician's orders

- Documentation per visit, documentation by each discipline involved in treatment plan, summaries, and other progress notes

- Comprehensive assessment (OASIS), plan of care, and case conference notes

- Consents and other legal documents

- Referral or transfer information from other facilities

- Discharge summaries

Information Pertaining to Hospice Care

Hospice care is similar to home care in that most services are provided to patients in their homes. However, hospices also may be located in other healthcare settings such as hospitals or long-term care facilities or in separate freestanding facilities. Hospice care is unique in that a hospice program provides **palliative care** to terminally ill patients and supportive services to patients and their families. This type of care focuses on symptom management (for example, pain) and patient comfort rather than life-prolonging measures.

When the patient is admitted to a hospice care program, his or her primary caregiver is identified. In addition, basic identification information, diagnoses, prognosis, attending physician, and emergency contact information are collected.

An interdisciplinary team establishes a plan of care, which is the foundation for the hospice services to be provided to the patient. The care plan is based on information collected in the physical and psychosocial assessments performed upon admission. The assessments are updated throughout the patient's participation in the program.

Documentation of a care plan review is required every thirty days. The hospice provider must prepare a summary when the patient is transferred between care settings (between hospital and home care, for example). Federal regulations require the hospice provider to follow the patient's care plan even when the patient receives inpatient services.

Federal regulations govern hospice providers, as do accreditation standards established by organizations such as JCAHO. Documentation requirements are based on federal regulations and accreditation standards, which are similar.

The payment rate for hospice services is based directly on the services provided and the level of care needed as documented in the health record. There are two basic episodes in hospice care. The first episode begins with the patient's admission to the program and ends when the patient dies, is discharged, or is transferred to another facility. The second begins with the patient's death and follows the family through the bereavement process until the survivors are discharged. Bereavement services can last as long as one year and must be documented.

Information Pertaining to Behavioral Healthcare

Behavioral healthcare is delivered in inpatient hospitals, outpatient clinics, physicians' offices, rehabilitation programs, and community mental health programs. Documentation reflects the type of facility and the level of care and services delivered. For example, an inpatient psychiatric hospital maintains documentation similar to an inpatient hospital in addition to documentation unique to behavioral health.

Following are the minimum documentation requirements unique to the behavioral health setting as established by JCAHO and federal regulations:

- Identification data

- Source of referral

- Reason for referral

- Patient's legal status

- All appropriate consents for admission, treatment, evaluation, and aftercare

- Admitting psychiatric diagnoses

- Psychiatric history

- Record of the complete patient assessment, including the complaints of others regarding the patient as well as the patient's comments

- Medical history, report of physical examination, and record of all medications prescribed

- Provisional diagnoses based on assessment that includes other current diseases as well as psychiatric diagnoses

- Written individualized treatment plan

- Documentation of the course of treatment and all evaluations and examinations

- Multidisciplinary progress notes related to the goals and objectives outlined in the treatment plan

- Appropriate documentation related to special treatment procedures

- Updates to the treatment plan as a result of the assessments detailed in the progress notes

- Multidisciplinary case conferences and consultation notes, which include date of conference or consultation, recommendations made, and actions taken

- Information on any unusual occurrences such as treatment complications, accidents or injuries to the patient, death of the patient, and procedures that place the patient at risk or cause unusual pain including restraints and seclusion

- Correspondence related to the patient, including all letters and dated notations of telephone conversations relevant to the patient's treatment

- Discharge or termination summary

- Plan for follow-up care and documentation of its implementation

- Individualized aftercare or posttreatment plan

CARF, the Council on Quality and Leadership in Support for People with Disabilities, and AOA also have standards for facilities that specialize in mental health, mental retardation, or developmental disabilities.

Information Pertaining to Rehabilitation Services

The documentation requirements for rehabilitation facilities vary because facilities range from comprehensive inpatient care to outpatient services or special programs. Health record documentation reflects the level of care and services provided by the facility.

Inpatient rehabilitation hospitals and rehabilitation units within hospitals are reimbursed by Medicare under a prospective payment system based on documentation. A **patient assessment instrument** (PAI) is completed shortly after admission and upon discharge. Based on the patient's condition, services, diagnosis, and medical condition, a payment level is determined for the inpatient rehabilitation stay.

Many rehabilitation facilities are accredited through CARF, although JCAHO or AOA also can be chosen. CARF requires the facility to maintain a single case record for any patient it admits. The documentation standard for the health record includes the following requirements:

- Identification data

- Pertinent history, including functional history

- Diagnosis of disability/functional diagnosis

- Rehabilitation problems, goals, and prognosis

- Reports of assessments and individual program planning

- Reports from referring sources and service referrals

- Reports from outside consultations and laboratory, radiology, orthotic, and prosthetic services

- Designation of a manager for the patient's program

- Evidence of the patient's or family's participation in decision making

- Evaluation reports from each service

- Reports of staff conferences

- Patient's total program plan

- Plans from each service

- Signed and dated service and progress reports

- Correspondence pertinent to the patient

- Release forms

- Discharge report

- Follow-up reports

Records of Healthcare Provided in Correctional Facilities

Correctional facilities often provide health services to inmates and thus maintain health records. These health records begin with the collection of certain baseline information obtained during the initial intake process. This information may include a history and physical, a chest x-ray, and laboratory testing as well as a dental examination and a psychological evaluation.

Additional information is added to the inmate's health record when he or she visits health services for treatment of illness or injury, therapy, or medication. Examples include interdisciplinary progress notes and physician's orders. Of note is the rule that inmates may not maintain their own over-the-counter medications. Thus, even these types of medications must be received from health services and documented in the health record.

Because some inmates are imprisoned for many years, paper records eventually may include numerous volumes. Therefore, health information staff must develop and adhere to procedures that keep the most current and comprehensive information readily available.

In some states, the inmate's original health record is transferred with the inmate when he or she moves to a different prison within the state system. As a result, HIM professionals in such states must work together to produce standardized policies, procedures, and formats. Federal facilities often have similar practices.

Correctional health services may choose to comply with the hospital accreditation standards of JCAHO or the standards developed by the American Correctional Association or the National Commission on Correctional Health Care.

Information Pertaining to End-Stage Renal Disease Service

Individuals with severe kidney disease requiring renal dialysis may be treated in outpatient settings of healthcare facilities, in independent dialysis centers, while residents of long-term care settings, or even in their own homes (self-dialysis). Medicare has specific **Conditions for Coverage** that apply to all these settings. The standards include criteria for record content as well as for record keeping.

Documentation begins with notification of patient rights. A unique component of that notification is inclusion of information on the facility's policy for hemodialyzer reuse. Treatment record elements include an interdisciplinary patient assessment and a plan of care with team members commonly consisting of a physician, nurse, social worker, registered dietitian, and the patient. Progress notes, laboratory test results, a discharge summary, and consents also must be found. Special emphasis is placed on recording the patient's nutritional, anemia, vascular access, transplant, and rehabilitation status, as well as social service interventions and dialysis dosages. Patient education and training are important for dialysis success and for continued service. Evidence of both must be documented.

Personal Health Records

A relatively new development, the **personal health record** has been defined by the AHIMA eHIM Personal Health Record Work Group (2005) as:

> an electronic, universally available, lifelong resource of health information needed by individuals to make health decisions

The personal health record is unique in that it is maintained and controlled by each individual and is a compilation of information obtained from healthcare providers as well as through personal discovery. It could be found on a personal computer, the web, desktop and Web, or portable devices. The Work Group also identified minimum common data elements (2005) as:

- Personal demographic information

- General medical information

- Allergies and drug sensitivities

- Conditions

- Hospitalizations

- Surgeries

- Medications

- Immunizations

- Clinical tests

- Pregnancy history

Because it is a lifelong record, information also could include:

- Information from providers

- Genetic information

- Personal, family, occupational, and environmental history

- Health plans and goals

- Health status of the individual

- Documentation of choices in relation to organ donation, durable power of attorney, and advance directives

- Charges paid for services and products

- Health insurance information

- Provider directory

Although health information professionals may not have direct contact with personal records, they serve as patient advocates and can play important support and educational roles. In addition, in the electronic record environment, patients have portals to communicate with practitioners via such methods as e-mails, their personal health records, patient questionnaires and surveys, and transferring clinical information (AHIMA e-HIM Task Force 2004). Policies need to be in place to determine how much and what type of information actually becomes part of the organization's health record.

Check Your Understanding 3.2

Instructions: Choose the most appropriate answer for the following questions.

1. ____ Which type of health record contains information about care provided prior to arrival at a healthcare setting and documentation of care provided to stabilize the patient?
   a. Ambulatory care
   b. Emergency care
   c. Long-term care
   d. Rehabilitative care

2. ____ Patient history questionnaires, problem lists, diagnostic tests results, and immunization records are commonly found in which type of record?
   a. Ambulatory care
   b. Emergency care
   c. Long-term care
   d. Rehabilitative care

3. _____ The ambulatory surgery record contains information most similar to _____.
   a. Physician office records
   b. Emergency care records
   c. Hospital operative records
   d. Hospital obstetric records

4. _____ Which standardized tool is used to assess Medicare-certified rehabilitation facilities?
   a. Outcomes and Assessment Information Set (OASIS)
   b. Resident assessment protocol (RAP)
   c. Patient assessment instrument (PAI)
   d. Minimum Data Set (MDS)

5. _____ Records in which of the following settings would not include an interdisciplinary care plan?
   a. Long-term care
   b. End-stage renal disease
   c. Hospice care
   d. Ambulatory care

6. _____ Portions of a treatment record may be maintained in a patient's home in which two types of settings?
   a. Hospice and behavioral health
   b. Home health and end-stage renal disease
   c. Obstetric and gynecologic care
   d. Rehabilitation and correctional care

7. _____ A patient's legal status, complaints of others regarding the patient, and reports of restraints or seclusion would be found most frequently in which type of health record?
   a. Rehabilitative care
   b. Ambulatory care
   c. Behavioral health
   d. Personal health record

8. _____ Paper records may require thinning in which two settings?
   a. Home health and hospice
   b. Rehabilitation and end-stage renal disease
   c. Ambulatory care and behavioral health
   d. Long-term care and correctional services

Documentation Standards

The importance of documentation to the quality of direct patient care cannot be over-emphasized. Documentation represents the primary communication among multidisciplinary caregivers for efficient and effective initial treatment, for continuing care, and for the evidence that care and treatment occurred.

Moreover, documentation promotes understanding of the whole patient in the long term. Health information management (HIM) professionals provide a valuable service in helping healthcare organizations to establish reasonable documentation policies and procedures. A well-executed approach satisfies numerous needs and interests, including those of the provider, the healthcare consumer, and external parties.

Internally, timely and effective documentation has a number of indirect benefits beyond patient care. Performance improvement and risk management activities rely heavily on health record documentation. These activities result in direct improvements in patient care and operational processes. In addition, healthcare organizations use cumulative health data as the basis for making decisions on future services. (Risk management is discussed further in chapter 11; performance improvement is discussed in chapter 12.)

Health record documentation also is reviewed by external organizations. Regulatory agencies use documentation as a tool to measure the quality of services before granting accreditation or **certification** to healthcare organizations. Third-party payers depend on documentation as proof that chargeable services were actually received. The legal system searches the written record for evidence. It is generally assumed that a service that was not documented was not done.

Basic Principles of Health Record Documentation

The basic principles of health record documentation apply to both paper-based and electronic patient records. The principles address the uniformity, accuracy, completeness, legibility, authenticity, timeliness, frequency, and format of health record entries. The American Health Information Management Association (AHIMA) has developed the following general documentation guidelines (Smith and Dougherty 2001):

- Every healthcare organization should have policies that ensure the uniformity of both the content and the format of the health record. The policies should be based on all applicable accreditation standards, federal and state regulations, payer requirements, and professional practice standards.

- The health record should be organized systematically in order to facilitate data retrieval and compilation.

- Only individuals authorized by the organization's policies should be allowed to enter documentation in the health record.

- Organizational policy and/or medical staff rules and regulations should specify who may receive and transcribe verbal physician's orders.

- Health record entries should be documented at the time the services they describe are rendered.

- The authors of all entries should be clearly identified in the record.

- Only abbreviations and symbols approved by the organization and/or medical staff rules and regulations should be used in the health record.

- All entries in the health record should be permanent.

- Errors in paper-based records should be corrected according to the following process: Draw a single line in ink through the incorrect entry. Then print the word *error* at the top of the entry along with a legal signature or initials and the date, time, and reason for change and the title and discipline of the individual making the correction. The correct information is then added to the entry. Errors must never be obliterated. The original entry should remain legible, and the corrections should be entered in chronological order. Any late entries should be labeled as such.

- Any corrections or information added to the record by the patient should be inserted as an addendum (a separate note). No changes should be made in the original entries in the record. Any information added to the health record by the patient should be clearly identified as an addendum.

- The HIM department should develop, implement, and evaluate policies and procedures related to the quantitative and qualitative analysis of health records.

(Quantitative and qualitative analysis are discussed in chapters 8 and 12.)

At the present time, accreditation organizations and regulatory agencies are still developing specific documentation guidelines for EHRs. In cases where no guidelines exist, HIM practitioners continue to apply basic documentation principles to every medium. However, the type of medium, paper or electronic, may require that specific details be handled differently to achieve the same documentation goals. For example, the method used to make corrections and amendments in EHRs may be different from the method used for paper-based records.

A number of laws, regulations, and standards requiring minimum levels of documentation exemplify the importance of high-quality documentation outside the organization as well as within. Healthcare organizations must comply in order to maintain licensure within their states, to remain certified for federal program reimbursement, to maintain current accreditation status with external agencies, and to avoid fines.

When developing documentation policies and practices, the healthcare organization is usually obligated to simultaneously follow legal, regulatory, and accreditation directives that pertain to its particular facility type within its geopolitical area. Generally, following the strictest directives that apply ensures adequate compliance. In all cases, the ultimate goal is quality of care for patients in every healthcare environment.

Significant overlap exists among the documentation requirements of accrediting bodies and federal and state regulations and laws. Although overlap may exist, differences among the standards must be recognized. When determining its policies, the organization must evaluate all relevant standards. Documentation requirements are usually recorded in medical staff rules and regulations and become a component of medical staff membership requirements

Even with best efforts, it can be difficult to sort through multiple documentation directives. HIM professionals must turn to legal counsel for guidance when circumstances are unusual.

Accreditation Organizations

Many healthcare organizations seek public recognition through accreditation with recognized accrediting bodies. This status signifies that the facility has met patient care and other standards for providing high-quality care. In some cases, it also allows facilities to participate in programs that affect their financial status, such as Medicare and Medicaid, Medical Resident Programs, and other training programs. Organizations seeking accreditation must meet specific documentation standards. Periodic surveys and detailed record review by the accrediting body evaluate how well the organization is complying with documentation standards.

Healthcare organizations voluntarily seek accreditation from a variety of private, not-for-profit accreditation organizations. Different types of organizations are accredited by different accreditation organizations.

Joint Commission on Accreditation of Healthcare Organizations

A number of healthcare settings are eligible for JCAHO accreditation, including hospitals (acute, critical care, children's, psychiatric, and rehabilitation), ambulatory care organizations, behavioral health organizations, home care including hospice providers, long-term care facilities, healthcare networks, clinical laboratories, and office-based surgery practices. Additional specialty settings are eligible for JCAHO certificate programs. Examples include disease-specific programs and primary stroke centers.

Beginning with its acute hospital standards in 2004, JCAHO initiated a new process called Shared Visions–New Pathways in its accreditation reviews. Among other changes, the survey focus moved from survey monitors every three years to a philosophy of continuous improvement and continuous standard compliance. Standards were streamlined and survey paperwork reduced, midcycle reviews were initiated, facility monitoring of sentinel (unexpected) events was encouraged, and following the hospital experience of selected patients (tracer methodology) during its surveys was instituted. Each accreditation standard is now accompanied by a rationale and steps to meet the standard called elements of performance. The scoring method also is new (Clark 2004).

JCAHO recognizes the appropriateness of applying documentation standards consistently across the healthcare continuum and has identified a number of common standards that apply to all healthcare settings. Frequently, these core expectations are supplemented by additional standards that represent the specific requirements of different settings and services. For example, a teaching hospital that hosts medical education programs for residents would be evaluated on its compliance with standards for supervision of residents, in addition to common standards and standards specific to acute care settings.

Many standards that apply to health records are found in accreditation manual sections called Management of Information. However, other sections that address rights and responsibilities of facilities, patient care, medication management, and responsibilities of the medical and nursing staffs, among others, also include pertinent information. To ensure compliance with all health information standards, review of all sections and monitoring all that are found is important. This concept applies to standards of other accreditation organizations as well. JCAHO also has addressed errors in interpretation of abbreviations commonly used in health records by publishing a prohibited abbreviation list. The abbreviations noted on the list should not be found in the patient health records of their accredited health providers.

American Osteopathic Association

AOA first initiated its hospital accreditation program to ensure the quality of residency programs for doctors of osteopathy. Today, AOA accredits a number of additional healthcare organizations and facilities, including laboratories, ambulatory care/ambulatory surgery, behavioral health, substance abuse, physical rehabilitation medicine, and critical care. Documentation standards are both broad as they pertain to common documentation requirements and specific as they address specialty services.

Accreditation Association for Ambulatory Healthcare

AAAHC has established standards that are similar to common acute care documentation practices. The standards emphasize summaries for enhancing the continuity of care. This is especially important for the ambulatory patient. For example, summaries of past surgeries, diagnoses, and problems are helpful in transferring history information to new treatment settings for complex cases.

Commission on Accreditation of Rehabilitation Facilities

CARF accredits programs and services in medical rehabilitation, assisted-living, behavioral health, adult day-care, and employment and community services. Health record documentation is used to evaluate procedural issues surrounding special circumstances in the treatment and handling of patients and clients.

National Committee for Quality Assurance

NCQA began accrediting managed care organizations in 1991. The NCQA's standards focus on patient safety, confidentiality, consumer protection, access to services, service quality, and continuous improvement. More recently, NCQA expanded its program to include other types of organizations, such as preferred provider organizations.

Other Accreditation Groups

A number of other organizations accredit specific types of healthcare facilities. For example, the Commission for the Accreditation of Birth Centers accredits those groups and the Community Health Accreditation Program of the National League for Nursing accredits home healthcare agencies. Standards that affect health record content can be found in the guidelines for all accreditation programs.

Medicare and Medicaid Programs

The Medicare Conditions of Participation or Conditions for Coverage apply to a variety of healthcare organizations that participate in the Medicare program. In other words, participating organizations receive federal funds from the Medicare program for services provided to patients and thus must follow the Medicare Conditions of Participation. The regulations vary according to setting and address documentation conditions that must be met to continue participation. Standards currently exist for hospitals, SNFs, home health agencies, hospices, rehabilitation facilities, ambulatory surgery centers, clinics in rural areas, and some behavioral health providers. Additionally, Conditions for Coverage of Suppliers of End Stage Renal Disease (ESRD) Services standards apply to dialysis centers.

Medicare recognizes some accreditation organizations as having standards that sufficiently cover the related Conditions of Participation. After reviewing standards of accrediting groups that seek this recognition, Medicare may award them **deemed status.** As long as a healthcare setting maintains active accreditation by an accreditation body with deemed status, separate Medicare surveys are not required. For all other settings, surveys are performed. This task is often contracted to state government health reviewers.

Medicaid programs are funded jointly by federal and state governments but are administered by the individual states. Thus, Medicaid guidelines vary from state to state. Similar to Medicare participation, facilities are often required to meet federal Conditions of Participation or Coverage to receive these funds.

State Regulating Agencies

Individual states pass legislation and mandate regulations that affect how healthcare organizations within them operate and care for patients. The nature of such regulations varies from state to state.

Compliance with state licensing laws is required in order for healthcare organizations to begin or remain in operation within their states. To continue licensure, organizations must demonstrate their knowledge of, and compliance with, documentation regulations.

Check Your Understanding 3.3

Instructions: Choose the most appropriate answer for the following questions.

1. _____ Which of the following is not an accrediting organization?
   a. Accreditation Association for Ambulatory Healthcare
   b. American Osteopathic Association
   c. National Committee for Quality Assurance
   d. Centers for Medicare and Medicaid Services

2. _____ An accrediting organization is awarded deemed status by Medicare. This means that facilities receiving accreditation under its guidelines do not need to _____.
   a. Meet licensure standards
   b. Undergo Medicare certification surveys
   c. Undergo accreditation surveys
   d. Meet Medicare certification standards

3. _____ Which group focuses on accreditation of managed care and preferred provider organizations?
   a. Accreditation Association for Ambulatory Healthcare
   b. National Committee for Quality Assurance
   c. Commission on Accreditation of Rehabilitation Facilities
   d. Joint Commission on Accreditation of Healthcare Organizations

4. _____ Which of the following regulations would most likely contain information on who is authorized to document in a patient's record?
   a. Facility rules and regulations
   b. Accreditation standards
   c. Licensure standards
   d. Conditions of Participation

5. _____ Which of the following groups has instituted a health record–prohibited abbreviation list?
   a. National Committee for Quality Assurance
   b. Joint Commission on Accreditation of Healthcare Organizations
   c. American Osteopathic Association
   d. Centers for Medicare and Medicaid Services

Format of the Health Record

Health records are maintained in two basic formats, paper based or electronic. Records are referred to as hybrid if they have some paper and some electronic components. Today, most healthcare facilities are working toward an EHR system.

Traditional (Paper-Based) Health Records

The traditional paper-based health record has several limitations. One limitation is the need to adhere to a strict record format. Unlike the true EHR in which computer screen views can be tailored to the needs of the end user, the paper-based record does not allow for individual customization.

The EHR allows the system administrator to limit access to information, restructure information, and highlight key information that the end user may need. In contrast, the paper-based record lacks such flexibility. Because the paper-based record is lengthy and difficult to handle, management most often chooses to keep it in a single format that all end users can agree on. The greater the number of end users, the more important it is to follow a defined format.

Accreditation standards and state licensure regulations require every provider to develop specific guidelines on how the information in health records is to be arranged in its particular facility. State laws, regulations, and accreditation standards also require specific content elements.

As mentioned in chapter 2, three major types of paper-based health record are in use today: the **source-oriented health record,** the **problem-oriented health record,** and the **integrated health record.** It is important to realize, however, that no hard and fast rules exist for arranging the elements of a health record. The healthcare provider is free to select the arrangement that best suits its needs. For example, some ambulatory health organizations arrange the materials in active records in one way and closed records in another (AHIMA 2001).

Source-Oriented Health Records

In the source-oriented health record, documents are grouped together according to their point of origin. That is, laboratory records are grouped together, radiology records are grouped together, clinical notes are grouped together, and so on. Thus, physicians' progress notes for a single episode of patient care would be arranged in either chronological or reverse chronological order and placed together in the patient's health record.

The result is that those individuals charged with filing reports in the paper-based health record can do so easily simply by looking at the source and date of the report. However, the end users of information filed in the record do not have as easy a time. To follow or record information on the patient's course of treatment, they must search by date of occurrence in each of the groups of information (that is, laboratory, radiology, and every group of clinical notes). The more departments a facility has, the more sections a source-oriented health record can have. It is left to the end user to tie together information from the various sections of the record to get a picture of the entire course of treatment.

Problem-Oriented Health Records

The problem-oriented health record is better suited to serve the patient and the end user of the patient information. The key characteristic of this format is an itemized list of the patient's past and present social, psychological, and medical problems. Each problem is indexed with a unique number.

In addition to a problem list, each problem-oriented health record contains a database, the initial care plan, and progress notes. The database is formatted much like the source-oriented health record and contains the following information:

- Chief complaint

- Present illness(es)

- Social history

- Medical history

- Physical examination

- Diagnostic test results

The initial plan serves as an overall road map for addressing each of the patient's problems. The plans are numbered to correspond to the problems they address.

The patient's healthcare provider uses progress notes to document how the patient's problems are being treated and how he or she is responding to treatment. Each progress note is labeled with the unique number assigned to the problem being addressed. Some providers also use a SOAP format for their problem-oriented progress notes. A subjective (S) entry relates significant information in the patient's words or from the patient's point of view. Objective (O) data includes factual information such as laboratory findings or provider observations. Professional conclusions reached from evaluation of the subjective or objective information make up the assessment (A), and any comments on or changes in plans (P) complete the framework. An example of a SOAP note can be found in figure 3.15. Not all SOAP components must be entered in every note. If the SOAP framework is used, only pertinent parts are documented. This problem-indexing system allows the healthcare provider to easily follow the patient's course of treatment regarding any specific problem. Ideally, other elements of the health record (for example, physician's orders) also would be numbered according to the problems they address.

Integrated Health Records
The third major type of paper-based health record is the integrated health record. The integrated health record is arranged so that the documentation from various sources is intermingled and follows strict chronological order. The advantage of the integrated format is that it is easy to follow the course of the patient's diagnosis and treatment. The disadvantage is that the format makes it difficult to compare similar information.

Strengths and Weaknesses of Paper-Based Health Records
The ultimate goal of every health record is to facilitate communication. A well-designed, well-maintained paper-based health record can significantly improve communication among healthcare providers and other health information end users. As the quality of healthcare services has advanced, so has the quality of health records. Advances in standardized format, standardized medical terminology, and improved information capture and delivery have improved the quality and value of the health record.

Figure 3.15.   Example of a SOAP progress note

SOAP PROGRESS NOTE

Identification Number

Medical Record Number

| Last Name | First Name | Middle Initial |

Date of Birth

DATE	DEPARTMENT	PROGRESS NOTES
7-28-89	INT MEDICINE	#1 Diabetes Mellitus
		S: Occasionally gets hungry. No insulin reactions. Says she is following diet.
		O: Adequately controlled. FBS 110 mg %, urine sugar, no acetone.
		A: Insulin-dependent diabetes, controlled.
		P: Continue 40 units NPH insulin daily, 1,200 calorie diet, return visit in 2 weeks.
		#6 Hypertension
		S: No headaches, dizziness, etc.
		O: BP 140/90, (RA sitting); pulse 80
		A: BP satisfactory
		P: Continue with Diuril, 500 mg once daily. Return visit in 2 weeks.

Still, the paper-based health record has several weaknesses. Various quality, standardization, and timeliness issues need to be addressed and resolved. For example, the average health record is needed by approximately 150 end users. However, the paper-based health record can be viewed by only one user at a time and in only one place at a time. Thus, the valuable information recorded in the health record is often unavailable to individuals who need it.

Further, paper-based health records can be difficult to update. An active record of a patient receiving care moves often from provider to provider within the healthcare facility. The individual(s) responsible for updating its content must hand-carry paper documents to wherever the record is located in order to file them or wait until the record is returned. The result is that updates may be delayed.

Finally, paper-based health records are fragile and susceptible to damage from water, fire, and the wear and tear of daily use. They also can easily be misplaced or misfiled. For most organizations, it would be prohibitively expensive and difficult to maintain duplicate copies of paper health records as backups.

Electronic (Computer-Based) Health Records

The EHR can be seen as the natural evolution of the health record. By design, it not only addresses many of the paper-based health record's existing problems but also presents new capabilities. The discussion here focuses on the impact of the EHR on the generation of record content whereas a much broader description and analysis of the EHR is presented in chapter 4.

Definition of the Electronic Health Record

Although work is under way, there currently is no widely accepted definition for the EHR. As a result, it is often described in relation to the functions it should perform. Mon (2004b) provides this summary list as described by the Institute of Medicine:

- Collect clinical, administrative, and financial data at the point of care. When combined with alerts and evidence, this integrated view of patient data helps clinicians make better decisions.

- Exchange data more easily among providers to facilitate continuity of care.

- Measure clinical process improvement and outcomes, compare them against benchmarks, and facilitate clinical trails and research.

- Report health data to public health, regulatory agencies, and accreditation bodies to more quickly detect and monitor disease outbreaks, measure population health status, and assist with bioterrorism surveillance.

- Support enterprise-wide management reporting and other administrative and financial (for example, revenue cycle management) processes.

In fact, in July 2004, using the IOM's work as a foundation, a national standards group called Health Level Seven (HL7) introduced a list of about 130 different functions that would help define an EHR. Refinement of the functions will come as they receive rigorous review. However, the content of the record itself will continue to be based on the standards and regulations presented earlier in this chapter with amplification as other approved functions are determined.

Technological Basis of the Electronic Record

A number of technologies support EHR systems. Some of these technologies are discussed briefly in the following sections; health information systems and technology are discussed in detail in chapters 16 through 19.

Databases and Database Management Systems

Most electronic records are organized according to one of two unique data base models—the centralized record and the distributed record—or a mix of the two models. In the centralized model, patient health information and data are stored in a single central computer system. In the distributed model, patient health information and data are located in department-based computer systems or subsystems. Whichever model is used, it is important that the systems be able to communicate and share data elements.

Image Processing and Storage

The traditional paper-based health record included few photographs and diagnostic images. However, with the introduction of **imaging technology,** it is now possible to combine health record text files with diagnostic imaging files. This development has created the multimedia health record.

Electronic imaging solves many of the problems associated with traditional record keeping. For example, because the actual images never leave the control of the system administrator, lost files are no longer a problem. In addition, medical imaging allows more than one end user to view a document at the same time. Further, the digitized files make it possible to transfer images to remote locations quickly and easily.

Text Processing

Retrieving a single piece of information from a paper record can require a lot of time and effort. Many organizations have attempted to improve retrieval processes by standardizing chart formats or flagging documents to assist in locating key pieces of information. Although such methods are helpful, they have not completely resolved the problem of information retrieval.

The introduction of electronic applications has further improved text searching and retrieval because files now can be indexed. The introduction of database systems using query language applications has allowed end users to perform text searches and retrievals. The ability of computer applications to identify key words and phrases found in textual data has improved the ability to retrieve key pieces of information from the record.

However, progress in implementing this technology in healthcare has been delayed by the lack of a uniform vocabulary. Some of the early developers have said that a medical term can be expressed many different ways within a single organization. Even so, some progress is being made in the standardization of medical language. (See chapter 4.)

Data Input

Creating a workable data capture process has proved to be one of the major challenges facing EHR implementers. Transcription remains the most common type of data input mechanism. The end user either inputs the information or dictates it in report style to be transcribed.

Alternative data capture tools are being developed or refined to address the challenge of creating workable data capture processes.

Among these technologies are the following:

- Continuous voice recognition
- Optical character readers
- Bar code readers
- Document imaging
- Automated templates
- Structured data entry

In an ideal situation, the individual responsible for providing the service or treatment enters the data into the database at or near the time the service or treatment occurs. When recorded, the information is immediately available to all end users on a need-to-know basis.

Data Retrieval

The ultimate goal of any EHR system is to quickly deliver useful health information to the end user in the location where it is most needed. When developing a data retrieval system, the most effective approach considers the end user's needs. Designs must consider:

- *Presentation of data:* What is the most effective way to present the information— via text, graphs, or tables?

- *Need to know:* What information does the end user need to quickly understand the patient's condition and progress?

- *Quick-search capabilities:* What is the most effective way to enable the end user to retrieve factual information easily and quickly?

- *Analytical capabilities:* What is the best method to enable the end user to analyze and compare a full range of patient data, from historic information to current information?

Data Exchange and Vocabulary Standards

In the current healthcare information system (IS) environment, there are hundreds of IS vendors, limited industry IS standardization, and widespread use of proprietary software and technology. Healthcare professionals, managers, policy makers, regulators, and educators often struggle to share information among different computer systems. The problem faced by everyone wishing to share information is the lack of standardization. And in situations where IS standards do exist, there is a problem with noncompliance with existing standards. The slow progress toward industry standardization was a major contributing factor behind passage of the HIPAA legislation. Unlike industries such as banking and air travel, healthcare has been slow to accept standardization.

Recently, efforts toward the development of healthcare IS standards have gained momentum. Today, a number of standards organizations are working to develop IS standards for healthcare organizations, including:

- Health Level Seven (HL7)
- American Society for Testing and Materials (ASTM)

- The Institute of Electronic and Electrical Engineers (IEEE)

- American College of Radiologists/National Electrical Manufacturers Association (ACR/NEMA)

- International Standards Organization (ISO)

- Systematized Nomenclature of Medicine (SNOMED)

- National Library of Medicine (NLM)

- Unified Medical Language System (UMLS)

(AHIMA Workgroup on Core Data Sets 2004).

System Communications and Networks
The evolution of widespread networks of healthcare providers called integrated delivery systems (IDSs) and the initiation of voluntary regional health information organizations (RHIOs) have added another dimension to the EHR. By nature, the healthcare industry depends heavily on information. For an IDS or an RHIO to succeed, healthcare professionals must be able to readily communicate and transmit information to many different locations, sometimes across organizational lines.

Because of the importance of system communications and networks, IS administrators in healthcare must manage a number of existing and evolving communications technologies as well as balance the needs and wants of multiple end users. This variation in needs requires system administrators to juggle many technologies or to limit technology choices to only a few.

The various communication technology options include the following:

- Wireless

- Internet

- Extranet

- Broadband Internet

- Client server networks

- Fiber optics

- Application service providers

EHR Implementation: Benefits and Challenges
The benefits of EHR systems are obvious. For example, well-designed EHR systems:

- Make it possible to access information quickly and easily

- Allow multiple users to access the same information at the same time

- Permit view customization

- Increase ease of maintenance and updates

- Process large and difficult tasks quickly

- Permit ready access to volumes of professional resource information
- Maintain duplicate copies of information that can be retrieved should the originals be lost or damaged

Before EHR systems are successfully implemented, sizable challenges must be overcome. Among these challenges are the following:

- Lack of a clear definition
- Difficulty meeting the needs of multiple end users
- Lack of standardization
- Potential threat to privacy and security
- Development and implementation costs
- Organizational and behavioral resistance

Progress is being made in a number of these areas because of federal initiatives and cooperation among affected organizations.

Lack of a Clear Definition
Healthcare professionals can usually reach a consensus on a general description of an EHR. However, beyond that there are many unanswered questions. The current EHR lacks a common data model, a common set of data elements, a common vocabulary, and a common structure, although efforts are under way in a number of these areas. (See chapter 4.)

Difficulty Meeting the Needs of Multiple End Users
The ultimate goal of EHR developers is to create a system that is user-friendly. Such a system would be centered on users, networked across care settings, and specialized in terms of use and circumstances.

However, being all things to all end users creates a real challenge for system designers. For example, certain end-user specifications cannot coexist in the same application. The greater the amount of variation, the greater the complexity of the application programs. Moreover, as users learn more about computers, they place additional demands on system designers. Despite these challenges, user participation in computer system design and implementation is a prerequisite to success.

Lack of Standardization
The modern American consumer can purchase a toaster in any appliance store and be assured that it will plug into a wall socket as long as the wall socket is in the United States. This ability to use any toaster in any wall socket is the result of planned standardization. However, this level of standardization does not currently exist for the EHR, although the development of standards has been identified as a priority by the federal government. In 2005, the Certification Commission for Healthcare Information Technology, a private sector, voluntary effort was initiated. The group's first task is to develop standards to be applied to information technology products seeking certification for EHR use in the United States. It will use the HL7 functionality standards as a starting point (Mon 2004a). (See also chapter 4.)

Potential Threat to Privacy and Security
The characteristics that make the EHR a powerful tool also directly affect the privacy and security of the information contained within the system. The challenge is to find the balance between access and restriction. It would be easy to blame threats to privacy and security on the electronic record, but privacy and security issues have been around long before computerized records were introduced. Moreover, technology is not the only challenge to ensuring privacy and security. The challenges posed by society, human nature, policy, procedure, and legislation also must be taken into consideration.

Development and Implementation Cost
An important barrier to purchasing and installing EHR systems is cost. Many organizations would prefer to maintain the status quo rather than spend hundreds of thousands of dollars on a new system. In many cases, the benefits of the EHR system would more than justify the purchase and installation costs. However, uncertainty about the cost-to-benefit ratio of installing an EHR system prevents many organizations from committing to system implementation. Organizations must consider not only the software and hardware purchase costs, but also the staff training costs involved in EHR system implementation.

Organizational and Behavioral Resistance
Finally, healthcare professionals must realize that organizational change occurs more slowly than technological change. Working with practitioners to change long-standing habits is a challenge. Incremental steps must be encouraged and celebrated. The technology is available now and standards are being addressed, but organizations must develop their own time line for implementation that involves their specific provider population.

Hybrid Health Records

One method of overcoming some of the EHR hurdles is for the healthcare setting to move in steps from paper-based systems to full EHR adoption. If planned appropriately, this allows the facility to thoroughly investigate the needs of its users and gradually address the weaknesses and challenges of an EHR. A record in this type of system is referred to as a hybrid health record.

Definition of the Hybrid Health Record
In a series of practice briefs on hybrid records, the AHIMA e-HIM Workgroup used the following description (2003b):

> A hybrid health record is a system with functional components that:
> - include both paper and electronic documents
> - use both manual and electronic processes

On the basis of this description, a hybrid record has many formats. For example, one facility may have laboratory and other diagnostic reports reported electronically, but the remainder on paper. This facility may take an EHR step by scanning all the paper documents upon patient discharge to make a full record accessible electronically for subsequent users. Another organization may have most record components generated electronically by providers as care is delivered, scan all other documents that are not part of the system, and have alerts and reminders that assist in clinical and care decision support.

Transitions in Record Practices

Hybrid records are positive steps toward the EHR, but they also create special challenges. Both manual and computer processes must be supported, policies and procedures are needed for both types of systems, and appropriate safeguards must be in place for privacy and security of both systems. A definition of what constitutes a record in each system must be developed. As the transition occurs, it also is important to regularly update system descriptions, including the location of all care documents, so that patient health information remains readily available to users. The AHIMA e-HIM Workgroup (2003) suggests a matrix for this step and provides an example. (See table 3.4.)

As the electronic system develops, different versions of documents may exist and these also must be monitored and logged for both legal and practice purposes. Additionally, the AHIMA e-HIM Task Force (2004) describes in detail changes in health information processes and procedures that are required as a record transitions from paper to hybrid to fully electronic formats.

Examples of Hybrid Systems

Many different types of healthcare organizations use hybrid systems. The following sections present some actual applications.

Physician Office Systems

Kaiser Permanente-Colorado is a large medical network located in the Denver-Boulder area. The network consists of 17 medical offices, 600 physicians, 2,500 staff, and 350,000 members. Network executives report that 25,000 health records must be delivered across its 100-square-mile service area every day.

To address this challenge, Kaiser Permanente-Colorado implemented a networkwide EMR. This system is based primarily on electronic imaging system technology. Before introduction of the EMR, the 152 HIM staff members spent 90 percent of their time tracking down and delivering paper records. Today, they spend most of their time scanning documents and cataloging them for reference within the electronic system.

Implementation of the new system has resulted in a reduction in the number of HIM staff members to seventy-five. Not surprisingly, many of the eliminated positions were medical record couriers. However, through careful planning, all the displaced employees have found new jobs within the network. The most significant change in terms of care delivery is that two physicians involved in the care of the same patient now can view the patient's records at the same time and consult with each other immediately (Burgess et al. 1999, 33).

Ambulatory Record Systems

Hall Health Primary Care Center (HHPCC) is a community-based primary care center at the University of Washington in Seattle. By the mid-1990s, HHPCC had outgrown its paper-based health record system. It had become difficult to share information among the University of Washington Academic Medical Center, HHPCC, and the multiple clinics that served patients daily.

In December 1995, HHPCC began implementing its new electronic system one clinic at a time. The women's clinic was chosen as the first site for implementation because it was the smallest, with only four clinicians. The implementation process began with the automation of progress notes. Some time later, scanner technology was introduced.

Table 3.4. Hybrid health record legal source legend

Organization's Name
HYBRID HEALTH RECORD
LEGAL SOURCE LEGEND

Report/Document Types	LHR Media Type (P)aper/ (E)lectronic	Source System Application (nonpaper)	Electronic Storage Start Date	Stop Printing Start Date
Admission History & Physical	P/E	System 1	1/1/2002	1/1/2003
Attending Admission Notes	P			
Physician Orders	E			
Inpatient Progress Notes	P			
Discharge Summary	E	System 1	1/1/2002	4/1/2002
Inpatient Transfer Note	E	System 1	1/1/2002	
Outpatient Progress Notes	P			
Clinical Laboratory Results— (Preliminary/Interim)	E	System 2	1/1/1999	1/1/1999
Clinical Laboratory Results (Final)	E	System 2	1/1/1999	1/1/2000
Radiology Reports	E	System 3	7/1/2003	
Care Flow Sheets	E	System 1	6/1/2003	
Medication Records	E	System 1	7/1/2003	
Clinical Consult Reports	E	System 1	1/1/2002	
Pre-operative, Pre-procedure Notes	P			
Pathology Reports	E	System 2	1/1/1999	1/1/2000
Organ/Tissue Donation or Transplants	P			
Patient Problem List (Summary List)	E	System 1	8/1/2003	
Urgent Care and Emergency Records	P			
Consents[1]	E	System 4	TBD	
Advance Directive				
Correspondence[1]	E	System 4	TBD	
Pre-operative Anesthetic Assessments and Plans	P			
Intra-operative Documentation	P			
Post-Operative Documentation	P			
Brief Post-Operative Note	P			
Surgical Operative Reports	E	System 1	1/1/2002	

[1]Scanned electronic documents
Source: AHIMD 2003.

HHPCS soon discovered that it faced many challenges, including:

- Software incompatibility

- Provider resistance

- Changes in work flow

- Too much paper

However, as a result of the implementation, HHPCC has seen many benefits and improvements, including:

- Improved chart legibility

- Ability to integrate practice guidelines

- Increased access by multiple users

- Reduced duplication of services

- No more lost charts

- Improved communication

- Access to professional resources

Using the computer-based record changed the way that HHPCC worked. Changes occurred at all levels (Burgess et al. 1999, 33). In some cases, employees saw changes in their job descriptions and were required to learn new skills.

Hospital Systems
For the 570-bed Stanford University Medical Center in Palo Alto, California, the move to an electronic record was a gradual one. The medical center began by installing imaging technology and scanning for all the medical records produced by the system. Later, it added a clinical data repository. Next, the center addressed clinical results reporting and physician order entry. "If you come to our medical records room now, all you will see is space, as there is no longer a file room," reports Russ Peckenpaugh, interim chief information officer.

The electronic record implementers at Stanford have found that some of the greatest challenges they face are cultural, organizational, and even psychological. Computer-based record implementation at Stanford created a strong partnership between the IS department and the HIM department. The HIM staff members found that they became more IS sophisticated as they focused on how the "customers" use the information (Burgess et al. 1999, 33).

Department of Veterans Affairs
Physical size is the most glaring difference between the electronic implementation efforts at the Department of Veterans Affairs and the work being done at the organizations discussed above. The Veterans Health Administration (VHA) encompasses 173 medical centers, 450 outpatient clinics, 131 nursing homes, and 39 domiciliaries (group homes). To be successful, the electronic record system had to capture and exchange data throughout the

nationwide organization, as well as with other government entities. For the VHA system to be all things to everyone, flexibility and portability had to be key characteristics.

The developers of this EHR focused on the VHA's three main missions: patient care, research, and education. In the area of patient care, the EHR system fosters coordinated care among providers at different locations, improves the legibility of records, and enhances the timeliness of information access. In support of research activities, the EHR system offers standardized data and improved data accuracy. Finally, the EHR system enhances the VHA's educational programs by increasing communication among staff, residents, and interns. It also enables the use of decision support tools and enhances the efficiency of clinical management.

Check Your Understanding 3.4

Instructions: Choose the most appropriate answer for the following questions.

1. _____ Which type of health record includes both paper and computerized components?
   a. Hybrid
   b. Electronic
   c. Problem oriented
   d. Source oriented

2. _____ Which of the following is not an advantage of an EHR over a paper-based record?
   a. Allows customization to user needs
   b. Permits multiple users at the same time
   c. Enables duplicate copies to be made easily
   d. Requires privacy and security measures

3. _____ In an integrated health record, documentation by health professionals is organized _____.
   a. In sections by type of professional
   b. In sections by problem number
   c. Intermixed in date sequence
   d. Depends on facility policy

4. _____ The patient indicates that her pain is worse. In which part of a SOAP note would this information be recorded?
   a. Subjective
   b. Objective
   c. Assessment
   d. Plan

5. _____ Which of the following electronic record technological capabilities would allow an x-ray to be sent to a physician in another state?
   a. Database management
   b. Image processing
   c. Text processing
   d. Vocabulary standards

6. _____ Which of the following is true of paper-based records?
   a. They are susceptible to damage from fire or floods.
   b. They lack standardization.
   c. They are easy to access and update.
   d. They require a limited number of personnel to process.

7. ____ A definition of what constitutes a record, recording where each component is located, and noting dates of format changes are particularly important in ____.
   a. Electronic records
   b. Integrated records
   c. Paper records
   d. Hybrid records

8. ____ In a problem-oriented health record, problems are organized by ____.
   a. Letter
   b. Number
   c. Patient name
   d. Body system

9. ____ Health Level Seven (HL7) has developed guidelines that address which aspect of the electronic record?
   a. A standard vocabulary
   b. Network communication standards
   c. Definition of functions
   d. Overcoming resistance

10. ____ Which type of data input mechanism is commonly used in both paper and electronic environments?
    a. Voice recognition
    b. Transcription
    c. Bar code readers
    d. Automated templates

Real-World Case

When St. James Hospital began developing its electronic record, system designers set out to capture every bit of information available. The unofficial goal of the implementation team was to compile all available health information into a single system and provide the means to deliver the information instantaneously to end users on demand. However, the large volumes of information, overcrowded computer screens, and lack of uniform structure soon proved overwhelming for the system's end users. Their feedback called for useful information formatted in a usable structure.

In response to end-user frustration, designers took a hard look at the information that was being captured. They considered the following questions:

- How is health information formatted and structured?

- How long is health information retained?

- What information is purged from the system?

- What health information is archived?

- How much control should end users have over the information they are allowed to access?

Summary

The records maintained by healthcare providers for patients—no matter the illness or healthcare setting—all contain similar information (for example, chief complaint/reason for visit, history and physical or assessment and plan, progress notes, diagnostic test results, and orders). However, some settings and medical specialties have documentation requirements that are unique to their fields.

Accreditation standards, state and federal laws, and facility policies all affect the content of the health record. Although standards and policies must be complied with, facilities should not lose sight of the primary purpose of the health record: to facilitate effective patient healthcare. Facilities must organize and maintain health records in a way that ensures that the information in them is complete and easy to retrieve. The end result is that healthcare providers can use the information effectively to make wise treatment decisions.

HIM technicians are often positioned within their employment settings to significantly influence established documentation practices. Their knowledge of quality coding principles clarifies the impact of documentation on reimbursement. Their experience in performance improvement clarifies the impact of documentation on the quality and continuity of patient care. And their expertise in release-of-information functions clarifies the impact of documentation on liability issues.

Bringing order to chaos is the primary justification for formalizing the content and structure of the health record. Health records that lack structure are of little use to the healthcare providers who use the information in them to make decisions about patient care. Thus, for health information to be useful, it must be expressed in a vocabulary that end users understand and organized in a predictable format. It also must provide details specific to the problem being addressed. In addition, the information must be current, legible, and accurate.

The challenge for EHR system designers is to develop computer systems that are flexible, accessible, and portable enough to meet the unique needs of every healthcare provider, administrator, researcher, educator, and policy maker.

References

Abdelhak, Mervat. 2001. *Health Information: Management of a Strategic Resource,* 2nd ed. Philadelphia: W. B. Saunders Company.

Abraham, Prinny Rose. 2001. *Documentation and Reimbursement for Home Health and Hospice Programs.* Chicago: AHIMA.

Accreditation Association for Ambulatory Health Care. 1993. *Accreditation Handbook for Ambulatory Health Care.* Skokie, IL: AAAHC.

AHIMA e-HIM Personal Health Record Work Group. 2005. The role of the personal health record in the EHR. *Journal of American Health Information Management Association* 76(7):64A–D.

AHIMA e-HIM Task Force. 2004 (October). The strategic importance of electronic health records management. *Journal of American Health Information Management Association* 75(9):80C–E.

AHIMA e-HIM Work Group. 2003 (October). The complete medical record in a hybrid EHR environment. Chicago: AHIMA.

AHIMA Workgroup on Core Data Sets as Standards for the EHR. 2004 (September). E-HIM strategic initiative: Core data sets, appendix A: Core data sets as standards for the EHR, part 2: Healthcare standards organizations. *Journal of American Health Information Management Association* 75(8):68A–D.

Amatayakul, Margret, K. 2004. *Electronic Health Records: A Practical Guide for Professionals and Organizations,* 2nd ed. Chicago: AHIMA.

American Academy of Pediatrics and American College of Obstetricians and Gynecologists. 1992. *Guidelines for Perinatal Care.* Elk Grove Village, IL: AAP.

American College of Obstetricians and Gynecologists. 1996. *Standards for Obstetric-Gynecologic Services.* Washington, DC: ACOG.

American Health Information Management Association. 2005. *Documentation and Reimbursement for Behavioral Healthcare Services.* Chicago: AHIMA.

American Health Information Management Association. 2001. *Ambulatory Care Documentation,* rev. ed. Chicago: AHIMA.

American Health Information Management Association. 2001. *Long-Term Care Health Information Practice and Documentation Guidelines.* Chicago: AHIMA.

American Society of Anesthesiologists. 1988. *Documentation of Anesthesia Care.* Park Ridge, IL: ASA.

Benson, Dale S., et al. 1988 (June). Quality ambulatory care: The role of the diagnostic and medication summary lists. *Quality Review Bulletin* 6:197.

Burgess, B., K. Wager, F. Wickham Lee, R. Glorioso, and L. Bergstrom. 1999 (June). Clinics go electronic: Two stories from the field. *Journal of American Health Information Management Association* 70(6):42–46.

Clark, Jean S. 2004. *Documentation for Acute Care.* Chicago: AHIMA.

Cofer, Jennifer. 1994. *Health Information Management,* 10th ed. Berwyn, IL: Physicians' Record Company.

Hughes, Gwen. 2001. Practice brief: Redisclosure of patient information. Chicago: AHIMA.

Institute of Medicine. 1997. *The Computer-Based Patient Record: An Essential Technology for Health Care,* rev. ed. Washington, DC: National Academy Press.

James, Ella. 2004. *Documentation and Reimbursement for Long-Term Care.* Chicago: AHIMA.

Joint Commission on Accreditation of Healthcare Organizations. 2004. *Comprehensive Accreditation Manual for Hospitals: The Official Handbook.* Oakbrook Terrace, IL: JCAHO.

Joint Commission on Accreditation of Healthcare Organizations. 2000. *Accreditation Manual for Ambulatory Health Care.* Oakbrook Terrace, IL: JCAHO.

Marrelli, Tina M. 2001. *Handbook of Home Health Standards and Documentation Guidelines for Reimbursement.* St. Louis: Mosby.

Mon, Donald T. 2004a (October). Defining the differences between the CPR, EMR, and EHR. *Journal of American Health Information Management Association* 75(9):74–75,77.

Mon, Donald T. 2004b (Nov.-Dec.). Next steps for the EHR draft standard: Core functionality and conformance criteria key for accreditation. *Journal of American Health Information Management Association* 75(10):50–51.

National Committee for Quality Assurance. 1996. *Standards for Managed Care Organizations.* Washington, DC: NCQA.

Smith, Cheryl M. 2001. Practice brief: Documentation requirements for the acute care inpatient record. *Journal of American Health Information Management Association* 72(3):56A–G.

Chapter 4
Electronic Health Records

Margret Amatayakul, MBA, RHIA, CHPS, CPHIT, CPEHR, FHIMSS

Learning Objectives

- To introduce the concept and evolution of the electronic health record (EHR)
- To identify and define terms associated with EHRs
- To relate the various initiatives local, regional, and national adoption of EHR and health information technology (HIT)
- To describe the current state of EHR adoption and the technologies that help transition to the EHR
- To discuss EHR challenges and the supporting roles of health information management professionals in addressing them, especially with respect to privacy, security, and legal aspects
- To develop an appreciation for the planning and implementation aspects of EHRs
- To provide examples of EHR systems as they may be implemented in various types of care settings

Key Terms

Acceptance testing

Access controls

Accredited Standards Committee X12N (ASC X12N)

Admissibility

American National Standards Institute (ANSI)

Ancillary systems

Architecture

ASTM International

Audit trail

Authentication

Best of breed

Best of fit

Certification Commission on Health Information Technology (CCHIT)

Chart conversion

Client/server architecture

Clinical data repository (CDR)

Clinical data warehouse (CDW)

Clinical decision support (CDS)

Clinical information system (CIS)

Computer output to laser disk (COLD)

Computer output to laser disk/enterprise report management (COLD/ERM)

Computerized provider order entry (CPOE)

Computers on wheels (COWs)

Contextual

Continuity of care record (CCR)

Controlled vocabulary

Data comparability

Data conversion

Data dictionary

Data exchange standards

Database management system (DBMS)

Digital dictation

Digital images

Discrete data

Disease management (DM)

Document imaging

Dual core (vendor strategy)

Electronic data interchange (EDI)

Electronic document/content management (ED/CM)

Electronic document management system (EDMS)

Electronic health record (EHR)

Electronic medication administration record (EMAR)

Electronic prescribing (e-Rx)

Electronic signature authentication (ESA)

Encoded

Ethernet

Evidence-based medicine

Extranet

Health information exchange (HIE)

Health information technology (HIT)

Health Insurance Portability and Accountability Act of 1996 (HIPAA)

Health Level Seven (HL7)

Hospital information system (HIS)

Hospitalist

Human–computer interface

Hybrid record

Integration testing

Integrity

Interoperability

Intranet

Issues management

Local area network (LAN)

Mainframe architecture

Medicare Modernization Act of 2003 (MMA)

Message format standards

Migration path

Mirrored processing

National Council for Prescription Drug Programs (NCPDP)

National Drug Codes (NDC)

National health information infrastructure (NHII)

National health information network (NHIN)

National Library of Medicine (NLM)

Natural language processing (NLP)

Patient care charting system

Pay for performance (P4P)

Pay for quality (P4Q)

Personal digital assistant (PDA)

Pharmacy benefits manager (PBM)

Picture archiving and communications system (PACS)

Point of care (POC)

Portals

Practice management system (PMS)

Primary care physicians (PCP)

Protected health information (PHI)

Quality improvement organization (QIO)

Record locator service (RLS)

Redundant arrays of independent (or inexpensive) disks (RAID)

Regional health information organization (RHIO)

Relational database

Request for proposal (RFP)

Server redundancy

Speech recognition

Standard vocabulary

Storage area network (SAN)

Storage management software

Stress testing

System build

System testing

Textual

Unit testing

Uses and disclosures

Web services architecture (WSA)

Wide area network (WAN)

Wireless local area network (WLAN)

Workflow

Introduction

As discussed in chapter 3, there are many interpretations of what makes up **electronic health records** (EHRs). Moreover, several different terms are used to describe the various forms of the EHR. In many cases, the terms reflect different approaches to achieving the ultimate vision of the EHR. The term *computer-based patient record* (CPR), first used in the 1980s, reflects some of the first attempts to automate essential functions such as alerts, medication administration, and orders communication. CPRs were implemented primarily in the hospital setting. In the 1990s, the term *electronic medical record* (EMR) was used to describe systems that integrated dictation, transcription, and **document imaging** with previous CPR functions. Both inpatient and outpatient settings used EMR systems, but there was little information exchange between physician office and inpatient acute electronic record systems. The EHR has the same features of CPRs and EMRs, but its functionality goes beyond such things as alerts, medication administration, and order communication. When fully realized, the EHR will provide seamless information interchange among providers at all levels of the healthcare continuum and provide support for fully integrated evidence-based medicine and embedded clinical terminology to assist with documentation.

This chapter discusses these approaches and explores various components of EHRs in depth. The overarching vision for the EHR is important to bear in mind as the path to achieving the vision is studied. The EHR is not so much a single computer system as it is a complex system of coordinating hardware, software, people, policies, and processes in support of patient care.

Theory into Practice

The EHR vision includes use of the EHR at the point of care for clinical decision support (CDS). This means that clinicians interact directly with the system as they care for patients. It entails documenting directly into the system, having the system combine these data with other data, and making the data available for the system to process into reminders and alerts.

Consider the scenario where a diabetic patient, John, moves to a new city, logs on to the Internet to review report cards from local **primary care physicians** (PCPs), and selects a physician who appears to have strong outcomes in diabetes and positive patient satisfaction scores. John schedules an appointment via the physician's Web site and is given a user ID and a password to enter pertinent medical history information. John asks his hometown physician to send information to this new PCP, which the physician does, adhering to the standard **continuity of care record** (CCR) content specifications. The CCR prepopulates the new PCP's EHR with a current problem list, recent laboratory results, and other objective data. Additionally, the medication history is prepopulated with medications the patient is taking, which have been identified by linking to information available from the **pharmacy benefits manager** (PBM) that John's health plan uses. John also can upload selected data from his PHR, such as diet, over-the-counter medications being taken, and other information relating to compliance with the diabetic treatment regimen, identifying which medications are actually being taken and on what schedule.

When John visits the new PCP, data previously entered will be validated and updated. The new PCP decides to put John on a strict smoking-cessation program and exercise routine, with plans to adjust medications according to John's vital signs and blood sugar levels, which will be taken automatically and monitored remotely. All is going well when John has an accident at work that requires a visit to the emergency department, subsequent admission to the hospital, and outpatient physical therapy. All his providers, however, are members of a **regional health information organization** (RHIO); thus, each provider has immediate access to the specific information needed to treat John throughout his care.

At the hospital, a **hospitalist** (a physician dedicated to hospital-based care services) is able to reconcile all of John's medications in accordance with JCAHO requirements and to select medications that have been screened against John's known allergies and order only needed diagnostic studies thanks to accessibility to previous information. This helps keep costs down and reduces John's discomfort. In selecting the physical therapy referral, the hospitalist has access to John's health plan benefits information, so no time is wasted in arranging for physical therapy to begin. During John's hospitalization, his PCP can monitor the impact of the accident on John's diabetes and make appropriate adjustments. After John is discharged and in physical therapy, the health plan can observe that he is no longer following the prescribed exercise routine and can notify the physician to follow up with a modified regimen during recovery. John can access tailored instructions for this exercise routine that superimpose his picture on the instructions so that it is clear how to avoid further injury. In addition, each provider John encounters throughout this episode of care follows up with him on the smoking-cessation program, motivating him to keep from smoking.

The Ideal Electronic Health Record System

The ideal EHR system is generally considered one that captures data from any number of computer systems in the healthcare organization and is used at the **point of care** (POC) to support clinical decision making. Some of these computer systems might include registration, admission, discharge, transfer (R-ADT) systems, patient accounting systems, encoders, and **ancillary systems** such as laboratory, radiology, and pharmacy information systems, billing systems, surgery scheduling systems, and many others. Large healthcare organizations such as hospitals may have hundreds of systems, sometimes from many different vendors. The EHR would eventually compile data from all these systems into a special kind of database.

Depending on where the patient receives care, POC can be a hospital bedside or a physician office's examining room. It also may mean information available to a caregiver at a patient's home or on a mobile device a healthy person carries to track personal wellness data.

Supporting clinical decision making means the EHR helps physicians, nurses, and other healthcare providers, as well as patients themselves, make decisions about patient care. This includes providing documentation of clinical findings and procedures; active reminders for medication administration; suggestions for prescribing less expensive, but equally effective, drugs; protocols for certain health maintenance procedures; alerts that a duplicate lab test is being ordered; and countless other decision-making aids for all stakeholders in the care process.

Despite having many information systems, most hospitals and other healthcare delivery organizations today do not have systems that require physicians, nurses, and other clinicians to enter data into the computer system while performing patient care activities. Much of this information is still handwritten or dictated for trancriptionists to turn into typed reports. The vision for the EHR is that such information will be captured electronically, including **digital images** of voice recordings, documents, or print files, and **discrete data** coming directly from ancillary systems or entered by the clinician at the POC. Discrete data are data elements that can be processed by the computer (for example, lab values, medication dosage, patient temperature, and so on). In the EHR vision, discrete data would be entered by healthcare providers using computer screen templates allowing them to point or click from choices or drop-down menus or typing certain characters to generate a macro representing a word or phrase. Each individual data element would be represented in the computer by a special code to be used in making comparisons, trending results, and supplying clinical reminders and alerts. This process is known as **clinical decision support** (CDS). For example, many laboratory information systems can graph a series of results so that a clinician can study the results of a treatment regimen over time. Medication orders can be entered and drugs compared with a known list of patient allergies, contraindications with other drugs, and even results of laboratory tests to determine potential adverse effects of a given drug for a patient.

For physician practices, the number and types of source systems that can supply data to the EHR may be fewer, but potentially more dispersed. A physician practice may have a scheduling system, a patient registration system, and a billing system, sometimes combined into one **practice management system** (PMS). External laboratories or imaging centers may send diagnostic studies reports and clinical images to the physician practice. The physician practice can connect with other specialty providers and one or more hospitals to exchange discharge summaries, current medication lists, and other information to support the continuity of patient care, perhaps through a CCR system. Moreover, the patient is a source of information, and through personal health records (PHRs) is becoming a more direct source for electronic data capture.

The CCR is a description of the content that physicians have agreed should be included in patient referrals. In the past, when a physician referred a patient to another physician, he or she frequently dictated a letter to describe the case. There was no consistency across physicians as to what they might describe or leave out in such letters. The CCR standard recommends specific categories of information to include in referral letters.

The CCR standard was developed by the ASTM E31 Committee on Health Informatics in conjunction with the Massachusetts Medical Society, Healthcare Information Management and Systems Society (HIMSS), and the American Academy of Family Physicians (AAFP). The developers of the standard stress that the CCR is not an EHR. It may be a subset of an EHR; or, if an organization does not yet have an EHR, it may be generated through dictation, scanned documents, or data from various source systems.

Health plans have long received health information via claims and claims attachments. Health plans are beginning to compile EHRs on individuals and to use them to support **disease management,** frequently contacting the physician when it appears that a patient with a chronic illness may not be seeking appropriate medical attention or complying with a treatment regimen.

Evolution of the Electronic Health Record

Achieving the ideal EHR system is very much a journey. There has been increased emphasis on EHRs since 2003 when President Bush included their promotion in an executive order to create an Office of the National Coordinator for Health Information Technology (ONC); however, the concept of an EHR is not new.

The earliest efforts to address **clinical information systems** (CISs) occurred in the mid-1960s. Clinical data are textual and contextual, making it difficult to develop systems that can collect and process these data effectively and efficiently. Healthcare data are largely **textual** because clinicians describe patient conditions in narrative form. Narrative data also depend on context or situation to make the data meaningful. For example, when a patient is described as "having a red face," but the situation is not explained, we do not know whether the patient is embarrassed, angry, hot, burned, or has a rash.

As a result of the difficulty in developing complex information systems that could handle textual and **contextual** data, the automation process of healthcare data started with simpler financial and administrative systems, such as patient registration, census, and billing. The healthcare delivery system is fragmented by departments within an organization and across the continuum of care. As a result, information systems initially focused on solving departmental and institutional business-related functions like those in other industries, such as materials and inventory management. Consequently, information systems to manage pharmacy inventory or lab specimen collection mimicked similar systems in other industries.

Evolution

By the mid-1980s, the Institute of Medicine (IOM) identified that new technologies should be considered for improving the state of medical records. A committee formed to make recommendations and produced a report in 1991 entitled *The Computer-based Patient Record: An Essential Technology for Health Care*. The concept of a CPR was an important result of the report, changing the thinking about the purpose, characteristics, and features of the medical record.

The report generated considerable interest, sparking the establishment of an organization dedicated to promoting CPRs and an awards program that recognizes exemplary implementations of CPRs (the Davies Recognition Program) now under the auspices of the Health Information Management and Systems Society (HIMSS). However, lack of federal funding and leadership, high development costs, and immature technologies hampered implementation of its recommendations. This led to haphazard approaches by vendors and providers to begin automating more of the medical record.

Document Imaging Systems

In an attempt to get as much medical record information online as possible, many hospitals turned to document imaging and COLD systems. Document imaging systems involve scanning documents created on paper and making their images available on a computer monitor. **COLD (computer output to laser disk)** systems capture print images of lab results and other documents that are in stand-alone electronic systems and make them available for viewing on a computer monitor. **Digital dictation** systems also became popular, where the dictation files could be accessed for listening prior to being transcribed.

Today, some hospitals use **speech recognition** systems where dictation automatically converts to text on a screen. Dictators themselves can make any necessary corrections or transcriptionists can listen and make corrections. Such systems permit clinicians to continue using paper-based processes for their day-to-day clinical functions but enhance the ability to gain access to information, which has been a major problem with paper-based records.

Document imaging systems have become more sophisticated and today are called **electronic document management systems** (EDMSs). They can manage many types of digital documents, including e-mails and electronic faxes. When EDMSs are well indexed, certain content within the documents can be uniquely retrieved. **Electronic document/ content management** (ED/CM) systems, for example, may include bar coding on the forms to identify specific content, such as the name of the form (for example, medication administration record [MAR], emergency services report) or part of a form, such as the section of a history and physical exam containing allergy information. When information on a patient's allergies is needed, it can be selected for viewing.

Workflow support also has been added to EDMSs. This means that the EDMS facilitates various functions that must be performed often simultaneously or in a specific sequence. For example, upon patient discharge, a notification is sent to an analyst that the record is ready for analysis and coding. The analyst can retrieve the electronic images and analyze and code the patient stay. When the coding is completed, a notification is sent to financial services for the next function to be performed. Because the images are in electronic form, patient care areas for follow-up by quality departments or any other locations that require access can also access them.

Simultaneously, the chart deficiency system can identify what documents require signature by which physicians and make them available at any computer workstation for electronic signature. **Electronic signature authentication** (ESA) systems require the author to sign onto the system using a user ID and password, review the document to be signed, and indicate approval. The system annotates that the review and approval took place by the specified individual at the date and time performed.

Another approach to EHR taken by some vendors and providers focuses on capturing and processing discrete data. Such approaches have been especially prevalent since the IOM released its study on medication errors in 2000. The IOM's study, *To Err Is Human,* identified that tens and possibly hundreds of thousands of errors occur in the U.S. healthcare system every day and sent a lightning bolt throughout the industry. Since the initial report, the IOM has generated a series of reports called the *Quality Chasm.* In 2003, the IOM report entitled *Patient Safety: Achieving a New Standard for Care* addressed many of the standardization issues that were needed to improve patient safety through the use of the EHR and, in a report appended to the work, defined the key capabilities of an EHR system. (See figure 4.1.) These key capabilities were then incorporated into a standard for EHR system functionality by the **Health Level Seven** (HL7) standards development organization. (See figure 4.2.)

Stages of EHR

As stated earlier, the EHR is not so much a single computer system as it is a complex system of coordinating hardware, software, people, policies, and processes in support of patient care. The ideal EHR system is generally considered one that captures data from multiple sources and is used at the point of care to support clinical decision making.

Today, EHR systems are generally based on the use of a **clinical data repository** (CDR), a special kind of database that manages data from different source systems in the hospital or other provider setting. CDRs can process discrete data from various ancillary systems, such as laboratory, pharmacy, and radiology systems. They also can process paper document images and clinical images such as those from **picture archiving and communication systems** (PACS). However, merely having a CDR does not equate with having an EHR. When CDRs are used with CDS systems and software that aids data capture and presentation, they are generally considered to have the components of an EHR.

Even with a CDR, a CDS, and presentation software, however, the system may not be a comprehensive EHR. For example, a CDR may only contain data from some, but not all, of the hospital's various ancillary departments because either some systems cannot produce data for the repository or some departments may not have an information system.

Figure 4.1.   IOM key capabilities of an EHR system

1. Health information and data
2. Results management
3. Order entry/management
4. Decision support
5. Electronic communication and connectivity
6. Patient support
7. Administrative processes
8. Reporting and population health management

Source: Adapted from Kohn 2000.

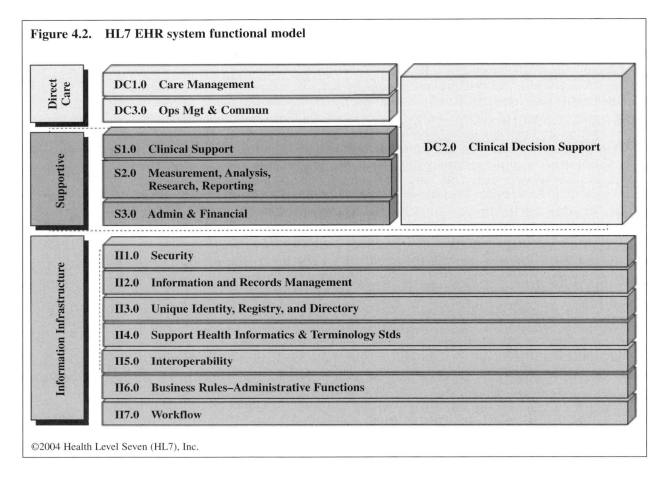

Figure 4.2.   HL7 EHR system functional model

Direct Care

DC1.0   Care Management

DC3.0   Ops Mgt & Commun

Supportive

S1.0   Clinical Support

S2.0   Measurement, Analysis, Research, Reporting

S3.0   Admin & Financial

DC2.0   Clinical Decision Support

Information Infrastructure

II1.0   Security

II2.0   Information and Records Management

II3.0   Unique Identity, Registry, and Directory

II4.0   Support Health Informatics & Terminology Stds

II5.0   Interoperability

II6.0   Business Rules–Administrative Functions

II7.0   Workflow

©2004 Health Level Seven (HL7), Inc.

In addition, not all clinicians may be ready to enter data directly into the EHR. For example, some hospitals have adopted **electronic medication administration record** (EMAR) systems (sometimes using computer-generated paper MAR forms, POC devices, or bar-coding systems) but have not yet adopted **computerized provider order-entry** (CPOE) systems that allow physicians to enter medication or other orders and receive clinical advice about drug dosages, contraindications, or other clinical decision support.

Nurses and allied health professionals may use **patient care charting systems** for documenting assessments and progress notes, but physicians may not use them for their notes. Alternatively, some hospitals have introduced CPOE systems, but not EMAR or patient care charting. Finally, CDS systems may be in various stages of sophistication.

Transition State

In general, several EHR components may exist in varying degrees in many healthcare delivery settings, but comprehensive EHR systems have yet to be realized, especially in most hospitals or other provider settings. The result is a hybrid record situation. A **hybrid record** is part electronic and part paper. Although this is clearly a transition state, the reality is that the hybrid record is complicated to manage and the transition from a paper to an electronic system may take a long time. Typical issues involved in managing a hybrid record include identification of storage media, printing issues, release of information (ROI) coordination, signature of both paper and electronic records, identification of users, and identification of the components of both the legal record and the designated record set.

There are various approaches to managing the hybrid record. Each organization must identify its legal record, authorized users, and contributors, as well as the circumstances under which clinicians and staff may print all or a portion of a record. The problem with this, however, is that some physicians may forget or not be interested in accessing the electronic information. As a result, they might print paper copies that end up in the paper chart. The printouts are often images of the screens and not a consolidated set of data on a form. For example, every lab result may print out on a separate page, adding tremendous bulk to the paper record. When it is unclear whether the electronic version is maintained as the official source, copies may be printed unnecessarily, adding to the workload of file clerks. Even more seriously, if any of the printouts have had annotations made on them and someone else is relying on only the electronic source of information, errors—and ultimately potential harm to the patient—could result.

Many hospitals attempting to overcome the patient safety issues of hybrid records have decided to continue printing everything routinely, even though some of the information is available electronically. This assists clinicians in gaining access to information that may not always be readily available, but it still increases the workload of the health information management (HIM) department, especially as the printouts are generally lengthier than their paper form counterparts.

The PHR is in a similar transition. It may be found in five different forms: paper based, personal electronic based, Web based (portal), hybrid personal electronic/Web based, and portable device based. PHRs are further defined as "tethered," or integrated with an existing EHR such as a hospital or clinic system, or "untethered," a stand-alone application the patient-owner develops and maintains. PHRs have been somewhat popular with patients, especially those with chronic illnesses, but are not popular with all providers. This is changing considerably as the importance of a PHR in a disaster situation is recognized. In addition, more and more EHR systems are able to generate PHRs so that provider and patient can have a copy. It is likely that a standard will be developed around the content and portability of such records, as none exists today.

Check Your Understanding 4.1

Instructions: Complete the following exercises.

1. _____ Early efforts to automate the content of the medical record were called _____.
   a. Clinical information systems
   b. Electronic medical records
   c. Hospital information systems
   d. Hybrid record systems

2. _____ A transition technology used by many hospitals to increase access to medical record content is _____.
   a. CPR
   b. EDMS
   c. ESA
   d. PACS

3. _____ Systems used by nurses and physicians to document assessments and findings are called _____.
   a. Computerized provider order entry
   b. Electronic medical records
   c. Electronic medication administration record
   d. Patient care charting

4. _____ A clinical data repository (CDR) is _____.
   a. An archive technology to back up and store data
   b. A database to manage data from multiple sources
   c. An electronic health record
   d. A location for storing and retrieving medical images

5. _____ When a print image of discrete data in an information system is sent to a repository for user viewing, the process is called _____.
   a. COLD
   b. Document imaging
   c. Digital dictation
   d. EDMS

6. _____ Which of the following represents a standard for EHR functionality?
   a. HL7 EHR System Functional Model
   b. IOM Key Capabilities of EHR System
   c. Office of the National Coordinator for Health Information Technology
   d. Patient Safety: Achieving a New Standard for Care

7. _____ When was the concept of clinical computing first conceived?
   a. 1960s
   b. 1991
   c. 1996
   d. 2003

Initiatives and Framework for the Electronic Health Record

How long the transition will take from paper to a fully operational EHR is uncertain. Some suggest the industry has been in transition for more than forty years and that it will take that much more time to reach a totally interoperable state where health information is fully automated and can be exchanged safely and securely.

Federal Government Initiatives

The 1991 IOM study urged adoption of EHRs within a decade. More than a decade after that, President Bush laid out a twelve-year EHR adoption plan. The federal government initiatives focus on a strategic national agenda for **health information exchange** (HIE). RHIOs are proposed to begin the process of HIE, at least among providers in a community that support a general referral network. Various models are currently being established. Figure 4.3 describes two such models that have already formed and have begun exchanging health information. In general, RHIOs require some specific form of governance, policies and procedures for exchanging health information, security utilities, and a **record locator service** (RLS) that would point to where a given patient may have health information using probability equations.

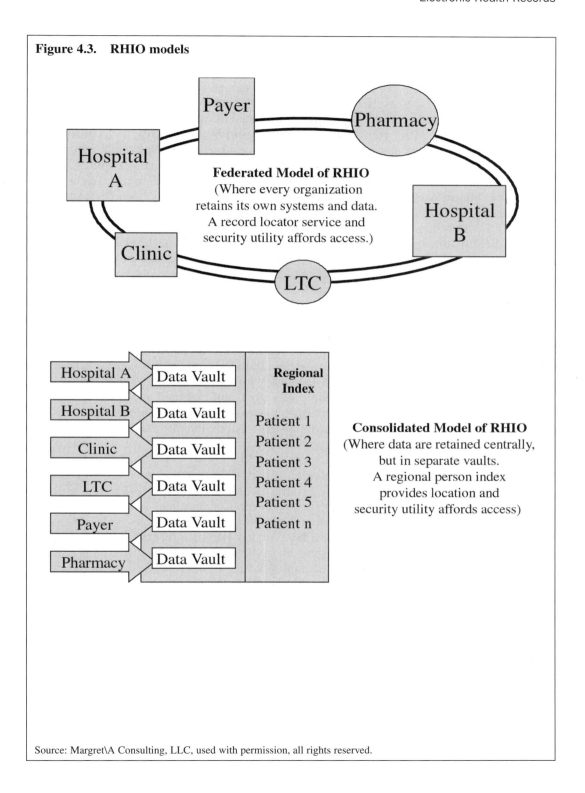

Figure 4.3. RHIO models

Federated Model of RHIO
(Where every organization retains its own systems and data. A record locator service and security utility affords access.)

Consolidated Model of RHIO
(Where data are retained centrally, but in separate vaults. A regional person index provides location and security utility affords access)

Under the **Health Insurance Portability and Accountability Act** (HIPAA) **of 1996,** RHIO members may be considered part of an organized healthcare arrangement. They would make their membership in the RHIO known through the notice of privacy practices (NPP) they distribute to patients. Because providers within such a community often have very different levels of readiness to exchange data electronically, **interoperability** (the ability to send data from one system to a different system and still retain its meaning) is a critical component to achieving success. Many RHIOs are hoping to begin by identifying the location where information may exist and then use more traditional means of accessing the information until there is greater deployment of EHRs in each environment and better interoperability.

At the national level, RHIOs would need to be linked together in the event a patient moves, falls ill, or is injured outside his or her community. Additionally, there is a need to study public health data, certainly to reduce the risk of epidemics, but also as part of Homeland Security.

In 2001, the National Committee on Vital and Health Statistics (NCVHS) proposed a **national health information infrastructure** (NHII) that would be a set of technologies, standards, applications, systems, values, and laws that support all facets of provider healthcare, individual health, and public health. A comprehensive knowledge-based network of interoperable systems of clinical, personal, and public health information would improve decision making by making health information available when and where it is needed. (See figure 4.4.)

In 2004, ONC released a request for information to seek ideas on how such a national health information network (NHIN) might be developed. A NHIN would provide the technology to support the NHII. The goal was to establish a privately financed consortium wherein the federal government would facilitate work and assist in identifying services, including standards, to ensure that public policy goals are executed and rapid adoption of interoperable EHRs is advanced. Numerous responses were received, including a collaborative response from virtually all the associations representing interest in HIE. It is anticipated that over the course of the coming years, much more will become known about the NHIN as it starts to take shape.

The federal government also has several initiatives under way to promote standards development and to pilot-test them. The Federal Health Architecture (FHA) is an effort to improve coordination and collaboration across federal government agencies and departments on government **health information technology** (HIT) solutions and investments. Within the framework of the FHA, the Consolidated Health Informatics (CHI) initiative is addressing the specific standards-setting interests. Approximately twenty-three federal agencies are involved in developing a recommended list of interoperability and **data comparability** (that is, vocabulary) standards and actually using them in their individual agency health data enterprise **architecture** to build new systems or to modify existing ones.

Check Your Understanding 4.2.

Instructions: Match technology in column B to concepts in column A.

A.	Concepts		B.	Technology
	____ 1.	RHIO	a.	Data comparability
	____ 2.	CHI	b.	Record locator service
	____ 3.	HIE	c.	Interoperability
	____ 4.	NHII	d.	EHR services
	____ 5.	NHIN	e.	Knowledge-based network

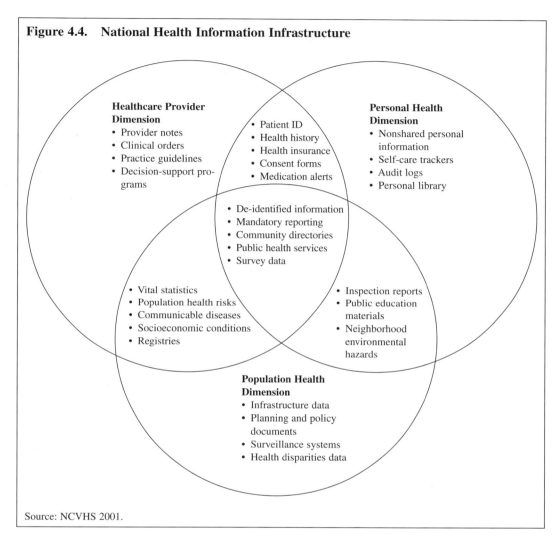

Figure 4.4.   National Health Information Infrastructure

Healthcare Provider Dimension
- Provider notes
- Clinical orders
- Practice guidelines
- Decision-support programs

- Patient ID
- Health history
- Health insurance
- Consent forms
- Medication alerts

Personal Health Dimension
- Nonshared personal information
- Self-care trackers
- Audit logs
- Personal library

- De-identified information
- Mandatory reporting
- Community directories
- Public health services
- Survey data

- Vital statistics
- Population health risks
- Communicable diseases
- Socioeconomic conditions
- Registries

- Inspection reports
- Public education materials
- Neighborhood environmental hazards

Population Health Dimension
- Infrastructure data
- Planning and policy documents
- Surveillance systems
- Health disparities data

Source: NCVHS 2001.

Local Efforts and Challenges

Clearly, many stakeholders are involved in advancing adoption of the EHR. On a more practical, local level, EHR vendors, health plans, provider organizations, healthcare professionals, and patients themselves play important roles.

EHR Vendors

Growing interest among providers has led to concerns that vendors may not be keeping up with the demand or do not have the capacity to implement all the systems desired. The laws of supply and demand are very evident in EHR system development. In the past, vendors who attempted to supply more than the industry was ready for found they could not sell their products. They either went out of business or refocused their efforts on enhancing ancillary systems or EHR components. When there is a sudden shift in demand, vendors often cannot respond quickly enough, resulting in frustrated consumers.

Many vendors are working to address the more sophisticated requirements laid out by the HL7 EHR system functional requirements and to overcome interoperability issues. Several vendors who sell **hospital information systems** (HISs), which are the traditional financial and operational systems used in hospitals, are moving into the EHR market and looking for ways to support physician practices in an integrated delivery network (IDN). Some vendors have been more successful than others in bridging the differences between workflow in acute care and ambulatory care environments. Likewise, vendors that have traditionally sold PMSs that support patient scheduling, registration, and billing to physician practices are looking at integrating EHR functionality into their products.

Because of the variability in products, the private sector recently initiated an effort to certify products. Called the **Certification Commission on Health Information Technology** (CCHIT), the effort would evaluate and test EHR products against specific criteria, drawn from the HL7 standard EHR system functionality. Initial development is focusing on EHR products for small physician practices because these practices are believed to be the most at risk for selecting products that do not live up to their expectations. The federal government is watching this project very closely. It is possible that any incentives given to providers for adoption of EHRs would only be given to providers that use certified products. Add in here that the CCHIT has won the contract from the Department of Health and Human Services (HHS) for evaluation of compliance certification. The contract includes "develop(ing) criteria and evaluation processes for certifying EHRs and the infrastructure or network components through which they interoperate" (HHS 2005).

Health Plans

Comprehensive EHR systems, whether built for hospitals or physician practices, are expensive, and providers want help, often from health plans and the federal government, paying for the systems. Health plans are starting to look at various forms of incentives, such as **pay for performance** (P4P) or **pay for quality** (P4Q), where EHRs would be used to support data collection and the reporting of clinical outcomes. Those with better outcomes could receive additional reimbursement or be eligible for grants or other subsidies to support further HIT efforts.

The Centers for Medicare and Medicaid Services (CMS), the nation's largest payer, has introduced public reporting in hospitals in return for full reimbursement. CMS is planning a similar program for physician practices called Doctor's Office Quality—Information Technology (DOQ-IT), which is administered by the **quality improvement organizations** (QIOs) in each state. DOQ-IT is providing consultative assistance in selecting and implementing EHRs in small primary care clinics. Some health plans have attempted to give away hardware and software (especially to physician practices) to encourage the use of electronic systems. As an incentive, the health plan may provide access to data in support of disease management and care management.

Healthcare Professionals

Physicians, nurses, and allied health professionals are in the middle of the journey to EHR. Some have had experience with EHRs; others have never even used a computer.

The Veterans Administration (VA) hospitals have an EHR system, and many physicians who have recently completed their training at a VA hospital are accustomed to it. Moreover, medical specialty societies and payers are encouraging physicians to adopt EHRs. Because EHR systems available for physician practices are more self-contained with fewer source systems from which to integrate data, they tend to be more comprehensive. Some hospitals have actually found that physicians are demanding the same level of functionality in the hospital systems that exists in their practice systems, often with the hospital unable to move that rapidly to such sophistication.

If interest is not strong in physician practices for a total EHR, some start off by introducing mobile devices, such as **personal digital assistants** (PDAs), which provide medication reference information in electronic form. They may graduate from there to using the PDA for **electronic prescribing** (e-Rx). Electronic prescribing is when a prescription is written from a PDA or other computer and an electronic fax or when an actual **electronic data interchange** (EDI) transaction is generated that transmits the prescription directly to the retail pharmacy's information system. Today, more than 80 percent of the major chain pharmacies can accept such transactions, although fewer than 10 percent of all physician practices have acquired electronic prescription writing capability.

Some physicians have acquired what is termed "EHR-lite" systems. These systems are less expensive and have only basic functionality that permits data capture and perhaps E&M coding support.

Still, many practices are struggling with even achieving interest in an EHR, let alone gaining adoption by all physicians. These physicians are even less likely to want to adopt CPOE or patient care charting at the hospital. Some physicians view such systems as requiring them to perform clerical functions previously performed by health unit coordinators or unit clerks. Without a strong value proposition in the form of CDS and true downstream savings in reducing calls from nursing or the pharmacy, CPOE and patient care charting can be a hard sell.

Many nurses and allied health professionals recognize the productivity and patient safety gains from an EHR and seek employment in organizations with such systems. However, many others have virtually no computer skills and have even less opportunity than physicians to learn about potential systems.

Hospitals often start their clinical staff on e-mail and **intranet** use as a way to provide training. Some also believe that getting nurses started on EHR system components paves the way for physician use.

Patients

Until now, patients have had little interaction with EHRs. Those who are computer savvy may recognize the benefits of EHRs but are often unaware whether EHRs are being used. In fact, many patients assume that because a computer is in the registration area, everything else is computerized. Alternatively, patients may be fearful of EHRs and not fully understand the privacy and security protections put into these systems. They may see news stories about patient data being inadvertently e-mailed to others and assume (sometimes correctly) that the systems are not as secure as they could be.

The idea of allowing patient-generated data into the EHR is emerging. Some systems do allow patients to log on to a Web site from home or a kiosk in a provider's waiting room and to enter data using a context-specific template. The provider reviews and validates the information, and it becomes part of the patient record.

The personal health record (PHR) is a relatively new concept that encourages patients to take an active role in their health information. Although PHRs are not widely available, efforts are being made to educate the public about them. The PHR is an electronic, universally available, lifelong resource of health information needed by individuals to make health decisions. Patients own and manage the information in the PHR, which comes from both healthcare providers and the individual. The PHR is maintained in a secure and private environment, with the patient determining rights of access. It is separate from and does not replace the legal record of any provider (AHIMA 2005). The vision is that in the future, PHRs will be a valuable asset to patients and families, enabling them to integrate and manage their healthcare information through secure, standardized tools.

In many cases, the laws of supply and demand are at work here also. Because provider organizations have been closed systems having virtually no direct electronic communication with the outside world, a high degree of security for such communication has not been required. But, again, as heightened interest in e-mailing physicians, gaining access to data through patient **portals** (special Web pages that offer secure access and entry of data upon authorization of the owner of the page), use of wireless devices, and PHRs on flash drives the size of coins suddenly become available, vendors may not be as ready to supply the security desired or needed. Likewise, healthcare organizations may not appreciate the need for heightened security when their "official" systems do not support external communication, but their physicians and patients are using newer technology.

Check Your Understanding 4.3.

Instructions: Indicate whether the following statements are true or false (T or F).

1. _____ The Certification Commission on Health Information Technology will provide P4P incentives for adoption of EHRs.

2. _____ Electronic prescribing is accomplished most effectively through electronic data interchange.

3. _____ EHR systems designed for physician offices are much less comprehensive than those developed for hospitals.

4. _____ Most physicians want to adopt CPOE to ensure that their orders are legible.

5. _____ In general, patients are comfortable with EHRs because they know they have solid information security services.

Technologies That Support Electronic Health Records

Technologies that support EHRs include databases; data exchange standards and vocabulary standards; image processing, storage, and workflow systems; data retrieval technology; data capture technology text processing; system communications and networks; and workstations.

Databases

A database is an organized collection of data. Most database systems in use today are relational databases. A **relational database** stores data in predefined tables that contain rows and columns similar to a spreadsheet. The kinds of data that can be stored in a relational database are currency, real numbers, integers, and strings (characters of data). Each table is a set of rows and columns that relate to one another. Rows represent a single record, such as for a given patient. Each column has a unique name and the content within it must be of the same type. For example, there may be columns for patient name, age, diagnosis, allergies, blood pressure, and so on. Because no single table can contain every piece of data collected about a patient, several tables are usually created and related to one another in a variety of ways. Many tables are relatively stable, that is, they contain information that does not change frequently, such as a table of all physicians on the medical staff and their credentials. Other tables are being populated (updated) constantly with new information, such as those that collect the lab results for a given patient over the course of a hospitalization.

Database management systems (DBMSs) are software that organize, provide access to, and otherwise manage a database. For example, there may be three tables, one containing patient demographics, another containing physician information, and the third containing lab results. When these are related, it is unnecessary to repeat information from one table to another. A specific patient is linked to a specific physician and to the lab results that apply.

Although the relational database is the basic form of database used today, it can be designed in a number of different and highly sophisticated ways. Some databases are designed to handle many individual transactions. In healthcare, examples of clinical transactions would be the retrieval of a lab result for a given patient, the entry of a medication order for a given patient, and the posting of vital signs for a given patient. Databases that are optimized to perform such transactions are often called CDRs (discussed earlier).

Other forms of databases are optimized to perform analysis of data on many different things at one time. When used to analyze a large set of clinical data, these databases are called **clinical data warehouses** (CDWs). For example, a researcher interested in understanding what combinations of medications have the greatest impact on a particular disease entity could analyze data from many different patients more easily in a CDW.

Although databases "store" data, "storage" of data usually refers to the media, location, and length of time the databases are retained. Repositories and warehouses may be stored anywhere for any period of time. It is the nature of the data that determines the **retention** schedule and location of the storage, not the database structure. Databases can store both discrete data (for example, documents or x-rays) and/or indexed parts of images.

Figure 4.5 illustrates some of these database concepts. In this very simple example, a patient demographic table is linked to the physician table and both are linked to a results

Figure 4.5.   Relational databases

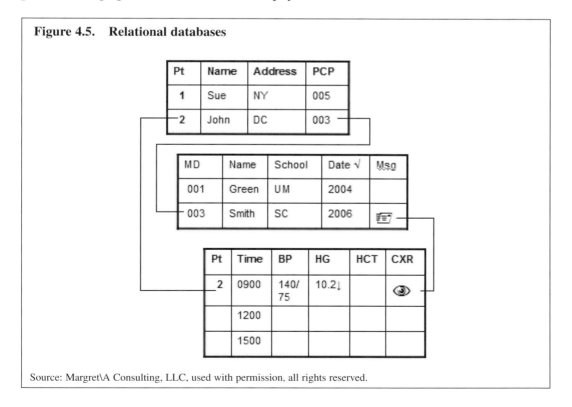

table. In this case, Dr. Smith is John's PCP. If the physician table were used for messaging, Dr. Smith could be alerted that there is a new result and that the new result may be an image of a chest x-ray for John. Discrete data elements also are recorded in the results table, including blood pressure and hemoglobin results taken at 9:00 a.m. Note that the hemoglobin results have been marked with a down arrow, indicating that this is a low result. This would have been processed by the results being compared with yet another table of normal values (not shown).

Data Exchange Standards

Because different databases may reside in different systems but need to be used together, **data exchange standards** and vocabulary standards are needed. For example, the patient and physician tables illustrated in figure 4.5 may both be in one database in one system, but the results table may be a separate database in another system. There are two primary ways the two databases in the different systems can relate to one another. One way is by one system sending a copy of data needed by the other system to it. Unless the same vendor created the two systems and their databases can be integrated, an interface is required. An interface is a special program where specific data are identified as needing to be exchanged and then rules about how those data are structured are applied. This is illustrated in figure 4.6, where one system sends the patient's name and medical record number from one table and the physician's name and date credentialed from the other table all to the other system. As illustrated, this process results in duplicate data in both systems, but this is necessary because whoever is using the results table will likely not have access to the other system or will not want to access it.

Figure 4.6. Data exchange

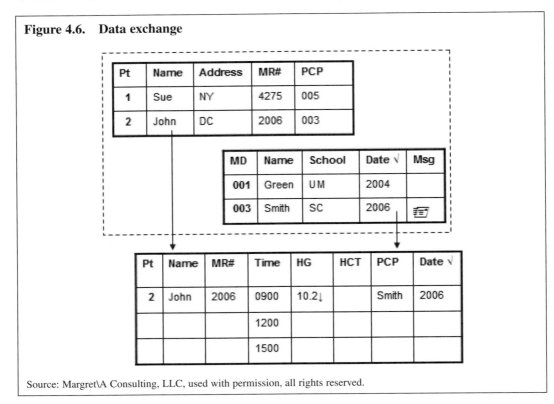

Data exchange as illustrated in figure 4.6 has to be planned carefully and requires data exchange standards to make sure the interface is written correctly and the exchange of data occurs reliably. These data exchange standards are also called **message format standards** or interoperability standards. They are protocols (predefined ways to do something) that describe how data need to be recorded in a database in any system in order to be sent to another system. For example, when John's medical record number (2006) is transferred to the new system, it must be interpreted as the medical record number and cannot be interpreted as the date the PCP's credentials expire (which also happens to be 2006). Data exchange standards provide a protocol that distinguishes between "medical record number" and "date credential expires."

The second way databases in different systems can be related is through a repository. A repository allows all data tables to be brought together through the use of standard interoperability protocols. Figure 4.5 illustrates this concept when all the tables were housed within the single repository.

When a hospital or other provider has many systems and wants one system to process data from multiple systems, only a repository will provide that functionality. It collects the data from many different systems and allows all the various tables to be related. It may be thought of as a super database, or database of databases. For example, the results table in figure 4.6 contains only lab values. It does not contain vital signs or the x-ray image included in the results table in figure 4.5. This is because lab results would be contained in a lab system, vital signs would be contained in a nurse charting system, and x-ray images would be contained in a PACS. A repository, however, is able to collect these data in one location so that they can be used in meaningful ways to support clinical decision making. For example, it is possible to graph lab results against vital signs.

Data exchange standards are developed by organizations devoted to their creation. The most common data exchange standards used in the U.S. healthcare system are:

- Health Level Seven (HL7) is a family of standards. Initially and currently in its Version 2.x standards, it primarily aids the exchange of data among hospital systems and, more recently, physician practices and other types of provider systems.

- Digital Imaging and Communications in Medicine (DICOM) helps exchange clinical images such as x-rays, CT scans, and so on.

- **National Council for Prescription Drug Programs** (NCPDP) enables the communication of retail pharmacy eligibility inquiries and claims (as mandated by HIPAA) and more recently provides a standard for the exchange of prescriptions from a physician practice electronic prescribing system directly to the retail pharmacy's information system (that has been proposed for use under the Medicare Part D drug program).

- **American National Standards Institute (ANSI) Accredited Standards Committee X12 Insurance Subcommittee (ASC X12N)** provides standards for hospital, professional, and dental claims, eligibility inquiries, electronic remittance advice, and other standards (as mandated by HIPAA).

- **ASTM International** (formerly known as the American Society for Testing and Materials) Committee E31 Health Informatics has developed guidelines primarily for various EHR management processes. Its most recent work has been to develop the standard content for the CCR standard in conjunction with several medical specialty societies and other groups.

The need for data exchange standards in healthcare is especially important because so many different systems are used. Unfortunately, not all vendors have been good about adopting data exchange standards. Some believe the only way to keep market share is to have a highly proprietary set of systems so that customers are dependent on buying additional systems from only that vendor. Furthermore, because data exchange standards are generally created in a group process often including competing vendors, the standards themselves may reflect only the minimal requirements everyone can agree on. The EHR initiatives discussed earlier in this chapter are urging vendors to adopt more open systems that use common standards and to develop better standards.

Data Comparability Standards

To date, data exchange standards have been limited to exchanging whatever data were sent from one system to another. There was no reconciliation that the vocabulary used in one system was the same in the other system. In other words, although the types and formats of the data elements were standardized (for example, medical record number [must contain 4 digits] versus date credential expires [expressed as YYYY]), the data values themselves were not standardized. Ensuring that the meaning of a term is consistent across all users is especially important in healthcare and is referred to as data comparability. Most recently, the industry has come to realize that for one clinical system to use another clinical system's data, terms must have the same meaning. Semantics is the term used to describe the fact that the value of the data in the message has a standardized meaning. When a message format standard specifies the vocabulary with which the data are **encoded,** the functionality is called semantic interoperability. HL7 Version 3 has begun to embed vocabulary references into its message format standard.

The vocabulary used in an EHR system should, at a minimum, be a **controlled vocabulary.** A controlled vocabulary means that a specific set of terms in the EHR's data dictionary may be used and that a central authority approves any additions or changes. A controlled vocabulary is essential to ensure common meaning for all users. For example, if the term *fall* is currently used in a template for physical therapists to describe the reasons for a patient's injury, but a group of nurses want to add *slip* as a synonym, there should be consensus that these two terms mean the same thing. Otherwise, when any one group wants to perform analysis on the data and does not realize that *fall* and *slip* are used as synonyms, only part of the data may be retrieved for the analysis.

A **standard vocabulary** is developed through a process that confirms consensus on the meaning of the terms included in the vocabulary. Standard vocabularies help achieve data comparability. Although standards may be recognized in many ways, the most important way is for the standards development organization to be accredited by ANSI. All the data exchange standards identified above are accredited by ANSI and/or its international counterpart. However, standardization also can come about through widespread use. For example, many people recognize the Microsoft Windows operating system as a standard operating system, although it has not been ANSI accredited.

Until recently, most healthcare vocabularies have been proprietary or unique to the vendor who develops the EHR. They may be controlled vocabularies because they may require approval for modification, but they are not standardized vocabularies. A controlled vocabulary may become a standard vocabulary through common usage, but more preferably when it is recognized as an ANSI standard. The SNOMED vocabulary, for example, is a recognized ANSI standard.

For example, when physicians enter data into a history and physical exam template, the data variables may be encoded with the SNOMED vocabulary. SNOMED International (formerly known as the Systematized Nomenclature of Human and Veterinary Medicine) was originally developed by the College of American Pathologists (CAP) in the 1960s. Initially it was a robust set of multi-axial codes that could identify the topography, morphology, etiology, and function associated with pathological specimens. Although becoming the standard vocabulary for pathology because of its widespread use, SNOMED has also become ANSI accredited as a formal standard. It has subsequently grown into the most comprehensive effort to standardize vocabulary for the representation of medical knowledge, and incorporates microglossaries that address nursing and other ancillary terminology. It has been licensed from CAP by the **National Library of Medicine** (NLM) so that it is now freely available to vendors as the basis for clinical data dictionaries in EHR systems. The NLM has also mapped SNOMED to other vocabularies and classification systems, such as ICD-9-CM and ICD-10. Such mapping should permit data encoded via SNOMED in an EHR system to be converted to other code systems for other purposes, such as ICD for reimbursement.

It is important to distinguish between vocabulary and classification. *Vocabulary* refers to the set of all terms that may be used in a language whereas *classification* is a grouping of the terms into various categories, such as all diseases of the respiratory system or all procedures performed by anesthesiologists.

To promote adoption of a single set of standard vocabularies, several components of the federal government recognize SNOMED and the following other vocabularies as important:

- Logical Observation Identifiers, Name and Codes (LOINC), developed by the Regenstrief Institute, provides names and codes for laboratory test results and other observations.

- Normalized notations for clinical drugs (RxNorm) developed jointly between the NLM and the Veterans Health Administration provides descriptions of medications in clinical form.

- The Universal Medical Device Nomenclature System (UMDNS) developed by the Emergency Care Research Institute provides standard terminology for medical devices.

In addition to these so-called recommended vocabularies, nearly 150 healthcare vocabularies and classification systems may be used in EHR systems or other health information technology. Some are widely used, such as the **National Drug Codes** (NDC) for maintaining inventories of drugs in pharmacies or Current Procedural Terminology (CPT) used to code physician services for reimbursement. Others are less widely used or are used for very specific purposes. For example, Alternative Link is a vocabulary and code system for integrative care that codes concepts for billing and research from alternative and complementary medicine, such as acupuncture and aromatherapy. Medcin is a computer-based nomenclature developed and maintained by Medicomp Systems, Inc. It is widely used for the recording of history and physical exam findings.

Electronic Document/Content Management

Although it may seem ideal to capture and use only discrete data in an EHR system, it is neither realistic nor practical. Narrative information is necessary to express unique information, and paper-based forms and digital images of documents will exist for some time to come. Many healthcare organizations start their journey to the EHR using various forms of document imaging and digital document management to automate paper records to make them more readily accessible to clinicians.

Technology that manages digital images is electronic document/content management (ED/CM) and **computer output to laser disk/enterprise report management** (COLD/ERM). These systems incorporate a variety of technologies. Document imaging systems scan existing documents and store them for viewing through a computer workstation. As documents are scanned, they are indexed, assigning a description of the document and key contents for later retrieval. Documents that have been entered into an electronic transcription system or outputted in report-formatted digital documents, such as laboratory results from a laboratory information system, can be COLD-fed into a repository for viewing. The benefit of document imaging is greatly enhanced access to documents.

However, when content management and workflow tools are added to the document imaging, the flow of work can be managed and many forms of documents can be accessible together, including the scanned and COLD-fed documents as well as e-mail, instant messages, Web pages, and so on. Workflow tools, for example, can not only provide access to scanned charts to coders at home, but also different categories of charts can be directed to different coders and volumes managed. Not all workflow systems can support both administrative (for example, coding and release of information) and clinical functions (for example, viewing the scanned documents in the emergency department).

Clinical images are "pictures" generated by medical devices such as x-rays, EKG monitors, and so on. Storage of these pictures is called PACS (picture archiving and communications systems). Clinical images from PACS can be viewed through standard monitors if great detail is not required. Diagnostic-quality viewing of such images requires special monitors with very high resolution and/or full-motion video capability. Because of their ability to be enlarged, rotated, and several images viewed simultaneously, many radiologists find PACS superior to standard radiology film.

Data Retrieval Technology

Because most HISs used today are primarily data retrieval systems, technology to support this functionality is quite mature. Retrieval technology may be as basic as a lookup, where a query is made to access certain data from a specific system, for example, a lab result on a certain patient from the laboratory information system. The desired patient may be selected from a list or by entering his or her name and/or medical record number. Navigational tools permit the user to select a specific data element, to make a customized table, or even to graph results.

More sophisticated retrieval technologies enable a user to access several different types of data from different source systems through a single application screen. Hence, a medication list may be viewed from the same application screen as the lab results. There may be windows for different types of data from different sources, or predesigned or customizable screens may permit viewing of a specific user's preferred set of data. The most sophisticated retrieval technology, coupled with a CDR, permits not only viewing of data by type, but also manipulation of several different types of data, such as plotting lab results on a graph against medication administered, vital signs, and so on.

One disadvantage to using a computer to view information is the inability to "flip" quickly through multiple "pages" of data. Clinicians have learned to rapidly scan a patient's record to both get an overall picture of the patient and find specific data. Although this capability is available in a computer through specific search features, color, and other navigational tools, these are not yet everyday tools used by clinicians. Eventually, everyone will use such tools as second nature.

An important characteristic of retrieval technologies is that the screen layout can be customized to the user's preference. Many EHR systems display a tailored screen based on the user's log-on. Thus, when Dr. Jones logs on, his personally preferred screen layout is displayed. The ability to drill down to greater detail also is important; but, again, caution must be applied to avoid having too many pathways to the data. Moreover, research has shown that three levels of screen layers are about the most anyone can use effectively.

Color, animation, icons, and sound are important screen design and data retrieval tools. Color can be very helpful in navigating a screen to find desired data, but the number of people (especially men) who are color-blind must be considered. Color should never be relied on solely for any critical alerts that are attempting to be conveyed; instead, alerts should be accompanied by a special icon, animation, and/or sound. Icons can be very effective in guiding users, but they must be large enough to see clearly and be very intuitive. Unfortunately, few standard symbols can be used in creating icons for HISs. Of all the navigational elements available, sound may be the least used in healthcare because of the many medical devices that routinely emit sounds and have special sound alarms.

Data Capture Technology

With the exception of possibly the most current generation of users, most clinicians have never learned to type and consider typing or any other form of keyboard use to be a clerical function. Even clinicians who are willing and able to type still often find data entry on a computer more challenging and time-consuming than handwriting or dictating.

Unfortunately, no ideal solution has yet been found to support data capture effectively for all users in all environments. However, there are a few key considerations. Most important, data entry must return value to the user. If the user can obtain decision support at the time of data entry that is valuable, he or she is more likely to perform data entry. Clinicians are more inclined to do data entry when they can see that the direct result of their data entry is a benefit to their subsequent work (for example, if the system automatically generates tailored instructions for the patient when discharge information is entered). If data entry is even perceived to take longer than traditional recording, even when its purpose is laudable (such as to have more legible data to improve patient safety), it will be a hard sell.

Several technologies can help make data capture easier. Collectively, these are often called **human-computer interfaces.** They include:

- *Discrete data entry through point-and-click fields, drop-down menus, structured templates, or macros:* These make data entry and processing easier. Devices supporting such data entry include the mouse, light pens, and touch screens.

- *Speech and handwriting recognition:* Speech recognition can be very effective in certain situations when data entry is fairly repetitive and the vocabulary used is fairly limited. As speech recognition improves, it is becoming a replacement for dictation. In some cases, the user reviews the speech as it is being converted to type and makes any needed corrections; in other cases, the speech is sent to a special device where it generates type for another individual to review and edit. Handwriting recognition is similar to speech recognition, where the system is "taught" to recognize a user's handwriting. Some tablet computers have been able to convert handwriting to type fairly successfully, but because of the need for somewhat greater precision than normal handwriting, most tablet computers are used today to capture and retain the handwriting.

- *Handheld and wireless devices:* Handheld devices, such as tablet computers and PDAs, may use any of the other forms of data entry, from keying and selecting from a list to speech and handwriting recognition. Although their use is growing in popularity, they still are not necessarily the answer for everyone. Tablets are generally easy for mobile professionals to have readily available, although they are still fairly heavy. PDAs may be limited in terms of the volume of data they can store and their processing capabilities. Moreover, the size of both the screen and the keypad may be smaller than desirable. Unless tablets or PDAs are wireless, their ability to communicate or link to primary information systems is limited to when they are docked to a workstation. Handheld devices can run out of power, requiring extra batteries and charging. However, handheld devices are ideal for certain limited functions, such as for writing prescriptions or capturing a home health data set; and as they are becoming more sophisticated and wireless, they are becoming very popular. Still, many healthcare organizations find it just as effective to mount a notebook computer to a cart and move it with the user. These are affectionately called **COWs** (computers on wheels). For the less mobile healthcare professional, desktop computer workstations are still the mainstay.

- *Direct data capture from a medical device attached to a patient:* This is yet another important means of capturing certain kinds of data, such as vital signs. Special medical devices (such as a pacemaker) can even be connected to a standard telephone for capturing data or checking on the device's status from a remote location.

- *Patient data entry:* Incorporating patient-generated data into the EHR discussed previously is just now starting to be used. In the past, providers have been somewhat reluctant to incorporate patient-generated information. There were misunderstandings that the patients could access and change the entire content of the provider's records. There also were misperceptions that the information may be too voluminous or erroneous. As patients continue to be seen by an ever-increasing number of providers, however, it is now recognized that they are the only source of at least where all their information is located, if not what the information is.

- *Natural language processing (NLP):* Considered a special form of data entry, NLP is the capability of a computer to apply very sophisticated mathematical and probabilistic formulas to narrative text and convert them to structured data. Although text processing is becoming more feasible, the technology has a long way to go before it can be used routinely.

Clinical Decision Support

A lot of importance has been placed on the role of CDS in EHRs. CDS systems directly address patient safety and healthcare quality improvement issues. They also aid in bringing value to the user. CDS systems depend on analytical tools that process discrete data in many sophisticated ways. Special analytical tools include reminders and alerts, clinical guideline advice, benchmarking, expert system resources, and diagnostic or procedural investigative tools. CDS systems often depend on an elaborate set of rules, or logical pathways, to trigger reminders or to direct data through a pathway. These rules may be defined by the healthcare organization using them, or they may be acquired from the EHR vendor, via subscription to a knowledge base (such as a drug knowledge base [DKB]), or through associations, government agencies, and/or health plans that compile the results of research into best practice guidance. **Evidence-based medicine,** then, is the practice of medicine utilizing guidance-based information gleaned from research studies.

System Communication and Networks

The backbone of an EHR obviously is the hardware and software on which the system runs. The term *architecture* refers to the configuration, structure, and relationships of all components of a computer system. Three main types of architecture are used in creating an EHR:

- **Mainframe architecture** uses a single large computer to process data received from terminals into which data are entered. Mainframe systems tend to be considered legacy systems because they are the configuration of older applications. In general, mainframe architecture is limited in its ability to support the extensive transaction processing required of an EHR.

- **Client/server** (C/S) **architecture** uses a combination of computers to capture and process data. Server computers are powerful processors. They typically house all the application software and store all active data captured by all the clients throughout the network. They then "serve" multiple client computers, which have less powerful processors (and in some cases have minimal processing capability of their own, in which case they are called thin clients).

- **Web services architecture** (WSA) is an emerging architecture that utilizes Web-based tools to permit communication among different software applications.

Whatever architecture is deployed, the intent is to share data among different users. In the mainframe architecture, every terminal (which was not a computer) had to connect directly to the mainframe computer to send and receive data, so this architecture generally was not considered a network. When one computer is linked to another computer, however, a network exists. Network devices link computers to one another and one network to another.

- **Local area networks** (LANs) using hardwire cable transmit data securely at very high speeds throughout a building, campus, or small geographic area.

- **Wireless local area networks** (WLANs) utilize radio waves or microwaves to transmit data without cable. These are becoming increasingly popular as their security and reliability have improved. Two standards make local wireless transmissions possible: the IEEE 802.11 and Bluetooth. Healthcare may use this technology to "beam" data from one device to another using infrared light waves. The devices must have IrDA (infrared data) ports and be in close proximity with a direct line of site. Another communication technology using radio waves is radio frequency identification (RFID). RFID is similar to bar code technology, RFID scanning can be done at greater distances than bar code scanning. It is being tried for patient identification in medication administration.

- **Wide area networks** (WANs) where data are transmitted across wide geographic areas generally depend on telephone lines to transmit data. Depending on the type of phone service, the number and type of lines leased from the telephone company, and the size of the data to be transmitted, speeds and level of security can vary.

Every network operates by conforming to an agreed-upon format for transmitting data. This format is called a protocol, and it aids data transmission by establishing standards for indicating the start and end of a message, by performing error checking to ensure the data are transmitted correctly, and, in some cases, by compressing the data to make them easier to transmit. There are a variety of protocols to choose from, each with its own advantages and disadvantages. One of the most popular protocols for LANs is **Ethernet.** To be able to use different protocols, the computer system must be set up to enable use of each desired protocol.

Many healthcare organizations are beginning to be interested in using the Internet protocol, TCP/IP (Transmission Control Protocol/Internet Protocol), to simplify their networking and to take advantage of Web-based technology. A WAN that uses TCP/IP is called an **extranet.** Intranets and extranets operate in very much the same way as the Internet but belong only to the organization setting them up and are accessible only by those authorized to access them.

Storage Technology

The volume of data captured by information systems in general, and EHRs in particular, is enormous. There is a growing expectation that data should be accessible in real time for very long periods of time. As clinicians become dependent on the computer for all their data needs, they will not tolerate downtime or delays for retrieving archived data.

As a result, managing data storage is an increasingly important issue. Unlike in the past when data were retained online for only a few days after discharge and backups were stored on tape, an EHR virtually demands that data be retained online forever and be instantaneously retrievable and backed up continuously.

A storage device is a machine that contains nothing but storage media. Tape drives are the oldest form of storage device and are rapidly becoming obsolete. Disk drives are the most common storage device today. Disk technology, however, has moved rapidly from magnetic disks to optical disks of many different forms. Many servers contain optical disk drives that can store very large volumes of data. Storing data on the same server used to process data slows response time. As a result, disks are being arrayed in **redundant arrays of independent (or inexpensive) disks,** called RAID, so that a great volume of data can be stored. Storage devices also are being organized into their own **storage area networks** (SANs) so that they can be accessible from any server in the network. When such technology is deployed, however, **storage management software** must be available to manage the SAN, to keep track of where data are stored, and to move older data to less expensive, but still accessible, storage locations. Storage management is becoming an entire domain within information systems management.

Data must be available continuously. As noted, when paper as a backup no longer exists in a paperless EHR environment, users must be assured that the computer system is available to them at all times. To achieve such availability, an EHR should have **server redundancy** accomplished through **mirrored processing.** This means that as data are entered and processed by one server, they are entered and processed simultaneously by a second server. Should the primary server crash, the system should be designed to "fail over" to the second server and can continue processing as if, at least from the user's point of view, nothing had happened. Obviously, the servers must be monitored; and when the primary server goes down, someone must be ready to repair or replace it as rapidly as possible. Most organizations do not invest in yet a third redundant server.

Thus, although storage media are cheap and healthcare has had a tendency to store all electronic data, storage management is becoming a more expensive proposition. The introduction of an EHR should trigger a review of the organization's retention schedule with an eye toward enabling a realistic retention schedule for electronic data. Another element of the retention schedule should be the retention of metadata, including both **audit trails** and the "data about data" that supports the **data dictionary.** As noted in the earlier discussion of CDS systems, it is important to manage how discrete data are captured and used. For example, it was noted that a discrete data element could be established originally as mandatory for documentation but be changed to optional. A smart attorney could require evidence of when the change took place to substantiate that the organization either did not change it or changed it at a point in time relative to an event under investigation.

Check Your Understanding 4.4

Instrucions: Distinguish between the following pairs of terms.

1. A clinical data repository (CDR) and a clinical data warehouse (CDW)
2. Data exchange standards and data comparability standards
3. A data dictionary and metadata
4. Controlled vocabulary and standard vocabulary
5. Vocabulary and classification
6. Discrete data and digital images
7. Speech recognition and natural language processing
8. Database management system and clinical decision support system
9. Distinguish between local area network and intranet
10. Radio frequency identification and high-density trunk lines

Instructions: Match the focus in column B to the data exchange or vocabulary standard in column A.

A. Standard		B. Focus	
_____ 1.	ASC X12N	a.	Clinical images
_____ 2.	LOINC	b	Clinical drug names
_____ 3.	.HL7	c.	Physician services
_____ 4.	NCPDP	d.	Drug inventory
_____ 5.	RxNorm	e.	Complementary medicine
_____ 6.	DICOM	f.	History and physical exam findings
_____ 7.	Medcin	g.	Prescriptions
_____ 8.	CPT	h.	Data exchange
_____ 9.	NDC	i.	Hospital claims
_____ 10.	Alternative Link	j.	Lab results

Creation of Electronic Health Record Systems

Creating an EHR system for a hospital or even a physician practice requires extensive planning and organizational commitment. Figure 4.7 illustrates the steps required to successfully determine organizational readiness for an EHR, develop strategic and tactical plans, select a vendor, implement and maintain the system, and ensure ongoing value. These steps are similar to those discussed in chapter 17.

Readiness Assessment

Although virtually everyone recognizes the benefits to be derived from EHRs, there are significant barriers to their acquisition and use. These barriers actually may first include an appreciation for what an EHR actually is. Executives, physicians and other clinicians, and even sometimes IT staff whose experience may be limited to financial and administrative

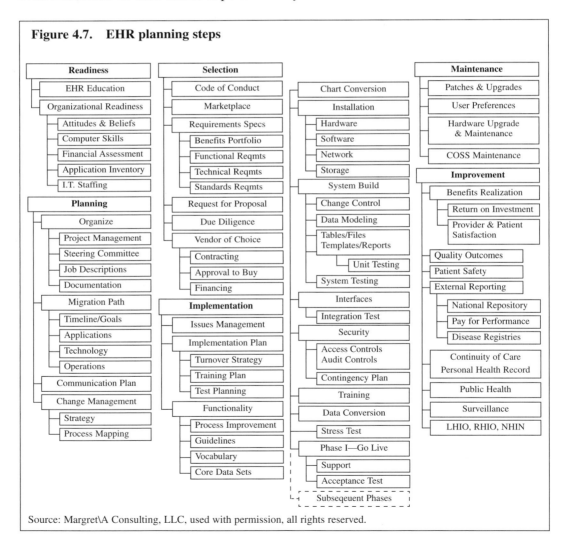

Figure 4.7.   EHR planning steps

Source: Margret\A Consulting, LLC, used with permission, all rights reserved.

systems may need an EHR education. It can often be helpful to conduct an attitudes and beliefs survey that pinpoints issues concerning EHR understanding and concerns. Education then can be directed specifically to the issues identified.

Cost is often cited as the biggest barrier to EHR adoption. EHR systems are undoubtedly expensive. In addition to the direct expenditures for the system, cost issues include the total cost of ownership, return on investment and other forms of benefits, and financing.

The cost of an EHR system for a hospital is difficult to generalize because hospitals do not purchase a single system. Rather, they integrate source systems into a repository and acquire other applications that collectively comprise the EHR. Moreover, costs vary over time. Estimates to acquire the hardware, software, and human resources to fully implement an EHR range from three to four million dollars for a small community hospital with generally a single vendor, ten to fifteen million dollars or more for a small to medium-sized community hospital with a **best-of-breed** situation, to upwards of $100 million for a large IDN. For physician offices, the cost is somewhat easier to estimate because the system being purchased is generally more self-contained. For very small practices (one to three physicians), an EHR may cost around $10,000 per physician (Monegain 2005). Costs go up as the practice increases in size because of the increase in complexity. Generally, there are more source systems to interface and practices often want greater customizability and more comprehensive functionality. Costs for such systems range from $25,000 to $50,000 or more per physician (also depending on whether a PMS is acquired or replaced as part of the EHR acquisition).

Benefits of EHR Implementation

The benefits of EHRs are often difficult to quantify. The primary benefits are quality and patient safety. However, other benefits do produce specific financial payback. For example, hospitals will realize the impact of the EHR system on the clerical workforce, admissions personnel, billers, transcriptionists, couriers, and other support staff. Storage of paper charts should be reduced (although as previously noted this depends on the hybrid record situation and may even increase). Although nurses are rarely, if ever, eliminated, overtime and temporary staff costs may be reduced or eliminated. The impact on nursing is related much more to productivity and reduced need to perform fewer administrative functions.

Hospitals also generally find improvements in charge capture, can reduce the number of repetitive tests, and realize savings from the use of lower-cost drugs. Still, the greatest impact is seen in the reduction of errors that ultimately affect the hospital's finances through better positioning for contracting and the improved likelihood of better accreditation and licensure outcomes.

Many of these same benefits apply to physician offices. Some offices find that they can see more patients because of productivity improvements. Others are able to add professional staff using paper storage space to enhance revenues to the group. Level of service (E&M) coding support generally improves revenues from two to three percent to as much as 20 to 30 percent, depending on the quality of coding performed prior to EHR adoption and sometimes the specialty of the practice.

Benefits, however, must be weighed against not only the cost of the EHR, but also other factors that go into the total cost of ownership. For example, more staff trained in health informatics may be necessary. Other IT support staff needs may increase or have to be outsourced. Even the most rudimentary of EHR systems require some effort to implement. The process of system build, which is the creation of data dictionaries, tables, decision support rules, templates for data entry, screen layouts, and reports, is enormous and time-consuming. The system has to undergo extensive testing. Adoption of an EHR system requires considerable process mapping and workflow analysis and redesign. Training is required for everyone, even for those who may have used another EHR system, because each system is not only different, but every implementation is different due to differences in source systems, customizations, and organizational preferences. Finally, because an EHR is a clinical system, it must be kept up to date with the latest evidence-based medicine, new and recalled drugs, new terms for new diseases, and new processes and workflows brought about by external factors such as reimbursement or patient needs.

Benefits of EHR Implementation

Still other barriers to EHR adoption are those related to the people who are stakeholders in the process. Executive support often goes hand in hand with costs, benefits, and financing issues. If executives are not on board, they are unlikely to fully commit to the level of funding needed, the creation and support of policies to ensure system adoption, and a culture that recognizes the importance of the EHR. EHR adoption is crucial to their success and depends less on the actual hardware and software than on the associated people, policy, and process components.

EHR adoption among clinicians is clearly the most critical element in a successful implementation. Clinicians include physicians, nurses, pharmacists, technicians, therapists, and all others who use clinical information. Although each type of clinician may be challenged in special ways, the support of physicians will likely be the most challenging to gain, followed by the support of nurses, who are the ones who will need the most training.

Patients should not be discounted in the people factor. They are frequently concerned about security and privacy issues. Today's information systems have typically been secured by virtue of the fact that they contain minimal patient data, few people know how to use them, and they are closed systems. They do not connect to the outside world. As use and users expand, security must be enhanced to better protect privacy. On the other hand, however, security measures must not be so onerous as to make EHRs even more formidable to learn and use.

Finally, many people are concerned about potential legal and regulatory matters. Many states have not adopted specific statutes relating to EHRs; others have updated their statutes to address electronic health information in general. Still other states are generally silent on whether health information is in paper or electronic form because the statutes are old and generally assume paper. Although every organization needs to review its own statutes, it is generally believed that EHRs are legally acceptable.

Some portions of EHRs may need to be converted to paper or signed on paper in certain circumstances and in certain states. For example, state boards of pharmacy generally control the form and format of a prescription. Standards for electronic prescribing are regulated by the federal government through the introduction of payment for outpatient drugs for Medicare beneficiaries under Part D, created by the **Medicare Modernization Act of 2003** (MMA). However, a few states do not permit electronic prescriptions, and until they change their statutes, electronic prescribing systems will not be adopted in these states.

Planning

When a decision is made to move forward with an EHR, it is important to put resources into planning. Virtually everyone who has conducted an EHR project has wished they had spent more time on planning. Planning includes organizing the project, developing a **migration path,** communicating to stakeholders, and developing a strategy and plan to manage change.

Most organizations create an EHR steering committee to engage all the various stakeholders. This ensures that the EHR planning is comprehensive and also starts the process of introducing change and gaining buy-in. In addition to the EHR steering committee, various domain teams, implementation teams, and other such groups are formed as the need for more specific focus arises.

The EHR project also needs support staff other than just IT staff. Certainly, the project needs a project manager. (A very large project might need a project management office.) Project managers ensure that the steps in the project are performed and coordinate the various committees and vendor staff. Project plans, budgets, staff resource utilization, issues logs, change control records, installation manuals, user manuals and training tools, and various forms of communications about the project are just one part of the overall documentation needed in developing an EHR project. Job descriptions also should be available for all persons filling new positions and may be helpful in describing the roles played on various committees.

Developing a migration path to describe the strategic approach to EHR is an often-overlooked planning activity. A migration path is a strategic plan that outlines the major components to be implemented. It should describe the phases over which the organization intends to implement its EHR components. In addition, each phase should have specific goals.

A good way to construct an EHR migration path is to list all the current applications, technology, and operations the organization has in place or is starting to roll out. Each phase can be populated with plans for subsequent rollout of applications, technology, and operations to support them. Figure 4.8 illustrates a sample migration path. The plan for the hospital in this illustration extends over three phases. The hospital has separated technology into three

Figure 4.8.   Sample EHR migration path

Phases	Current	Phase 1	Phase 2	Phase 3
Applications	ADT MPI Digital dictation Abstracting Encoder Pt accts Lab Pharmacy Radiology Materials mgt Strategic planning Order communication	Outpt Registration Electronic signature Record tracking EMAR PACS Nurse charting	E-registration E-MPI Document Imaging Speech recognition CPOE Physician charting	 Integrated RIS CDSS
Database	Vendor proprietary	Drug Knowledge all terminals		
Network	Upgrade license	E-mail for MDs		
Interfaces	One vendor	Connect w/Ref Lab	Connect Pharmacy to CPOE	
Operations	EHR Steering Manual pathways development and approval	Physician champion MPI clean up	Process Mapping	

categories: database, network, and interfaces. It should be noted that this is an example of a plan and is not necessarily the right plan for everyone. The nature of the current applications and technical infrastructure needs to be considered. The readiness of the organization's clinicians to adopt various types of applications plays an important role in what the migration path will look like. But the key point of an EHR migration path is that it is an overarching plan that everyone can understand and follow.

EHR Selection

When the major elements of planning are in place, the organization usually begins the process of selecting a vendor. Many hospitals already have purchased HIS systems from one or more vendors and often will consider one of their current vendors as the primary source for an EHR. Even so, however, it is still worth "going to market" to ensure that the vendor actually can supply what is needed. When most systems are from one vendor, the situation is often called **best of fit.** Using the best-of-fit solution can be a major investment in either replacing all the source systems from a new vendor or finding the EHR components that will work with the applications from the current vendor.

Many organizations find that their HIS vendor does not provide the level of EHR sophistication they desire and are looking to interface their HIS applications with clinical applications from another vendor. Sometimes called **dual core,** in this vendor strategy one vendor primarily supplies the financial and administrative applications and another vendor primarily supplies the clinical applications. Alternatively, hospitals may have applications from many different vendors, often called best of breed, meaning that a system was selected for each application that was considered to be the best in its class. Because so many different systems are difficult to manage, organizations with a best-of-breed strategy also are migrating to dual core to reduce the number of disparate systems.

Whatever vendor strategy is deployed, a selection process has a fairly well defined set of steps. (See chapter 15 for more on the selection process.) Briefly, the marketplace of possible vendors is scanned, and a list of those most likely to fit the current environment is identified. The organization develops requirement specifications, often including a description of the benefits it hopes to achieve with the EHR, the specific functional requirements desired (often using the HL7 EHR System Functional Model as a guide), the technical requirements for the system to fit into the current infrastructure, and any standards requirements, such as for data exchange and vocabulary. This information is compiled into a **request for proposal** (RFP) document and sent to vendor candidates, who respond with a detailed proposal.

Because an EHR is a major investment, the organization should undertake two critical steps. First, it should develop (or review) its code of conduct that spells out its ethical principles surrounding vendor selection. The EHR marketplace is highly competitive, and the organization will want to avoid any appearance of improprieties. Second, the organization should observe due diligence. Due diligence involves thoroughly reviewing the vendors' proposals, conducting product demonstrations, visiting sites where the product is already installed, calling references, and investigating the vendors' business practices. The organization must be assured that not only will the EHR function as expected, but that the vendor will do a good job implementing it, provide appropriate support when there are problems, keep it current, and remain in business.

Most organizations require the EHR steering committee to recommend a specific vendor to executive leadership, who then approves the move toward contract negotiation.

When satisfactory terms are negotiated, executive leadership also must approve the signing of the contract. Often a contract negotiation team is used to negotiate the contract and legal counsel reviews it. Of course, financing must be secured prior to signing the contract.

Implementation Activities

EHR implementation varies with the type of EHR acquired. Implementation strategies and plans vary by vendor as well as by the component being implemented. For example, one vendor's product may allow extensive customization so that **system build** becomes a huge process whereas another vendor's product may not be so customizable. Implementing CPOE versus EMAR or any other component that might be acquired in a hospital has different challenges. For example, CPOE requires that the various ancillary systems for which orders are written be able to receive data from the CPOE system. If a CPOE system is acquired with minimal decision support, a repository may not be needed. However, if there is extensive decision support about what drugs are best, the price of diagnostic studies, and so on, a repository may be needed. A more robust pharmacy information system also may be needed. Every component that may be implemented for an EHR has its own set of issues.

Addressing Issues Management
One important element in planning an implementation is addressing **issues management.** Issues will always arise. For example, hardware may not be delivered on time, a server may be delivered dead on arrival, the EHR vendor's implementation team may not fix a system problem correctly the first time, or an interface may not work when it is tested. An issues log should be maintained, and the project manager should ensure that every issue is resolved or relegated to the appropriate person.

Developing an Implementation Plan
The organization needs to develop an implementation plan for the EHR. The vendor usually supplies a generic plan for how it likes to implement the EHR. It is important to harmonize the vendor's plan outlining the various details it must address with the organization's plan, which will include some of the same tasks in addition to other ones. The implementation plan should include a turnover strategy that describes which nursing unit or clinic site will implement the system first and whether the implementation will run parallel with the paper processes for a while. In addition, the organization should have a training plan and a test plan.

Actual implementation may take place in several parts. Although shown sequentially in figure 4.7, the steps often take place simultaneously or in a series of cycles. Functional implementation entails making sure the EHR functions exist and are implemented, including process improvement, use of clinical guidelines or pathways, vocabulary adoption, and core data set incorporation. Attention to functionality is a precursor to system build, where a data model is often developed and the specific tables, files, templates, and reports are designed and tested. Teams may work on each of these areas or domain teams organized by user or clinical specialty may work on all the areas together for their domain.

Effecting Chart Conversion
Another critical implementation activity is **chart conversion.** Chart conversion is the process whereby data from the paper chart are converted into electronic form. This may be accomplished by abstracting certain data from the paper chart and entering them into the new EHR, scanning certain existing documents, or a combination of both. This is important

when current data are needed for subsequent care (for example, in an outpatient or ambulatory environment such as a clinic or physician practice).

In the hospital, chart conversion varies significantly according to the type of component being implemented. For example, it may be appropriate where patients with multiple admissions to abstract their medication history information into the CPOE system. Depending on the availability of source systems, some of these data may already exist in another system, so **data conversion,** rather than chart conversion, is required. Data conversion ensures that data in one system can be converted over to the new system. For example, an existing pharmacy information system may be upgraded and the data contained in it need to be converted to the upgraded system. Patients who are currently inpatients will have data in various systems that may need to be converted into the new EHR system.

Establishing the Technical Infrastructure

To undertake system build, chart conversion, and data conversion, the technical infrastructure must be in place. Hardware, software, network infrastructure, and storage need to be installed, and interfaces may have to be written. Security considerations must be addressed (discussed in the next section). As each phase of installation takes place, testing should be performed. **Unit testing** ensures that each data element is captured, recorded, and processed appropriately within a given application. **System testing** then tests that the various parts of the applications work together within a single system. **Integration testing** ensures that the interfaces between applications and systems work. **Stress testing** is performed toward the end of implementation to ensure that the actual number, or load, of transactions that would be performed during peak hours can be performed. At the conclusion of all testing and some time after go-live, **acceptance testing** is performed. This may be a review all tests performed, assurance that all issues have been resolved, and some measure of adoption. Acceptance testing usually triggers the final payment for the system and when a maintenance contract becomes effective.

Training Users to Use the System

Users must be trained to use the system. Generally, a set of "super users" are trained by the vendor, who, in turn, either train all staff users in the organization, or are available to support new users as the system goes live. Training must include not only formal training, but also context-sensitive help screens and user reference manuals and even "cheat sheets."

Implementation of the system, even with successful adoption, is not the end of the process. In fact, it is the beginning of the maintenance mode, where regular upgrades need to be implemented, user preferences need to be accommodated, hardware upgrades and maintenance are performed, and the clinical decision support logic, rules, and knowledge sources are kept current. (And, if benefits are occurring, the organization should celebrate.) Organizations may conduct formal financial benefits realization studies to make sure their return on investment is achieved and/or conduct provider and/or patient satisfaction surveys. With recent emphasis on patient safety and quality, especially relating to P4P or P4Q initiatives, there is more interest in evaluating quality and patient safety outcomes. Hospitals have recently started to perform external reporting to national repositories, and physician practices will likely follow in a few years.

Evaluting That Goals Are Met

Finally, evaluating that the goals of the EHR system are met is an important, but often-overlooked, step. Few organizations conduct formal benefits realization studies because they are time-consuming and because EHRs take a long time to implement. Still, it is important to understand that benefits are occurring; if they are not, corrective action should be taken.

Check Your Understanding 4.5

Instructions: Put the steps in creating an EHR system in the sequence in which they are generally performed, from beginning to end.

1. Turnover strategy   _____

2. Due diligence   _____

3. Migration path   _____

4. Chart conversion   _____

5. Integration test   _____

6. Training   _____

7. Request for proposal   _____

8. System build   _____

9. Issues management   _____

10. Change control   _____

Information Management in an Electronic Environment

The electronic environment presents many new roles for HIM professionals. AHIMA has done a tremendous amount of work in identifying, describing, sponsoring training for, and introducing these new roles to HIM professionals and the facilities for whom HIM professionals work, as well as those organizations that accredit and license those facilities. AHIMA envisions HIM professionals as data analysts, information brokers, data set developers, data miners, workflow analysts, data security managers, database administrators, and in many other capacities that support EHRs. Not only do HIM professionals have the expertise to fill these roles, but they also have demonstrated an appreciation for data quality, confidentiality, and data security that is unparalleled in any other healthcare profession.

Data Quality

In 1998, AHIMA developed a data quality management model. (See figure 4.9.) Appreciating the various characteristics of data quality is essential to making the EHR work. Chapter 2 discussed the elements of data quality and its importance to patient care. Likewise, the EHR depends on data that are complete and accurate to function appropriately.

Confidentiality and Privacy

Every individual has private information he or she does not share with anyone, including innermost thoughts, dreams, and feelings. When private information is shared with someone else, a condition called confidentiality is established. Sometimes confidential

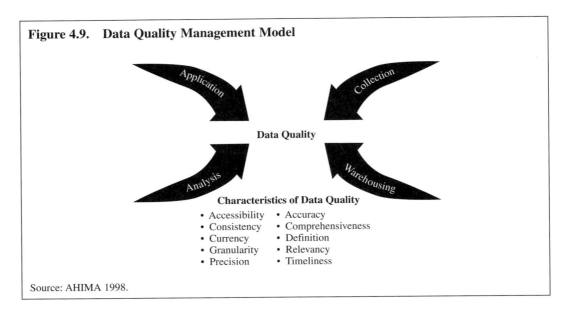

Figure 4.9.   Data Quality Management Model

Data Quality

Characteristics of Data Quality

- Accessibility
- Consistency
- Currency
- Granularity
- Precision

- Accuracy
- Comprehensiveness
- Definition
- Relevancy
- Timeliness

Source: AHIMA 1998.

information is written down or placed into a computer system. Security measures are put into place to ensure that only those to whom the individual has given permission can access confidential information. Security measures also protect the **integrity** of the information so that it is not altered in any way and ensure its availability so that it is accessible when needed for subsequent care and other legitimate purposes. Because of the multiple types of protection needed for health information, HIPAA used the term **protected health information** (PHI) to recognize the nature of confidential information that organizations covered by the law (covered entities) must protect.

An EHR system can afford better security for PHI because **access controls,** audit trails, **authentication** systems, and other measures exist where they do not in a paper environment. Attention to confidentiality and privacy is not new. The Hippocratic Oath has directed physician protection of private information for centuries. Moreover, every provider has instituted security measures as part of his or her standard business practice. HIM professionals have long been considered the custodians of medical records and have managed disclosures through ROI functions for many years.

HIPAA Privacy and Security Requirements

HIPAA privacy requirements include specific policies and procedures on **uses and disclosures** of PHI, individuals' privacy rights with respect to their information (including the right to receive a notice of privacy practices [NPP], to access their PHI, to request restrictions or amendments, and to receive an accounting of disclosures), and privacy management. Although most of HIPAA's privacy requirements are accomplished through administrative and operational activities, EHR technology can assist in carrying out a number of the privacy standards.

For example, because patients have the right to request restrictions on who may use and disclose PHI, special access provisions should be in place that limit access to perhaps only the creator of the data or those few users given special authorization. In the paper environment, restrictions may have been accomplished by putting a special note on the chart cover, which may not be very effective when many individuals are involved in treating a patient and have access to all parts of the medical record. An EHR places highly effective controls on specific categories of information for specific categories of people who may access the information.

In another example, when patients request confidential communication, there needs to be a way to notify providers that an alternate address or phone number must be used to contact the patient concerning certain information. Again, a note on the chart cover may be the only available solution in the paper environment, but a flag that pops up on a computer screen or that automatically routes calls or correspondence would provide much greater assurance that the patient's request is being carried out. Many technical measures are available to help protect patient privacy.

HIPAA's security requirements are generally more technical than the privacy requirements, but they also require the establishment of policy on how to apply the technical tools. Using the example, again, of access controls, a policy will need to be established on how access is authorized, who establishes the access controls, and what each user is authorized to access. Access profiles are established as a matter of policy. For example, some hospitals decide to control nurse access to patient information by the floor on which the nurse is working. Within nursing, there may be controls on who may view information and who may view and enter information. Laboratory technicians may be given access only to those patients for whom a laboratory test order has been placed. Their access may be limited to viewing only certain information about the patient, such as diagnosis and current medications, and entering information only into the laboratory component of the information system. (Chapters 15 and 19 discuss HIPAA privacy and security requirements in additional detail.)

Retention and Admissibility

Retention and admissibility of information in the electronic environment is an important information management component. Healthcare organizations have long been concerned with record retention because paper records consume so many resources to manage and store. How long a record must be retained is determined by state statute and individual organizational requirements. Generally, states allow records to be destroyed seven to ten years from the time the record was created. The exception is minors' records, which must be kept until some period of time after the minors reach the age of majority as specified in the state. Some organizations prefer to keep their records longer, perhaps for educational or research purposes.

Electronic records, however, are easy to store. They consume very little space and, until recently (because we have been accumulating so much information), they have required little management. As a result, many organizations are keeping electronic records virtually forever. However, even absent the need to manage the location of information within a storage system, other issues need to be addressed.

One issue relates to the permanence and durability of the medium on which the electronic information is stored. Although paper can fade and deteriorate, it does so at a relatively known rate and usually is durable for a much longer period of time than the records are required to be kept. Because some of the computer media that EHRs are stored on are so new, their permanence may be unknown, or at least not trusted. Studies have been done on the permanence and durability of electronic media, but many are still uneasy about this.

As a result, contingency plans should be developed that address how and where EHRs are stored, where backups are stored, and how to periodically test their ability to be restored. Some organizations go so far as to make new copies of the backups periodically so that their permanence and durability are assured. HIM professionals should take an active role in managing retention of EHRs, just as they do in managing the retention of paper-based records.

Admissibility is another, related issue. Many courts admit into evidence paper records generated from EHR systems under best evidence rules. However, as the EHR becomes less a reflection of its former paper-based form and more a series of processes on data, what can be printed out from an EHR may not look very much like the paper-based medical records of the past. In a few cases, courts have permitted records to be retrieved and displayed from their EHR systems to be admissible as evidence. Thus, a computer that can access the EHR system must be brought into the court and possibly projected for viewing. HIM professionals need to keep current with what is permitted in their state. For the most part, however, there will be a transition period where it may be necessary to have adjustments made in the printout capability to generate an appropriate record to take to court. A "printable version" may be necessary. However, HIM professionals also need to keep an open mind that so long as the printout contains all the information, even though it may not appear exactly in the same form as in the paper record, it should be acceptable in court.

Future Directions in Information Technology

Every eighteen months, some form of the technology becomes obsolete or at least is replaced with new technology. When one considers the fate of the floppy disk as an example, it is clear that the future of HIM professionals is one of continuous need. Each change in technology presents new challenges that a background in health information management can support.

Exactly what the future holds is, of course, uncertain. General trends suggest that devices will get smaller and more user-friendly. Data processing will become more and more sophisticated. Today's speech and handwriting recognition are far better than they used to be and will likely get better. Natural language processing, where it is possible to extract discrete data from narrative data, also will continue to get better. In fact, all the effort put into screen design to capture discrete data will no longer be necessary if natural language processing really succeeds in the years to come.

Much of the new technology today is coming from Internet and Web-based technologies. The tools available to present dynamic, context-driven information to users are only just beginning to be invented. If it is feasible today to conduct a search on the Web for a specific topic that yields not only national, but also international, results in different languages, it is certainly conceivable that health information can be made available to any provider with a legitimate need to know and protected from individuals without a legitimate need for it.

Even as the promise of the future draws near, the challenges are ever present and must be addressed. Hackers with all sorts of new malware and spyware will continue to exploit systems, especially when humans make decisions not to protect them to their fullest extent or create workarounds to avoid hassles. In some cases, it seems as though systems are needed to protect humans from themselves. Still, the power of information technology will only continue to grow, especially in healthcare, which is one of the last frontiers for its adoption.

Check Your Understanding 4.6

Instructions: What term does each of the following statements define?

1. _____ Determination of the appropriate level of security controls given the organization's specific environment.

2. _____ Ensuring that appropriate backup, disaster recovery, and emergency mode operations are in place in the event of a disruption to data.

3. _____ A contract that ensures that persons not covered under HIPAA will protect health information.

4. _____ Proof of identity of an individual or entity.

5. _____ Control that stipulates who may have access to what data.

6. _____ Acceptance as evidence in a court that a document represents the actual document.

7. _____ A security service that allows data to be transmitted through a secure tunnel in the Internet.

8. _____ Auditing data for use in clinical decision support.

9. _____ The fact that data have not been altered or destroyed as they are saved on electronic media or transmitted electronically.

Real-World Case

Community Hospital has a single-vendor hospital information system (HIS) that provides typical financial and administrative information systems services, including laboratory, radiology, and pharmacy information systems and order-entry/results review. Other ancillary departments such as dietary, physical therapy, nursing, and others are not online. The hospital participates in a cardiac care registry but abstracts data from their paper charts to contribute to the registry. The health plans servicing the community are starting to offer incentives for use of health information technology if positive patient outcomes can be identified. Community hospital is considering acquiring a CPOE system to reduce medication errors.

Physicians who are affiliated with Community Hospital have expressed interest in acquiring EHR systems for their practices but are waiting for the hospital to make a vendor decision concerning CPOE. They believe that if they acquire an EHR from the same vendor as the hospital, they will be able to write orders from their offices for patients who are in the hospital, have better access to the information they need to monitor their patients, and be able to tap into other providers' EHR systems when they are covering in the emergency department.

The hospital and representative physicians are reviewing vendor products but are confused by what various vendors are telling them. One vendor has suggested that the hospital does not have the type of pharmacy information system that would support CPOE and thus would have to also buy a new pharmacy system. A vendor selling EDMS has suggested scanning and COLD feeding all the current chart forms from all provider settings into one repository so that they would be readily available when needed in an emergency. In the meantime, a couple of physicians purchased a stand-alone electronic prescribing device. They can send prescriptions to the major chain pharmacies in the community, but not to the community pharmacy, nor are they told they can get an interface written between the device and the clinical pharmacy in the hospital that would be needed for CPOE.

Summary

Many hospitals and physician offices are in the throes of analyzing their current information systems environment and assessing how to move forward to achieve an electronic health record (EHR). An EHR is a major investment, a complex undertaking, and involves all the organization's stakeholders, especially clinicians. The EHR also is touching others in the healthcare community, including payers, employers, and, most important, patients who are demanding EHR adoption to increase patient safety and quality healthcare. Many employers are looking for insurers to "incentivize" the adoption of the EHR and are starting to look at P4P or P4Q models that help support system acquisition.

Ensuring that data can be collected from all the various source systems and that there are applications to provide reminders and alerts when needed most by the clinician is a laudable goal and may "sound" easy. However, such an undertaking requires hardware and software that adhere to standards for interoperability and data comparability, as well as active engagement of all potential users, appropriate policies for adoption and use, and change management to use the computer to improve processes. Implementing an EHR is a clinical transformation; it truly changes how clinicians think and act.

Most hospitals cannot migrate to such systems overnight, which results in hybrid records that challenge the HIM professional's skills in managing the two worlds of paper and computer. Moreover, some are concerned that the electronic systems may not be receiving the data quality attention previously given paper records and which is even more acutely needed in the electronic environment. Such challenges point to the enhanced need for HIM professionals to understand and lead their organization's adoption of health information technology.

References

Advance Extra. 2003 (September). Point-of-care technologies. *ADVANCE for Health Information Executives.* Available online from advanceforhie.com.

AHIMA e-HIM Work Group on Health Information in a Hybrid Environment. 2003 (October). Complete medical record in a hybrid EHR environment. Available online from ahima.org.

AHIMA Work Group on Electronic Health Records Management. 2004 (October). The strategic importance of electronic health records management: Checklist for transition to the EHR. *Journal of American Health Information Management Association* 75(9):80C–E. Available online from ahima.org.

AHIMA Work Group on Electronic Health Records Management. 2004 (October). The strategic importance of electronic health records management, appendix A: Issues in electronic health record management. *Journal of American Health Information Management Association* 75(9): Web extra. Available online from ahima.org.

Amatayakul, Margret K. 2004. *Electronic Health Records: A Practical Guide for Professionals and Organization,* 2nd ed. Chicago: American Health Information Management Association.

Amatayakul, Margret K., and Steven S. Lazarus. 2005. *Electronic Health Records: Transforming Your Medical Practice.* Denver, CO: Medical Group Management Association.

American Health Information Management Association. 2005. The role of the personal health record in the EHR. *Journal of American Health Information Management Association* 76(7):64A-D.

American Health Information Management Association. 2003 (August 15). A vision of the e-HIM future. *Journal of American Health Information Management Association:* supplement. Available online from ahima.org.

American Health Information Management Association. 1998 (June). Practice brief: Data quality management model. *Journal of American Health Information Management Association* 69(6).

Andrew, William F., and Robert B. Bruegel. 2005 (May 1). An exclusive look at the EHR system market-place: 2005 EHR systems review. *ADVANCE for Health Information Executives.* Available online from advanceforhie.com.

Belmont, Carol. 2003 (July 1). White paper: Clinical documentation. HCT Project vol. 1. San Francisco: Montgomery Research.

Connecting for Health. 2005 (February). Linking health care information: Proposed methods for improving care and protecting privacy. Working Group on Accurately Linking Information for Health Care Quality and Safety. Available online from connectingforhealth.org.

Connecting for Health. 2004 (October). Financial, legal, and organizational approaches to achieving electronic connectivity in healthcare. Working Group on Financial, Organizational, and Legal Sustainability of Health Information Exchange. Available online from connectingforhealth.org.

Connecting for Health. 2003 (July 1). The Personal Health Working Group Final Report. Available online from connectingforhealth.org.

Evans, Celwyn C. 2005. Healthcare technology project ownership. *Journal of Healthcare Information Management* 19(1):34–38.

Feldbaum, James, and Karen Fuller. 2005 (July). CPOE has arrived: Will your institution lead, follow or just get out of the way? *Healthcare Informatics,* pp. 20–22. Available online from healthcare-informatics.com.

Gillespie, Greg. 2000 (January). Online clinical guidelines help trim costs. *Health Data Management,* pp. 39–53. Available online from healthdatamanagement.com.

Health and Human Services. 2005 (Oct. 6). Press release: HHS Awards Contracts to Advance Nationwide Interoperable Health Information Technology. Available online from hhs.gov/news/press/2005pres/20051006a.html.

Health Level Seven. EHR-System Functional Model, draft standard for trial use. Available online from hl7.org/ehr.

Monegain, B. 2005 (March). EHRs seen coming down in price. *Healthcare IT News.* Available online from healthcareitnews.com/story.cms?id=2705.

Kohn, Linda T., Corrigan, Janet M. and Donaldson, Molla S., editors. Committee on Quality of Health Care in America, Institute of Medicine. 2000. *To Err Is Human: Building a Safer Health System.* Washington, DC: The National Academies Press.

Institute of Medicine. 2003. *Key Capabilities of an Electronic Health Record System, Letter Report. Patient Safety: Achieving a New Standard of Care.* Washington, DC: The National Academies Press.

Institute of Medicine. 1997, 1991. *The Computer-Based Patient Record: An Essential Technology for Health Care.* Washington, DC: National Academies Press.

Lormand, Jared. 2005 (August). Bringing patient safety technology to the bedside. *Health Management Technology,* pp. 24-27. Available online from healthmgttech.com.

Miller, Randolph A., et al. 2005 (July/August). Clinical decision support and electronic prescribing systems: A time for responsible thought and action. *Journal of the American Medical Informatics Association* 12(4):403–409.

National Committee on Vital and Health Statistics. 2001 (December 19). Information for health: A strategy for building the national health information infrastructure. Available online from ncvhs.hhs.gov/reports.

President's Information Technology Advisory Committee. 2004 (June). Revolutionizing health care through information technology. Available online from nitrd.gov.

Standards for Privacy of Individually Identifiable Health Information and Security Standards for the Protection of Electronic Protected Health Information, 45 CFR Parts 160 and 164. Health Insurance Portability and Accountability Act of 1996.

Thompson, Tommy G., and David J. Brailer. 2004 (July 21). The decade of health information technology: Delivering consumer-centric and information-rich health care, framework for strategic action. Available online from hhs.gov/healthit/framework.html.

Westin, Alan F. 2005 (July/August). Public attitudes toward electronic health records. America's Health Insurance Plans. Available online from ahip.org.

Chapter 5
Healthcare Data Sets

Kathleen M. LaTour, MA, RHIA, FAHIMA

Learning Objectives

- To describe the purpose of healthcare data sets
- To explain the importance of healthcare data sets and standards
- To identify the common health information standardized data sets
- To explain the need for electronic data and data interchange standards
- To explain the healthcare data needs in an electronic environment
- To discuss how data standards are developed
- To identify well-known standards that support electronic health record (EHR) systems
- To discuss how data standards support the development of EHR systems
- To identify prominent health information standards development organizations
- To recognize the impact of the Health Insurance Portability and Accountability Act of 1996 (HIPAA) on the development of health informatics standards
- To explain the relationship of core data elements to healthcare informatics standards in electronic environments
- To describe current federal initiatives to support EHR development and to create a national health information network

Key Terms

American College of Radiology-National Electrical Manufacturers Association (ACR-NEMA)

American National Standards Institute (ANSI)

American Society for Testing and Materials (ASTM)

ASTM Standard E1384-02a

Community Health Dimension (CHD)

Consolidated Health Informatics initiative (CHI)

Continuity of care record (CCR)

Core data elements/core content

Core measure

Data dictionary

Data elements

Data Elements for Emergency Department Systems (DEEDS)

Data set

Department of Health and Human Services (HHS)

Digital Imaging and Communication in Medicine (DICOM)

Electronic data interchange (EDI)

Essential Medical Data Set (EMDS)

Extensible markup language (XML)

Health Plan Employer Data and Information Set (HEDIS)

Healthcare provider dimension (HPD)

Health information exchange (HIE)

Healthcare information standards

Hospital discharge abstract system

Identifier standards

Inpatient

Institute of Electrical and Electronics Engineers (IEEE)

Medicare prospective payment system

Minimum Data Set for Long Term Care-Version 2.0 (MDS 2.0)

National Alliance for Health Information Technology (NAHIT)

National Center for Health Statistics (NCHS)

National Committee on Vital and Health Statistics (NCVHS)

National Information Infrastructure-Health Information Network Program (NII-HIN)

National provider identifier (NPI)

Office of the National Coordinator of Health Information Technology (ONC)

ORYX initiative

Outcomes and Assessment Information Set (OASIS)

Outpatient

Personal health dimension (PHD)

Privacy standards

Security standards

Social Security number (SSN)

Standards development organizations (SDOs)

Structure and content standards

Transaction standards

Uniform Ambulatory Care Data Set (UACDS)

Uniform Hospital Discharge Data Set (UHDDS)

Unique physician identification number (UPIN)

Unique identification number

Vocabulary standards

Introduction

Data and information pertaining to individuals who use healthcare services are collected in virtually every setting where healthcare is delivered. As noted in other chapters, data represent basic facts and measurements. In healthcare, these facts usually describe specific characteristics of individual patients. The term *data* is plural. Although the singular form is *datum,* the term that is frequently used to describe a single fact or measurement is **data element.** For example, age, gender, insurance company, and blood pressure are all data elements concerning a patient. The term *information* refers to data that have been collected, combined, analyzed, interpreted, and/or converted into a form that can be used for specific purposes. In other words, data represent facts; information represents meaning.

In healthcare settings, data are stored in the individual's health record whether that record is in paper or electronic format. The numerous data elements in the health record are then combined, analyzed, and interpreted by the patient's physician and other clinicians. For example, test results are combined with the physician's observations and the patient's description of his or her symptoms to form information about the disease or condition that is affecting the patient. Physicians use both data and information to diagnose diseases, develop treatment plans, assess the effectiveness of care, and determine the patient's prognosis.

Data about patients can be extracted from individual health records and combined as aggregate data. Aggregate data are used to develop information about groups of patients. For example, data about all of the patients who suffered an acute myocardial infarction during a specific time period could be collected in a database. From the aggregate data, it would be possible to identify common characteristics that might predict the course of the disease or provide information about the most effective way to treat it. Ultimately, research using aggregated data might be used for disease prevention. For example, researchers identified the link between smoking and lung cancer by analyzing aggregate data about patients with a diagnosis of lung cancer; smoking cessation programs grew from the identification of the causal effect of smoking on lung cancer and a variety of other conditions.

History of Healthcare Data Collection

The first known efforts to collect and use healthcare data to produce meaningful statistical profiles date back to the seventeenth century. In the early 1600s, Captain John Graunt gathered data on the common causes of death in London. He called his study the Bills of Mortality. However, few systematic efforts were undertaken to collect statistical data about the incidence and prevalence of disease until the mid-twentieth century, when technological developments made it possible to collect and analyze large amounts of healthcare data.

Modern efforts at standardizing healthcare data began in the 1960s. At that time, healthcare facilities began to use computers to process larger amounts of data than could be handled manually. The goal was to make comparisons among data from multiple providers. It soon became evident that healthcare organizations needed to use standardized, uniform data definitions in order to arrive at meaningful data comparisons.

The first data standardization efforts focused generally on hospitals and specifically on hospital discharge data and the intent of the efforts was to standardize definition of key data elements commonly collected in hospitals. Discharge data were collected in **hospital discharge abstract systems.** These systems used databases compiled from aggregate data on all the patients discharged from a particular facility. The need to compare uniform discharge data from one hospital to the next led to the development of **data sets,** or lists of recommended data elements with uniform definitions.

Today, hospitals and other healthcare organizations collect more data and develop more information than ever before. Moreover, data and information from the health records of individual patients are used for more purposes than ever before. The demand for information is coming from users within the organizations as well as from external users such as third-party payers, government agencies, accreditation organizations, and others. The extensive use of information within and across organizational boundaries demands standards that promote interoperable electronic interchange of data and information. Information standards are critical in the migration to electronic health records (EHRs), as described in chapter 4.

Data Sets in the Electronic Environment

The data sets originally developed to support uniform data collection are inadequate for an electronic environment, and many public and private organizations have been actively engaged in the process of developing **healthcare information standards** to support EHR development and information interchange. Healthcare information standards development is a dynamic process that evolves on a continuous basis as key players in the standards development community negotiate, refine, and revise standards. The critical importance of healthcare information standards has been recognized in recent federal initiatives including the **Consolidated Health Informatics** (CHI) **initiatives** as well as efforts of the **Office of the National Coordinator of Health Information Technology** (ONC).

According to the **National Committee on Vital and Health Statistics** (NCVHS) in its initial 2000 report titled *Toward a National Health Information Infrastructure,* "if information in multiple locations is to be searched, shared, and synthesized when needed, we will need agreed-upon information guardians that can exchange data with each other . . . we will need equitable rules of data exchange so that competitors (within or between healthcare provider systems, health information management companies, or health Web services) will be willing to connect and share data" (NCVHS 2000).

Developing Standardized Data Sets and Standards

This chapter describes the initial efforts at developing standardized data sets for use in different types of healthcare settings, including acute care, ambulatory care, long-term care, and home care. It explores the recent national initiatives related to interoperability and connectivity of healthcare information systems that will support widespread implementation of EHRs. It also explains the work of developing a national health information network that will improve patient care, increase safety, and assist clinical and administrative decision making.

It is essential that the HIM professional understand the purpose, content, and importance of healthcare data sets and standards. HIM professionals work with many of these data sets on the job. In the years to come, the roles of the HIM professional will be influenced and likely change as standards continue to develop.

Theory into Practice

In a large Midwestern health system, the director of health information services leads the system's clinical data standards committee. The committee recently decided to develop a **data dictionary** as a first step toward implementing an EHR system.

Data dictionaries include the following components:

- A list of data elements collected in individual health records

- Definitions of the data elements

- Descriptions of the attributes of each data element

- Specifications for the size of the data field in the information system

- Descriptions of the data views to be accessed by various users

The committee began the process with what it considered to be a simple data element: patient gender. Committee members looked at the two standard references for patient data sets in acute care settings: the **Uniform Hospital Discharge Data Set** (UHDDS) and the **Uniform Ambulatory Care Data Set** (UACDS). Both data sets indicated that gender should be recorded as either "male" or "female." However, this either-or choice presented a problem.

The healthcare system included a number of hospitals and clinics. One of the hospitals offered a gender re-identification program that treated patients who were in the process of transitioning from one gender to the other. Another hospital provided neonatal intensive care services for a large geographical region. Some of the infants treated in the neonatal intensive care unit had been born with congenital defects that made it difficult to determine their gender.

During discussions of the problem, the clinical laboratory representative on the committee stressed the importance of documenting the gender of every patient. She explained that the normal range for most laboratory tests varies by gender. This information was a surprise to many committee members.

After the committee's initial discussion, the health information management director agreed to research other data sets and standards. He found that recent healthcare information standards for electronic and computer-based patient records recommended using four gender descriptors: male, female, undetermined, and unknown.

The committee decided to adopt the four descriptors for gender. In the data collection process, if the term *undetermined* or *unknown* were selected, the individual doing data entry would be referred to another screen that would explain the data choice in more detail and include another data element to describe the patient's genitalia.

The challenges the committee faced in defining this relatively simple data element raised its awareness of how difficult it would be to adequately define every data element to be included in the new EHR system. The committee members gathered information on every available healthcare data set and healthcare information standard and carefully compared the data definitions recommended. They discovered that implementation of the EHR system would be a huge project. However, they were committed to the process because it would improve the quality of the data collected in the system. The collection of consistent, reliable, and valid data would improve administrative and clinical decision making and make it possible to perform meaningful performance improvement comparisons.

Standardized Healthcare Data Sets

The idea of data standardization became widely accepted during the 1960s. Under the leadership of the **National Center for Health Statistics** (NCHS) and the National Committee on Vital and Health Statistics (NCVHS) in collaboration with other organizations, data sets were developed for a variety of healthcare settings. Data sets for acute care, long-term care, and ambulatory care were the first to be created. Healthcare data sets have two purposes. The first is to identify the data elements that should be collected for each patient. The second is to provide uniform definitions for common terms. The use of uniform definitions ensures that data collected from a variety of healthcare settings will share a standard definition.

Standardizing data elements and definitions makes it possible to compare the data collected at different facilities. For example, when data are standardized, the term *admission* means the same thing at City Hospital and at University Hospital. Because both hospitals define *admission* in the same way, they can be compared with each other on such things as number of admissions and percentage of occupancy. The **National Alliance for Health Information Technology** (NAHIT) has compiled a comprehensive list of current health-related standards in its Alliance Standards Directory. Available online at hitsdir.org, the directory overviews the extent of the many standards used in the healthcare industry.

Comparison data are used for many purposes, including external accreditation, internal performance improvement, and statistical and research studies. However, data sets are not meant to limit the number of data elements that can be collected. Most healthcare organizations collect additional data elements that have meaning for their specific administrative and clinical operations.

The following are data sets that the HIT professional will most likely encounter in his or her daily work.

Uniform Hospital Discharge Data Set

In 1969, a conference on hospital discharge abstract systems was sponsored jointly by NCHS, the National Center for Health Services Research and Development, and Johns Hopkins University. Conference participants recommended that all short-term general hospitals in the United States collect a minimum set of patient-specific data elements. They also recommended that these data elements be included in all databases compiled from hospital discharge abstract systems. They called the list of patient-specific data items the Uniform Hospital Discharge Data Set (UHDDS).

The purpose of the UHDDS is to list and define a set of common, uniform data elements. The data elements are collected from the health records of every hospital **inpatient** and later abstracted from the health record and included in national databases. Most short-term, general hospitals in the U.S. collect patient-specific data in the format recommended by the UHDDS.

In 1974, the federal government adopted the UHDDS as the standard for collecting data for the Medicare and Medicaid programs. When the Prospective Payment Act was enacted in 1983, UHDDS definitions were incorporated into the rules and regulations for implementing diagnosis-related groups (DRGs). A key component was the incorporation of the definitions of principal diagnosis, principal procedure, and other significant procedures into the DRG algorithms. As a result, accurate DRG assignment depends on accurate selection and coding of the principal diagnosis and principal procedure and the appropriate sequencing of other significant diagnoses and procedures. NCVHS revised the UHDDS in 1984, and the new UHDDS was adopted for all federal health programs in 1986.

The UHDDS has been revised several times since 1986. The current version includes the recommended data elements shown in figure 5.1, pp. 164–65.

Uniform Ambulatory Care Data Set

Ambulatory care includes medical and surgical care provided to patients who return to their homes on the same day they receive care. The care is provided in physicians' offices, medical clinics, same-day surgery centers, **outpatient** hospital clinics and diagnostic departments, emergency treatment centers, and hospital emergency departments. Patients who receive ambulatory care services in hospital-based clinics and departments are referred to as outpatients.

Since the 1980s, the number and the length of inpatient hospitalizations have gone down dramatically. At the same time, the number of healthcare procedures performed in ambulatory settings has gone up. There are several reasons for this trend, including:

- Technological improvements in diagnostic and therapeutic procedures and the development of short-acting anesthetics have made it possible to perform many medical and surgical procedures in ambulatory facilities. Surgical procedures that once required inpatient hospitalization and long recovery periods now are being performed in same-day surgery centers.

- Third-party payers have extended coverage to include most procedures performed on an outpatient basis.

- The **Medicare prospective payment system** limits reimbursement for inpatient care and, in effect, encourages the use of ambulatory and/or outpatient care as an alternative to more costly inpatient services.

Like hospitals, ambulatory care organizations depend on having accurate data and information. A standardized data set to guide the content and structure of ambulatory health records and data collection systems in ambulatory care was needed.

Figure 5.1.   UHDDS data elements

Data Element	Definition/Descriptor
01. Personal identification	The unique number assigned to each patient within a hospital that distinguishes the patient and his or her hospital record from all others in that institution.
02. Date of birth	Month, day, and year of birth. Capture of the full four-digit year of birth is recommended.
03. Sex	Male or female
04. Race and ethnicity	04a. Race American Indian/Eskimo/Aleut Asian or Pacific Islander Black White Other race Unknown 04b. Ethnicity Spanish origin/Hispanic Non-Spanish origin/Non-Hispanic Unknown
05. Residence	Full address of usual residence Zip code (nine digits, if available) Code for foreign residence
06. Hospital identification	A unique institutional number across data collection systems. The Medicare provider number is the preferred hospital identifier.
07. Admission date	Month, day, and year of admission.
08. Type of admission	Scheduled: Arranged with admissions office at least 24 hours prior to admission Unscheduled: All other admissions
09. Discharge date	Month, day, and year of discharge.
10 & 11. Physician identification • Attending physician • Operating physician	The Medicare unique physician identification number (UPIN) is the preferred method of identifying the attending physician and operating physician(s) because it is uniform across all data systems.
12. Principal diagnosis	The condition established after study to be chiefly responsible for occasioning the admission of the patient to the hospital for care.
13. Other diagnoses	All conditions that coexist at the time of admission or that develop subsequently or that affect the treatment received and/or the length of stay. Diagnoses that relate to an earlier episode and have no bearing on the current hospital stay are to be excluded.
14. Qualifier for other diagnoses	A qualifier is given for each diagnosis coded under "other diagnoses" to indicate whether the onset of the diagnosis preceded or followed admission to the hospital. The option "uncertain" is permitted.
15. External cause-of-injury code	The ICD-9-CM code for the external cause of an injury, poisoning, or adverse effect (commonly referred to as an E code). Hospitals should complete this item whenever there is a diagnosis of an injury, poisoning, or adverse effect.

Figure 5.1. *(Continued)*

Data Element	Definition/Descriptor
16. Birth weight of neonate	The specific birth weight of a newborn, preferably recorded in grams.
17. Procedures and dates	All significant procedures are to be reported. A significant procedure is one that is: • Surgical in nature, or • Carries a procedural risk, or • Carries an anesthetic risk, or • Requires specialized training. The date of each significant procedure must be reported. When more than one procedure is reported, the principal procedure must be designated. The principal procedure is one that is performed for definitive treatment rather than one performed for diagnostic or exploratory purposes or was necessary to take care of a complication. If there appear to be two procedures that are principal, then the one most closely related to the principal diagnosis should be selected as the principal procedure. The UPIN must be reported for the person performing the principal procedure.
18. Disposition of the patient	• Discharged to home (excludes those patients referred to home health service) • Discharged to acute care hospital • Discharged to nursing facility • Discharged home to be under the care of a home health service (including a hospice) • Discharged to other healthcare facility • Left against medical advice • Alive, other; or alive, not stated • Died All categories for primary and other sources are: • Blue Cross/Blue Shield • Other health insurance companies • Other liability insurance • Medicare • Medicaid • Worker's Compensation • Self-insured employer plan • Health maintenance organization (HMO) • CHAMPUS • CHAMPVA • Other government payers • Self-pay • No charge (free, charity, special research, teaching) • Other
19. Patient's expected source of payment	Primary source Other sources
20. Total charges	All charges billed by the hospital for this hospitalization. Professional charges for individual patient care by physicians are excluded.

In 1989, NCVHS approved the Uniform Ambulatory Care Data Set (UACDS). The committee recommended its use in every facility where ambulatory care is delivered. Several of the data elements that make up the UACDS are similar to those used in the UHDDS. For example, the UACDS data elements that describe the personal identifier, residence, date of birth, gender, and race/ethnicity of the patient are the same as the definitions in the UHDDS. The reason for keeping the same demographic data elements is to make it easier to compare data for inpatients and ambulatory patients in the same facility.

The UACDS also includes data elements specific to ambulatory care, such as the reason for the encounter with the healthcare provider. Additionally, it includes optional data elements to describe the patient's living arrangements and marital status. These data elements (shown in figure 5.2) are unique to the UACDS. Ambulatory care practitioners need information about the living conditions of their patients because patients and their families often need to manage at-home nursing care (such as activity restrictions after a surgical procedure). Hospital staff members provide such nursing services in acute care settings.

The goal of the UACDS is to improve data comparison in ambulatory and outpatient care settings. It provides uniform definitions that help providers analyze patterns of care. The data elements in the UACDS are those most likely to be needed by a variety of users. Unlike the UHDDS, the UACDS has not been incorporated into federal regulations. Therefore, it is a recommended, rather than a required, data set. In practical terms, it has been subsumed by other data definition efforts, most notably the **core data elements** recommended as part of the national health information network (NHIN) described later in this chapter.

Minimum Data Set for Long-Term Care and Resident Assessment Protocols

Uniform data collection is likewise important in the long-term care setting. Long-term care incorporates the healthcare services provided in residential facilities for individuals who are unable to live independently because of a chronic illness or disability. Long-term care facilities also provide dietary and social services as well as housing and nursing care. To participate in the Medicare and Medicaid programs, long-term care facilities must develop a comprehensive functional assessment for every resident. From this assessment, a nursing home resident's plan of care is developed.

The **Minimum Data Set for Long-Term Care-Version 2.0** (MDS 2.0) is a federally mandated standard assessment form used to collect demographic and clinical data on nursing home residents. It consists of a core set of screening and assessment elements based on common definitions. To meet federal requirements, long-term care facilities must complete an MDS for every resident at the time of admission and at designated reassessment points throughout the resident's stay.

The MDS uses some of the same data elements and definitions used in other data sets. However, it is far more extensive and includes more clinical data than either the UHDDS or the UACDS. The data collected via the MDS are used to develop care plans for residents and to document placement at the appropriate level of care.

The MDS organizes data according to twenty main categories. Each category includes a structured list of choices and/or responses. The use of structured lists automatically standardizes the data that are collected. The major categories of data collected in the MDS include:

1. Demographic information
2. Identification and background information

Figure 5.2.   UACDS data elements

Data Element	Definition/Descriptor
Provider identification, address, type of practice	Provider identification: Include the full name of the provider as well as the unique physician identification number (UPIN). Address: The complete address of the provider's office. In cases where the provider has multiple offices, the location of the usual or principal place of practice should be given. Profession: • Physician including specialty or field of practice • Other (specify)
Place of encounter	Specify the location of the encounter: • Private office • Clinic or health center • Hospital outpatient department • Hospital emergency department • Other (specify)
Reason for encounter	Includes, but is not limited to, the patient's complaints and symptoms reflecting his or her own perception of needs, provided verbally or in writing by the patient at the point of entry into the healthcare system, or the patient's own words recorded by an intermediary or provider at that time.
Diagnostic services	Includes all diagnostic services of any type.
Problem, diagnosis, or assessment	Describes the provider's level of understanding and the interpretation of the patient's reasons for the encounter and all conditions requiring treatment or management at the time of the encounter.
Therapeutic services	List by name all services done or ordered: • Medical (including drug therapy) • Surgical • Patient education
Preventive services	List by name all preventive services and procedures performed at the time of the encounter.

Disposition	The provider's statement of the next step(s) in the care of the patient. At a minimum, the following classification is suggested:
	1. No follow-up planned
	2. Follow-up planned
	  • Return when necessary
	  • Return to the current provider at a specified time
	  • Telephone follow-up
	  • Returned to referring provider
	  • Referred to other provider
	  • Admit to hospital
	  • Other

3. Cognitive patterns

4. Communication/hearing patterns

5. Vision patterns

6. Mood and behavior patterns

7. Psychosocial well-being

8. Physical functioning and structural problems

9. Continence in past fourteen days

10. Disease diagnoses

11. Health conditions

12. Oral/nutritional status

13. Oral/dental status

14. Skin condition

15. Activity pursuit patterns

16. Medications

17. Special treatments and procedures

18. Discharge potential and overall status

19. Assessment information

20. Therapy supplement for Medicare PPS

The data collected by the MDS are used to develop a RAP (resident assessment proto-col) summary for each resident. The MDS provides a structured way to organize resident information and develop a resident care plan. Problems identified through the assessment process are documented, and a RAP is triggered. For each triggered RAP, the facility must describe the following factors:

- Nature of the condition (may include presence or lack of objective data and sub-jective complaints)

- Complications and risk factors that affect the decision to proceed to care planning

- Factors that must be considered in developing individualized care plan interventions

- Need for referrals/further evaluation by appropriate healthcare professionals

Nursing home personnel use the data from the MDS and RAP to plan, carry out, and assess the care given to individual residents. Other practice settings, such as rehabilitation and post–acute care, are considering versions of the MDS for use in patient assessment, but to date none has been implemented. The **Department of Health and Human Services** (HHS) is in the process of developing MDS Version 3.0. The original target date for implementation was 2003, but as of mid-2005, Version 3.0 had not been implemented and no new implementation date had been published.

Because the MDS is used nationwide to collect data about residents in long-term care facilities, the data can and will be used as a basis for identifying and assessing resident safety and quality improvement activities in nursing homes. For example, MDS data can give valuable information about the incidence of falls and their impact on the care of nursing home residents. From those data, prevention measures can be developed and implemented to address a common and significant problem in elderly care.

Outcomes Assessment Information Set

In 1999, the Health Care Financing Administration (HCFA) (renamed the Centers for Medicare and Medicaid Services [CMS]) implemented a standardized data set for use in the home health industry. The **Outcomes and Assessment Information Set** (OASIS) is designed to gather data about Medicare beneficiaries who are receiving services from a home health agency. OASIS includes a set of core data items that are collected on all adult home health patients. The data are used in measuring patient outcomes to assess the quality of home healthcare services. Under the prospective payment program for home health, OASIS data are used as the basis of reimbursement for home heath services.

OASIS data are grouped into the following categories:

- Demographics and Patient History
- Living Arrangements
- Supportive Assistance
- Respiratory
- Neurological
- Psychological
- Integument
- Pain
- Activities of Daily Living (ADLs)/Instrumental Activities of Daily Living (IADLs)
- Medications
- Elimination Status
- General Information
- Emergent Care

Data collected through OASIS are used to assess the patient's ability to be discharged or transferred from home care services. They also are used to evaluate the quality and outcome of services given to the patient.

Data Elements for Emergency Department Systems

Emergency and trauma care in the United States are very sophisticated. Emergency services represent a large part of healthcare delivery. As services increase, it is more and more important to collect relevant aggregate data about emergency and trauma care. Many states require the reporting of trauma cases to state agencies.

In 1997, the Centers for Disease Control and Prevention (CDC) through its National Center for Injury Prevention and Control (NCIPC) published a data set called **Data Elements for Emergency Department Systems** (DEEDS). The purpose of this data set is to support the uniform collection of data in hospital-based emergency departments and to reduce incompatibilities in emergency department records.

DEEDS recommends the collection of 156 data elements in hospitals that offer emergency care services. As with the UHDDS and UACDS, this data set contains recommendations on both the content and the structure of the data elements to be collected. The data are organized into the following eight sections:

- Patient identification data

- Facility and practitioner identification data

- Emergency department payment data

- Emergency department arrival and first-assessment data

- Emergency department history and physical examination data

- Emergency department procedure and result data

- Emergency department medication data

- Emergency department disposition and diagnosis data

DEEDS incorporates national standards for **electronic data interchange** (EDI), so its implementation in an EHR system can make possible communication and integration with other information systems (NCIPC 1997).

Essential Medical Data Set

The **Essential Medical Data Set** (EMDS) was created as a complement to DEEDS. It was developed as part of the **National Information Infrastructure-Health Information Network Program** (NII-HIN) in 1997. EMDS gives healthcare providers a concise medical history data set for each individual patient. The goal is to enhance the effectiveness of emergency care. EMDS is different from DEEDS in that DEEDS is designed to collect data about a specific emergency encounter whereas EMDS is designed to create a health history for an individual patient.

EMDS is intended for use in EHR systems. During the course of an emergency, the emergency department's information system queries a data repository for the patient's past medical history. Documentation for the visit is recorded according to the DEEDS format, and the data are sent to a regional data repository when the emergency care episode is complete.

Emergency care often has a critical impact on patient survival. Therefore, it is important to collect standardized, comparable data. These data then can be used to assess the effectiveness of treatment modalities, response time, and patient survival rates.

Trauma registries and statewide trauma database systems have grown incrementally over the past several years. State departments of public health as well as the federal agencies involved in oversight of emergency care are interested in statistical data on the efficacy of emergency treatment. Collecting standardized data in the emergency care system is fundamental to meaningful analysis of information about emergency care.

Standardized Data Collection Efforts

The following three initiatives do not represent the development and dissemination of information standards, but each does collect and use standardized data in assessing utilization, quality, and cost of healthcare for selected populations. As such, they are worth addressing in this chapter.

Health Plan Employer Data and Information Set

The **Health Plan Employer Data and Information Set** (HEDIS) is sponsored by NCQA. HEDIS is a set of standard performance measures designed to provide healthcare purchasers and consumers with the information they need to compare the performance of managed healthcare plans.

HEDIS is designed to collect administrative, claims, and health record review data. It collects standardized data about specific health-related conditions or issues so that the success of various treatment plans can be assessed and compared. HEDIS data form the basis of performance improvement (PI) efforts for health plans. They also are used to develop physician profiles. The goal of physician profiling is to positively influence physician practice patterns.

HEDIS contains more than fifty measures related to conditions such as heart disease, cancer, diabetes, asthma, chlamydia infection, smoking cessation, and menopause counseling. It includes data related to patient outcomes and data about the treatment process used by the clinician in treating the patient.

Standardized HEDIS data elements are abstracted from health records in clinics and hospitals. The health record data are combined with enrollment and claims data and analyzed according to HEDIS specifications.

An example of a focus area for HEDIS is diabetes care and treatment. Other examples of HEDIS clinical measures include:

- Adolescent immunizations
- Smoking cessation programs
- Antidepressant medication management
- Breast cancer screening
- Cholesterol screening after a heart attack
- Prenatal care during the first trimester

Health plans often release data from HEDIS studies publicly to document substantial positive effects on the health of their clients. Results are compared over time and with data from other sources. From the data, health plans determine opportunities for PI and develop potential interventions.

HEDIS is an example of a population-based data collection tool. It illustrates the need for developing standardized data definitions and uniform collection methods. It also emphasizes the importance of data quality management.

Core Measures for ORYX

The Joint Commission on Accreditation of Healthcare Organizations (JCAHO) is one of the largest users of healthcare data and information. Its primary function is the accreditation of hospitals and other healthcare organizations. In 1997, JCAHO introduced the **ORYX initiative** to integrate outcomes data and other performance measurement data into its accreditation processes. (The initiative was named ORYX after an African animal that can be thought of as a different kind of zebra.) The goal of the initiative is to promote a comprehensive, continuous, data-driven accreditation process for healthcare facilities.

The ORYX initiative uses nationally standardized performance measures to improve the safety and quality of healthcare. The program's objectives include:

- Establishing a national comparative database to support benchmarking, health services research, and internal PI activities

- Fostering standardization of performance measures

- Encouraging the use of evidence-based treatment protocols

The goal of the ORYX initiative is to develop data sets for each core measure so that data collection can be standardized among all healthcare facilities. The **core measures** are based on selected diagnoses/conditions such as diabetes mellitus, the outcomes of which can be improved by standardizing care. They include the minimum number of data elements needed to provide an accurate and reliable measure of performance. Core measures rely on data elements that are readily available or already collected. Current ORYX core measure studies are explored in chapter 17.

National Health Information Network

As discussed above, the standardized collection of common data elements can provide valuable information about the effectiveness of interventions and treatments for specific diseases. Healthcare providers are able compare their success rates with those of other providers to determine areas for performance improvement. This type of analysis can provide critical information that will eventually have a positive impact on clinical outcomes.

In 1998, NCVHS produced a concept paper that discussed a conceptual model of a nationwide network of health information (NCVHS 1998). In 2001, NCVHS began to explore the feasibility of a national health information infrastructure (NHII) that would allow the electronic exchange of health information. (As the initiative developed, the term *national health information network* [NHIN] replaced the term *national health information infrastructure* [NHII].) The goal of the initiative was to offer a technology solution that would increase patient safety, reduce medical errors, increase efficiency and effectiveness of health care, and contain costs (Mon 2005).

The initiative launched an industry-wide discussion on how to exchange information electronically in a secure and standardized fashion (Mon 2005). The need for standards to facilitate the definition, collection, exchange, and use of data and information was obvious. However, there are diverging opinions on how to accomplish the objective and, to date, there is no consensus on a single method of developing this information network. However, many key public and private organizations are actively working on making the concept of a national health information network a reality.

In late 2004, ONC used input from the healthcare industry on how to develop and adopt national **health information exchange** (HIE). ONC issued a series of three-year government contracts focused on the four key areas identified by the healthcare industry as key to HIE development: EHR certification, data standards, NHIN architecture, and privacy and security (Carol 2005). In November 2005, contracts were awarded to public and private groups to address three of the key areas:

- A contract was awarded to the Certification Commission for Health Information Technology (CCHIT) to develop criteria and evaluation processes to certify EHRs and the infrastructure or network components through which they interoperate.

- The **American National Standards Institute** (ANSI) was awarded a contract to convene the National Health Information Technology Panel to bring together U.S. standards organizations and others to develop, test, and evaluate a process for bringing together a set of health information technology (IT) standards that will support interoperability among healthcare software applications, especially EHRs.

- The Health Information Security and Privacy Collaboration was charged with working collaboratively with the National Governors Association and industry experts to develop privacy and security solutions.

An additional contract to develop a NHIN architecture will be awarded at a later time. (For more information visit www.hhs.gov/news/press/2005press/20051006a.html.)

According to the NCVHS report titled *Information for Health: A Strategy for Building the National Health Information Infrastructure,* the NHII includes not just technologies but, more important, values, practices, relationships, laws, standards, systems, and applications that support all facets of individual health, healthcare, and public health (NCVHS 2001). The report stresses how important national health information standards are in supporting connectivity and interoperability.

Past efforts at standards development have been diverse with little industry leadership and little federal influence. There has been minimal coordination of efforts among **standards development organizations** (SDOs). This has resulted in fragmented and, in some cases, competing standards. Under the NHIN initiative, efforts are focused on creating standards that define a universal language of health information and to maintain that universality as NHIN development and EHR implementation move forward. A key principle of the NHIN is that the ideal is to collect information only once at the point of care. This is an important principle because many users need data for many purposes both during and after the episode of care.

As noted in chapter 4, efforts in NHIN development led to President George W. Bush issuing Executive Order 13335 in April 2004. This order called for widespread interoperable EHRs within ten years and established ONC. The directive to the national coordinator was to develop and implement a strategic plan to guide the nationwide implementation of interoperable health information technology (HIT) in both the public and private sectors (Thompson and Brailer 2004). ONC was given responsibility for moving forward the already existing NHII initiative; in fact, it was ONC that replaced the term *NHII* with the more contemporary term *NHIN.*

As currently envisioned, the NHIN will be composed of a "network of networks" that will be built incrementally using Internet technology with particular emphasis on data confidentiality and security. A key element is that the network is private and secure and built on patient control and authorization. Personal information would remain with the healthcare provider and be accessed and exchanged only as needed and with proper authorization (Kloss 2005a).

The NHIN has supported and, in fact, given impetus to the development of local or regional health information organizations (RHIOs) as discussed in chapter 4. RHIOs also are referred to as regional health information networks (RHINs), community health information networks, and, most recently, health information exchanges (HIEs). At the time of this writing, it appeared that the term *subnetwork organization* (SNO) might replace the term *RHIO*. An RHIO is a networked community (with the community defined at the local or regional level) that includes physician offices, hospitals, nursing homes, pharmacies, and, in some cases, payers, vendors, and other healthcare-related agencies. The purpose of an RHIO is to give regional healthcare providers access to clinical information for all patients in the defined region across a decentralized technology environment. As noted in chapter 4, there are several models for RHIOs, but no one accepted model. To date, each RHIO has developed in response to local and regional needs and each operates independently, in both choice of network design and access model. The goals of RHIOs are consistent with those of NHINs: improved quality of care, increased patient safety, reduction of medical errors, improved efficiency, and cost savings.

NHIN Dimensions and Core Data Elements

To support the development of networked health information systems, NHIN defines three dimensions of the infrastructure that provide a means for conceptualizing the capture, storage, communication, processing, and presentation of information for each group of information users. A set of core data elements has been developed for each dimension as part of the NCVHS report titled *Toward a National Health Information Infrastructure* (NCVHS 2000). The three dimensions are as follows:

- **Personal health dimension (PHD):** Core content of the PHD will be controlled by the individual in both the initial input of data and the ability to edit personal data. The issues relating to patient input of data into the provider record and the ability to edit the provider record is still under discussion in the industry and no final recommendations have been agreed on. Individuals will select data elements that are relevant to their specific age, gender, health history, health and wellness concerns, and other factors. The core content in table 5.1 represents a minimum data set; the intent of NHIN is to develop standards for a personal health record and a data dictionary that supports a consistent format that will allow healthcare providers to access the data as needed and authorized by the individual.

- **Healthcare provider dimension (HPD):** The HPD includes information captured during the patient care process and concurrently integrates it with clinical guidelines, protocols, and selected information the provider is authorized to access from the personal health record, as well as information from the CHD that is relevant to the patient's care (NCVHS 2000). The HPD would be useful to providers in any and all care settings. Core content of the HPD is shown in table 5.2.

- **Community health dimension (CHD):** The CHD acknowledges the importance of population-based health data and resources that are necessary to improve public health. These data will help public health professionals to identify public health threats, assess population health, focus programs and policies on well-defined health problems, inform and educate individuals about health issues, evaluate programs and services, conduct research to address health issues, and perform other public health services (NCVHS 2000). Core content of the CHD is identified in table 5.3. In subsequent publications this is also referred to as the population health dimension.

These dimensions are graphically represented in figure 4.4, page 127.

According to the Nova Scotia Department of Health, core data sets are "sharable electronic patient demographic and essential 'persistent' clinical information necessary to provide informed medical care" (AHIMA 2004). Data sets provide the means to record and communicate the most relevant and timely facts about a patient's health information and healthcare (AHIMA 2004).

The transition from paper to EHRs necessitates the transition from legacy data sets toward a comprehensive core data set that maps back to EHR functions (AHIMA 2004).

Table 5.1. Core content of the PHD

Personal Health Record	• Personal identification information • Emergency contact information • Lifetime health history; summary of caregiver records from all sources of care, including immunizations, allergies, family history, occupational history, environmental exposures, social history, medical history, treatments procedures, medication history, outcomes • Lab results, e.g., EKGs; or links to results, e.g., MRI results at a radiology department data warehouse, digital images of biopsy slides, or digital video of coronary angiography • Emergency care information, e.g., allergies, current medications, medical/surgical history summary • Provider identification and contact information • Treatment plans and instructions • Health risk factor profile, recommended clinical preventative services, and results of those services • Health insurance coverage information
Other Elements	• Correspondence: records of patient–provider communication, edits made to PHR, or concerns about accuracy of information in health care provider medical records • Instructions about access by other persons and institutions • Audit log of individuals/institutions who access electronic records • Self-care trackers: nutrition, physical activity, medications, dosage schedules • Personal library of quality health information resources • Healthcare proxies, living wills, and durable power of attorney for health care
Elements from the Community Health Dimension	• Local public health contact information • Local healthcare services (e.g. walk-in clinics) • Environmental measures and alerts pertinent to an individual's home, neighborhood, school, and workplace

Source: NCVHS 2000.

Table 5.2.	Core content of the HPD
Patient Record Elements	• Personal identification information • Sociodemographic identifiers (gender, birthday, age, race/ethnicity, marital status, living arrangements, education level, occupation) • Health insurance information (including covered benefits) • Legal consents or permissions • Referral information • Correspondence • Patient history information (may include longitudinal history from PHD, immunizations, allergies, current medications) • Stated reason for visit • External causes of injury/illness • Symptoms • Physical exams • Assessment of patient signs and symptoms • Diagnoses • Laboratory, radiology, and pharmacy orders • Laboratory results • Radiological images and interpretations • Record of alerts, warnings, and reminders • Operative reports • Vital signs from ICU • Vital signs from PHD • Treatment plans and instructions • Progress notes • Functional status • Discharge summaries • Instructions about access • Audit log of individuals who accessed patient record • Patient amendments to patient record • Provider notes, such as knowledge of patient, patient-provider interactions, patient's access to services
Other Elements That Support Clinical Practice Elements from the Community Health Dimension	• Protocols, practice guidelines • Clinical decision-support programs • Referral history Depending on the patient, the HCPD would include additional contextual information necessary for understanding, treating, and planning the care of the patient: • Aggregate data on the health care of community members • Community attributes affecting health (e.g., economic status and population age • Community health resources (e.g., home health services) • Community health (e.g., possible environmental hazards at home, work, school, or in the community at large)
Source: NCVHS 2000.	

Table 5.3. Core content of the CHD	
Public Health Data	• Infant mortality, immunization levels, and communicable disease rates • Environmental, social, and economic conditions • Measures related to public health infrastructure, individual healthcare providers, and healthcare institutions • Other summary measures of community health • Registries • Disease surveillance systems • Survey data • Data on Healthy People objectives and Leading Health indicators
Information from the HCPD (with personally identifiable information removed except under legally established public health protocols and strict security)	• Health status and outcomes, health events, health risks, health behaviors, and other individual characteristics • Healthcare utilization and access, health insurance status • Health care of community members
Other Elements	• Directories of community organizations and services • Planning, evaluation, and policy documents • Compendia of laws and regulations • Material to support public education campaigns • Practice guidelines and training materials for public health officials
Source: NCVHS 2000.	

Check Your Understanding 5.1

Instructions: Choose the most appropriate answer for the following questions.

1. _____ When did modern methods at standardizing healthcare data begin?
   a. 1900s
   b. 1960s
   c. 1980s
   d. 2000s

2. _____ Which of the following is designed to collect a minimum set of data about inpatients?
   a. DRGs
   b. NCHS
   c. UACDS
   d. UHDDS

3. _____ Which of the following is used to collect data about ambulatory care patients?
   a. DRGs
   b. MDS
   c. ORYX
   d. UACDS

4. _____ Which of the following is used to collect data about long-term care residents?
   a. NCHS
   b. MDS
   c. UACDS
   d. UHDDS

5. _____ Which of the following provides a structured way to develop a long-term care resident care plan?
   a. MDS
   b. OASIS
   c. UACHDS
   d. UHDDS

6. _____ Which of the following is used to gather data about Medicare beneficiaries receiving home care?
   a. MDS
   b. NCHS
   c. OASIS
   d. UHDDS

7. _____ Which of the following best describes the DEEDs data set?
   a. Uses data for home health outcomes research
   b. Collects data about hospital emergency encounters
   c. Uses data for inpatient analysis
   d. Collects data for ambulatory care

8. _____ Which of the following is a set of performance measures used to compare the performance of healthcare plans?
   a. DEEDS
   b. HEDIS
   c. ORYX
   d. UHDDS

9. _____ Which of the following is associated with the JCAHO?
   a. HEDIS
   b. MDS
   c. OASIS
   d ORYX

10. _____ Which of the following is charged with establishing a plan for development of widespread interoperable EHR systems?
    a. HIT
    b. NHII
    c. NHIN
    d. ONC

Standards for Electronic Data and Electronic Data Interchange

The original uniform data sets such as the UHDDS and the UACDS were created for use in paper-based (manual) health record systems. They were not designed to accommodate the data needs of the current healthcare delivery system or the demands of EHRs and clinical information systems.

The NHIN initiative has clearly identified the need to develop standards that allow data to be easily, accurately, and securely communicated electronically among various computer systems. This is referred to as interoperability. Without standards for interoperability, EHRs and the NHIN will not realize their full benefits (Thompson and Brailer 2004).

Many types of standards are being developed to support the EHR and the NHIN vision. Some involve defining data structure and content, others specify technical approaches for transmitting data, and still others provide rules for protecting the privacy and security of data.

Data Needs in an Electronic Environment

As discussed in chapter 4, healthcare organizations often have several different computer systems operating at the same time. For example, a hospital's laboratory system might be entirely separate from its billing system. In fact, the various departments of large healthcare organizations often use different operating systems and are serviced by different vendors. In addition to operating multiple systems, it is an ongoing challenge to integrate information from legacy (older) systems operating on old platforms with state-of-the art information systems.

Healthcare organizations must integrate data that originate in various databases within facilities as well as in databases outside the facility. They also must be able to respond to requests to transfer data to other facilities, payers, accrediting and regulating agencies, quality improvement organizations, and other information users. These goals can only be accomplished when every database system is either operating on the same platform or using common standards.

Healthcare Information Standards

Healthcare information standards describe accepted methods for collecting, maintaining, and/or transferring healthcare data among computer systems. These standards are designed to provide a common language that makes it easy to:

- Exchange information
- Share information
- Communicate within and across disciplines and settings
- Integrate disparate data systems
- Compare information at a regional, national, and international level
- Link data in a secure environment

Having the ability to exchange, share, communicate, integrate, compare, and link data is important to healthcare delivery. These activities make possible important activities such as:

- Disease surveillance
- Health and healthcare population monitoring
- Outcomes research
- Decision making and policy development

The long-term vision is to enhance the comparability, quality, integrity, and utility of health information from a wide variety of public sources through uniform data policies and standards (NCVHS 2001).

As mentioned earlier, the Certification Commission for Health Information Technology is developing functional standards and criteria for certification of EHR products.

Because there are hundreds of standards, it is impossible to discuss them all in this chapter. A few of the better-known standards that HIT professionals may work with are presented in the following sections.

Standards Development

Developing healthcare standards is a complex process in which many organizations are involved. These organizations are referred to as standards development organizations (SDOs). HL7 and ASTM, for example, are both accredited SDOs. Table 5.4 provides a list of several organizations that are actively involved in developing standards for health-related information management.

Both private organizations and government agencies are involved in standards development. Many standards are created through a voluntary consensus process that involves identifying the need for the standard, negotiating its content, and drafting a proposed version. The final standard is published after undergoing a comment and revision period.

Because so many organizations are developing standards, there needs to be coordination. Therefore, some organizations play key roles in coordinating the efforts of other SDOs. ANSI is one example. It coordinates the development of voluntary standards in a variety of industries, including healthcare. Most SDOs in the United States are members of ANSI.

The United Nations International Standards Organization (ISO) coordinates international standards development. ANSI represents the U.S. at the ISO.

Types of Standards

Many types of standards are necessary to implement EHRs and a health information technology infrastructure that supports connectivity, interoperability, and seamless data interchange. Some of these types of standards include the following:

- **Structure and content standards** establish and provide clear and uniform definitions of the data elements to be included in EHR systems. They specify the type of data to be collected in each data field, the width of each field length, and the attributes of each data field, all of which are captured in data dictionaries.

- *Functionality standards* define the components that an EHR needs to support the functions for which it was designed. HL7 draft standards (discussed below) for an EHR were developed in 2004 and, at the time of publication, were being tested in the healthcare industry.

- *Technical standards* complement content and structure and vocabulary standards and are the next step in making interoperability possible. Technical standards provide the rules, often called protocols, of how these data are actually transmitted from one computer system to another.

Placing a standard in one category is often difficult. This is because some standards can be classified in more than one way. For example, LOINC can be classified as both a terminology standard and a standard for EHRs.

Table 5.4.   Standards development organizations

Organization	Types of Standards	Description
Accredited Standards Committee X12 Data Interchange Standards Association (DISA) 333 John Carlyle Street, Suite 600 Alexandria, VA 22314 Telephone: (703) 548-7005 www.disa.org	Electronic data interchange for billing transactions The committee's particular area of focus has been computer-to-computer communications between healthcare providers and third-party payers	Chartered in 1979 by ANSI, the X12N subcommittee develops and maintains X12 standards, interpretations, and guidelines. X12N is one of the standards for EDI that is specified in the regulations of the Health Insurance Portability and Accountability Act of 1996. Subgroups of X12N include: *WEDI: Workgroup on Electronic Data Interchange* WEDI has been the prime mover in the development of insurance industry standards. In 1995, WEDI became a private standards advocacy group. *HIBCC: Health Industry Business Communications Council*
American College of Radiology— **National Electrical Manufacturers Association** **(ACR-NEMA)** American College of Radiology 1891 Preston White Drive Reston, VA 20191 Telephone: (703) 648-8900 www.acr.org National Electrical Manufacturers Association 1300 N. Seventeenth Street, Suite 1847 Rosslyn, VA 22209 Telephone: (703) 841-3200 www.nema.org	Exchange of digitized images	ACR is a professional association, and NEMA is a trade association. They have worked collaboratively to develop the Digital Imaging and Communications in Medicine (DICOM) standard, which promotes a digital image communications format and facilitates development by the American College of Radiology of picture archive and communications systems. DICOM may be used for electronic exchange of x-rays, computed tomography (CT), magnetic resonance imaging (MRI), ultrasound, nuclear medicine, and other radiology images. Work is under way to support other diagnostic images.
American Society for Testing and Materials (ASTM) 100 Barr Harbor Drive West Conshohocken, PA 19428 Telephone: (610) 832-9585 www.astm.org	Multiple health informatics standards, including clinical content of patient records, exchange of messages about clinical observations, data security and integrity, healthcare identifiers, data modeling, clinical laboratory systems, Arden syntax (a coding system), and system functionality	Organized in 1898, the ASTM is one of the largest SDOs in the world. It provides a forum for vendors, users, consumers, and others to develop standards for a wide range of materials, products, systems, and services. It is composed of more than 140 subcommittees or working groups identified as E31 and E32. Since 1990, Committee E31 on Healthcare Informatics has developed standards for health information and health information systems. Standard E1384, discussed earlier, is a product of the E31 subcommittee of ASTM.
Health Level Seven (HL7) 3300 Washtenaw Avenue, Suite 227 Ann Arbor, MI 48104 Telephone: (734) 677-7777 www.hl7.org	Electronic interchange of clinical, financial, and administrative information among disparate health information systems	HL7 is an ANSI-accredited SDO. Level 7 refers to the highest level of the Open System Interconnection (OSI) model of the International Standards Organization. The HL7 standard addresses issues that occur within the seventh, or application, layer.
Institute of Electrical and Electronics Engineers (IEEE) 445 Hoes Lane P.O. Box 1331 Piscataway, NJ 08855-1331 Telephone: (732) 981-0060 www.ieee.org	Medical device information and general informatics format	The IEEE's Medical Data Interchange Standard (MEDIX) is a standard set of hospital system interface transactions based on the ISO standards for all seven layers of the OSI model. Another IEEE standard for a medical information bus (MIB) links bedside instruments in critical care with health information systems.
National Council on Prescription Drug Programs (NCPDP) 4201 N. Twenty-fourth Street, Suite 365 Phoenix, AZ 85016 Telephone: (602) 957-9105 www.ncpdp.org	Data interchange and processing standards for pharmacy transactions	The NCPDP has defined standards for transmitting prescription information from pharmacies to payers for prescription management services and for receiving approval and payment information back in near-real time. Other standards address adverse drug reactions and utilization review.

Adapted from Brandt 2000, p. 39.

Standards That Support EHRs

The standards discussed below support EHR systems in some way.

Health Level Seven

Mentioned briefly in chapter 4, HL7 is a not-for-profit SDO. It provides standards, guidelines, and methodologies that make data exchange possible among hospitals, physician practices, and other types of provider systems. For example, the standards consist of rules for transmitting demographic data, orders, patient observations, laboratory results, history and physical observations, and findings. They also include message rules for appointment scheduling, referrals, problem list maintenance, and care plans.

HL7 developed the HL7 Electronic Health Record System (EHR-S) Functional Model and Standards that addresses the content and structure of an EHR (HL7.org). Figure 4.2, p. 122, shows the HL7 EHR-S Functional Model. The purpose of the functional model is to provide a foundation for common understanding of possible functions of EHR systems (Shafarman and Van Hentenryck 2004).

The HL7 Clinical Document Architecture (CDA) provides an exchange model for clinical documents (such as discharge summaries and progress notes) and brings the healthcare industry closer to the realization of an EHR. The CDA standard makes documents machine-readable so that they can be easily processed electronically. It also makes documents human-readable so that they can be retrieved easily and used by the people who need them.

American Society for Testing and Materials (ASTM) E31 Committee

The **American Society for Testing and Materials** (ASTM) is an SDO that develops standards for a variety of industries in the United States. The ASTM Technical Committee on Healthcare Informatics E31 is charged with the responsibility for developing standards related to the EHR. E31 works through subcommittees assigned to various aspects of this endeavor. An example is the Health Information Transcription and Documentation Committee (E31.22), which recently developed two new standards: E2344 Standard Guide for Data Capture through the Dictation Process, and E2364 Standard Guide for Speech Recognition Products in Health Care (Tessier 2004)

ASTM Standard E1384-02a identifies the content and structure for EHRs. The scope of this standard is intended to cover all types of healthcare services, including acute care hospitals, ambulatory care, skilled nursing facilities, home healthcare, and specialty environments (ASTM 2005).

As mentioned in chapter 4, ASTM Committee 31 currently is focused on the **continuity of care record** (CCR) initiative, which is categorized as Electronic Health Records standard E31.28. The CCR standard is a core data set of relevant current and past information about a patient's health status and healthcare treatment. It was created to help communicate that information from one provider to another for referral, transfer, or discharge of the patient or when the patient wishes to create a personal health record (ASTM 2005).

The CCR contains the following elements (ASTM 2005):

- Patient administrative and clinical data

- Basic information about the patient's payer

- Advance directives

- Patient's sources of support
- Patient's current functional status
- Problems
- Family history
- Social history
- Alerts
- Medications
- Medical devices or equipment need by the patient
- Immunization history
- Vital signs (as appropriate)
- Results of laboratory, diagnostic, and therapeutic results
- Diagnostic and therapeutic procedures
- Encounters
- Plan of care
- Healthcare providers

Because both ASTM and HL7 are involved in developing standards for EHRs, the two organizations have negotiated a memorandum of understanding to bring ASTM's CCR initiative into line with HL7's EHR functionality and CDA standards. In a report issued in October 2005, the HL7 board of directors issued a report on progress in this initiative, stating: "The Continuity of Care Record. . . is rich in functionality and clinical utility. From a technical implementation perspective, however, it has not achieved the same degree of readiness for standardization. . . We hope to continue to work with ASTM toward a common solution that leverages the strengths of both organizations" (HL7 2005).

Identifier Standards

Identifier standards recommend methods for assigning unique identification numbers to individuals, including patients, healthcare providers (physicians, dentists, and so on), corporate providers (healthcare organizations), and healthcare vendors and suppliers. Identifiers usually use a combination of numeric or alphanumeric characters, such as a hospital number or a billing number. At present, most identifiers are used only within one facility or within a single healthcare system. HIPAA regulations require development of **unique identification numbers** that can be used across information systems. As standards development efforts move forward, one of the biggest privacy and security issues is how to identify a patient and link the patient's information among providers while controlling access to patient information (Carol 2005).

At present, there is no consensus on a standard method of identifying individuals. Much of the controversy relates to use of the **Social Security number** (SSN) as the identifier for patients. The Social Security Administration is adamant in its opposition to using the SSN for purposes other than those identified by law. The American Health Information

Management Association (AHIMA) is in agreement on this issue due to privacy, confidentiality, and security issues related to use of the SSN.

As an alternative to use of the SSN as a unique patient identifier, there have been proposals to develop a unique healthcare identifier number. For a variety of reasons, primarily related to confidentiality and security, these proposals have not been widely endorsed.

The most commonly used provider identifier is the **unique physician identification number** (UPIN). The UPIN was originally created by CMS for use by physicians who bill for services provided to Medicare patients.

In 1993, CMS initiated the National Provider Identification Initiative to develop a provider identification system to meet Medicare and Medicaid needs and, ultimately, the needs of all users. The work group investigated all existing identifiers and designed a new **national provider identifier** (NPI). The NPI uses an eight-character alphanumeric identifier. CMS is working on implementing the NPI for the Medicare program. It announced a system whereby all healthcare providers, including Medicare providers, can apply for a new identifier known as the NPI starting in May 2005. The CMS letter to providers indicates that all providers must be using the NPI by May 23, 2007.

Clinical Representation Standards

Clinical representation standards include classification systems, vocabularies, terminologies, lab and clinical observation codes (LOINC), and drug codes, as well as standards for information modeling and metadata.

Vocabulary standards establish common definitions for medical terms to encourage consistent descriptions of an individual's condition in the health record. Various synonymous medical terms are often used in different areas of the country. In fact, medical terminology can vary among physicians working in the same organization, depending on where and when each physician was trained and which medical specialty he or she practices. For example, one physician might describe a patient's diagnosis as Parkinson's disease, another might describe it as Parkinsonism, and a third might use the term *paralysis agitans* to describe it. All three terms are correct, but using the terms interchangeably could adversely affect data quality. In addition, data comparison among the physicians' patients would be difficult, if not impossible.

The use of clinical classification codes (for example, CPT and ICD-9-CM codes) to represent health-related conditions and procedures is common in healthcare. The use of standardized, uniform terminology is critical to accurate coding. Vocabulary standards not only provide guidance in code selection, but they also establish common definitions and standard representations of textual data that can be used as a basis for future automated coding systems.

The development of vocabularies, terminologies, and classification systems as well as drug codes, laboratory and clinical observation codes, information modeling, and metadata are explored thoroughly in chapter 6.

ASC X12N

One of the purposes of HIPAA's Administrative Simplification rules was to standardize information exchange; and in August, 2000, HHS published regulations for electronic transactions. These regulations apply to transactions that occur among healthcare providers and healthcare plans and payers (Rode 2001). The long-term goal of the transaction standards is to allow providers and plans or payers to seamlessly transfer data back and forth with little intervention. To do this, HHS has adopted the electronic transaction standards of ASC X12 Insurance Subcommittee (Accredited Standards Committee Health Care Task group (X12N).

The standards adopted for EDI are called ANSI ASC X12N and include:

- Professional/institutional X12N 837 Healthcare Claim Transactions, version 4010

- X12N 835 Health Care Claim (HCC) Payment/Advice (or remittance advice, RA) transactions

- X12N 837 Coordination of Benefits (COB) transactions

To implement the HIPAA Administrative Simplification provisions, the above transaction standards are included under part 162 of title 45 of the Code of Federal Regulations (CFR) as the standard for processing electronic healthcare claims, coordination of benefits, and RA transmissions.

Laboratory Logical Observation Identifier Name Codes
LOINC is a well-accepted set of standards that represents laboratory data for ordering lab tests and reporting results including the electronic exchange of clinical laboratory results. It is managed by the Regenstrief Institute in Indianapolis.

Institute of Electrical and Electronics Engineers 1073
The **Institute of Electrical and Electronics Engineers** (IEEE) 1073 provides for open-systems communications in healthcare applications, primarily between bedside medical devices and patient care information systems, optimized for the acute care setting. The IEEE 1073 series was adopted as a federal health information interoperability standard for EDI (NAHIT 2005).

Digital Imaging and Communications in Medicine
Through a cooperative effort between the **American College of Radiology and the National Electronic Manufacturers Association** (ACR-NEMA), **Digital Imaging and Communication in Medicine** (DICOM) was originally created to permit the interchange of biomedical image wave forms and related information. These organizations define the health record to include not only textual, coded, and numeric information (linguistic), but also a detailed, structured record of image-related information (Bidgood 1997).

DICOM is used by most medical professions that use imaging within the healthcare industry, such as cardiology, dentistry, endoscopy, mammography, ophthalmology, and orthopedics. DICOM was adopted as the federal health information interoperability messaging standard for imaging in March 2003 (NAHIT 2005).

Medication Standards
Medications are used extensively to prevent and treat medical conditions. Physicians, payers, and pharmacies communicate with one another to ensure that correct medications are prescribed, administered, and reimbursed. Research studies are frequently conducted to determine the efficacy of various drugs; recent events relative to the removal of certain categories of drugs from the market due to unforeseen adverse effects has focused attention on medication issues and underscored the need for accurate and accessible information about medications.

A number of standards have been developed to address medication and drug issues. Among these are the National Drug Directory (NDC), which lists all drugs manufactured, prepared, propagated, compounded, or presented by a drug establishment registered under the Federal Food, Drug, and Cosmetic Act. The National Council for Prescription Drug Programs (NCPDP) creates and promotes data interchange standards for the pharmacy services sector of healthcare. Seventy thousand pharmacies are given a unique identifying number for interactions with federal agencies and third-party payers.

Privacy and Security Standards

HIPAA mandated the adoption of privacy and security protection for identifiable health information. HIPAA **privacy standards** have been implemented throughout the healthcare industry. (See chapter 15.)

Security standards ensure that patient-identifiable health information remains confidential and protected from unauthorized disclosure, alteration, or destruction. Effective security standards are especially important in computer-based environments because patient information is accessible to many users in many locations.

Security standards, including access controls, audit controls, integrity, person or entity authentication, and transmission are addressed in detail in chapter 19 as they relate to the EHR. Many SDOs, most notably, ASTM and HL7, have developed security standards, but no single standard currently addresses all the HIPAA provisions.

Check Your Understanding 5.2

Instructions: Choose the best answer for each of the following questions.

1. _____ Which of the following provides a foundation for a common understanding of EHR functions?
   a. ANSI
   b. DICOM
   c. HL7
   d. LOINC

2. _____ Which of the following best describes an SDO?
   a. Coordinates standards groups
   b. Develops standards
   c. Develops data sets
   d. Develops best practices

3. _____ Which of the following provides standards for transmitting clinical documents such as discharge summaries?
   a. CDA
   b. NHIN
   c. OASIS
   d. ORYX

4. _____ Which of these could be used best to create a personal health record?
   a. CDA
   b. CCR
   c. HL7
   d. ORYX

5. ____ Which of the following is considered to be an identifier standard?
   a. CDA
   b. CCR
   c. HL7
   d. UPIN

6. ____ Which of the following is true about the SSN?
   a. Should be used as a unique health identifier
   b. Poses little data security threat as a unique identifier
   c. Is supported by the SSA for use as a patient identifier
   d. Should not be used as a unique patient identifier

7. ____ Which of the following are considered to be clinical representation standards?
   a. ASC X12
   b. CDA
   c. CPT
   d. HL7

8. ____ Which of the following lists all drugs manufactured by a drug establishment under the Food, Drug and Cosmetic Act?
   a. DEED
   b. NCPDP
   c. NDC
   d. NHIN

Evolving Health Information Standards

The development of healthcare information standards is far from complete. The task is critically important to the development of EHR systems and, ultimately, to implementation of a national health information infrastructure. Leading standards groups are continuously working to reach consensus on a variety of standards, but many issues remain unresolved.

Development of Extensible Markup Language (XML)

Recent advances in standards development have occurred in the area of **extensible markup language** (XML). XML was developed as a universal language to facilitate the storage and transmission of data published on the Internet. Markup languages communicate electronic representations of paper documents to computers by inserting additional information into text (Sokolowski 1999). The best-known markup language is hypertext markup language (HTML), which is used to convert text documents into Internet-compatible format.

Real-World Case

In Winona, Minnesota, local healthcare providers and a healthcare information software vendor have developed a health information network that improves communication among patients and local physicians and other healthcare providers. The system relies on an already-existing high-speed network to provide interactive health records that can be used by local facilities, physicians, pharmacies, and patients. Patients are able to make appointments, check their health records for test results, and communicate with their physicians via the Internet. Physicians also are able to communicate with one another and with local hospitals, nursing homes, and clinics. The system was designed to ensure the security and confidentiality of data.

Because more than 60 percent of Winona residents use the Internet, the population is well prepared to use this health network to improve healthcare. Residents who do not own computers have access to computer labs in schools, libraries, and other public locations.

Baseline data for the project are gathered through health risk assessments, and patients gain access to the health information network via a sign-in process. The results of the health risk assessments provide a baseline of data about the community and allows the community to assess the impact of this project on its health status.

Summary

According to Brandt(2000), "the vision is clear: a longitudinal, or lifetime, health record for each person that is computer-based, secure, readily accessible when needed, and linked across the continuum of care [is needed]. In reality, we are a long way from that model." It is impossible to develop a longitudinal EHR that meets Brandt's specifications without standards that guide its development. The complexity of technology, the variations in computer platforms from one system to the next, and the different (and sometimes conflicting) data needs of users demand flexible health data/information systems. The systems must be able to store volumes of data in a standardized format, communicate across vendor-specific systems, and keep data in a secure manner that protects individual privacy and information confidentiality.

The need for standardized data definitions was recognized in the 1960s, and the National Committee on Vital and Health Statistics took the lead in developing uniform minimum data sets for various sites of care. As technology has driven the development of the data/information systems, the early data sets have been supplemented with healthcare information standards that focus on electronic health record (EHR) systems. A number of standards-setting organizations have been involved in developing uniform definitions, data fields, and views for health record content and structure. Standards for developing medical vocabularies, messaging/communications systems, and data/information security, privacy, and confidentiality are being created and implemented. These standards are dynamic and in constant development by various groups. Standards development generally takes place as a consensus-driven process among various interested parties. In most cases, implementation is voluntary. However, many groups are involved in standards development and competition exists among those groups. One of the major efforts of the Office of the National Coordinator (ONC) is standards harmonization that consolidates standards into a useful and accepted set of national information technology standards. ANSI will convene the Health Information Technology Standards Panel to address standards harmonization.

Some data sets and standards have been incorporated into federal law and are thus required for use by affected healthcare organizations. For example, in 1983, the standardized definitions of the Uniform Hospital Discharge Data Set were incorporated into the Prospective Payment Act (PL98-603) and are still required for reporting inpatient data for reimbursement under the Medicare program.

The Health Insurance Portability and Accountability Act of 1996 mandated incorporation of healthcare information standards into all electronic or computer-based health information systems. Of particular importance under HIPAA are transaction/messaging standards for communication of data across systems, privacy standards that protect individual privacy and confidentiality, security standards that ensure that data are accessed only by those who have a specific right to access them, and identifier standards that offer methods of identifying both individual patients and healthcare providers. The rules and regulations for HIPAA are still in development, and, to date, the transaction, privacy, and security standards have been implemented. Other standards are still under development.

The development of health information standards to support EHR development gained national support through recent federal initiatives aimed at developing a strategic plan to guide the nation's implementation of interoperable health information technology in both the public and private sectors. The Office of the National Coordinator of Health Information Technology has been given a mandate to advance the development, adoption, and implementation of healthcare information technology nationally through collaboration among public and private interests and to ensure that these standards are consistent with current efforts to set HIT standards for use by the federal government (Thompson and Brailer 2004).

Work will continue on the development of healthcare informatics standards well into the twenty-first century. It is a complex and dynamic task with constant activity in the development, modification, negotiation, and implementation process. The rapid growth of technology and the increasing need for healthcare data/information makes the task a daunting one. According to Kloss (2005), "the EHR is seen as essential for safe, effective care and a building block to wire the healthcare system. Now we need to better understand the prerequisites for interoperability so technology investments deliver on their promises. It is not sufficient to automate health records within organizations; there must be interconnectivity among providers and between providers and patients."

References

AHIMA Workgroup on Core Data Sets as Standards for the EHR. 2004 (September). Practice brief: E-HIM strategic initiative: core data sets. *Journal of American Health Information Management Association* 75(8):68A–D.

Amatayakul, M. 2002. Practice brief: The transactions extension: No reason to procrastinate. *Journal of American Health Information Management Association* 73(3):16A–C.

American Society for Testing and Materials. 2005. www.astm.org.

Bidgood, W. D., Jr. 1997. Documenting the information content of images. *Proceedings of the AMIA Annual Fall Symposium,* pp. 424–28.

Brandt, M. D. 2000. Health informatics standards: A user's guide. *Journal of American Health Information Management Association* 71(4):39–43.

Brandt, M. D. 1999. Standards for EHR content, systems, and data exchange. In *Electronic Health Records: Changing the Vision,* edited by G. F. Murphy et al. Philadelphia: W. B. Saunders Company.

Carol, R. 2005. Short-term forecast: Experts speak up on ONC's RFI, RFPs and the year ahead. *Journal of American Health Information Management Association* 76(9):42–44,46.48,50.

Dougherty, M. 2005. Understanding the EHR system functional model standard. *Journal of American Health Information Management Association* 76(2):64A–D.

Dougherty, M. 1999. Reimbursement. In *Long-Term Care Handbook: Resources for the Health Information Manager,* edited by Teresa Ganser. Chicago: American Health Information Management Association.

Food and Drug Administration Center for Drug Evaluation and Research. 2005. National Drug Code Frequently Asked Questions. Available online from www.fda.gov/cder/ndc.

Food and Drug Administration Center for Drug Evaluation and Research. 2002. CDER Data Standards Manual. Available online from www.fda.gov/cder/dsm.

Hanken, M. A., and K. Water, eds. 1994. *Glossary of Healthcare Terms.* Chicago: American Health Information Management Association.

Health Level 7. 2005. HL7.org.

Himlin, J. 2005. HL7s EHR technical committee enhances system functional model: New public comment to open this summer. Available online from HL7.org.

Health Information Systems Society. Available online from himss.org/content/files/StandardsInsight/2003/12-2003.pdf.

Kloss, L. 2005b. Standardized data: The difference for EHR solutions. *Journal of American Health Information Management Association* 76(2):23.

Kloss, L. 2005a. The NHIN comes into focus. *Journal of American Health Information Management Association* 76(3):23.

Linck, J. C. 1996. Patient and health care data. In *Health Information: Management of a Strategic Resource,* edited by M. Abdelhak et al. Philadelphia: W. B. Saunders Company.

Mon, D. T. 2005. An update on the NHIM and RHIOs. *Journal of American Health Information Management Association* 76(6):56–57, 59.

Morissey, J. 2000 (June 12). Minnesota town to get health data online. *Modern Healthcare.*

Murphy, G., and M. Brandt. 2001. Practice brief: Health informatics standards and information transfer: Exploring the HIM role. *Journal of American Health Information Management Association* 72(1):68A–D.

National Association for Health Information Technology. 2005. Alliance Standards Directory. Available online from www.hitsdir.org.

National Center for Injury Prevention and Control. 1997. *Data Elements for Emergency Department Systems, Release 1.0.* Atlanta: NCIPC.

National Committee on Vital and Health Statistics. 2001. *Information for Health: A Strategy for Building the National Health Information Infrastructure.* Washington, DC: HHS.

National Committee on Vital and Health Statistics. 2000. *Toward a Health Information Infrastructure: Interim Report.* Washington, DC: HHS

National Committee on Vital and Health Statistics. 1998. *Assuring a Health Dimension for the National Information Infrastructure.* Washington, DC: HHS

Peters, R. M. 2000. XML: Defining the transition from paper to digital records. *Journal of American Health Information Management Association* 71(1):34–38.

Pothen, D. J., and B. Parmanto. 2000. XML furthers CPR goals. *Journal of American Health Information Management Association* 71(9):24–29.

Rulon, V., and J. Sica. 1997. The evolution of HEDIS: 3.0 and beyond. *Journal of American Health Information Management Association* 68(6):32–39.

Rode, D. 2001. Understanding HIPAA transactions and code sets. *Journal of American Health Information Management Association* 72(1):26–32.

Shafarman, M., and K. Van Hentenryck. 2004 (September). HL7 makes headway on version 3. *Healthcare Informatics* 50.

Smith, D. A. 2001. Data transmission: A world of possibilities. *Journal of American Health Information Management Association* 72(5):26–27.

Sokolowski, R. 1999. XML makes its mark. *Journal of American Health Information Management Association* 70(10):21–24.

Tessier, C. 2004 (September). ASTM E31 committee. *Healthcare Informatics* 47.

Thompson, T. G., and D. J. Brailer. 2004. The decade of health information technology: Delivering consumer-centric and information-rich health care— framework for strategic action. Washington, DC: HHS. Available online from hhs.gov/healthit/documents/hitframework.pdf.

Chapter 6
Clinical Vocabularies and Classification Systems

Karen Scott, MEd, RHIA, CCS-P, CPC

Learning Objectives

- To discuss the history of the development of clinical vocabularies

- To understand the history, uses, and structure of ICD-9-CM, ICD-10, ICD-O-3, HCPCS, CPT, SNOMED CT, DSM-IV-TR, and nursing vocabularies

- To describe the coding process

- To identify the technology used in the coding process

- To understand the history, elements, policies, and procedures for corporate compliance

- To discuss new directions in clinical vocabularies

Key Terms

Classification system

Clinical vocabulary

Current Procedural Terminology (CPT)

Diagnostic and Statistical Manual of Mental Disorders, Fourth Revision, Text Revision (DSM-IV-TR)

E codes

Encoder

Healthcare Common Procedure Coding System (HCPCS)

Classification of Diseases, Ninth Revision, Clinical Modification (ICD-9-CM)

International Classification of Diseases, Tenth Revision, Clinical Modification (ICD-10-CM)

International Classification of Diseases, Tenth Revision, Procedure Coding System (ICD-10-PCS)

International Classification of Diseases for Oncology, Third Edition (ICD-O-3)

Morbidity

Mortality

Natural language processing (NLP)

Nomenclature

Nosology

Nursing vocabularies

Read Codes

Systemized Nomenclature of Medicine Clinical Terminology (SNOMED CT)

V codes

World Health Organization (WHO)

Introduction

Over the years, diseases and medical–surgical procedures have come to be known by different names. For example, Downs' syndrome is sometimes referred to as mongolism or trisomy 21. Clearly, the use of more than one term for the same disease makes it difficult to collect and retrieve information. In an effort to organize and standardize medical language, the healthcare industry has developed nomenclatures, classification systems, and clinical vocabularies.

In medicine, a **nomenclature** is a recognized system that lists preferred medical terminology. Nomenclatures, or "naming" system, such as CPT, also are referred to as *clinical terminology.* **Classification systems** group together similar diseases and procedures. They also organize related entities for easy retrieval. The ***International Classification of Diseases, Ninth Revision, Clinical Modification*** (ICD-9-CM), is an example of a classification system. **Clinical vocabularies** have been developed to create a list of clinical words or phrases with their meanings.

These systems facilitate the organization, storage, and retrieval of healthcare diagnostic and procedural data. Moreover, they aid in the development and implementation of computerized patient record systems. This chapter discusses the various nomenclatures, classification systems, and clinical vocabularies used in the healthcare industry today.

Theory into Practice

Hillcrest Health Care Clinic is a multispeciality group practice with clinics in five different locations. The office manager has determined that various editions of codebooks are being used throughout the practice to assign codes for reimbursement. She also noticed that many of the providers do not use codebooks at all but, instead, assign codes from a list prepared by their office staff. Such lists often contain incorrect codes, as do out-dated codebooks. The end result is incorrect code assignment, denied reimbursement, and erroneous database entries. Clearly, policies and procedures are needed to control the coding process.

History and Importance of Clinical Vocabularies

In the late 1800s, the Anatomical Society developed one of the first medical nomenclatures. In 1895, this international organization published the *Basle Nomina Anatomica*. This work initiated the standardization of anatomical terms used in medicine.

The first medical nomenclature to be universally accepted in the United States was developed by the New York Academy of Medicine and titled the *Standard Nomenclature of Disease and Operations*. In 1937, the American Medical Association (AMA) assumed the copyright and editing responsibility for this work and expanded it to include a nomenclature for procedures as well as diseases. The expanded work was published in one volume titled *Standard Nomenclature of Disease and Standard Nomenclature of Operations*.

ICD-9-CM is the most recognized classification system used today. It evolved from a classification developed by Dr. Jacques Bertillon. His system was published in 1893 as the *Bertillon Classification of Causes of Death*. In 1898, the American Public Health Association recommended that registrars in the United States, Canada, and Mexico use the Bertillon classification.

This classification system was revised throughout the early 1900s. In 1948, the **World Health Organization** (WHO) published the sixth revision of the system. The sixth revision included a classification for **morbidity** and **mortality** data. Throughout the 1900s, various healthcare associations and public health organizations representing numerous countries worked to create a standardized classification system for healthcare.

In 1975, representatives from numerous countries met in Geneva, Switzerland, to develop the *International Classification of Diseases* under the direction of WHO. Today, the ICD classification system is used throughout the world.

Development of these systems has helped to standardize terminology for the collection, processing, and retrieval of medical information. Additional systems of classification and nomenclatures are discussed later in this chapter.

Clinical Vocabularies

Users of clinical vocabularies can be divided into two main groups: clinical and administrative.

Clinical users are providers who use clinical vocabularies to collect, process, and retrieve data for clinical purposes. They use the vocabularies to support activities such as clinical research, disease prevention, and patient care. An example of a clinical user would be a physician who uses ICD-9-CM codes to track a patient's diagnostic history.

Administrative users include healthcare facilities, professional organizations, and government agencies. These groups use clinical vocabularies to support administrative, statistical, and reimbursement functions. An example of this is when ***Current Procedural Terminology*** (CPT) codes are used to report physician services to the Medicare program to determine reimbursement. The specific users of clinical vocabularies are discussed in the sections that follow.

The Health Insurance Portability and Accountability Act (HIPAA) required the establishment of electronic transactions and coding standards. In 2000, the Department of Health and Human Services (HHS), in accordance with HIPAA, established official medical coding set standards. To be in compliance with the HIPAA law, all covered entities are required to use the following official medical coding sets:

- *International Classification of Diseases, Ninth Revision, Clinical Modification* (ICD-9-CM), including the Official ICD-9-CM Guidelines for Coding and Reporting: Volumes 1 and 2 are used for reporting all diseases, injuries, impairments, other health problems and causes of such, an Volume 3 is used to report procedures performed on hospital inpatients.

- ***Healthcare Common Procedure Coding System,*** which includes *Current Procedural Terminology* (CPT): This system is used for reporting physician and other healthcare services, including all noninpatient procedures.

- *Current Dental Terminology, Code on Dental Procedures and Nomenclatures* (CDT): This system is used for reporting dental services.

- *National Drug Codes* (NDC): In the original ruling from Medicare, the NDC was designated as the official data set for reporting drugs used by pharmacies. However, this adoption was repealed in 2003. Currently, there is no official standard for reporting medications on pharmacy transactions.

International Classification of Diseases, Ninth Revision, Clinical Modification

The *International Classification of Diseases* (ICD) is a classification system for reporting medical diagnoses and procedures.

History

ICD-9-CM is one of the most common classification systems used in the United States today. It is an adaptation of the *International Classification of Diseases, Ninth Revision* (ICD-9), published by WHO in Geneva, Switzerland.

In the United States, the federal government, through the National Center for Health Statistics (NCHS), modified ICD-9 to create ICD-9-CM. ICD-9-CM was issued for use in the U.S. in 1978. The intent of this modification was to provide a classification system for morbidity data.

ICD-9-CM is maintained by four organizations known as the Cooperating Parties: NCHS, the American Hospital Association (AHA), the American Health Information Management Association (AHIMA), and the Centers for Medicare and Medicaid Services (CMS). The Cooperating Parties assume the following responsibilities:

- To serve as a clearinghouse to answer questions on ICD-9-CM

- To develop educational materials and programs on ICD-9-CM

- To work cooperatively in maintaining the integrity of ICD-9-CM

- To recommend revisions and modifications to current and future revisions of ICD

The work of the Cooperating Parties was supplemented by AHA's Editorial Advisory Board for *Coding Clinic,* which was composed of representatives of hospitals, heath data systems, and the federal government (NCVHS 1991).

Primarily, NCHS is responsible for updating the diagnosis classification (Volumes 1 and 2), and CMS is responsible for updating the procedure classification (Volume 3). AHIMA works to help provide training and certification, and the AHA maintains the Central Office on ICD-9-CM and publishes *Coding Clinic for ICD-9-CM,* which contains the Official Coding Guidelines and official guidance on the usage of ICD-9-CM codes.

In 1985, the ICD-9-CM Coordination and Maintenance Committee was established. Cochaired by representatives of NCHS and CMS, the committee is made up of advisors and representatives of all the Cooperating Parties. It meets twice a year to provide a public forum for discussing possible revisions and updates to ICD-9-CM. Discussions at these meetings are advisory only. The director of NCHS and the administrator of CMS determine all final revisions.

Purpose and Use

According to the Central Office on ICD-9-CM, ICD-9-CM has the following uses:

- Classifying morbidity and mortality information for statistical purposes

- Indexing hospital records by disease and operations

- Reporting diagnoses by physicians

- Storing and retrieving data

- Reporting national morbidity and mortality data

- Serving as the basis of diagnosis-related group (DRG) assignment for hospital reimbursement

- Reporting and compiling healthcare data to assist in the evaluation of medical care planning for healthcare delivery systems

- Determining patterns of care among healthcare providers

- Analyzing payments for health services

- Conducting epidemiological and clinical research

Overview of Structure

ICD-9-CM is published in three volumes. Volume 1 is known as the Tabular List. It contains the numerical listing of codes that represent diseases and injuries. Volume 2 is the Alphabetic Index. It consists of an alphabetic index for all the codes listed in volume 1. The Tabular List and Alphabetic Index for Procedures are published as volume 3. Volume 3 is not part of the international version of ICD-9. It is used only in the U.S. to report procedures performed on hospital inpatients.

Volume 1

Volume 1 of ICD-9-CM is divided into three subdivisions: classification of diseases and injuries, supplementary classifications, and appendixes.

The classification of diseases and injuries is divided into seventeen chapters. (See figure 6.1.) The chapters are organized by type of condition and anatomical system. For example, chapter 5, Mental Disorders, represents a chapter that groups diseases by type of condition. Chapter 6, Diseases of the Nervous System and Sense Organs, represents a chapter that groups diseases by anatomical system.

The chapters are further divided into sections. Sections are groups of three-digit code numbers. An example of a section in chapter 5 is the disease classification for organic psychotic conditions (290–294). (See figure 6.2.)

Sections are subdivided into categories. Categories represent a group of closely related conditions or a single disease entity. Category 290, Senile and presenile organic psychotic conditions, is an example of a category found in chapter 5.

Categories are further divided into subcategories. At this level, four-digit code numbers are used. Figure 6.2 provides an example of a subcategory: code number 290.1, Presenile dementia.

The most specific codes in the ICD-9-CM system are found at the subclassification level. Five-digit code numbers represent this level. In figure 6.2, code 290.10 represents a code at the subclassification level.

Two supplementary classifications are part of volume 1: the Supplementary Classification of Factors Influencing Health Status and Contact with Health Services (V codes)

Figure 6.1.   Chapter titles in the *ICD-9-CM Classification of Diseases and Injuries*

1. Infectious and Parasitic Diseases
2. Neoplasms
3. Endocrine, Nutritional, and Metabolic Diseases and Immunity Disorders
4. Diseases of the Blood and Blood-Forming Organs
5. Mental Disorders
6. Diseases of the Nervous System and Sense Organs
7. Diseases of the Circulatory System
8. Diseases of the Respiratory System
9. Diseases of the Digestive System
10. Diseases of the Genitourinary System
11. Complications of Pregnancy, Childbirth, and the Puerperium
12. Diseases of the Skin and Subcutaneous Tissue
13. Diseases of the Musculoskeletal System and Connective Tissue
14. Congenital Anomalies
15. Certain Conditions Originating in the Perinatal Period
16. Symptoms, Signs, and Ill-Defined Conditions
17. Injury and Poisoning

Figure 6.2. Example of an ICD-9-CM section

ORGANIC PSYCHOTIC CONDITIONS (290–294)

Includes: psychotic organic brain syndrome

Excludes: *nonpsychotic syndromes of organic etiology (310.0–310.9)*
psychoses classifiable to 295–298 and without
  impairment of orientation, comprehension, calculation,
  learning capacity, and judgment, but associated with
  physical disease, injury, or condition affecting the brain
  [e.g., following childbirth] (295.0–298.8)

290   Senile and presenile organic psychotic conditions
Code first the associated neurological condition

Excludes: *dementia not classified as senile, presenile, or arteriosclerotic*
    (294.10–294.11)
psychoses classifiable to 295–298 occurring in the senium
    without dementia or delirium (295.0–298.8)
senility with mental changes of nonpsychotic severity (310.1)
transient organic psychotic conditions (293.0–293.9)

290.0   Senile dementia, uncomplicated
Senile dementia:
  NOS
  simple type

Excludes: *mild memory disturbances, not amounting to dementia,*
    associated with senile brain disease (310.1)
senile dementia with:
    delirium or confusion (290.3)
    delusional [paranoid] features (290.20)
    depressive features (290.21)

290.1   Presenile dementia
Brain syndrome with presenile brain disease

Excludes: *arteriosclerotic dementia (290.40–290.43)*
dementia associated with other cerebral conditions
    (294.10–294.11)

290.10   Presenile dementia, uncomplicated
Presenile dementia:
  NOS
  simple type
290.11   Presenile dementia with delirium
Presenile dementia with acute confusional state
290.12   Presenile dementia with delusional features
Presenile dementia, paranoid type
290.13   Presenile dementia with depressive features
Presenile dementia, depressed type

and the Supplementary Classification of External Causes of Injury and Poisoning (E codes).

V codes are used to classify occasions when circumstances other than disease or injury are recorded as the reason for the patient's encounter with the healthcare provider. Such circumstances generally occur in one of the following three ways:

- When a person who is not currently sick encounters a health service provider for some specific reason, such as to act as an organ or tissue donor, to receive prophylactic vaccination, or to discuss a problem that in itself is not a disease or injury (for example, when a patient sees a physician for a measles vaccination)

- When a person with a known disease or injury, whether current or resolving, encounters the healthcare system for a specific treatment of that disease or injury (for example, when a patient seeks follow-up care for a previously applied cast)

- When some circumstance or problem influences the person's health status but is not in itself a current injury or illness (for example, when a patient has a personal history of smoking)

V codes are always alphanumeric codes. They are easy to identify because they begin with the alpha character *V* and are followed by numerical digits. An example is V15.04, Allergy to seafood.

E codes provide a means to classify environmental events, circumstances, and conditions as the cause of injury, poisoning, and other adverse effect. These codes must be used in addition to codes from the main chapters of ICD-9-CM. E codes provide additional information used by insurance companies, safety programs, and public health agencies to determine the causes of injuries, poisonings, or other adverse situations. Even though use of many E codes is optional, many facilities use them as secondary codes to identify the cause of accidents and injuries. Some states have mandated reporting of E codes in certain circumstances, such as in reporting head trauma.

E codes begin with the alpha character *E* and are followed by numerical characters. E925.0 represents the code for an accident caused by an electric current in domestic wiring and appliances.

The last subdivision of volume 1 consists of the appendixes. ICD-9-CM includes five appendixes:

Appendix A: Morphology of Neoplasms

Appendix B: Glossary of Mental Disorders

Appendix C: Classification of Drugs by American Hospital

Formulary Service List Number

Appendix D: Classification of Industrial Accidents According to Agency

Appendix E: List of Three-Digit Categories

Volume 2

The Index to Diseases and Injuries is printed as volume 2 of ICD-9-CM. Main terms appear alphabetically in the index by type of disease, injury, or illness. Subterms are indented under the main term. For example, the main term **Bradycardia** and the subterms for bradycardia appear as shown in figure 6.3.

Volume 3

The third volume of ICD-9-CM contains the tabular and alphabetic lists of procedures. The Tabular List of Procedures contains chapters organized according to anatomical system, except for the last chapter, Miscellaneous Diagnostic and Therapeutic Procedures. Figure 6.4 shows the procedure chapter titles. According to the HIPAA regulations, these codes are to be used only for inpatient hospital billing.

ICD-9-CM procedure codes are organized according to these chapters, and then the chapters are divided into two-, three-, and sometimes four-digit code numbers. All procedure codes are written with two digits to the left of the decimal point. Figure 6.5 provides an example of a tabular listing from the beginning of chapter 2, Operations on the Endocrine System (06–07).

The Alphabetic Index to Procedures is organized in the same manner as the Alphabetic Index to Diseases. Figure 6.6 shows an example of the alphabetic organization of procedures.

Figure 6.3.   Example of index entries for main terms and subterms in ICD-9-CM

Brachycephaly 756.0
Brachymorphism and ectopia lentis 759.89
Bradley's disease (epidemic vomiting) 078.82
Bradycardia 427.89
    chronic (sinus) 427.81
    newborn 763.83
    nodal 427.89
    postoperative 997.1
    reflex 337.0
    sinoatrial 427.89
      with paroxysmal tachyarrhythmia or tachycardia 427.81
      chronic 427.81
    sinus 427.89
    with paroxysmal tachyarrhythmia or tachycardia 427.81
      chronic 427.81
      persistent 427.81
      severe 427.81
    tachycardia syndrome 427.81
    vagal 427.89
Bradypnea 786.09
Brailsford's disease 732.3
    radial head 732.3
    tarsal scaphoid 732.5

Figure 6.4.   Chapter titles in the ICD-9-CM tabular list of procedures

1.   Operations on the Nervous System
2.   Operations on the Endocrine System
3.   Operations on the Eye
4.   Operations on the Ear
5.   Operations on the Nose, Mouth, and Pharynx
6.   Operations on the Respiratory System
7.   Operations on the Cardiovascular System
8.   Operations on the Hemic and Lymphatic System
9.   Operations on the Digestive System
10. Operations on the Urinary System
11. Operations on the Male Genital Organs
12. Operations on the Female Genital Organs
13. Obstetrical Procedures
14. Operations on the Musculoskeletal System
15. Operations on the Integumentary System
16. Miscellaneous Diagnostic and Therapeutic Procedures

Figure 6.5.   Example from the ICD-9-CM tabular list of procedures

06   Operations on thyroid and parathyroid glands
        Includes: incidental resection of hyoid bone
  06.0   Incision of thyroid field

  Excludes: *division of isthmus (06.91)*

  06.01   Aspiration of thyroid field
          Percutaneous or needle drainage of thyroid field

  Excludes: *aspiration biopsy of thyroid (06.11)*
                 drainage by incision (06.09)
                 postoperative aspiration of field (06.02)

  06.02   Reopening of wound of thyroid field
          Reopening of wound of thyroid field for:
             control of (postoperative) hemorrhage
             examination
             exploration
             removal of hematoma

  06.09   Other incision of thyroid field
          Drainage of hematoma   ⎫
          Drainage of thyroglossal tract ⎬
          Exploration: ⎬
             neck   ⎬ by incision
             thyroid (field)   ⎬
          Removal of foreign body   ⎬
          Thyroidotomy NOS   ⎭

  Excludes: *postoperative exploration (06.02)*
                 removal of hematoma by aspiration (06.01)

Figure 6.6.   Example of alphabetic entries in the ICD-9-CM index to procedures

Acromioplasty 81.83
    for recurrent dislocation of shoulder 81.82
    partial replacement 81.81
    total replacement 81.80
Actinotherapy 99.82
Activities of daily living (ADL)
    therapy 93.83
    training for the blind 93.78
Acupuncture 99.92
    with smouldering moxa 93.35
    for anesthesia 99.91
Adams operation
    advancement of round ligament 69.22
    crushing of nasal septum 21.88
    excision of palmar fascia 82.35

Check Your Understanding 6.1

Instructions: Use the following excerpt from the Alphabetic Index to complete the questions below.

Bacillary—see condition
Bacilluria 791.9
    asymptomatic, in pregnancy or puerperium 646.5
    tuberculous (*see also* Tuberculosis) 016.9
Bacillus—*see also* Infection, bacillus
    abortus infection 023.1
    anthracis infection 022.9
    coli
        infection 041.4
            generalized 038.42
            intestinal 008.00
        pyemia 038.42
        septicemia 038.42
    Flexner's 004.1
    fusiformis infestation 101
    mallei infection 024
    Shiga's 004.0
    suipestifer infection (*see also* Infection, Salmonella) 003.9
Back—*see* condition
Backache (postural) 724.5
    psychogenic 307.89
    sacroiliac 724.6

1.   List the first four main terms that appear in the excerpt.

    _____   _____   _____   _____

2.   List the first four subterms that appear under **Bacillus.**

    _____   _____   _____   _____

3.   Indicate whether each of the following codes represents a disease (D) or a procedure (P).
  a.   ____   99.82
  b.   ____   098.0
  c.   ____   301.51
  d.   ____   73.4
  e.   ____   844.0
  f.   ____   45.24

International Classification of Diseases, Tenth Revision, Clinical Modification

Established by WHO, the ICD system was designed to be totally revised at ten-year intervals. In the mid-1990s, WHO published the newest version of ICD; *International Statistical Classification of Diseases and Related Health Problems, Tenth Revision,* known as ICD-10. This revision is currently in use by many countries throughout the world and has been used in the U.S. to capture mortality statistics since 1999. However, studies in the U.S. determined that ICD-10 needed to be modified to capture data that would support our reimbursement system prior to implementation.

Purpose and Use

The Clinical Modification of ICD-10 is known as the ***International Classification of Diseases, Tenth Revision, Clinical Modification.*** According to NCHS, ICD-10-CM is the planned replacement for ICD-9-CM, volumes 1 and 2. This revision is considered to be an improvement over both ICD-9-CM and ICD-10, and was developed to contain a great many more codes and allow greater specificity than existing ICD code sets.

Overview of Structure

Although the traditional ICD structure remains, ICD-10-CM is a complete alphanumeric coding scheme. The former supplementary classification information (V and E codes) was incorporated into the main classification system with different letters preceding the numerical portions of the codes. ICD-10 contains new chapters, and several categories have been restructured and new features added to maintain consistency with modern medicine. The disease classification has been expanded to provide greater specificity at the sixth-digit level and with a seventh-digit extension.

A draft of ICD-10-CM is available from the NCHS Web site at cdc.gov/nchs/about/otheract/icd9/icd10cm.htm. A draft of official guidelines for ICD-10-CM has been developed and can be downloaded from cdc.gov/nchs/data/icd9/draft_i10guideln.pdf.

Examples of ICD-10-CM codes include the following:

* Malignant Neoplasm

    C34.1 Malignant neoplasm of upper lobe, bronchus or lung

    C34.10 Malignant neoplasm of upper lobe, bronchus or lung, unspecified side

    C34.11 Malignant neoplasm of upper lobe, right bronchus or lung

    C34.12 Malignant neoplasm of upper lobe, left bronchus or lung

* Diabetes

    E10.2 Type 1 diabetes mellitus with renal complications

E10.21 Type 1 diabetes mellitus with diabetic nephropathy

Type 1 diabetes mellitus with intercapillary glomerulosclerosis

Type 1 diabetes with intracapillary glomerulonephritis

E10.22 Type 1 diabetes mellitus with Ebstein's disease

E10.29 Type 1 diabetes mellitus with other diabetic renal complication

International Classification of Diseases, 10th Revision, Procedure Coding System

ICD-10-CM does not include a procedure volume. Thus, when the U.S. began planning to clinically modify WHO's ICD-10, it was determined that creating a separate volume for procedures would be insufficient. As a result, CMS contracted with 3M Health Information Systems to develop a separate procedure code system that would serve as a replacement for ICD-9-CM, Volume 3. This coding system is known as the *International Classification of Diseases, 10th Revision, Procedure Classification System,* or ICD-10-PCS.

Purpose and Use

According to CMS, the agency responsible for updating the procedure section of ICD-9-CM, the design of ICD-10-PCS included the following goals:

- To improve accuracy and efficiency of coding

- To reduce training effort

- To improve communication with physicians

Overview of Structure

ICD-10-PCS has no correlation to the ICD-10-CM structure. It consists of a multiaxial seven-character alphanumeric code structure. The ten digits 0 through 9 and the 24 letters A–H, J–N, and P–Z are characters used in ICD-10-PCS. Although this system has the capability and flexibility to replace all existing procedural coding systems, it is currently being recommended to replace only ICD-9-CM procedure codes (NCVHS 1991). Because of its unique structure, ICD-10-PCS is considered to be both complete and expandable.

Because many different and confusing names of procedures are in use in the medical field, each root procedure has been defined in ICD-10-PCS. This helps to clarify terms that currently have overlapping meaning, such as excision, resection, or removal.

Procedures are divided into sixteen sections related to general type of procedure (medical and surgical, imaging, and so on). All procedure codes have seven characters. The first character of the procedure code always specifies the section where the procedure is indexed. The second through seventh characters have a standard meaning within each section. In medical and surgical procedures, the seven characters are defined as follows:

1 = Section of the ICD-10-PCS system where the code resides

2 = The body system

3 = Root operation (such as excision, incision)

4 = Specific body part

5 = Approach used, such as intraluminal or open

6 = Device used to perform the procedure

7 = Qualifier to provide additional information about the procedure (for example, diagnostic versus therapeutic)

An example of an ICD-10-PCS code is 095HBYZ, Dilation Eustachian Tube, Right with Device NEC, Transorifice Intraluminal.

0	Surgical Section
9	Body System—Ear, nose, sinus
5	Procedure is a dilation
H	Eustachian tube, right
B	Transorifice intraluminal approach
Y	Device NEC
Z	No qualifier

The draft ICD-10-PCS code system and training manual are available online from cms.hhs.gov/paymentsystems/icd9/icd10.asp?

Implementation of ICD-10 in the U.S.

At the time of this writing, the National Committee on Vital and Health Statistics (NCVHS) had recommended that both ICD-10-CM and ICD-10-PCS be adopted as the national standards under the HIPAA electronic transactions and coding standards rule to replace the current uses of ICD-9-CM. The next step is for the government to publish a notice of proposed rulemaking in the *Federal Register*. After the required time frame for comments has passed, a final rule will be published with an effective date. The new coding system(s) would be implemented as the standard in a designated time frame (typically two years) from then to allow for training and the upgrading of coding systems.

Coders should begin to familiarize themselves with the new systems. The *Journal of American Health Information Management Association* and other publications are beginning to publish preparation articles that will enable coders to stay current and be prepared for the changes as they take effect. Extensive training sessions and coding materials are being developed to assist coders and facilities with this transition.

International Classification of Diseases for Oncology, Third Edition

The third edition of the *International Classification of Diseases for Oncology, Third Edition* (ICD-O-3) is a system used for classifying incidences of malignant disease. Hospitals use ICD-O-3 for several purposes, for example, to develop cancer registries. Cancer registries list all the cases of cancer diagnosed and treated in the facility.

History of ICD-O-3

WHO published the first edition of the *International Classification of Diseases for Oncology* (ICD-O) in 1976. It was developed jointly by the United States Cancer Institute and WHO's International Agency for Research on Cancer.

In 1968, the American Cancer Society published *Manual of Tumor Nomenclature and Coding* (MOTNAC). Also in 1968, WHO asked the International Agency for Research on Cancer to develop a chapter on neoplasms for the ninth revision of ICD. WHO decided to publish a supplemental neoplasm classification based on MOTNAC for ICD-9.

ICD-O-3 was published for use in coding cancers diagnosed in the United States after January 1, 2001.

Purpose and Use

Originally, ICD-O was developed to aid in the collection of information in the field of oncology. (Oncology is the study of neoplasms [new tissue], or tumors.) Its purpose is to provide a detailed classification system for coding the histology (morphology [structure]), topography (site), and behavior of neoplasms. The current version of ICD-O provides a detailed classification used by pathology departments, cancer registries, and healthcare providers who treat cancer patients.

Overview of Structure

A dual-axis classification is used in ICD-O-3 to code the topography and morphology of the neoplasm. These codes are identical or compatible with other coding classifications and nomenclatures. For example, the topography codes used in ICD-10 for malignant neoplasms are the same codes used in ICD-O-3.

The morphology codes identify the type of tumor found and its behavior. The morphology code numbers consist of the letter *M* followed by five digits. The first four digits identify the histological type of the neoplasm. The fifth digit identifies the behavior of the tumor. The following morphology codes for some leukemias provide an example:

Leukemias

M9891/3   Acute monocytic leukemia

M9895/3   Acute myeloid leukemia with multilineage dysplasia

M9896/3   Acute myeloid leukemia, AML1

M9897/3   Acute myeloid leukemia, MLL

The fifth-digit (behavior) codes that appear after the slash are used to indicate the following:

/0 Benign

/1 Uncertain whether benign or malignant, borderline malignancy

/2 Carcinoma in situ

    Intraepithelial

    Noninfiltrating

    Non-invasive

/3 Malignant, primary site

/6 Malignant, metastatic site

    Secondary site

/9 Malignant, uncertain whether primary or metastatic site

Check Your Understanding 6.2

Instructions: List the type of behavior for the tumors represented by the following codes.

1. _____ M8140/0

2. _____ M8490/6

3. _____ M8331/3

4. _____ M8120/2

Healthcare Common Procedure Coding System

HCPCS was originally called the HCFA Common Procedure Coding System. The name of the system was changed in 2001, when the Health Care Financing Administration (the agency that administered the Medicare and Medicaid programs) changed its name to the Centers for Medicare and Medicaid Services (CMS). HCPCS is used to report physicians' services to Medicare for reimbursement.

History of HCPCS

HCPCS (pronounced "Hick Picks") is a collection of codes and descriptors used to represent healthcare procedures, supplies, products, and services. When the Medicare program was first implemented in the early 1980s, the Health Care Financing Administration (HCFA) found it necessary to expand the HCPCS system because not all supplies, procedures, and services could be coded using the CPT system. An example of this shortcoming is durable medical equipment (DME). CPT does not contain codes for DME. Therefore, HCFA developed an additional level of codes to report supplies and services that are not in CPT (for example, DME).

Purpose and Use

In 1983, Medicare introduced HCPCS to promote uniform reporting and statistical data collection of medical procedures, supplies, products, and services. Most state Medicaid programs also use portions of the HCPCS coding system. Physicians and providers use HCPCS codes to report the services and procedures they deliver.

Overview of Structure

HCPCS is divided into two code levels or groups: I and II.

Level I

Level I codes are the AMA's CPT codes. These five-digit codes and two-digit modifiers are copyrighted by the AMA. CPT codes primarily cover physicians' services but are used for hospital outpatient coding as well. CPT codes are updated annually, effective January 1.

Level II

Level II codes, also called National Codes, are maintained by CMS. With the exception of temporary codes, level II codes are updated annually on January 1. Temporary codes begin with the letters *G, K,* or *Q.* Temporary codes are updated throughout the year. Level II also contains modifiers in the form of letters and alphanumeric characters.

Level II codes were developed to code medical services, equipment, and supplies that are not included in CPT. Today, when people refer to HCPCS codes, they are often referring to Level II codes; Level I codes are most often referred to merely as CPT. Technically,

HCPCS includes both Level I (CPT) and Level II codes. The codes are alphanumeric and start with an alphabetic character from A to V. The alphabetic character is followed by four numeric characters. The alphabetic character identifies the code section and type of service or supply coded. At times, Level II codes were designed to reflect code assignment based on Medicare payment regulations. Figure 6.7 shows the different code choices for patients undergoing a colonoscopy based on their medical necessity.

Figure 6.8 provides a list of the major sections in Level II.

Level II also contains modifiers that can be used with all levels of HCPCS codes, including CPT codes. The modifiers permit greater reporting specificity in reference to the main code. Sample level II modifiers appear in figure 6.9.

Figure 6.7.   CPT/HCPCS code choices for colonoscopy

Example:

Reason for Colonoscopy	Appropriate code
Problem, such as bleeding or polyps	CPT codes 45378–45392
Colorectal cancer screening, patient does not meet Medicare definition of high risk	G0121
Colorectal cancer screening, patient meets definition of high risk	G0105

Figure 6.8.   HCPCS Level II section titles

A0000–A0999	Transport Services Including Ambulance
A4000–A4899	Medical and Surgical Supplies
A9000–A9999	Administrative, Miscellaneous, and Investigational
B4000–B9999	Enteral and Parenteral Therapy
D0000–D9999	Dental Procedures
E0100–E9999	Durable Medical Equipment
G0000–G9999	Procedures/Professional Services (Temporary)
J0000–J8999	Drugs Other Than Chemotherapy
J9000–J9999	Chemotherapy Drugs
K0000–K9999	Orthotic Procedures
L5000–L9999	Prosthetic Procedures
M0000–M0009	Medical Services
P2000–P2999	Laboratory Tests
Q0000–Q9999	Temporary Codes
R0000–R5999	Domestic Radiology Services
S0009–S9999	Temporary National Codes
V0000–V2999	Vision Services
V5000–V5299	Hearing Services

Figure 6.9. Sample HCPCS Level II modifiers

–AA	Anesthesia services performed personally by anesthesiologist
–E1	Upper left eyelid
–E2	Lower left eyelid
–E3	Upper right eyelid
–E4	Lower right eyelid
–NU	New equipment
–QC	Single channel monitoring

Current Procedural Terminology, Version 4

As mentioned earlier, the CPT system is copyrighted and maintained by the AMA. There have been several major updates to the system since the original edition was published in 1966. Code updates are published annually and take effect every January 1.

History of CPT-4

CPT is a comprehensive descriptive listing of terms and codes for reporting diagnostic and therapeutic procedures and medical services. Currently, it is updated annually by the AMA's CPT Editorial Panel. This panel is composed of physicians and other healthcare professionals who revise, modify, and update the publication.

The Editorial Panel gets advice on revisions from the CPT Advisory Committee. This committee is nominated by the AMA House of Delegates and is composed of representatives from more than ninety medical specialties and healthcare providers. As defined by the AMA, the committee has three objectives:

- To serve as a resource to the Editorial Panel by giving advice on procedure coding and nomenclature as relevant to the member's specialty

- To provide documentation to staff and the Editorial Panel regarding the medical appropriateness of various medical and surgical procedures

- To suggest revisions to CPT

Purpose and Use

The purpose of CPT is to provide a system for standard terminology and coding to report medical procedures and services. CPT is one of the most widely used systems for reporting medical services to health insurance carriers. In addition, it is used for other administrative purposes, such as developing guidelines for medical care review. Organizations that collect data for medical education and research purposes also use CPT.

Today, CMS requires that CPT codes be used to report medical services provided to patients in specific settings. Starting in 1983, HCFA (now called the CMS) required that CPT be used to report services provided to Medicare Part B beneficiaries. In October 1986, HCFA required state Medicaid agencies to use CPT as part of the Medicaid Management Information System. As part of the Omnibus Budget Reconciliation Act, HCFA required in July 1987 that CPT be used for reporting outpatient hospital surgical procedures and ambulatory surgery center procedures. The most recent mandate for CPT use occurred with the final rule of the Health Insurance Portability and Accountability Act (HIPAA). HIPAA mandates that CPT be used as the required code set for physicians' services and other medical services such as physical therapy and most laboratory procedures.

Overview of Structure

The CPT codebook consists of an introduction, eight sections containing the codes, appendixes, and an index. Five digit codes are used, most are numeric, although specific sections include an alpha character. The eight sections include: evaluation and management services, anesthesia, surgery, radiology (including nuclear medicine and diagnostic ultrasound), pathology and laboratory, medicine, Category II and Category III codes.

Introduction

The introduction contains a list of the codebook section numbers and their sequences and instructions for use. Information that appears in the introduction applies to all sections of the codebook. A coder who is unfamiliar with CPT coding should read the introduction.

Symbols and punctuation marks are used to assist coders in correct usage of CPT codes. The symbols used in the CPT codebook are explained in the introduction and are found at the bottom of each page of the coding section of the book. For example, a bullet listed to the left of a code signifies that the code is new for that year's updated book.

Sections

The sections are as follows:

Evaluation and Management	99210–99499
Anesthesia	00100–01999
Surgery	10040–69990
Radiology	70010–79999
Pathology and Laboratory	80049–89399
Medicine	90281–99199
Category II Codes	0500F–4011F
Category III Codes	0003T–0088T

Each of these sections begins with guidelines containing specific instructions and definitions that are unique to the section. Coders must understand the information in the guidelines in order to code correctly from each section.

Category II and III Codes

According to CPT, Category II codes were designed as "supplemental tracking codes that can be used for performance measurement." Although these codes are optional, they can be used to provide greater specificity regarding a patient's visit and treatment details.

Category III codes were added to the CPT book to allow for temporary coding assignment for new technology and services that do not meet the rigorous requirements necessary to be added to the main section of the CPT book. The codes are not optional and should be used to report procedures performed. Codes in the Category III section are evaluated and added every six months. As Category I codes (codes ranging from 00100 to 99499) are created to describe new procedures, the corresponding temporary category III codes will be deleted from the CPT system.

Appendixes

Appendixes follow the last section of codes. The appendixes provide information to help the coder in the coding process. Appendix A provides a complete list of modifiers and their descriptions. Modifiers are written as two-digit codes that follow the main CPT codes.

For example, the two-digit modifier for prolonged evaluation and management services is –21.

Appendix B is a summary of the additions, deletions, and revisions that have been implemented for the current CPT edition. This appendix can be used to update information and data that contain CPT codes.

Appendix C provides clinical examples for codes found in the evaluation and management section (E/M) of the book. These examples can be used as a tool to assist the coder in reporting an E/M code.

Appendix D is a listing of CPT add-on codes. These codes must be preceded by a primary procedure code and would never be reported alone.

Appendix E is a summary of CPT codes that are exempt from modifier 51, and appendix F is a summary of CPT codes that are exempt from modifier 63.

Appendix G contains codes that include conscious sedation.

Appendix H is an alphabetic index of performance measures by clinical condition or type. This appendix was developed to provide further description of the codes found in the Category II section of CPT.

Appendix I contains genetic testing code modifiers used for reporting with lab procedures related to genetic testing.

Index

The index of the CPT codebook lists main terms alphabetically. Main term entries are of four types:

- Procedure or service
- Organ or other anatomic site
- Condition
- Synonym, eponym, or abbreviation

Main terms are followed by subterms. The subterms modify the main terms and are indented under them. Coders begin their search for the correct CPT code by checking the alphabetic index in the above order until finding a likely code to describe the procedure performed. The coder should then verify the code(s) selected in the main section of the codebook to be certain the code best describes the procedure(s) performed. Figure 6.10 shows a portion of the CPT index.

Figure 6.10.   Portion of the CPT index

Face

CT Scan	70486–70488
Lesion Destruction	17000–17004, 17280–17286
Magnetic Resonance Imaging (MRI)	70540–70543
Tumor Resection	21015

Face Lift   15824–15828

Facial Asymmetries
See Hemifacial Microsomia

Check Your Understanding 6.3

Instructions: List the section of the CPT codebook in which each of the following codes is located.

1. _____ 99311

2. _____ 90807

3. _____ 33470

4. _____ 01200

5. _____ 87551

6. _____ 77295

7. _____ 0071T

Systematized Nomenclature of Medicine

The **Systematized Nomenclature of Medicine Clinical Terminology** (SNOMED CT) is a controlled reference terminology. The American College of Pathologists (ACP) defines SNOMED CT as a systematized, multiaxial, and hierarchically organized nomenclature of medically useful terms.

History

ACP published the first edition of SNOMED in 1977. SNOMED is based on the Systematized Nomenclature of Pathology (SNOP), which was published by ACP in 1965 to organize information from surgical pathology reports. Because SNOP was widely used and accepted in the medical community, it was expanded as a nomenclature for other specialties.

Numerous versions of SNOMED have been published since 1977. The current version includes more than 150,000 terms that are used in countries throughout the world. SNOMED CT is the most comprehensive controlled vocabulary developed to date.

The updated version of SNOMED is SNOMED CT (clinical terms) is a "comprehensive multilingual clinical terminology tool providing the information framework for clinical decision making for electronic medical record" (Brouch 2003). This version is an adaptation of earlier versions of SNOMED and also contains the United Kingdom's National Health Service's Clinical Terms (previously known as **Read Codes**). Read Codes users are being migrated over to SNOMED CT.

In 2003, the Department of Health and Human Services "purchased a license for SNOMED CT, allowing all federal and private developers of [Electronic Health Record] EHR systems to freely incorporate the vocabulary system" (Giannangelo and Berkowitz 2005). Mapping between ICD-9-CM and SNOMED codes is being completed by the National Library of Medicine (NLM) to help vendors crosswalk between ICD-9-CM codes required for reimbursement and SNOMED CT's larger number of diagnostic terms.

Purpose and Use

In the field of medicine, two physicians may use two different terms for the same medical condition. This makes it difficult to gather and retrieve information. Standardized vocabulary is needed to facilitate the indexing, storage, and retrieval of patient information in an EHR. SNOMED CT creates a standardized vocabulary.

The Computer-based Patient Record Institute (CPRI) has studied the ability of current nomenclatures to capture information for EHRs. The institute has determined that

SNOMED CT is the most comprehensive controlled vocabulary for coding the contents of the health record and facilitating the development of computerized records.

Overview of Structure

Using SNOMED as a foundation, SNOMED CT presents data in a completely machine-readable format. According to SNOMED International, the core content data of SNOMED CT includes the following tables:

- Concepts
- Descriptions
- Relationships
- History

SNOMED CT has been mapped to ICD-9-CM as well as other commonly used vocabularies such as ICD-O3, ICD-10, and LOINC.

The core tables provide the framework for the organization. The concepts table lists every concept that appeared in earlier versions of SNOMED CT, starting with version 3. More than 366,000 concepts are organized into 18 hierarchies within the SNOMED CT system. Each concept, or fully specified name as listed on the table, is given a concept identifier.

Concepts are further identified by various terms or phrases that define them. The combination of a concept and a term is a description. Descriptions are given a Description ID.

Real-World Example

TheraDoc is a medical informatics company that produces software used for clinical decision support. One of its systems, Antibiotic Assistant, was designed to support the appropriate use of antibiotics. SNOMED CT was integrated into Antibiotic Assistant to allow the system to be integrated with other patient information systems in order to analyze possible drug interactions or adverse reactions to the medications. According to SNOMED International, TheraDoc's Antibiotic Assistant, powered by SNOMED CT, converts the raw data into usable information, dramatically reducing the time from recognition of a potential problem to intervention. Instead of having to track down information form various sources . . . the physician receives comprehensive information in real time as part of his daily routine, and is able to decide on an immediate course of action" (SNOMED International 2005).

Diagnostic and Statistical Manual of Mental Disorders, Fourth Edition, Text Revision

The American Psychiatric Association (APA) developed the ***Diagnostic and Statistical Manual of Mental Disorders*** (DSM) as a tool for providing a set of codes that could be used to aid in the collection of clinical data using stand-alone personal computers.

History of DSM-IV

The APA published the first edition of the DSM in 1952. The APA's Committee on Nomenclature and Statistics developed DSM from ICD. DSM-I contained a glossary of descriptions of mental disorders. DSM has been revised three times since 1952 and is now published as the fourth revision, or **DSM-IV-TR.** The updated text revision (TR) became effective in 2004 to maintain currency with updated clinical terms. There were very few coding changes in the DSM-IV-TR version.

To facilitate ease of use with ICD versions, the APA has worked closely with other organizations to make DMS-IV, ICD-9-CM, and ICD-10 fully compatible. All DSM-IV-TR codes are ICD-9-CM codes. This is even more important because the HIPAA law requires that valid ICD-9-CM codes be used for diagnostic purposes. According to the APA, "The DSM-IV is a diagnostic manual that employs the ICD-9-CM codes to assist the clinician medical record keeping. Because the DSM-IV-TR is a diagnostic manual, there are a number of subtypes and specifiers that are not codable to the ICD-9-CM" (2005).

Purpose and Use

The main purpose of DSM-IV-TR is to provide a means to record data on patients treated for substance abuse and mental disorders. DSM is used as a nomenclature that clinicians can reference to enhance their clinical practices and as a language for communicating diagnostic information. Clinicians use DSM to assign a diagnosis.

DSM contains a listing of the criteria for diagnosing each mental disorder and its key clinical manifestations. Mental conditions are evaluated along five axes.

Overview of Structure

The five axes used in DSM-IV-TR are:

Axis I	Clinical Disorders Other Conditions That May Be a Focus of Clinical Attention
Axis II	Personality Disorders Mental Retardation
Axis III	General Medical Conditions
Axis IV	Psychosocial and Environmental Problems
Axis V	Global Assessment of Functioning

Use of these axes by clinicians helps to establish a systematic evaluation of patient symptoms. This will lead to the establishment of diagnoses for the patient. The diagnoses then are given a code or codes that are the same as ICD-9-CM codes.

Read Codes

The Read Codes were developed in the United Kingdom during the 1980s. They were designed for use in computer-based formats.

History of Read Codes

Dr. James Read was a general medical practitioner in Loughborough, England. In 1982, he developed a set of alphanumeric codes for use on his office computer. The codes allowed him to record the most common diseases and conditions for which he saw patients. From 1982 to 1987, the Read Codes were expanded and produced a coding system for the recording of many areas of clinical care.

In 1987, the British Medical Association and the Royal College of General Practitioners established a work party to investigate classification systems that could be used in general medical practices. A year later, this group concluded that the Read Codes should become the standard code set for recording medical data in general practice. Therefore, the Royal College of General Practitioners adopted the Read Codes as the standard.

The United Kingdom's National Health Service (NHS) also began to use Read Codes in other parts of the NHS. In 1990, the U.K. Department of Health purchased the Read Codes. They became Crown Copyright, and the name changed to the NHS Codes.

After the NHS secured the copyright to the Read Codes, they formed the NHS Centre for Coding and Classification (CCC). The CCC is now responsible for developing and maintaining the Read Codes.

Purpose and Use

The purpose of the Read Codes was to provide a set of codes that could be used to aid in the collection of clinical data using stand-alone personal computers. The Read Codes translate clinical data into a file structure that is easily used with computers.

The codes also translate other information that has an impact on patient care. Information on patient occupations, therapeutic regimes, administrative data, and equipment information are some of the other types of information that the Read Codes translate. Thus, the Read Codes can be used in all aspects of healthcare to translate many types of clinical and nonclinical information.

Overview of Structure

The Read Codes are organized into chapters. Some of the main chapters in version 3 include:

Occupations

History and Observations

Disorders

Investigations

Operations and Procedures

Regimes and Therapies

Prevention

Causes of Injury and Poisoning

Tumor Morphology

These chapters are further divided into hierarchies of five bytes represented by alphanumeric characters. The numeric characters used are 0 through 9, and the alphabetical characters used are from *A* through *Z*. Theoretically, the design of the hierarchy of codes allows for 916,132,832 codes in version 3.

Nursing Vocabularies

The use of vocabularies is a relatively new concept in the field of nursing. Many nursing vocabularies are currently used to classify nursing diagnoses, interventions, and outcomes.

History of Nursing Vocabularies

Nursing vocabularies were developed to aid in the collection of data about nursing care. They serve as a way to document nursing care and to facilitate the capture of these data on computer systems. The American Nurses Association (ANA) has established a steering committee on databases to support clinical nursing practice. The committee has recommended use of a unified nursing language system in the nursing profession.

Purpose and Use

The ANA recognizes approximately thirteen standardized terminologies. These are developed by separate agencies for various purposes. These terminologies are described in table 6.1. All the classifications approved by the ANA are included in the Unified Medical Language System (UMLS).

Table 6.1. Widely used nursing vocabularies and classifications

Vocabulary or Classification System	Usage	Web Site
North American Nursing Diagnosis Association (NANDA) Taxonomy II	This classification is used to classify nursing diagnoses in all nursing settings. The NANDA multiaxial taxonomy is designed to provide a standardized nursing terminology to define patient responses, document care for reimbursement, and to allow for inclusion of nursing terminology in building clinical EHRs. (North American Nursing Diagnosis Association 2005).	nanda.org
Nursing Interventions Classifications (NIC) +	NIC is used to classify nursing interventions. Nursing interventions are any direct-care treatment that a nurse performs on behalf of the patient. These interventions are used to direct the care of patients.	nursing.uiowa.edu/centers/cncce/nic/nicoverview.htm
Nursing Outcomes Classification (NOC)	NOC is used to classify nursing outcomes. Nursing outcomes are the end result of care. They can measure quality of care, cost-efficiency, and progress of treatment.	nursing.uiowa.edu/centers/cncce/noc/index.htm
Home Health Care Classifications (HHCC)	HHCC contains two interrelated vocabularies used for classifying and documenting ambulatory and home health care. The HHCC of Nursing Diagnoses and the HHCC of Nursing Interventions are used.	sabacare.com
Nursing Management Minimum Data Set (NMMDS)	NMMDS captures nursing data for the comparison of patient outcomes.	nursing.uiowa.edu/nsa/nmmds.htm
OMAHA System	This classification is used to classify nursing diagnoses, interventions, and outcomes.	omahasystem.org/index.htm
SNOMED CT	SNOMED is a reference terminology for healthcare.	SNOMED.org
Perioperative Nursing Dataset (PNDS)	This data set is a standardized nursing vocabulary for use when patients undergo surgery. It allows for the capture of data from preadmission care until patient discharge.	aorn.org/research/pnds.htm
Clinical Care Classification (CCC)	The CCC is used to classify nursing diagnoses and outcomes, and interventions.	sabacare.com/
Patient Care Data Set	This terminology is now retired.	ncvhs.hhs.gov/990518t3.pdf
International Classification for Nursing Practice (2000) Information (ICNP)	ICNP provides data to influence decision-making, education, and health policy.	icn.ch/icnp_about.htm
Alternative Link	Alternative Link's ABC codes represent integrative healthcare products and services (complementary and alternative medicine).	alternativelink.com/ali/intro_altlink.html
Logical Observation Identifiers Names & Codes (LOINC)	LOINC is used to pool results—such as blood hemoglobin, serum potassium, or vital signs—for clinical care, outcomes management, and research.	regenstrief.org/loinc/

The nursing data sets and classification systems are developed to capture documentation on nursing care. They are designed to capture nursing diagnoses, interventions, and outcomes for acute, surgery, home, and ambulatory care settings.

According to the ANA, "A standardized vocabulary assists nurses to document care while providing a foundation for examining and evaluating the quality and effectiveness of that care. An information infrastructure provides the foundation for benchmarking, measuring and comparing outcome data, and evaluating the quality and effectiveness of care" (ANA 2002).

Overview of Structure

The various ANA-recognized standardized terminologies have different structures. Information on the specific structures can be found at the various Web sites listed in table 6.1 (p. 217).

Check Your Understanding 6.4

Instructions: Match the following classification systems with their functions.

1. _____ SNOMED CT

2. _____ Nursing vocabularies

3. _____ DSM-IV-TR

a. To document nursing care and to facilitate the capture of nursing information on computer systems
b. To provide a means to record information about patients treated for substance abuse and mental disorders
c. To aid in the collection of clinical data using stand-alone personal computers
d. To provide a system for coding the clinical services provided by physicians and other clinical professionals
e. To provide a controlled vocabulary for coding the contents of the patient record and for facilitating the development of computer-based patient records

---

The Coding Process

The coding process varies from organization to organization, but some standards, elements, and steps are common to almost all organizations.

Standards of Ethical Coding

In today's healthcare environment, coding plays an important role in the determination of reimbursement for healthcare facilities. AHIMA developed its Standards of Ethical Coding, last updated in December 1999. The standards were developed by AHIMA's Coding Policy and Strategy Committee and approved by its Board of Directors. The AHIMA standards are meant to serve as a guide for coding professionals. (See figure 6.11.)

Elements of Coding Quality

The coding function must be reviewed on an ongoing basis for consistency and accuracy. Audits should occur to review the codes selected by coders. Coding processes should be monitored for the following elements of quality:

- *Reliability:* The degree to which the same results are achieved consistently (that is, when different individuals code the same health record, they assign the same codes)

- *Validity:* The degree to which codes accurately reflect the patient's diagnoses and procedures

- *Completeness:* The degree to which the codes capture all the diagnoses and procedures documented in the health record

- *Timeliness:* The time frame in which the health records are coded

---

Figure 6.11.   AHIMA's Standards of Ethical Coding

1. Coding professionals are expected to support the importance of accurate, complete, and consistent coding practices for the production of quality healthcare data.

2. Coding professionals in all healthcare settings should adhere to the ICD-9-CM (International Classification of Diseases, 9th revision, Clinical Modification) coding conventions, official coding guidelines approved by the Cooperating Parties,* the CPT (Current Procedural Terminology) rules established by the American Medical Association, and any other official coding rules and guidelines established for use with mandated standard code sets. Selection and sequencing of diagnoses and procedures must meet the definitions of required data sets for applicable healthcare settings.

3. Coding professionals should use their skills, their knowledge of currently mandated coding and classification systems, and official resources to select the appropriate diagnostic and procedural codes.

4. Coding professionals should only assign and report codes that are clearly and consistently supported by physician documentation in the health record.

5. Coding professionals should consult physicians for clarification and additional documentation prior to code assignment when there are conflicting or ambiguous data in the health record.

6. Coding professionals should not change codes or the narratives of codes on the billing abstract so that meanings are misrepresented. Diagnoses or procedures should not be inappropriately included or excluded because payment or insurance policy coverage requirements will be affected. When individual payer policies conflict with official coding rules and guidelines, these policies should be obtained in writing whenever possible. Reasonable efforts should be made to educate the payer on proper coding practices in order to influence a change in the payer's policy.

7. Coding professionals, as members of the healthcare team, should assist and educate physicians and other clinicians by advocating proper documentation practices, further specificity, and resequencing or inclusion of diagnoses or procedures when needed to more accurately reflect the acuity, severity, and the occurrence of events.

8. Coding professionals should participate in the development of institutional coding policies and should ensure that coding policies complement, not conflict with, official coding rules and guidelines.

9. Coding professionals should maintain and continually enhance their coding skills, as they have a professional responsibility to stay abreast of changes in codes, coding guidelines, and regulations.

10. Coding professionals should strive for optimal payment to which the facility is legally entitled, remembering that it is unethical and illegal to maximize payment by means that contradict regulatory guidelines.

*The Cooperating Parties are the American Health Information Management Association, American Hospital Association, Centers for Medicare and Medicaid Services, and National Center for Health Statistics.

Coding Policies and Procedures

Every healthcare facility should establish coding policies and procedures that establish guidelines that coders should follow to ensure coding consistency. Using the coding guidelines established by organizations such as the AHA, the AMA, AHIMA, and state health information management association policies can be developed for coding consistency.

The AHA publishes the official guidelines for ICD-9-CM coding in a quarterly newsletter entitled *Coding Clinic*. The AMA publishes information regarding CPT codes in a newsletter entitled *CPT Assistant*. Both publications can be used as a basis for developing facility policies and procedures.

Steps in the Coding Process

For accurate coding to occur, the coder must have a complete health record on the patient. Each facility needs to define what constitutes a complete record. The coder must review the contents of the record to determine the patient's condition and the treatment and care he or she received.

For an inpatient record, the health record should contain the following documents prior to being coded: a face sheet, operative and procedural reports, pathology reports, and a discharge summary. The coder needs to review these documents to verify diagnoses and procedures.

After the record is reviewed, the coder selects the diagnoses and procedures that need to be coded and assigns appropriate code numbers. Codes then have to be sequenced according to Uniform Hospital Discharge Data Set (UHDDS) guidelines.

After the diagnoses and procedures are coded, the codes are entered into the facility's database. These data then become the foundation for statistical, reimbursement, and clinical information systems.

Quality Assessment for the Coding Process

Assessment of the coding process should occur through regular monitoring of coding accuracy. Monitoring is the ongoing internal review of coding practices conducted by an organization on a regular basis. A monitoring/audit program plan should be a written plan that outlines the objectives and frequency of the audits, the record selection process, the qualifications of auditors, and corrective actions the organization will take as a result of the audit findings.

Initially, a baseline audit should be performed. The audit should be a review of a large sample of the coding completed. It should include a sample of records coded by all coders for all types of services. Moreover, the sample should be representative of all physicians and types of cases treated by the organization. The baseline audit provides an overview of the organization's current coding practices.

The organization should conduct follow-up audits according to the schedule established in the monitoring/audit plan. Follow-up audits will provide ongoing monitoring of the coding process to ensure coding accuracy. The results of the audits also can be used to outline areas in which coder education and training are needed. Figure 6.12 is an example of a coding audit review sheet.

Figure 6.12.   Example of a coding audit review sheet

Coding Audit Review Sheet

Coder _____
Type of Review (IP,OP,ER) _____
Date of Review _____
Medical Record # _____
Discharge Date _____

Initial Codes Assigned	Reviewer's Recommendations

Principal Diagnosis
- A.   Chosen and coded correctly _____
- B.   Chosen correctly, coded incorrectly _____
- C.   Chosen incorrectly, coded correctly _____
- D.   Chosen and coded incorrectly _____

Secondary Diagnoses
- A.   Chosen and coded correctly _____
- B.   Chosen correctly, coded incorrectly _____
- C.   Chosen incorrectly, coded correctly _____
- D.   Chosen and coded incorrectly _____

Principal Procedure
- A.   Chosen and coded correctly _____
- B.   Chosen correctly, coded incorrectly _____
- C.   Chosen incorrectly, coded correctly _____
- D.   Chosen and coded incorrectly _____

Secondary Procedures
- A.   Chosen and coded correctly _____
- B.   Chosen correctly, coded incorrectly _____
- C.   Chosen incorrectly, coded correctly _____
- D.   Chosen and coded incorrectly _____

DRG
- A.   Chosen and coded correctly _____
- B.   Chosen correctly, coded incorrectly _____
- C.   Chosen incorrectly, coded correctly _____
- D.   Chosen and coded incorrectly _____

Note: A review sheet can also be constructed to monitor CPT coding information instead of DRG assignments.

Check Your Understanding 6.5

Instructions: Indicate whether the following statements are true or false (T or F)

1. ____ Coding plays an important role in the determination of reimbursement of healthcare facilities.
2. ____ The coding function must be reviewed on an ongoing basis for coding consistency and accuracy.
3. ____ The AMA publishes the official guidelines for CPT coding in its newsletter, *Coding Clinic.*
4. ____ Codes are sequenced in the patient's health record according to AHIMA's Standards of Ethical Coding.
5. ____ A baseline audit should include a sample of records coded by all coders for all types of services.

Coding Technology

Technology is changing many aspects of the health information profession. One of the primary areas where it has assisted in making jobs more efficient is in the area of coding. As early as the 1980s, information technology was applied to make the coding process more effective and efficient. The type of tool used to aid in the coding process is commonly referred to as an **encoder.** The development of other technologies, including **natural language processing** (NLP), will likely have an even greater impact on the coding process.

Encoders

Encoders for ICD were developed in the early 1980s. Over the subsequent years, greater sophistication has been built into these technology solutions. An encoder is computer software that helps the coding professional to assign codes. Initially, encoders were developed for assisting coders in assigning ICD-9-CM codes. Today, however, encoders include assistance with other coding systems.

The information science and technology behind the encoding software varies from vendor to vendor. Some encoders are built using expert system techniques such as rule-based systems. Other encoding software is more simplistic, merely automating a look-up function similar to the manual index in ICD or other coding classifications.

Encoders have many different types of interfaces, depending on the vendor. An interface can be defined as the total component of screens, navigation, and input mechanisms used to help the end user operate the encoding software. Some encoder systems have an interface that prompts the coder through a series of questions. As the coder answers the questions, the encoder leads the coder to codes for diagnoses and procedures.

Alternatively, other encoders allow coders to input classification codes directly into the system and then go through a series of edit checks to ensure that only allowable code numbers are entered. In more sophisticated software systems, the encoder also prompts the coder to review the sequencing of the codes that have been selected in order to optimize reimbursement.

Good encoding software should include edit checks to ensure data quality. For example, an inappropriate combination of codes or inconsistent data should be flagged for the coder's attention. Encoding software is frequently linked to other information systems applications. This includes direct links to DRG grouper software and billing systems.

The use of encoders has become a predominant tool in the HIM department, particularly in acute care facilities. Today, however, there is even a greater movement toward more complete computerization of the coding function using a supporting technology called natural language processing, or NLP. In an NLP system, digital text from online documents stored in the organization's information system is read directly by the software and then automatically coded. For example, the digital text in an online emergency department record would be interpreted automatically by the NLP system and, through the use of expert or artificial intelligence software, would automatically suggest appropriate code numbers.

This type of system will dramatically change the role of the coder from being a frontline interpreter and translator of textual data to being an editor, validator, or auditor of code assignments made automatically and electronically. NLP Computer-Assisted Coding (CAC) is in use predominantly in the outpatient setting, where repetitive tasks can be easily automated to free up the coder to focus on more complex chart review and coding assignment. (See figure 6.13.) The trend toward this type of information system use is expected to grow. According to the AHIMA e-HIM Work Group on Computer-Assisted Coding:

> As the transition to EHRs and the adoption of ICD-10-CM and ICD-10-PCS occur in the US, the detailed and logical structure of these systems will increase the use of CAC tools across many different domains. In addition, as CAC technology becomes increasingly sophisticated, there will be less demand for coding professionals to perform traditional clinical coding tasks. CAC software applications that assist coding professionals in their workflow by allowing them to review and edit a draft set of codes will require coding professionals to further develop skills and competencies in the clarification and scrutiny of data. Computer-assisted coding is a budding technology whose time has come, and it heralds a new era for coding professionals (2004, 48G).

Figure 6.13. Screen shot of computer-assisted coding program

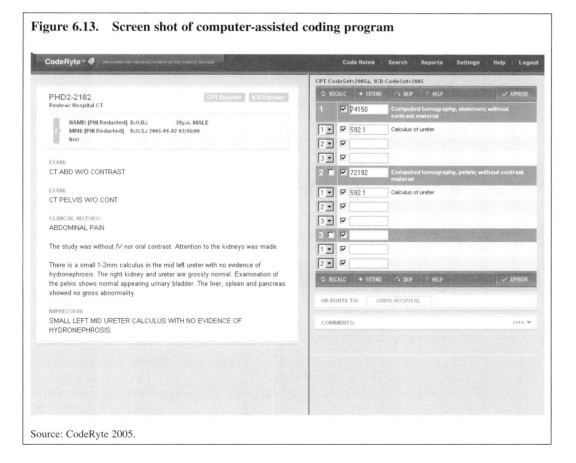

Source: CodeRyte 2005.

Other Technical Tools

In the early 1980s, the federal government implemented the Medicare prospective payment system (PPS) for inpatient reimbursement. Each patient is assigned to a diagnosis-related group (DRG) that determines the facility reimbursement amount. (See table 6.2.).

In the DRG system, patients are categorized into DRGs that represent cases that are medically similar with respect to diagnosis, treatment, and length of stay. ICD-9-CM diagnoses and procedure codes are used to determine placement into the DRG payment categories.

Similar to the DRG system, Medicare reimburses hospitals for outpatient services based on the Outpatient Prospective Payment System (OPPS), which categorizes patients into groups. These groups are known as Ambulatory Payment Classifications (APCs) according to the types of services commonly provided in that setting. Primarily, the CPT/HCPCS coding system is utilized to determine correct payment of services.

In both the DRG and APC groupings, coders enter the codes that have been selected into a computer program called a grouper. The grouper then assigns the patient's case to the correct group based on the ICD-9-CM and/or CPT/HCPCS codes. (See table 6.3 for an example of APC groupings.)

Check Your Understanding 6.6

Instructions: Indicate whether the following statements are true or false (T or F).

1. ____ An encoder is computer software that assists in determining coding accuracy and reliability.

2. ____ An interface is the total component of screens, navigation, and input mechanisms used to operate encoding software.

3. ____ Good encoding software should include edit checks.

4. ____ The NLP encoding system uses expert or artificial intelligence software to automatically assign code numbers.

5. ____ Diagnosis-related groups categorize patient cases that are medically similar with respect to diagnosis, treatment, and length of stay.

Coding and Corporate Compliance

Each year, it is estimated that millions of dollars of the U.S. healthcare industry budget is misappropriated because of fraudulent practices by healthcare organizations and providers. Through the Office of the Inspector General (OIG), the federal government establishes annual compliance plans for the healthcare industry. A compliance plan can be defined as a plan to ensure that a facility is providing and billing for services according to the laws, regulations, and guidelines that govern it. The goal of these plans is to help providers monitor their billing and coding practices to prevent fraud and abuse.

History of Corporate Compliance

The basis for prosecution of healthcare fraud and abuse is the Federal False Claims Act (FCA). This act was signed into law by Abraham Lincoln in 1863. Its original intent was to encourage private citizens during the Civil War to report fraudulent actions taken against the Union Army. Under this act, the government had to prove that an individual acted with specific intent to defraud the government.

DRG	FY 2006 postacute care transfer DRG	FY 2006 postacute care special pay transfer DRG	MDC	TYPE	DRG title	Relative weights	Geometric mean LOS	Arithmetic mean LOS
Table 6.2. Example of DRG groupings								
1	Yes	No	01	SURG	CRANIOTOMY AGE >17 W CC	3.4347	7.6	10.1
2	Yes	No	01	SURG	CRANIOTOMY AGE >17 W/O CC	1.9587	3.5	4.6
3	No	No	01	SURG	CRANIOTOMY AGE 0–17	1.9860	12.7	12.7
4	No	No	01	SURG	NO LONGER VALID	0.0000	0.0	0.0
5	No	No	01	SURG	NO LONGER VALID	0.0000	0.0	0.0
6	No	No	01	SURG	CARPAL TUNNEL RELEASE	0.7878	2.2	3.0
7	Yes	Yes	01	SURG	PERIPH & CRANIAL NERVE & OTHER NERV SYST PROC W CC	2.6978	6.7	9.7
8	Yes	Yes	01	SURG	PERIPH & CRANIAL NERVE & OTHER NERV SYST PROC W/O CC	1.5635	2.0	3.0
9	No	No	01	MED	SPINAL DISORDERS & INJURIES	1.4045	4.5	6.4
10	Yes	No	01	MED	NERVOUS SYSTEM NEOPLASMS W CC	1.2222	4.6	6.2
11	Yes	No	01	MED	NERVOUS SYSTEM NEOPLASMS W/O CC	0.8736	2.9	3.8
12	Yes	No	01	MED	DEGENERATIVE NERVOUS SYSTEM DISORDERS	0.8998	4.3	5.5
13	Yes	No	01	MED	MULTIPLE SCLEROSIS & CEREBELLAR ATAXIA	0.8575	4.0	5.0
14	Yes	No	01	MED	INTRACRANIAL HEMORRHAGE OR CEREBRAL INFARCTION	1.2456	4.5	5.8
15	Yes	No	01	MED	NONSPECIFIC CVA & PRECEREBRAL OCCLUSION W/O INFARCT	0.9421	3.7	4.6
16	Yes	No	01	MED	NONSPECIFIC CEREBROVASCULAR DISORDERS W CC	1.3351	5.0	6.5

Table 6.3.   Example of APC groupings

APC	Group Title	SI	Relative Weight	Payment Rate	National Unadjusted Copayment	Minimum Unadjusted Copayment
0001	Level I Photochemotherapy	S	0.3998	23.79	7.00	4.76
0002	Level I Fine Needle Biopsy/ Aspiration	T	0.9357	55.68	—	11.14
0003	Bone Marrow Biopsy/Aspiration	T	2.6756	159.23	—	31.85
0004	Level I Needle Biopsy/ Aspiration Except Bone Marrow	T	1.7771	105.76	22.36	21.15
0005	Level II Needle Biopsy/ Aspiration Except Bone Marrow	T	3.5834	213.25	71.59	42.65
0006	Level I Incision & Drainage	T	1.5100	89.86	21.76	17.97
0007	Level II Incision & Drainage	T	11.6717	694.59	—	138.92
0008	Level III Incision and Drainage	T	16.2953	969.75	—	193.95

In 1986, the FCA was amended to include provisions that eliminated the requirement that specific intent to defraud be proven. The law now has become the basis for prosecuting healthcare providers who knowingly present a false claim for payment to the government. Therefore, when a healthcare provider shows a pattern or practice of coding that results in overcharges to Medicare and Medicaid, that provider can be prosecuted.

To avoid fraudulent behaviors, healthcare providers need to develop compliance plans that ensure the establishment of internal controls. Since 1997, the OIG has released its compliance program guidelines for segments of the healthcare industry, including hospitals, home health agencies, clinical laboratories, third-party medical billing companies, and DME suppliers, hospices, nursing homes, and physicians' practices.

Elements of Corporate Compliance

Healthcare providers should use the compliance programs released by the OIG to develop and implement their own compliance programs. The guidelines outline elements that represent a plan that healthcare providers can follow. The various compliance program guidelines can be found on the OIG Web site at hhs.gov/oig.

Several basic elements required for corporate compliance programs were outlined in the OIG's "Compliance Program Guidance for Hospitals," published in the *Federal Register* on February 23, 1999. A supplemental plan for hospitals was published in the *Federal Register* on January 31, 2005. Corporate compliance programs for hospitals should include at least the following seven elements:

1.   The development and distribution of written standards of conduct, as well as written policies and procedures that promote the hospital's commitment to com-

pliance (for example, by including adherence to compliance as an element in evaluating managers and employees) and that address specific areas of potential fraud such as claims development and submission processes, code gaming, and financial relationships with physicians and other healthcare professionals

2. The designation of a chief compliance officer and other appropriate bodies (for example, a corporate compliance committee) charged with responsibility for operating and monitoring the compliance program and that report directly to the CEO and the governing body

3. The development and implementation of regular, effective education and training programs for all affected employees

4. The maintenance of a process, such as a hotline, to receive complaints and the adoption of procedures to protect the anonymity of complainants and to protect whistleblowers from retaliation

5. The development of a system to respond to allegations of improper/illegal activities and the enforcement of appropriate disciplinary action against employees who have violated internal compliance policies, applicable statutes, and regulations or federal healthcare program requirements

6. The use of audits and/or other evaluation techniques to monitor compliance and assist in the reduction of identified problem areas

7. The investigation and remediation of identified systemic problems and the development of policies that address the nonemployment or retention of sanctioned individuals

Each year, the OIG publishes a work plan that details areas of compliance it will be investigating for that year. Facilities should study this document carefully and plan their compliance and auditing projects to ensure that they are in compliance with identified target areas. The OIG work plan for 2005 can be found online at oig.hhs.gov/publications/docs/workplan/2005/2005%20Work%20Plan.pdf.

Policies and Procedures for Corporate Compliance

Policies and procedures for corporate compliance must be developed at the facility level and for the HIM department. The OIG outlines specific areas of concern that need to be addressed in facilities' policies. HIM professionals play an active role in the development of both HIM department and organization-wide policies.

In October 1999, AHIMA published a practice brief titled "Seven Steps to Corporate Compliance." Organizations should use the guidelines in this practice brief to develop specific HIM compliance plans. As recommended by AHIMA, HIM compliance policies and procedures should ensure that:

- All rejected claims pertaining to diagnosis and procedure codes are reviewed.

- Proper and timely documentation of all physician and other professional services is obtained prior to billing.

- Compensation for coders and consultants does not provide any financial incentive to code claims improperly.

- A process is in place for pre- and postsubmission review.
- The proper selection and sequencing of diagnoses occurs.
- The correct application of official coding rules and guidelines occurs.
- A process exists for reporting potential and actual violations.
- A process is in place for identifying coding errors.

Check Your Understanding 6.7

Instructions: Indicate whether the following statements are true or false (T or F).

1. _____ The federal Office of the Inspector General established compliance plans for the healthcare industry.

2. _____ The basis for prosecuting healthcare fraud and abuse is the Federal False Compliance Act.

3. _____ The OIG compliance programs offer guidelines that healthcare organizations can follow to establish their internal compliance programs.

4. _____ A corporate compliance program should include the development and implementation of education and training programs for all affected employees.

5. _____ HIM professionals are not involved in developing policies and procedures for corporate compliance.

New Directions in Clinical Vocabularies

As the number and sophistication of clinical vocabularies increase, there has been a significant movement toward research in understanding the fundamental elements and structures in both vocabularies and classification systems. One of the most farsighted endeavors toward bringing together the various medical vocabularies is the Unified Medical Language System (UMLS) project being conducted by the National Library of Medicine (NLM).

National Library of Medicine UMLS Project

The NLM established a research project in 1986. This long-range project is called the Unified Medical Language System (UMLS) project.

The purpose of the UMLS is to aid in the development of systems that help healthcare professionals retrieve and integrate electronic biomedical information from a variety of sources. UMLS uses three knowledge sources to make it easier for users to link separate information systems:

- The *metathesaurus* provides a uniform collection of more than one hundred biomedical/health-related vocabularies, coding systems, and classifications and links the different names used in the various vocabularies and classifications, such as SNOMED CT, LOINC, and RXNorm to a common concept.
- The *specialist lexicon* contains syntactic information for many terms. (For example, it lists the parts of speech, various forms of a word, and spelling variations of the terms within UMLS.)

- The *semantic network* provides a system for categorizing objects and identifying the relationships among various concepts.

The UMLS knowledge sources overcome retrieval problems that occur when different terminology and separate databases are used. They are currently being used in a variety of applications, including patient data creation, natural language processing, and information retrieval. The NLM maintains fact sheets describing the progress of this project on its Web site.

Development of the Nosologist Role

Nosology is the branch of medical science that deals with classification systems. A nosologist is a person who works with using and developing classification systems. The AHIMA Coding Futures Task Force envisions that the role of the coder will change dramatically over the next decade. At present, the coder's primary responsibility is the assignment of codes. In the future, the coder will become a nosologist responsible for the development, maintenance, and management of classification systems and vocabularies. A peek into this future role was provided in the following scenario as an outgrowth of the work of the Coding Futures Task Force (Johns 2000):

It's 2010 and a brave new world for coders.

Jane Smith, RHIT, CCS, is a health information technician and clinical coder who is now employed in the clinical nosology, or classification, department of Community Health System. Jane recognized some time ago that coding would become more and more automated in the future and that she could get a better job if she had a deeper understanding and broader knowledge of lexical technologies and medical vocabularies. She continued her education and landed an enviable and challenging position. Now she works with colleagues who have backgrounds in health information management, medical and nursing informatics, clinical sciences, computer science, and statistics.

Jane's nosology group works on various projects associated with merging and mapping overlapping clinical vocabularies to support development of the computer-based patient record, automated decision support, and outcomes analysis. With more than 25 different medical vocabularies in use in the system, overlapping terms are a tremendous problem—resulting in duplication and difficulty in translation and retrieval of data for patient care, research, and decision support.

The nosology group's current project involves comparing the output of two systems that use different approaches in merging and mapping clinical vocabularies. The group wants to evaluate how well these two systems can initially map terms from two selected vocabularies—LOINC and SNOMED CT. Jane's team wants to determine which of the two systems does a better job in merging the two clinical vocabularies. Jane, whose job title is now clinical nosologist, developed the initial research plan for the comparison. In preparation for the analysis, she reviewed system options and selected the best possible systems for the test.

When the team has finished its testing, it will be able to recommend whether the health system should purchase either of the two systems and incorporate it into the enterprise-wide clinical computing system. The result, ideally, will be more reliable, consistent, and accurate data for automated decision support systems and clinical information systems.

Like Jane's job, the health information industry is very different than what it was 10 years ago. Fast-moving technology has fed development of a complex web of players, from investors to healthcare teams and forward-thinking organizations who have anticipated technological breakthroughs and accordingly reengineered to capitalize on them.

A convergence of technology breakthroughs has made code assignments for patient care, billing, and research purposes essentially automatic. Coding specialists are still important, but rather than assign codes, they now analyze coded data for quality control and trends and maintain data mappings from vocabularies to classification systems.

Check Your Understanding 6.8

Instructions: Indicate whether the following statements are true or false (T or F).

1. _____ The UMLS project was initiated to bring together the various medical vocabularies.

2. _____ The metathesaurus, one of the UMLS knowledge sources, contains syntactic information for many terms.

3. _____ The UMLS knowledge sources are currently being used in natural language processing.

4. _____ A nosologist's primary responsibility is the assignment of diagnosis codes.

5. _____ In the future, coders will become nosologists.

Real-World Case

Can natural language processing be helpful to outpatient coders? NLP is a supporting technology that has reached an exciting stage of development. It holds a great deal of promise for assisting in further automation of the coding process. Although the technology holds great promise, it also faces a huge challenge because of the complexity and variability of human speech. However, promising new NLP products are beginning to emerge in certain medical arenas, such as emergency medicine. To validate the claims that an NLP system can improve coding accuracy, 3M Health Information Systems designed and performed a study of ICD-9-CM and CPT to determine how a NLP technology system matched up with real-world coders.

To determine whether an NLP automated system was as accurate at assigning ICD and CPT codes to emergency room records as experienced coders, the researchers evaluated 328 emergency room charts using both the NLP system and the experienced coders. The study results indicated that in the specialized arena of emergency medicine, the NLP system compared favorably to actual coders in assigning ICD and CPT codes. (This case was adapted from Warner [2000].) Since that time, other studies have shown that tools utilizing NLP have become increasingly more effective.

Summary

In recent decades, coding, classification, and vocabulary systems have grown in importance. This is clear in the critical role that coding now plays in the healthcare industry's reimbursement process and its use in research and quality assurance efforts.

Nomenclatures, classification systems, and clinical vocabularies were created to help organize healthcare data. In medicine, a nomenclature is a system that lists preferred medical terminology. A classification system groups together similar diseases and procedures and organizes related entities for easy retrieval.

The purpose and use of clinical classifications today are varied. For example, physicians use classifications such as ICD to classify morbidity and mortality information for statistical purposes, to index hospital records by disease and operations, and to report diagnoses. In addition, clinical classifications are used in the reporting and compilation of healthcare data to assist in evaluating medical care planning for healthcare delivery systems, determining patterns of care among healthcare providers, analyzing payments of healthcare services, and conducting epidemiological and clinical research studies.

Although ICD-9-CM is perhaps the most prominent classification system in use today, health information technicians use many other systems in their daily practice, such as CPT, HCPCS, ICD-O-2, DSM, and nursing vocabularies. The continued development of these and other classification systems and vocabularies reflects the complexity of describing the medical care process.

Every healthcare organization must have policies and procedures in place that set guidelines for managing the coding process and ensuring the consistency of the organization's coding output. Further, every organization should establish a monitoring/audit program to review and assess coding accuracy on a regular basis. Moreover, every organization should develop a corporate compliance plan that monitors its billing and coding activities to prevent fraudulent practices.

Finally, technological advances are having a tremendous impact on the coding process today and will likely have an even greater impact in the future. Important projects such as the Unified Medical Language System project conducted by the National Library of Medicine, coupled with the growth and maturity of automated coding and natural language processing systems, will revolutionize the coding function.

References

AHIMA e-HIM Work Group on Computer-Assisted Coding. 2004 (November–December). Delving into computer-assisted coding. *Journal of American Health Information Management Association* 75(10):48A–48H.

ANA Committee for Nursing Practice Information Infrastructure. 2005. Frequently Asked Questions: Standardized Terminologies. Available online from dlthede.net/CNPII/HomeStuff/FAQ.htm.

American Psychiatric Association. 2005. Frequently Asked Questions about DSM. Available online from www.psych.org/research/dor/dsm/dsm_faqs/faq81301.cfm.

Brouch, K. 2003 (July–August). AHIMA project offers insights into SNOMED, ICD-9-CM mapping process. *Journal of American Health Information Management Association* 74(7):52–55.

Centers for Medicare and Medicaid Services. 2003 (May). HIPAA Information Series: 4. Overview of Electronic Transactions and Code Sets, 1. Baltimore, MD: CMS.

CodeRyte. 2005. Natural Language Processing (NLP) Computer-Assisted Coding solution. Available online from coderyte.com.

Giannangelo, K., and L. Berkowitz. 2005 (April). SNOMED CT helps drive EHR success. *Journal of American Health In formation Management Association* 76(4):66–67.

Johns, M. 2000. A crystal ball for coding. *Journal of American Health Information Management Association* 71(8):26–33.

National Committee on Vital and Health Statistics. 1991 (June). *NCVHS 1990.* DHHS Publication No. (PHS) 91-1205. Hyattsville, MD: HHS. Available online from cdc.gov/nchs/data/ncvhs/nchvs90.pdf.

SNOMED International, n.d. SNOMED Clinical Terms (SNOMED CT). in *TheraDoc's Antibiotic Assistant Underlies Actionable Clinical Decision Support.* Available online from www.snomed.org.

Warner, H.R., Jr. 2000. Can natural language processing aid outpatient coders? *Journal of American Health Information Management Association* 71(8):78–81.

Chapter 7
Reimbursement Methodologies

Anita C. Hazelwood, MLS, RHIA, FAHIMA
Carol A. Venable, MPH, RHIA, FAHIMA

Learning Objectives

- To understand the historical development of healthcare reimbursement in the United States

- To describe current reimbursement processes, forms, and support practices for healthcare reimbursement

- To understand the difference between commercial health insurance and employer self-insurance

- To describe the purpose and basic benefits of the following government-sponsored health programs: Medicare Part A, Medicare Part B, Medicare Advantage, Medicaid, CHAMPVA, TRICARE, HIS, TANF, PACE, SCHIP, workers' compensation, and FECA

- To understand the concept of managed care and to provide examples of different types of managed care organizations

- To identify the different types of fee-for-service reimbursement methods

- To understand ambulatory surgery center rates

- To describe prospective payment systems

- To understand the purpose of the fee schedules, chargemasters, and auditing procedures that support the reimbursement process

Key Terms

Accept assignment

Accounts receivable

Accredited Standards Committee (ASC) X12, Electronic Data Interchange (ASC X12)

Acute care prospective payment system (PPS)

Administrative services only (ASO) contracts

Advance Beneficiary Notice (ABN)

All patient DRGs (AP-DRGs)

All patient refined DRGs (APR-DRGs)

Ambulatory payment classification (APC) system

Ambulatory surgery center (ASC)

American National Standards Institute (ANSI)

Attending Physician Statement (APS) (or COMB-1)

Auditing

Balance billing

Balanced Budget Refinement Act (BBRA)

Blue Cross and Blue Shield (BC/BS)

Blue Cross and Blue Shield Federal Employee Program (FEP)

Bundled payments

Capitation

Case-mix group

Case-mix group (CMG) relative weights

Case-mix index

Categorically needy eligibility groups (Medicaid)

Centers for Medicare and Medicaid Services (CMS)

Chargemaster

Civilian Health and Medical Program-Veterans Affairs (CHAMPVA)

Civilian Health and Medical Program of the Uniformed Services (CHAMPUS)

Claim

CMS-1500

Coinsurance

Comorbidity

Compliance

Compliance program guidance

Complication

Coordination of benefits (COB) transaction

Cost outlier

Cost outlier adjustment

CPT (Current Procedural Terminology)

Department of Health and Human Services (HHS)

Diagnosis-related groups (DRGs)

Discharge planning

Discounting

DRG grouper

Electronic remittance advice (ERA)

Emergency Maternal and Infant Care Program (EMIC)

Employer-based self-insurance

Episode-of-care (EOC) reimbursement

Exclusive provider organization (EPO)

Explanation of Benefits (EOB)

External reviews (audits)

Federal Employees' Compensation Act (FECA)

Fee schedule

Fee-for-service basis

Fiscal intermediary (FI)

Fraud and abuse

Geographic practice cost index (GPCI)

Global payment

Global surgery payment

Group health insurance

Group model health maintenance organization

Group practice without walls (GPWW)

Hard-coding

Health maintenance organization (HMO)

Health Plan Employer Data and Information Set (HEDIS)

Healthcare Common Procedure Coding System (HCPCS)

Healthcare provider

Home Assessment Validation and Entry (HAVEN)

Home health agency (HHA)

Home health prospective payment system (HH PPS)

Home health resource group (HHRG)

Hospice

Hospitalization insurance (HI) (Medicare Part A)

ICD-9-CM (International Classification of Diseases, Ninth Revision, Clinical Modification)

Indemnity plans

Independent practice association (IPA)

Indian Health Service (IHS)

Inpatient psychiatric facility (IPF)

Inpatient rehabilitation facility (IRF)

Inpatient Rehabilitation Validation and Entry (IRVEN)

Insured

Insurer

Integrated delivery system (IDS)

Integrated provider organization (IPO)

Long-term care hospital (LTCH)

Low-utilization payment adjustment (LUPA)

Major diagnostic category (MDC)

Major medical insurance (catastrophic coverage)

Managed care

Management service organization (MSO)

Medicaid

Medical foundation

Medical Group Management Association (MGMA)

Medically needy option (Medicaid)

Medicare

Medicare Advantage

Medicare carrier

Medicare fee schedule (MFS)

Medicare Summary Notice (MSN)

Medigap

Minimum Data Set 2.0 (MDS)

National Committee for Quality Assurance (NCQA)

National conversion factor (CF)

National Correct Coding Initiative (NCCI)

National Uniform Billing Committee (NUBC)

National Uniform Claim Committee (NUCC)

Network model health maintenance program

Network provider

Nonparticipating providers

Omnibus Budget Reconciliation Act (OBRA)

Outcome and Assessment Information Set (OASIS)

Out-of-pocket expenses

Outpatient code editor (OCE)

Outpatient prospective payment system (OPPS)

Packaging

Partial hospitalization

Payer of last resort (Medicaid)

Payment status indicator (PSI)

Per member per month (PMPM)

Per patient per month (PPPM)

Physician-hospital organization (PHO)

Point-of-service (POS) plan

Policyholder

Preferred provider organization (PPO)

Premium

Primary care manager (PCM)

Primary care physician (PCP)

Principal diagnosis

Principal procedure

Professional component (PC)

Programs of All-Inclusive Care for the Elderly (PACE)

Prospective payment system (PPS)

Public assistance

Relative value unit (RVU)

Remittance advice (RA)

Resident Assessment Instrument (RAI)

Resident Assessment Validation and Entry (RAVEN)

Resource Utilization Groups, Version III (RUG-III)

Resource-based relative value scale (RBRVS)

Respite care

Retrospective payment system

Revenue codes

Skilled nursing facility prospective payment system (SNF PPS)

Social Security Act

Staff model health maintenance organization

State Children's Health Insurance Program (SCHIP)

State workers' compensation insurance funds

Supplemental medical insurance (SMI) (Medicare Part B)

Tax Equity and Fiscal Responsibility Act of 1982 (TEFRA)

Technical component (TC)

Temporary Assistance for Needy Families (TANF)

Third-party payer

Traditional fee-for-service reimbursement

TRICARE

TRICARE Extra

TRICARE Prime

TRICARE Prime Remote

TRICARE Senior Prime

TRICARE Standard

UB-04

UB-92 (CMS-1450)

Unbundling

Upcoding

Usual, customary, and reasonable (UCR) charges

Voluntary Disclosure Program

Workers' compensation

Introduction

In the United States, the systems used to pay healthcare organizations and individual healthcare professionals for the services they provide are very complex. This complexity is due in part to the variety of reimbursement methods in use today as well as to strict requirements for detailed documentation to support medical **claims.** The government and other third-party payers also are concerned about potential **fraud and abuse** in claims processing. Therefore, ensuring that bills and claims are accurate and correctly presented is an important focus of healthcare **compliance.**

A reimbursement claim is a statement of services submitted by a **healthcare provider** (for example, a physician or a hospital) to a **third-party payer** (for example, an insurance company or **Medicare**). The claim documents the medical and/or surgical services that were provided to a specific patient during a specific episode of care. Accurate reimbursement is critical to the operational and financial health of healthcare organizations. In most healthcare organizations, health insurance specialists process reimbursement claims. Health information management (HIM) professionals also play an important role in healthcare reimbursement by:

- Ensuring that health record documentation supports services billed

- Assigning diagnostic and procedural codes according to patient record documentation

- Applying coding guidelines and edits when assigning codes or **auditing** for coding quality and accuracy

- Appealing insurance claims denials

This chapter reviews the history of healthcare reimbursement in the United States and explains the different reimbursement systems commonly used since the start of **prospective payment systems.** It then discusses a variety of healthcare reimbursement methodologies with a focus on Medicare prospective payment systems. Finally, it explains how reimbursement claims are processed and the support processes involved.

Theory into Practice

It is not uncommon to hear the phrase "if it wasn't documented, it wasn't done" in reference to health record documentation. In the context of reimbursement, this phrase means that when a healthcare provider (for example, a hospital) provides a service to a patient but fails to document the service in the patient's health record, that provider has no evidence to support a claim for the service. As a result, the third-party payer may deny the claim.

For example, a hospital submitted a claim for outpatient services totaling $1,950. When the third-party payer reviewed the claim, it might disallow $200 in charges for which there was no health record documentation. The payer then would recalculate the claim for a total payment of $1,750. The hospital would have lost $200 in revenue on this one case. However, if the hospital were underpaid $200 on every case because of incomplete documentation and there were 36,500 patient encounters per year, the potential revenue loss for one year would be $7,300,000!

History of Healthcare Reimbursement in the United States

Healthcare reimbursement in the United States has a long and complex history. Until the late 1800s, Americans paid their own healthcare expenses. Many people without the means to pay for care received charity care or no care at all. Over the past 100 years, a number of groups have attempted to develop systems that would ensure adequate healthcare for every American. But the development of prepaid insurance plans and third-party reimbursement systems did not follow a straight path. The result is the complicated reimbursement system in place today.

Campaigns for National Health Insurance

The American Association of Labor Legislation (AALL) began the campaign for health insurance in the United States with the creation of a committee on social welfare. The committee held its first national conference in 1913 and drafted model health insurance legislation in 1915. The proposed legislation limited coverage to the working class and others who earned less than $1,200 a year, and included their dependents. Coverage included the services of physicians, nurses, and hospitals; sick pay; maternity benefits; and a death benefit of $50 to pay for funeral expenses. Although the plan was supported by the American Medical Association (AMA), it was never passed into law.

During the 1930s, expanding access to medical care services became the focus of healthcare reforms. Hospital costs increased as the middle class used more hospital services. Medical care, especially hospital care, became a bigger item in family budgets. The Committee on the Cost of Medical Care (CCMC) was formed to address concerns about the cost and distribution of medical care. It was funded by eight philanthropic organizations, including the Rockefeller, Millbank, and Rosenwald foundations. It first met in 1926 and stopped meeting in 1932. The CCMC's published research findings demonstrated the need for additional healthcare services. The committee recommended that national resources be allocated for healthcare and that voluntary health insurance be provided as a means of covering medical costs. Like the AALL's earlier efforts, however, nothing came of the CCMC initiative.

In 1937, the Tactical Committee on Medical Care was formed. It drafted the Wagner National Health Act of 1939. The act supported a federally funded national health program to be administered by states and localities. The Wagner Act evolved from a proposal for federal grants-in-aid to a plan for national health insurance. The proposal called for compulsory national health insurance and a payroll tax. Although the proposed legislation generated extensive national debate, Congress did not pass it into law.

In 1945, the healthcare issue received the support of an American president for the first time when Harry Truman introduced a plan for universal comprehensive national health insurance. Proposed compromises included a system of private insurance for those who could afford it and public welfare services for the poor. Truman's plan died in a congressional committee in 1946.

After the Second World War, private insurance systems expanded and union-negotiated healthcare benefits served to protect workers from the impact of unforeseen healthcare expenses. The Hill-Burton Act (formally called the Hospital Survey and Construction Act) was passed in 1946. This health facility construction program was instituted under Title VI of the Public Health Service Act. The program was designed to provide federal grants for modernizing hospitals that had become obsolete due to a lack of capital investment during the Great Depression and the Second World War (1929 to 1945). The program later evolved to address other types of infrastructure needs. In return for federal funds, facilities agreed to provide medical services free or at reduced rates to patients who were unable to pay for their own care.

Congress first introduced a bill to fund coverage of hospital costs for Social Security beneficiaries in 1948. In response to criticism from the AMA, the proposed legislation was expanded to cover physician services. The concept of federal health insurance programs for the aged and the poor was highly controversial. It was not until 1965 that President Lyndon Johnson signed the law that created federal healthcare programs for the elderly and poor as part of his Great Society legislation (also called the War on Poverty).

Title XVIII of the **Social Security Act,** or Health Insurance for the Aged and Disabled, is commonly known as Medicare. Medicare legislation was enacted as one element of the 1965 amendments to the Social Security Act. Medicare is a health insurance program designed to complement the retirement, survivors, and disability insurance benefits enacted under Title II of the Social Security Act. It covered most Americans over the age of sixty-five when it was first implemented in 1966. In 1973, several additional groups became eligible for Medicare benefits, including those entitled to Social Security or Railroad Retirement disability cash benefits for at least twenty-four months, most persons with end-stage renal disease (ESRD), and certain individuals over sixty-five who were not eligible for paid coverage but elected to pay for Medicare benefits.

Medicaid was designed as a cost-sharing program between the federal and state governments. It pays for the healthcare services provided to many low-income Americans. The program became effective in 1966 under Title XIX of the Social Security Act. It allowed states to add health coverage to their **public assistance** programs for low-income groups, families with dependent children, the aged, and the disabled. Because Medicaid eligibility is based on meeting criteria other than income, today the program covers only about 40 percent of the population living in poverty.

The Medicare and Medicaid programs were originally the responsibility of the Department of Health, Education, and Welfare (predecessor to the **Department of Health and Human Services** [HHS]). The Social Security Administration (SSA) administered the Medicare program, and the Social and Rehabilitation Service (SRS) administered the Medicaid Program. In 1977, administration of Medicare and Medicaid was transferred to a newly created administrative agency within HHS, the Health Care Financing Administration (HCFA). HCFA's name was changed in 2001, and the agency is now called the **Centers for Medicare and Medicaid Services** (CMS).

The demand for medical services grew tremendously during the 1970s and early 1980s. As a result, health insurance premiums and the cost of funding Medicare and Medicaid programs skyrocketed. By the mid-1980s, both private and government-sponsored healthcare programs had instituted cost-control initiatives.

Since 1983, CMS has developed prospective payment systems (PPSs) to manage the costs of the Medicare and Medicaid programs. The PPS for inpatient acute care was the first to be implemented, followed by numerous others ranging from home health services to outpatient facility services. The most recently implemented system is for inpatient psychiatric facilities. Medicare and Medicaid reimbursement is discussed in more detail later in the chapter.

Private and self-insured health insurance plans also have implemented a number of cost-containing measures, most notably, **managed care** delivery and reimbursement systems. Managed care has virtually eliminated **traditional fee-for-service reimbursement** systems in just two decades. The implementation of managed care systems has had far-reaching effects on healthcare organizations and providers in every setting. However, hospitals have experienced the greatest financial pressure. Managed care is discussed in detail later in this chapter.

Development of Prepaid Health Plans

In 1860, Franklin Health Assurance Company of Massachusetts became the first commercial insurance company in the United States to provide private healthcare coverage for injuries that did not result in death. Within twenty years, sixty other insurance companies offered health insurance policies. By 1900, both accident insurance companies and life insurance companies were offering policies. These early policies covered loss of income and provided benefits for a limited number of illnesses (such as typhus, typhoid, scarlet fever, and smallpox).

Modern health insurance was born in 1929 when Baylor University Hospital in Dallas, Texas, agreed to provide healthcare services to Dallas schoolteachers. The hospital agreed to provide room, board, and certain ancillary services to the teachers for a set monthly fee of fifty cents. This plan is generally considered to be the first Blue Cross plan. Such plans were attractive to consumers and hospitals alike because they provided a way to ensure that patients would be able to pay for hospital services when they needed them. Payment was made directly to the hospital, not to the patient. In addition, coverage usually included a hospital stay for a specified number of days or for specific hospital services.

The Blue Cross plans contrasted with standard **indemnity plans** (insurance benefits provided in the form of cash payments) offered by private insurance companies that reimbursed (or indemnified) the patient for covered services up to a specified dollar limit. It was then the responsibility of the hospital to collect the money from the patient. Blue Shield plans were eventually developed by physicians. The plans were similar to Blue Cross plans except that they offered coverage for physicians' services.

Starting in the 1930s and continuing through the Second World War, traditional insurance companies added health insurance coverage for hospital, surgical, and medical expenses to their accident and life insurance plans. During the Second World War, **group health insurance** was offered as a way to attract scarce wartime labor. Group health insurance plans provide healthcare benefits to full-time employees of a company. This trend was strengthened by the favorable tax treatment for fringe benefits. Unlike monetary wages, fringe benefits were not subject to income or Social Security taxes. Therefore, a pretax dollar spent on health insurance coverage was worth more than an after-tax dollar spent directly on medical services. After the war, the Supreme Court ruled that employee benefits, including health insurance, were a legitimate part of the labor–management bargaining process. Health insurance quickly became a popular employee benefit.

Although early health insurance policies covered expenses associated with common accidents and illnesses, they were inadequate for coverage of extended illnesses and lengthy hospital stays. To correct this deficiency, insurance companies began offering **major medical insurance** coverage for catastrophic illnesses and injuries during the early 1950s. Major medical insurance provides benefits up to a high-dollar limit for most types of medical expenses. However, it usually requires patients to pay large deductibles. It also may place limits on charges (for example, room and board) and require patients to pay a portion of the expenses. **Blue Cross and Blue Shield** soon followed by offering similar plans.

Typically, the major medical insurance **policyholder** (or **insured**) paid a specified deductible (the amount the insured pays before the **insurer** assumes liability for any remaining costs of covered services). After the deductible had been paid, insured and insurer (third-party payer) shared covered losses according to a specified ratio, and the insured paid a **coinsurance** amount. Coinsurance refers to the amount the insured pays as a requirement of the insurance policy. For example, an insurance company may require the insured to pay a percentage of the daily costs for inpatient care.

According to the Washington Insurance Council (a nonprofit association of insurance companies and insurance professionals), by 1955, health insurance coverage continued to expand, and eventually 77 million Americans were covered by either an indemnity plan or a major medical plan. In subsequent years, insurance companies introduced high-benefit-level major medical plans, which limited **out-of-pocket expenses.** Out-of-pocket expenses are the healthcare expenses the insured is responsible for paying. After the insured has paid an amount specified in the insurance plan (that is, the deductible plus any copayments), the plan pays 100 percent of covered expenses. Such health insurance plans are common today and have been expanded to include coverage for advanced medical technology.

According to the U.S. Census Bureau, the percentage of people covered by health insurance in 2003 was 84.4 percent, lower than in previous years. (See table 7.1.)

The lack of health insurance for so many Americans continues to be a serious concern. Because of the financial constraints brought about by changes in Medicare/Medicaid and managed care reimbursement, many hospitals are no longer able to provide charitable services. As a result, underfunded and overcrowded public hospitals are struggling to provide services to uninsured patients who cannot pay for their own care. In addition, many uninsured patients delay seeking medical treatment until they are extremely ill, with long-term consequences for their own health and for the healthcare system. Thousands of patients with chronic diseases such as diabetes and asthma are brought to hospital emergency departments every day because they do not have access to basic healthcare services.

Table 7.1. Health insurance coverage status: 1987–2003

Year	Total U.S. Population (000)	Number Covered (000)	Percentage Covered
2003	288,280	243,320	84.4
2002	285,933	242,360	84.8
2001	282,082	240,875	85.4
2000	279,517	239,714	85.8
1999	274,087	231,533	84.5
1998	271,743	227,462	83.7
1997	269,094	225,646	83.9
1996	266,792	225,077	84.4
1995	264,314	223,733	84.6
1994	262,105	222,387	84.8
1993	259,753	220,040	84.7
1992	256,830	218,189	85.0
1991	251,447	216,003	85.9
1990	248,886	214,167	86.1
1989	246,191	212,807	86.4
1988	243,685	211,005	86.6
1987	241,187	210,161	87.1

Source: Based on U.S. Census Bureau information (www.census.gov/hhes/hlthins/historic/hihistt4.html).

One solution to the problem may be to expand government-sponsored healthcare programs. Another may be to create tax incentives to help individuals and small employers purchase private health insurance. For example, tax deductions could be offered to low-income people who buy their own insurance, or tax credits could be offered to small employers that offer health insurance coverage to employees.

Check Your Understanding 7.1

Instructions: Select the correct answer to complete each of the following statements.

1. _____ Prior to implementation of government programs like Medicare, the uninsured paid for healthcare services by:
   a. Receiving charity care
   b. Paying cash for services
   c. Going without healthcare services
   d. All of the above

2. _____ Prospective payment systems were developed by CMS to:
   a. Increase healthcare access
   b. Manage Medicare and Medicaid costs
   c. Implement managed care programs
   d. Eliminate fee-for-service programs

3. _____ Table 7.1 shows that the percentage change in health insurance coverage from 2002 to 2003 is:
   a. .1%
   b. .4%
   c. 1.0%
   d. 1.4%

4. _____ The government agency that administers the Medicaid and Medicare programs is:
   a. HCFA
   b. DHHS
   c. CMS
   d. SSA

5. _____To increase wartime labor during the Second Wold War, employers began offering:
   a. Private indemnity plans
   b. Group health insurance
   c. Prospective payment systems
   d. Out-of-pocket reimbursement

Healthcare Reimbursement Systems

Before the widespread availability of health insurance coverage, individuals were assured access to healthcare only when they were able to pay for the services themselves. They paid cash for services on a retrospective **fee-for-service basis,** in which the patient was expected to pay the healthcare provider after a service was rendered. Until the advent of managed care, **capitation,** and other PPSs, private insurance plans and government-sponsored programs also reimbursed providers on a retrospective fee-for-service basis.

Fee-for-service reimbursement is now rare for most types of medical services. Today, some form of health insurance covers most Americans and most health insurance plans compensate providers according to predetermined discounted rates rather than fee-for-service charges. However, some types of care are not covered by most health insurance plans and are still paid for directly by patients on a fee-for-service basis. Cosmetic surgery is one example of a medical service that is usually not considered medically necessary and is not covered by most insurance plans. Many insurance plans limit coverage for psychiatric services, substance abuse treatment, and the testing and correction of vision and hearing.

Commercial Insurance

Most Americans are covered by private group insurance plans tied to their employment. Typically, employers and employees share the cost of such plans. Two types of commercial insurance are commonly available: private insurance and **employer-based self-insurance.**

Private Health Insurance Plans

Private commercial insurance plans are financed through the payment of **premiums.** Each covered individual or family pays a preestablished amount (usually monthly), and the insurance company sets aside the premiums from all the people covered by the plan in a special fund. When a claim for medical care is submitted to the insurance company, the claim is paid out of the fund's reserves. Before payment is made, the insurance company reviews every claim to determine whether the services described on the claim are covered by the patient's policy. The company also reviews the diagnosis codes provided on the claim to ensure that the services provided were medically necessary. Payment then is made to either the provider or the policyholder.

When purchasing an insurance policy, the policyholder receives written confirmation from the insurance company when the insurance goes into effect. This confirmation document usually includes a policy number and a telephone number to be called in case of medical emergency. An insurance policy represents a legal contract for services between the insured and the insurance company.

Most insurance policies include the following information:

- What medical services the company will cover

- When the company will pay for medical services

- How much and for how long the company will pay for covered services

- What process is to be followed to ensure that covered medical expenses are paid

Employer-Based Self-Insurance Plans

During the 1970s, a number of large companies discovered that they could save money by self-insuring their employee health plans rather than purchasing coverage from private insurers. Large companies have large workforces, and so aggregate (total) employee medical experiences and associated expenses vary only slightly from one year to the next. The exception to this is during periods of rapid inflation in healthcare charges. The companies understood that it was in their best interest to self-insure their health plans because yearly expenses could be predicted relatively accurately.

The cost of self-insurance funding is lower than the cost of paying premiums to private insurers because the premiums reflect more than the actual cost of the services provided to beneficiaries. Private insurers build additional fees into premiums to compensate them for assuming the risk of providing insurance coverage. In self-insured plans, the employer assumes the risk. By budgeting a certain amount to pay its employees' medical claims, the employer retains control over the funds until such time as medical claims need to be paid.

Employer-based self-insurance has become a common form of group health insurance coverage. Many employers enter into **administrative services only (ASO) contracts** with private insurers and fund the plans themselves. The private insurers administer self-insurance plans on behalf of the employers.

Not-for Profit Healthcare Plans

Community-based, non-investor owned healthcare plans have existed for decades in the United States. These healthcare plans are referred to as not-for-profit and non-profit plans. However, since the 1990s there has been substantial growth of investor or for-profit health plans. In fact, many non-profit plans have converted to investor-owned plans in recent years. The conversion of non-profit health plans to for-profit status and the growth of for-profit healthcare plans have sparked a great deal of debate.

A primary difference between non-profit and for-profit entities is where their excess revenues are directed (American Nursing Association 1997). In a for-profit health plan, like any other stock company, excess revenues are distributed to shareholders. In non-profit entities, excess revenues are not distributed to shareholders, but are retained for future internal investments. The literature regarding the comparative benefits, quality of care and performance of nonprofit versus for-profit healthcare entities differs. Some studies indicate that for-profit health plans provide lower quality care and poorer performance than non-profit plans (Himmelstein et al. 1999; Schneider et al. 2005). Others indicate little or no difference between the two (Kim et al. 2004).

Blue Cross and Blue Shield Plans

Blue Cross and Blue Shield (BC/BS) plans, also known as the Blues, were the first prepaid health plans in the United States. Originally, Blue Cross plans covered hospital care and Blue Shield plans covered physicians' services. Prior to 1994, the national Blue Cross/Blue Shield Association required member plans to operate as nonprofit plans. Today, however, several Blue Cross/Blue Shield plans have converted to a for-profit status.

The first Blue Cross plan was created in 1929. In 1939, a commission of the American Hospital Association (AHA) adopted the Blue Cross national emblem for plans that met specific guidelines. The Blue Cross Association was created in 1960, and the relationship with the AHA ended in 1972.

The first Blue Shield plan was created in 1939, and the Associated Medical Care Plans (later known as the National Association of Blue Shield Plans) adopted the Blue Shield symbol in 1948. In 1982, the Blue Cross Association and the National Association of Blue Shield Plans merged to create the Blue Cross and Blue Shield Association.

Today, the Blue Cross and Blue Shield Association includes over sixty independent, locally operated companies with plans in fifty states, the District of Columbia, and Puerto Rico. The Blues offer health insurance to individuals, small businesses, seniors, and large employer groups. In addition, federal employees are eligible to enroll in the **BC/BS Federal Employee Program (FEP)** (also called the BC/BS Service Benefit Plan). The plan offers the two products to federal employees:

- A **preferred provider organization** (PPO) plan, in which healthcare providers provide healthcare services to members of the plan at a discounted rate

- A **point-of-service (POS) plan,** in which subscribers are encouraged to select providers from a prescribed network but are allowed to seek healthcare services from providers outside the network at a higher level of copay.

Government-Sponsored Healthcare Programs

The federal government administers several healthcare programs. The best known are Medicare and Medicaid. The Medicare program pays for the healthcare services provided to Social Security beneficiaries sixty-five years old and older as well as people with permanent disabilities, people with end-stage renal disease, and certain other groups of individuals. State governments work with the federal Medicaid program to provide healthcare coverage to low-income individuals and families

In addition, the federal government offers three health programs to address the needs of military personnel and their dependents as well as native Americans. The **Civilian Health and Medical Program-Veterans Affairs (CHAMPVA)** provides healthcare services for dependents and survivors of disabled veterans, survivors of veterans who died from service-related conditions, and survivors of military personnel who died in the line of duty. **TRICARE** (formerly CHAMPUS, the Civilian Health and Medical Program-Uniformed Services) provides coverage for the dependents of armed forces personnel and retirees receiving care outside a military treatment facility. The **Indian Health Service** (IHS) provides federal health services to American Indians and Alaska natives.

Medicare

The original Medicare program was implemented on July 1, 1966. In 1973, Medicare benefits were expanded to include individuals of any age who suffered from a permanent disability or end-stage renal disease.

For Americans receiving Social Security benefits, Medicare automatically provides **hospitalization insurance (HI) (Medicare Part A).** It also offers voluntary **supplemental medical insurance** (SMI) (Medicare Part B) to help pay for physicians' services, medical services, and medical–surgical supplies not covered by the hospitalization plan. Enrollees pay extra for Part B benefits. To fill gaps in Medicare coverage, most Medicare enrollees also supplement their benefits with private insurance policies. These private policies are referred to as **Medigap** insurance. The Balanced Budget Act (BBA) of 1997, to expand the options for participation in private healthcare insurance, established **Medicare Advantage** (formerly Medicare+Choice).

According to CMS, approximately 19 million Americans were enrolled in the Medicare program in 1966. In 2005, approximately 40 million people were enrolled in Parts A and/or B of the Medicare program, and 6.4 million of the enrollees participated in a Medicare Advantage plan.

Medicare Part A
Medicare Part A is generally provided free of charge to individuals age sixty-five and over who are eligible for Social Security or Railroad Retirement benefits. Individuals who do not claim their monthly cash benefits are still eligible for Medicare. In addition, workers (and their spouses) who have been employed in federal, state, or local

government for a sufficient period of time qualify for Medicare coverage beginning at age sixty-five.

Similarly, individuals who have been entitled to Social Security or Railroad Retirement disability benefits for at least twenty-four months and government employees with Medicare coverage who have been disabled for more than twenty-nine months are entitled to Part A benefits. This coverage also is provided to insured workers (and their spouses) with end-state renal disease as well as to children with end-stage renal disease. In addition, some otherwise-ineligible aged and disabled beneficiaries who voluntarily pay a monthly premium for their coverage are eligible for Medicare Part A.

The following healthcare services are covered under Medicare Part A: inpatient hospital care, long-term care, skilled nursing facility (SNF) care, home health care, and **hospice** care. (See table 7.2.) Inpatient hospital care and long-term care are paid for under Medicare Part A when such care is medically necessary. An initial deductible payment is required for each hospital admission, plus copayments for all hospital days following day sixty within a benefit period.

Each benefit period begins the day the Medicare beneficiary is admitted to the hospital and ends when he or she has not been hospitalized for a period of sixty consecutive days. Inpatient hospital care is usually limited to ninety days during each benefit period. There is no limit to the number of benefit periods covered by Medicare hospital insurance during a beneficiary's lifetime. However, copayment requirements apply to days sixty-one through ninety. When a beneficiary exhausts the ninety days of inpatient hospital care available during a benefit period, a nonrenewable lifetime reserve of up to a total of sixty additional days of inpatient hospital care can be used. Copayments are required for such additional days.

SNF care is covered when it occurs within thirty days of a three-day-long or longer acute hospitalization and is certified as medically necessary. The number of SNF days provided under Medicare is limited to 100 days per benefit period, with a copayment required for days 21 through 100. Medicare Part A does not cover SNF care when the patient does not require skilled nursing care or skilled rehabilitation services.

Care provided by a **home health agency** (HHA) may be furnished part-time in the residence of a homebound beneficiary when intermittent or part-time skilled nursing and/or certain other therapy or rehabilitation care is needed. Certain medical supplies and durable medical equipment (DME) also may be paid for under the Medicare home health benefit.

The Medicare program requires the HHA to develop a treatment plan that is periodically reviewed by a physician. Home health care under Medicare Part A has no limitations on duration, no copayments, and no deductibles. For DME, beneficiaries must pay 20 percent coinsurance, as required under Medicare Part B.

Terminally ill persons, whose life expectancies are certified by their attending physician to be six months or less, may elect to receive hospice services. To qualify for Medicare reimbursement for hospice care, patients must elect to forgo standard Medicare benefits for treatment of their terminal illnesses and agree to receive only hospice care. When a hospice patient requires treatment for a condition that is not related to his or her terminal illness, however, Medicare does pay for all covered services necessary for that condition. The Medicare beneficiary pays no deductible for hospice coverage but does pay coinsurance amounts for drugs and inpatient **respite care.** (Respite care is any inpatient care provided to the hospice patient for the purpose of providing primary caregivers a break from their care-giving responsibilities.)

Table 7.2   Medicare Part A benefit period, beneficiary deductibles and copayments, and Medicare payment responsibilities according to healthcare setting

Healthcare Setting	Benefit Period	Patient's Responsibility	Medicare Payments
Hospital (Inpatient)	First 60 days	$912 annual deductible	All but $912
	Days 61–90	$228 per day	All but $228/day
	Days 91–150 (these reserve days can be used only once in the patient's lifetime)	$456 per day	All but $456/day
	Beyond 150 days	All costs	Nothing
Skilled Nursing Facility	First 20 days	Nothing	100% approved amount
	Days 21–100	$114 per day	All but $114 per day
	Beyond 100 days	All costs	Nothing
Home Health Care	For as long as patient meets Medicare medical necessity criteria	Nothing for services, but 20% of approved amount for durable medical equipment (DME)	100% of the approved amount, and 80% of the approved amount for DME
Hospice Care	For as long as physician certifies need for care	Limited costs for outpatient drugs and inpatient respite care	All but limited costs for outpatient drugs and inpatient respite care
Blood	Unlimited if medical necessity criteria are met	First 3 pints unless you or someone else donates blood to replace what you use	All but first 3 pints per calendar year

Source: Adapted from *Medicare and You* 2005.

Medicare Part B

Medicare Part B (supplemental medical insurance) covers the following services and supplies:

- Physicians' and surgeons' services, including some covered services furnished by chiropractors, podiatrists, dentists, and optometrists; and services provided by the following Medicare-approved practitioners who are not physicians: certified registered nurse anesthetists, clinical psychologists, clinical social workers (other than those employed by a hospital or an SNF), physician assistants, and nurse practitioners and clinical nurse specialists working in collaboration with a physician

- Services in an emergency department or outpatient clinic, including same-day surgery and ambulance services

- Home health care not covered under Medicare Part A

- Laboratory tests, x-rays, and other diagnostic radiology services, as well as certain preventive care screening tests
- Ambulatory surgery center (ASC) services in Medicare-approved facilities
- Most physical and occupational therapy and speech pathology services
- Comprehensive outpatient rehabilitation facility services and mental healthcare provided as part of a partial hospitalization psychiatric program when a physician certifies that inpatient treatment would be required without the partial hospitalization services (A partial hospitalization program offers intensive psychiatric treatment on an outpatient basis to psychiatric patients, with an expectation that the patient's psychiatric condition and level of functioning will improve and that relapse will be prevented so that re-hospitalization can be avoided.)
- Radiation therapy, renal dialysis and kidney transplants, and heart and liver transplants under certain limited conditions
- DME approved for home use, such as oxygen equipment, wheelchairs, prosthetic devices, surgical dressings, splints, and casts, walkers, and hospital beds needed for use in the home
- Drugs and biologicals that cannot be self-administered, such as hepatitis B vaccines and immunosuppressive drugs (plus certain self-administered anticancer drugs)
- Preventive services such as bone mass measurements, cardiovascular screening blood tests, colorectal cancer screening, diabetes services, glaucoma testing, Pap test and pelvic exam, prostate cancer screening, screening mammograms, and vaccinations (flu, pneumococcal, hepatitis B)
- Inpatient hospitalizations when part A benefits have been exhausted

To be covered, all Medicare Part B services must be either documented as medically necessary or covered as one of several prescribed preventive benefits. Part B services also are generally subject to deductibles and coinsurance payments. (See table 7.3.) Certain medical services and related care are subject to special payment rules, for example:

- Deductibles for administration of blood and blood products
- Maximum approved amounts for Medicare-approved physical or occupational therapy services performed in settings other than hospitals
- Higher cost-sharing requirements, such as those for outpatient psychiatric care

The following healthcare services are usually not covered by Medicare Part A or B and are only covered by private health plans under the Medicare Advantage program:

- Long-term nursing care
- Custodial care
- Dentures and dental care
- Eyeglasses
- Hearing aids
- Most prescription drugs

Table 7.3. Medicare Part B benefit deductibles and copayments, and Medicare payment responsibilities according to type of service

Type of Service	Benefit	Deductible and Copayment	Medicare Payment
Medical Expenses	Physicians' services, inpatient and outpatient medical and surgical services and supplies, and durable medical equipment (DME)	$110 annual deductible, plus 20% of approved amount after deductible has been met, except in outpatient setting	80% of approved amount (after patient has paid $110 deductible)
	Mental health care	50% of most outpatient care	50% of most outpatient care
	Occupational, physical, and speech therapy	20% of the first $1500 and all charges thereafter	80% of first $1500
Clinical Laboratory Services	Blood tests, urinalysis, and more	Nothing	100% of approved amount
Home Health Care	Intermittent skilled care, home health aide services, DME and supplies, and other services	Nothing for home care service 20% of approved amount for DME	100% of approved amount 80% of approved amount for DME
Outpatient Hospital Services	Services for diagnosis and/or treatment of an illness or injury	$110 annual deductible, plus a coinsurance amount for *each service* received during an outpatient visit. For *each* outpatient service received, the coinsurance amount cannot be greater than the Medicare Part A inpatient hospital deductible. The coinsurance amount is based on 20% of the national median charge for services in the ambulatory payment classification associated with the service. Charges for items or services that Medicare does not cover	Payment based on ambulatory patient classifications/outpatient prospective payment system
Blood	Unlimited if medical necessity criteria are met	First 3 pints (if met under Part B, does not have to be met again under Part A)	All but first 3 pints

Source: Adapted from *Medicare & You* 2005.

Medicare Advantage

Medicare Advantage provides expanded coverage of many healthcare services. Although any Medicare beneficiary may receive benefits through the original fee-for-service program, most beneficiaries enrolled in both Parts A and B can choose to participate in a Medicare Advantage plan instead. Organizations that offer Medicare Advantage plans must meet specific requirements as determined by CMS.

Primary Medicare Advantage products include the following types of plans:

- *Managed care plans:* In a managed care plan, patients can only go to doctors, specialists, or hospitals on the plan's list, which is referred to as a network, except in an emergency. Patients also may have to choose a primary care doctor and be referred to see a specialist, but pay lower copayments and receive extra benefits.

- *PPO plans:* In a PPO plan, patients use doctors, specialists, and hospitals in the plan's network and can go to doctors and hospitals not on the list, usually at an additional cost. Patients do not need referrals to see doctors or go to hospitals that are not part of the plan's network and may pay lower copayments and receive extra benefits.

- *Private fee-for-service plans:* These plans allow beneficiaries to go to any doctor or hospital that accepts the terms of the plan's payment. The private company, rather than the Medicare program, decides how much it will pay and how much patients pay for services rendered.

- *Medicare specialty plans:* Medicare specialty plans provide more focused healthcare for specific people, such as those with congestive heart failure, diabetes or end-stage renal disease.

Medicare Prescription Drug, Improvement and Modernization Act

The Medicare Prescription Drug, Improvement and Modernization Act, also known as the Medicare Reform Bill, was signed into law by President George W. Bush on December 8, 2003. This legislation provides seniors and individuals with disabilities with a prescription drug benefit, more choices, and better benefits under Medicare.

Out-of-Pocket Expenses and Medigap Insurance

Medicare beneficiaries who elect the fee-for-service option are responsible for charges not covered by the Medicare program and for various cost-sharing aspects of Parts A and B. These liabilities may be paid by the Medicare beneficiary; by a third party, such as an employer-sponsored health plan or private Medigap insurance; or by Medicaid, when the person is eligible.

Medigap is private health insurance that pays, within limits, most of the healthcare service charges not covered by Medicare Parts A and/or B. These policies must meet federal and state laws.

The payment share for beneficiaries enrolled in Medicare Advantage plans is based on the cost-sharing structure of the specific plan they select. Most plans have lower deductibles and coinsurance than are required of Medicare fee-for-service beneficiaries. Such beneficiaries pay the monthly Part B premium and may pay an additional plan premium, depending on the plan.

For hospital care covered under Medicare Part A, a fee-for-service beneficiary's payment share includes a one-time deductible amount payable at the beginning of each benefit period. For 2005, the deductible was $912. This deductible covers the beneficiary's part of the first sixty days of each inpatient hospital stay. When continued inpatient care is needed beyond the sixty days, additional coinsurance payments ($228 per day in 2005) are required through the ninetieth day of a benefit period. Each Part A beneficiary also has a lifetime reserve of sixty additional hospital days that may be used when the covered days within a benefit period have been exhausted. Lifetime reserve days may be used only once, and coinsurance payments ($456 per day in 2005) are required.

For SNF care covered under Part A, Medicare fully covers the first twenty days in a benefit period. For days 21 through 100, a copayment ($114 per day in 2005) is required. Medicare benefits expire after the first 100 days of SNF care during a benefit period.

Home health care services require no deductible or coinsurance payment by the beneficiary.

For any Part A service, the beneficiary is responsible for paying fees to cover the first three pints or units of nonreplaced blood per calendar year. The beneficiary has the option of paying the fee or arranging for the blood to be replaced by family and friends.

Most beneficiaries covered by Medicare Part A pay no premiums. Eligibility is generally earned through the work experience of the beneficiary or of his or her spouse. In addition, most individuals over sixty-five who are otherwise ineligible for Medicare Part A coverage can enroll voluntarily by paying a monthly premium when they also enroll in Part B.

For Part B (table 7.3), the beneficiary's payment share includes:

- One annual deductible ($110 in 2005)
- Monthly premiums ($78.20 per month in 2005)
- Coinsurance payments for Part B services (usually 20 percent of medically allowable charges)
- Any deductibles for blood products
- Certain charges above approved charges (for claims not on assignment)
- Payment for any services that are not covered by Medicare

Check Your Understanding 7.2

Instructions: Select the best answer for the following statements.

1. _____ Private health insurance is a type of:
   a. Commercial insurance
   b. Federal insurance
   c. Military insurance
   d. State insurance

2. _____ A health insurance plan in which providers give healthcare services to members of the plan at a discounted rate is called:
   a. ASO plan
   b. Medigap plan
   c. POS plan
   d. PPO plan

3. _____ The healthcare plan that provides coverage for the dependents of armed forces personnel and retirees receiving care outside a military treatment facility is:
   a. ASO
   b. IHS
   c. PPO
   d. TRICARE

4. _____ A plan in which subscribers are encouraged to select providers from a prescribed network but are allowed to seek healthcare services from providers outside the network at a higher level of copay is called:
   a. ASO
   b. POS
   c. PPO
   d. TRICARE

5. ____ Medicare Part A provides:
   a. Dental insurance
   b. Hospitalization insurance
   c. Outpatient insurance
   d. All of the above

6. ____ Medicare Part B covers:
   a. Services in an emergency department
   b. Ambulatory surgery center services
   c. Services in an outpatient clinic
   d. All of the above

7. ____ Medicare coverage applies to:
   a. Individuals age 65 and over
   b. Individuals who are disabled
   c. Individuals who undergo chronic kidney dialysis for end-stage renal disease
   d. All of the above

8. ____ This is private health insurance that pays, within limits, most of the healthcare service charges not covered by Medicare Parts A and/or B:
   a. POS
   b. PPO
   c. Medigap
   d. TRI CARE

Medicaid

Title XIX of the Social Security Act enacted Medicaid in 1965. The Medicaid program pays for medical assistance provided to individuals and families with low incomes and limited financial resources. Individual states must meet broad national guidelines established by federal statutes, regulations, and policies to qualify for federal matching grants under the Medicaid program. Individual state medical assistance agencies, however, establish the Medicaid eligibility standards for residents of their states. The states also determine the type, amount, duration, and scope of covered services; calculate the rate of payment for covered services; and administer local programs.

Medicaid policies on eligibility, services, and payment are complex and vary considerably among states, even among states of similar size or geographic proximity. Therefore, an individual who is eligible for Medicaid in one state may not be eligible in another. In addition, the amount, duration, and scope of care provided vary considerably from state to state. Moreover, Medicaid eligibility and/or services within a state can change from year to year.

Medicaid Eligibility Criteria

Low income is only one test for Medicaid eligibility. Other financial resources also are compared against eligibility standards. These standards are determined by each state according to federal guidelines.

Generally, each state is allowed to determine which groups Medicaid will cover. Each state also establishes its own financial criteria for Medicaid eligibility. However, to be eligible for federal funds, states are required to provide Medicaid coverage to certain individuals. These individuals include recipients of federally assisted income maintenance payments, as well as related groups of individuals who do not receive cash payments. The federal **categorically needy eligibility groups** include:

- Individuals eligible for Medicaid when they meet requirements for **Temporary Assistance for Needy Families** (TANF)

- Children below age six whose family income is at or below 133 percent of the federal poverty level (FPL) (the income threshold established by the federal government)

- Pregnant women whose family income is below 133 percent of the FPL (services are limited to those related to pregnancy-related medical care)

- Supplemental Security Income (SSI) recipients in most states

- Recipients of adoption or foster care assistance under Title IV-E of the Social Security Act

- Specially protected groups (typically individuals who lose their cash assistance due to earnings from work or from increased Social Security benefits, but who may keep Medicaid for a period of time)

- Infants born to Medicaid-eligible pregnant women

- Certain low-income Medicare beneficiaries

States also have the option of providing Medicaid coverage to other categorically related groups. Categorically related groups share the characteristics of the eligible groups (that is, they fall within defined categories), but the eligibility criteria are somewhat more liberally defined. A **medically needy option** also allows states to extend Medicaid eligibility to persons who would be eligible for Medicaid under one of the mandatory or optional groups except that their income and/or resources are above the eligibility level set by their state. Individuals may qualify immediately or may "spend down" by incurring medical expenses that reduce their income to or below their state's income level for the medically needy.

In 1996, Congress passed the Personal Responsibility and Work Opportunity Reconciliation Act (also known as welfare reform). The act made restrictive changes in the eligibility requirements for SSI coverage. These changes also affected eligibility for participation in the Medicaid program.

The welfare reform act also affected a number of disabled children. Many lost their SSI benefits as a result of the restrictive changes. However, their eligibility for Medicaid was reinstituted by the BBA.

In addition, the welfare reform act repealed the open-ended federal entitlement program known as Aid to Families with Dependent Children (AFDC). TANF, which replaced AFDC, provides states with grant money to be used for time-limited cash assistance. A family's lifetime cash welfare benefits are generally limited to a maximum of five years. Individual states also are allowed to impose other eligibility restrictions.

Medicaid Services

To be eligible for federal matching funds, each state's Medicaid program must offer medical assistance for the following basic services:

- Inpatient hospital services
- Outpatient hospital services

- Emergency services

- Prenatal care

- Vaccines for children

- Physicians' services

- SNF services for persons aged twenty-one or older

- Family planning services and supplies

- Rural health clinic services

- Home health care for persons eligible for skilled nursing services

- Laboratory and x-ray services

- Pediatric and family nurse practitioner services

- Nurse-midwife services

- Federally qualified health center (FQHC) services and ambulatory services performed at an FQHC that would be available in other settings

- Early and periodic screening and diagnostic and therapeutic services for children under age twenty-one

States also may receive federal matching funds to provide some of the optional services, the most common being:

- Diagnostic services

- Clinic services

- Prescription drugs and prosthetic devices

- Transportation services

- Rehabilitation and physical therapy services

- Prosthetic devices

- Home care and community-based care services for persons with chronic impairments

The BBA also called for implementation of a state option called **Programs of All-Inclusive Care for the Elderly** (PACE). PACE provides an alternative to institutional care for individuals fifty-five years old or older who require a level of care usually provided at nursing facilities. It offers and manages all of the health, medical, and social services needed by a beneficiary and mobilizes other services, as needed, to provide preventive, rehabilitative, curative, and supportive care.

PACE services can be provided in day healthcare centers, homes, hospitals, and nursing homes. The program helps its beneficiaries to maintain their independence, dignity, and quality of life. PACE also functions within the Medicare program. Individuals enrolled in PACE receive benefits solely through the PACE program.

Medicaid–Medicare Relationship

Medicare beneficiaries who have low incomes and limited financial resources also may receive help from the Medicaid program. For persons eligible for full Medicaid coverage, Medicare coverage is supplemented by services that are available under their state's Medicaid program according to their eligibility category. Additional services may include, for example, nursing facility care beyond the 100-day limit covered by Medicare, prescription drugs, eyeglasses, and hearing aids. For those enrolled in both programs, any services covered by Medicare are paid for by the Medicare program before any payments are made by the Medicaid program because Medicaid is always the **payer of last resort.** Table 7.4 provides a comparison of the Medicare and Medicaid programs.

State Children's Health Insurance Program

The **State Children's Health Insurance Program** (SCHIP) (Title XXI of the Social Security Act) is a program initiated by the BBA SCHIP (sometimes referred to as the Children's Health Insurance Program, or CHIP), which allows states to expand existing insurance programs to cover children up to age nineteen. It provides additional federal funds to states so that Medicaid eligibility can be expanded to include a greater number of children.

SCHIP became available on October 1, 1997, and is jointly funded by the federal government and the states. Following broad federal guidelines, states establish eligibility and coverage guidelines and have flexibility in the way they provide services. Recipients in all states must meet three eligibility criteria:

- They must come from low-income families.
- They must be otherwise ineligible for Medicaid.
- They must be uninsured.

Table 7.4. Comparison of Medicare and Medicaid programs

Medicare	Medicaid
Health insurance for people age 65 and older, or people under 65 who are entitled to Medicare because of disability or are receiving dialysis for permanent kidney failure	Health assistance for people of any age
Administered through fiscal intermediaries, insurance companies under contract to the government to process Medicare claims	Administered by the federal government through state and local governments following federal and state guidelines
Medicare regulations are the same in all states	Medicaid regulations vary from state to state
Financed by monthly premiums paid by the beneficiary and by payroll tax deductions	Financed by federal, state and county tax dollars
For people age 65 and over, eligibility is based on Social Security or Railroad Retirement participation. For people under age 65, eligibility is based on disability. For people who undergo kidney dialysis, eligibility is not dependent on age	Eligibility based on financial need
Beneficiary responsible for paying deductibles, coinsurance or copayments, and Part B premiums	Medicaid can help pay Medicare deductible, coinsurance or copayment, and premiums
Hospital and medical benefits; preventive care and long-term care benefits are limited	Comprehensive benefits include hospital, preventive care, long-term care, and other services not covered under Medicare such as dental work, prescriptions, transportation, eyeglasses, and hearing aids

States are required to offer the following services:

- Inpatient hospital services
- Outpatient hospital services
- Physicians' surgical and medical services
- Laboratory and x-ray services
- Well-baby/child care services, including age-appropriate immunizations

Check Your Understanding 7.3

Instructions: Select the best answer for the following statements.

1. _____ Title XVIII of the Social Security Act Amendment of 1965 is also known as:
    a. Medicare
    b. Medicaid
    c. Medigap
    d. SCHIP

2. _____ Medicaid eligibility standards are established by:
    a. Center of Medicare and Medicaid Services
    b. Department of Health and Human Services
    c. Individual states
    d. Federal Government

3. _____ To be eligible for federal matching funds, each state's Medicaid program must offer medical assistance for:
    a. Inpatient hospital services
    b. Prenatal care
    c. Vaccines for children
    d. All of the above

4. _____ This program pays for medical assistance to individuals and families with low incomes and limited financial resources:
    a. Medicaid
    b. Medicare Part A
    c. Medicare Part B
    d. PACE

5. _____ This program provides additional federal funds to states so that Medicaid eligibility can be expanded to include a greater number of children:
    a. Medicaid
    b. Medigap
    c. SCHIP
    d. PACE

TRICARE

TRICARE is a healthcare program for active-duty members of the military and other qualified family members. CHAMPUS-eligible retirees and their family members as well as eligible survivors of members of the uniformed services also are eligible for TRICARE.

The idea of medical care for the families of active-duty members of the uniformed military services dates back to the late 1700s. It was not until 1884, however, that Congress directed Army medical officers and contract surgeons to care for the families of military personnel free of charge.

There was very little change in the provision of medical care to members of the military and their families until the Second World War, when the military was made up mostly of young men who had wives of childbearing age. The military medical care system could not handle the large number of births or the care of young children. So, in 1943, Congress authorized the **Emergency Maternal and Infant Care Program** (EMIC). The program provided maternity and infant care to dependents of service members in the lowest four pay grades.

During the early 1950s, the Korean conflict also strained the capabilities of the military healthcare system. As a result, the Dependents Medical Care Act was signed into law in 1956. Amendments to the act created the **Civilian Health and Medical Program of the Uniformed Services** (CHAMPUS) in 1966.

During the 1980s, the search for ways to improve access to top-quality medical care and at the same time control costs led to implementation of CHAMPUS demonstration projects in various parts of the country. The most successful of these projects was the CHAMPUS Reform Initiative (CRI) in California and Hawaii. Initiated in 1988, the CRI offered military service families a choice in the way their military healthcare benefits could be used. Five years of successful operation and high levels of patient satisfaction persuaded Department of Defense officials that they should extend and improve the CRI concepts as a uniform program nationwide.

The new program, known as TRICARE, was phased in nationally by 1998. Expansion to overseas military bases will soon be complete. TRICARE offers three options: **TRICARE Prime, TRICARE Extra,** and **TRICARE Standard.**

TRICARE Prime

Of the three options, TRICARE Prime provides the most comprehensive healthcare benefits at the lowest cost. Military treatment facilities, for example, military base hospitals, serve as the principal source of healthcare, and a **primary care manager** (PCM) is assigned to each enrollee.

Two specialized programs supplement TRICARE Prime. **TRICARE Prime Remote** provides healthcare services to active-duty military personnel stationed in the United States in areas not served by the traditional military healthcare system. (Active-duty personnel include members of the Army, Navy, Marine Corps, Air Force, Coast Guard, and active National Guard.) **TRICARE Senior Prime** is a managed care demonstration program designed to serve the medical needs of military retirees who are sixty-five years old or over and their dependents and survivors.

TRICARE Extra

TRICARE Extra is a cost-effective preferred provider network (PPN) option. Healthcare costs in TRICARE Extra are lower than for TRICARE Standard because beneficiaries must select physicians and medical specialists from a network of civilian healthcare professionals working under contract with TRICARE. The healthcare professionals who participate in TRICARE Extra agree to charge a preestablished discounted rate for the medical treatments and procedures provided to participants in the plan.

TRICARE Standard

TRICARE Standard incorporates the services previously provided by CHAMPUS. TRICARE Standard allows eligible beneficiaries to choose any physician or healthcare provider.

It pays a set percentage of the providers' fees, and the enrollee pays the rest. This option permits the most flexibility but may be the most expensive for the enrollee, particularly when the provider's charges are higher than the amounts allowed by the program.

CHAMPVA

The Civilian Health and Medical Program-Veterans Affairs (CHAMPVA) is a healthcare program for dependents and survivors of permanently and totally disabled veterans, survivors of veterans who died from service-related conditions, and survivors of military personnel who died in the line of duty. CHAMPVA is a voluntary program that allows beneficiaries to be treated for free at participating VA healthcare facilities, with the VA sharing the cost of covered healthcare services and supplies. Because of the similarity between CHAMPVA and TRICARE (which replaced CHAMPUS), people sometimes confuse the two programs. However, CHAMPVA is separate from TRICARE and there are distinct differences between them.

Indian Health Service

The provision of health services to native Americans originally developed from the relationship between the federal government and federally recognized Indian tribes. This relationship was established in 1787. It is based on Article I, Section 8, of the U.S. Constitution. It has been given form and substance by numerous treaties, laws, Supreme Court decisions, and executive orders.

The IHS is an agency within the HHS. It is responsible for providing healthcare services to American Indians and Alaska natives. The American Indians and Alaska natives served by the IHS receive preventive healthcare services, primary medical services (hospital and ambulatory care), community health services, substance abuse treatment services, and rehabilitative services. Secondary medical care, highly specialized medical services, and other rehabilitative care are provided by IHS staff or by private healthcare professionals working under contract with the IHS.

A system of acute and ambulatory care facilities operates on Indian reservations and in Indian and Alaska native communities. In locations where the IHS does not have its own facilities or is not equipped to provide a needed service, it contracts with local hospitals, state and local healthcare agencies, tribal health institutions, and individual healthcare providers.

Workers' Compensation

Most employees are eligible for some type of **workers' compensation** insurance. Workers' compensation programs cover healthcare costs and lost income associated with work-related injuries and illnesses. Federal government employees are covered by the **Federal Employees' Compensation Act** (FECA). Individual states pass legislation that addresses workers' compensation coverage for nonfederal government employees. Some states exclude certain workers, for example, business owners, independent contractors, farm workers, and so on. Texas employers are not required to provide workers' compensation coverage.

Federal Workers' Compensation Funds

In 1908, President Theodore Roosevelt signed legislation to provide workers' compensation for certain federal employees in unusually hazardous jobs. The scope of the law was narrow, and its benefits were limited. The 1908 law represented the first workers' compensation program to pass the test of constitutionality applied by the U.S. Supreme Court.

FECA replaced the 1908 statute in 1916. Under FECA, civilian employees of the federal government are provided medical care, survivors' benefits, and compensation for lost wages. The Office of Workers' Compensation Programs (OWCP) administers FECA as well as the Longshore and Harbor Workers' Compensation Act of 1927 and the Black Lung Benefits Reform Act of 1977.

FECA also provides vocational rehabilitation services to partially disabled employees. Employees who fully or partially recover from their injuries are expected to return to work. FECA does not provide retirement benefits.

State Workers' Compensation Funds

According to the American Association of State Compensation Insurance Funds (AASCIF), state workers' compensation insurance was developed in response to the concerns of employers. Before state workers' compensation programs became widely available, employers faced the possibility of going out of business when insurance companies refused to provide coverage or charged excessive premiums. Legislators in most states have addressed these concerns by establishing **state workers' compensation insurance funds** that provide a stable source of insurance coverage and serve to protect employers from uncertainties about the continuing availability of coverage. Because state funds are provided on a nonprofit basis, the premiums can be kept low. In addition, the funds provide only one type of insurance: workers' compensation. This specialization allows the funds to concentrate resources, knowledge, and expertise in a single field of insurance.

State workers' compensation insurance funds do not operate at taxpayer expense because, by law, the funds support themselves through income derived from premiums and investments. As nonprofit departments of the state or as independent nonprofit companies, they return surplus assets to policyholders as dividends or safety refunds. This system reduces the overall cost of state-level workers' compensation insurance. Numerous court decisions have determined that the assets, reserves, and surplus of the funds are not public funds but, instead, the property of the employers insured by the funds.

In states where state funds have not been mandated, employers purchase workers' compensation coverage from private carriers or provide self-insurance coverage.

Check Your Understanding 7.4

Instructions: Select the best answer for the following statements.

1. _____ A healthcare program for active duty members of the military and other qualified family members:
   a. HIS
   b. Medicare
   c. Medicaid
   d. TRICARE

2. _____ This program provides the most comprehensive health care benefits at lowest cost for active duty members of the military and other qualified family members:
   a. CHAMPVA
   b. TRICARE prime
   c. TRICARE extra
   d. TRICARE standard

3. _____ A health care program for dependents and survivors of permanently and totally disabled veterans:
   a. CHAMPUS
   b. CHAMPVA
   c. IHS
   d. TRICARE

4.   ____ Agency responsible for providing healthcare services to American Indians and Alaskan
            natives:
            a.   CHAMPUS
            b.   CHAMPVA
            c.   IHS
            d.   TRICARE

5.   ____ Insurance that covers healthcare costs and lost income associated with work-related
            injuries:
            a.   CHAMPVA
            b.   Medicare
            c.   Medicaid
            d.   Workers compensation

6.   ____ FECA covers:
            a.   Individuals 65 years and older
            b.   Individuals with low incomes
            c.   Federal employees
            d.   State employees

Managed Care

Healthcare costs in the United States rose dramatically during the 1970s and 1980s. As a result, the federal government, employers, and other third-party payers began investigating more cost-effective healthcare delivery systems. The federal government decided to move toward PPSs for the Medicare program in the mid-1980s. Prospective payment as a reimbursement methodology is discussed later in this chapter. Commercial insurance providers looked to managed care.

Managed care is the generic term for prepaid health plans that integrate the financial and delivery aspects of healthcare services. In other words, managed care organizations work to control the cost of, and access to, healthcare services at the same time that they strive to meet high-quality standards. They manage healthcare costs by negotiating discounted providers' fees and controlling patients' access to expensive healthcare services. In managed care plans, services are carefully coordinated to ensure that they are medically appropriate and needed.

The cost of providing appropriate services also is monitored continuously to determine whether the services are being delivered in the most efficient and cost-effective way possible.

Since 1973, several pieces of federal legislation have been passed with the goal of encouraging the development of managed healthcare systems. (See table 7.5.) The Health Maintenance Organization Assistance Act of 1973 authorized federal grants and loans to private organizations that wished to develop **health maintenance organizations** (HMOs). Another important advancement in managed care was development of the **Health Plan Employer Data and Information Set** (HEDIS) by the **National Committee for Quality Assurance** (NCQA).

The NCQA is a private, not-for-profit organization that accredits, assesses, and reports on the quality of managed care plans in the United States. It worked with public and private healthcare purchasers, health plans, researchers, and consumer advocates to develop HEDIS in 1989. HEDIS is a set of standardized measures used to compare managed care plans in terms of the quality of services they provide. The standards cover areas such as plan membership, utilization of and access to services, and financial indicators. The goals of the program include:

- To help beneficiaries make informed choices among the numerous managed care plans available

- To improve the quality of care provided by managed care plans

- To help the government and other third-party payers make informed purchasing decisions

Table 7.5. Federal legislation relevant to managed care

Year	Legislative Title	Legislative Summary
1973	Federal Health Maintenance Organization Assistance Act of 1973 (HMO Act of 1973)	• Authorized grants and loans to develop HMOs under private sponsorship • Defined a federally qualified HMO (certified to provide healthcare services to Medicare and Medicaid enrollees) as one that has applied for and met federal standards established in the HMO Act of 1973 • Required most employers with more than 25 employees to offer HMO coverage when local plans were available
1974	Employee Retirement Income Security Act of 1974 (ERISA)	• Mandated reporting and disclosure requirements for group life and health plans (including managed care plans) • Permitted large employers to self-insure employee healthcare benefits • Exempted large employers from taxes on health insurance premium
1982	Tax Equity and Fiscal Responsibility Act of 1982 (TEFRA)	• Modified the HMO Act of 1973 • Created Medicare risk programs, which allowed federally qualified HMOs and competitive medical plans that met specified Medicare requirements to provide Medicare-covered services under a risk contract • Defined risk contract as an arrangement among providers to provide capitated (fixed, prepaid basis) healthcare services to Medicare beneficiaries • Defined competitive medical plan (CMP) as an HMO that meets federal eligibility requirements for a Medicare risk contract but is not licensed as a federally qualified plan
1981	Omnibus Budget Reconciliation Act of 1981 (OBRA)	• Provided states with flexibility to establish HMOs for Medicare and Medicaid programs • Resulted in increased enrollment
1985	Preferred Provider Health Care Act of 1985	• Eased restrictions on preferred provider organizations • Allowed subscribers to seek healthcare from providers outside the PPO
1985	Consolidated Omnibus Budget Reconciliation Act of 1985 (COBRA)	• Established an employee's right to continue healthcare coverage beyond scheduled benefit termination date (including HMO coverage)
1988	Amendment to the HMO Act of 1973	• Allowed federally qualified HMOs to permit members to occasionally use non-HMO physicians and be partially reimbursed
1989	Health Plan Employer Data and Information Set (HEDIS)—developed by National Committee for Quality Assurance (NCQA)	• Created standards to assess managed care systems in terms of membership, utilization of services, quality, access, health plan management and activities, and financial indicators
1994	HCFA's Office of Managed Care established	• Facilitated innovation and competition among Medicare HMOs

CMS offers several managed care options to Medicare and Medicaid enrollees. It began collecting HEDIS data from Medicare managed care plans in 1996.

Several kinds of managed care plans are available in the United States, including:

- Health maintenance organizations (HMOs)
- Preferred provider organizations (PPOs)
- **Point-of-service (POS) plans**
- **Exclusive provider organizations** (EPOs)
- **Integrated delivery systems** (IDSs)

Health Maintenance Organizations

An HMO is a prepaid voluntary health plan that provides healthcare services in return for the payment of a monthly membership premium. HMO premiums are based on a projection of the costs that are likely to be involved in treating the plan's average enrollee over a specified period of time. If the actual cost per enrollee were to exceed the projected cost, the HMO would experience a financial loss. If the actual cost per enrollee turned out to be lower than the projection, the HMO would show a profit. Because most HMOs are for-profit organizations, they emphasize cost control and preventive medicine.

Today, most employers and insurance companies offer enrollees some type of HMO option. The benefit to third-party payers and enrollees alike is cost savings. Most HMO enrollees have significantly lower out-of-pocket expenses than enrollees of traditional fee-for-service and other types of managed care plans. The HMO premiums shared by employers and enrollees also are lower than the premiums for other types of healthcare plans.

HMOs can be organized in several different ways, including the **group model HMO,** the **independent practice association** (IPA), the **network model HMO,** and the **staff model HMO.**

Group Model HMOs

In the group model HMO, the HMO enters into a contract with an independent multi-specialty physician group to provide medical services to members of the plan. The providers usually agree to devote a fixed percentage of their practice time to the HMO. Alternatively, the HMO may own or directly manage the physician group, in which case the physicians and their support staff would be considered its employees.

Group model HMOs are closed-panel arrangements. In other words, the physicians are not allowed to treat patients from other managed care plans. Enrollees of group model HMOs are required to seek services from the designated physician group.

Independent Practice Associations

IPAs are sometimes called individual practice associations. In the IPA model, the HMO enters into a contract with an organized group of physicians who join together for purposes of fulfilling the HMO contract but retain their individual practices. The IPA serves as an intermediary during contract negotiations. It also manages the premiums from the HMO and pays individual physicians as appropriate. The physicians are not considered employees of the HMO. They work from their own private offices and continue to see other patients. The HMO usually pays the IPA according to a prenegotiated list of discounted fees. Alternatively, physicians may agree to provide services to HMO members for a set prepaid capitated payment for a specified period of time. Capitation is discussed later in this chapter.

The IPA is an open-panel HMO, which means that the physicians are free to treat patients from other plans. Enrollees of such HMOs are required to seek services from the designated physician group.

Network Model HMOs

Network model HMOs are similar to group model HMOs except that the HMO contracts for services with two or more multispecialty group practices instead of just one practice. Members of network model HMOs receive a list of all the physicians on the approved panel and are required to select providers from the list.

Staff Model HMOs

Staff Model HMOs directly employ physicians and other healthcare professionals to provide medical services to members. Members of the salaried medical staff are considered employees of the HMO rather than independent practitioners. Premiums are paid directly to the HMO, and ambulatory care services are usually provided within the HMO's corporate facilities. The staff model HMO is a closed-panel arrangement.

Preferred Provider Organizations

PPOs represent contractual agreements between healthcare providers and a self-insured employer or a health insurance carrier. Beneficiaries of PPOs select providers such as physicians or hospitals from a list of participating providers who have agreed to furnish healthcare services to the covered population. Beneficiaries may elect to receive services from nonparticipating providers but must pay a greater portion of the cost (in other words, higher deductibles and copays). Providers are usually reimbursed on a discounted fee-for-service basis.

Point-of-Service Plans

POS plans are similar to HMOs in that subscribers must select a **primary care physician** (PCP) from a network of participating physicians. (The PCP is usually a family or general practice physician or an internal medicine specialist.) The PCP acts as a service gatekeeper to control the patient's access to specialty, surgical, and hospital care as well as expensive diagnostic services.

POS plans are different from HMOs in that subscribers are allowed to seek care from providers outside the network. However, the subscribers must pay a greater share of the charges for out-of-network services. POS plans were created to increase the flexibility of managed care plans and to allow patients more choice in providers.

Exclusive Provider Organizations

EPOs are similar to PPOs except that EPOs provide benefits to enrollees only when the enrollees receive healthcare services from **network providers.** In other words, EPO beneficiaries do not receive reimbursement for services furnished by nonparticipating providers. In addition, healthcare services must be coordinated by a PCP. EPOs are regulated by state insurance departments. (In contrast, HMOs are regulated by state departments of commerce or departments of incorporation.)

Integrated Delivery Systems

An IDS is a healthcare provider made up of a number of associated medical facilities that furnish coordinated healthcare services. Most IDSs include a number of facilities that provide services along the continuum of care, for example, ambulatory surgery centers, physicians' office practices, outpatient clinics, acute care hospitals, SNFs, and so on.

Integrated delivery systems can be structured according to several different models, including:

- **Group practices without walls** (GPWWs)
- **Integrated provider organizations** (IPOs)
- **Management service organizations** (MSOs)
- **Medical foundations**
- **Physician–hospital organizations** (PHOs)

Group Practices without Walls

A GPWW is an arrangement that allows physicians to maintain their own offices, but to share administrative, management, and marketing services (for example, medical transcription and billing) for the purpose of fulfilling contracts with managed care organizations.

Integrated Provider Organizations

An IPO manages and coordinates the delivery of healthcare services performed by a number of healthcare professionals and facilities. IPOs typically provide acute care (hospital) services, physicians' services, ambulatory care services, and skilled nursing services. The physicians working in an IPO are salaried employees. IPOs are sometimes referred to as delivery systems, horizontally integrated systems, health delivery networks, accountable health plans, integrated service networks (ISNs), vertically integrated plans (VIPs), and vertically integrated systems.

Management Service Organizations

MSOs provide practice management (administrative and support) services to individual physicians' practices. They are usually owned by a group of physicians or a hospital.

Medical Foundations

Medical foundations are nonprofit organizations that enter into contracts with physicians to manage the physicians' practices. The typical medical foundation owns clinical and business resources and makes them available to the participating physicians. Clinical assets include medical equipment and supplies, and treatment facilities. Business assets include billing and administrative support systems.

Physician-Hospital Organizations

PHOs, previously known as medical staff–hospital organizations, provide healthcare services through a contractual arrangement between physicians and hospital(s). PHO arrangements make it possible for the managed care market to view the hospital(s) and physicians as a single entity for the purpose of establishing a contract for services.

Check Your Understanding 7.5

Instructions: Select the best option for the following statements.

1. ____ This model of HMO is created when physicians join together in an organized group for the purposes of fulfilling a contract but retain individual practices:
   a. Group
   b. Independent practice
   c. Network model
   d. Staff

2. ____ This model of HMO employs physicians and other healthcare professionals to provide healthcare services to members
   a. Group
   b. Independent practice
   c. Network
   d. Staff

3. ____ In this model healthcare services are contracted with two or more multispecialty group practices instead of just one:
   a. Group
   b. Independent practice
   c. Network
   d. Staff

4. ____ In this HMO contract, providers usually agree to devote a fixed percentage of their practice time to the HMO:
   a. Group
   b. Independent practice
   c. Network
   d. Staff

5. ____ Premiums are paid directly to this type of HMO, and services are usually provided within corporate facilities:
   a. Group
   b. Independent practice
   c. Network
   d. Staff

6. ____ This nonprofit organization contracts with physicians to manage their practices and owns clinical/business resources that are made available to participating physicians:
   a. Exclusive provider organization
   b. Group practice without walls
   c. Management service organization
   d. Medical foundation

7. ____ This arrangement provides practice management services to individual physicians' practices:
   a. Exclusive provider organization
   b. Integrated delivery system
   c. Management service organization
   d. Point-of-service plan

8. ____ In this arrangement physicians maintain their offices but share administrative services:
   a. Exclusive provider organization
   b. Group practice without walls
   c. Management service organization
   d. Medical foundation

9. ____ This organization manages and coordinates the delivery of healthcare services performed by a number of healthcare professionals and facilities and its physicians are salaried employees:
   a. Group practice without walls
   b. Integrated delivery system
   c. Integrated provider organization
   d. Management service organization

10. ____ This arrangement makes it possible for the managed care market to view hospitals and physicians as a single entity for the purpose of contracting services:
    a. Management service organization
    b. Medical foundation
    c. Physician-hospital organization
    d. Point-of-service plan

Healthcare Reimbursement Methodologies

As mentioned earlier in this chapter, about 85 percent of Americans are covered by some type of private prepaid health plan or federal healthcare program. Therefore, third-party payers rather than actual recipients of services pay for most healthcare expenses in the United States. The recipients can be considered the "first parties" and the providers the "second parties." Third-party payers include commercial for-profit insurance companies, nonprofit and for-profit Blue Cross and Blue Shield organizations, self-insured employers, federal programs (Medicare, Medicaid, SCHIP, TRICARE, CHAMPVA, and IHS), and workers' compensation programs.

Providers charge their own determined amounts for services rendered. However, providers are rarely reimbursed this full amount because third-party payers may have a unique reimbursement methodology. For example, commercial insurance plans usually reimburse healthcare providers under some type of **retrospective payment system.** The federal Medicare program uses **prospective payment systems** (PPSs). In retrospective payment systems, the exact amount of the payment is determined after the service has been delivered. In a PPS, the exact amount of the payment is determined before the service is delivered.

Fee-for-Service Reimbursement Methodologies

Fee-for-service reimbursement methodologies issue payments to healthcare providers on the basis of the charges assigned to each of the separate services that were performed for the patient. **Chargemasters** are used to list the individual charges for every element entailed in providing a service (for example, surgical supplies, surgical equipment, room and board, nursing care, respiratory therapy, pharmaceuticals, medical equipment, and so on). The total bill for an episode of care represents the sum of all the itemized charges for every element of care provided. Independent clinical professionals such as physicians and psychologists who are not employees of the facility issue separate itemized bills to cover their services after the services are completed or on a monthly basis when the services are ongoing.

Before prepaid insurance plans became common in the 1950s and the Medicare and Medicaid programs were developed in the 1960s, healthcare providers sent itemized bills directly to their patients. Patients were held responsible for paying their own medical bills. When prepaid health plans and the Medicare/Medicaid programs were originally developed, they also based reimbursement on itemized fees.

Traditional Fee-for-Service Reimbursement

In traditional fee-for-service (FFS) reimbursement systems, third-party payers and/or patients issue payments to healthcare providers after healthcare services have been provided (for example, after the patient has been discharged from the hospital). Payments are based on the specific services delivered. The fees charged for services vary considerably by the type of services provided, the resources required, and the type and number of healthcare professionals involved.

For example, the charges for a typical visit to a physician's office might include a fee for the physician's consultation and examination and a charge for blood tests performed by the lab personnel in the physician's office. The physician's overhead expenses (rent, equipment, utilities, payroll, taxes, and so on) are included in his or her fee schedule.

Obviously, the charges for heart transplantation surgery would be much higher. These would include the professional fees of the surgeons, the surgeons' assistants, and the anesthesiologist. In addition, these charges would include hospital charges for surgical supplies and equipment, nursing care, postoperative and rehabilitative services, room and board, drugs and surgical dressings, and much more. As for the physician's charges, the hospital's overhead expenses would be built in to the hospital's fee schedule. In these examples, the total charges for the trip to the physician's office might be less than $125, but the total charges for the heart surgery might well exceed $150,000, depending on the geographic location of the facilities that provided the services.

Payments can be calculated on the basis of actual billed charges, discounted charges, prenegotiated rate schedules, or **usual, customary, and reasonable charges (UCR).** Usual, customary, and reasonable charges are based on the amount considered to represent reasonable compensation for the service or procedure in a specific area of the country. For example, the charge for particular service may be higher in a large city than in a rural town.

Typically, in the traditional fee-for-service payment methodology, the third-party payer reimburses providers according to charges that are calculated after the healthcare services have been rendered (for example, after the patient has been discharged from the hospital). First, an employee of the healthcare facility analyzes the patient's health record and assigns appropriate diagnostic and procedural codes to represent the facts as documented in the health record. (In hospitals, HIM personnel assign these codes. In other settings, nurses, physicians, trained administrative staff, and/or HIM professionals may perform coding. Facilities also may enter into contracts with coding vendors.)

After the codes have been assigned, the billing department takes over the process. It follows these general steps:

1. The provider's billing department itemizes the services provided to the patient as represented by the procedural codes assigned to the case.

2. It then assigns a fee to each service from the provider's standard fee schedule or chargemaster.

3. It applies the charges to the patient's account.

4. It transmits the detailed claim to the patient's third-party payer and sends an itemized account of the billed services to the patient.

Some third-party payers pay only the maximum allowable charges as determined by the plan. Maximum allowable charges may be significantly lower than the provider's billed charges. Some payers issue payments on the basis of usual, customary and reasonable charges. Commercial insurance and Blue Cross/Blue Shield plans often issue payments based on prenegotiated discount rates and contractual cost-sharing arrangements with the patient.

For many plans, the health plan and the patient share costs on an 80:20 percent arrangement. The portion of the claim covered by the patient's insurance plan would be 80 percent of allowable charges. After the third-party payer transmits its payment to the provider, the provider's billing department issues a final statement to the patient. The statement shows the amount for which the patient is responsible (in this example, 20 percent of allowable charges).

The traditional FFS reimbursement methodology is still used by many commercial insurance companies for visits to physicians' offices.

Managed Fee-for-Service Reimbursement

Managed FFS reimbursement is similar to traditional FFS reimbursement except that managed care plans control costs primarily by managing their members' use of healthcare services. Most managed care plans also negotiate with providers to develop discounted **fee schedules.** Managed FFS reimbursement is common for inpatient hospital care. In some areas of the country, however, it also is applied to outpatient and ambulatory services, surgical procedures, high-cost diagnostic procedures, and physicians' services.

Utilization controls include the prospective and retrospective review of the healthcare services planned for, or provided to, patients. For example, a prospective utilization review of a plan to hospitalize a patient for minor surgery might determine that the surgery could be safely performed less expensively in an outpatient setting. Prospective utilization review is sometimes called precertification.

In a retrospective utilization review, the plan might determine that part or all of the services provided to a patient were not medically necessary or were not covered by the plan. In such cases, the plan would disallow part or all of the provider's charges and the patient would be responsible for paying the provider's outstanding charges.

Discharge planning also can be considered a type of utilization control. The managed care plan may be able to move the patient to a less intensive, and therefore less expensive, care setting as soon as possible by coordinating his or her discharge from inpatient care.

Episode-of-Care Reimbursement Methodologies

Plans that use **episode-of-care (EOC) reimbursement** methods issue lump-sum payments to providers to compensate them for all the healthcare services delivered to a patient for a specific illness and/or over a specific period of time. EOC payments also are called

bundled payments. Bundled payments cover multiple services and also may involve multiple providers of care. EOC reimbursement methods include capitated payments, global payments, global surgery payments, Medicare ambulatory surgery center rates, and Medicare PPSs.

Capitation

Capitation is based on per-person premiums or membership fees rather than on itemized per-procedure or per-service charges. The capitated managed care plan negotiates a contract with an employer or government agency representing a specific group of individuals. According to the contract, the managed care organization agrees to provide all the contracted healthcare services that the covered individuals need over a specified period of time (usually one year). In exchange, the individual enrollee and/or third-party payer agrees to pay a fixed premium for the covered group. Like other insurance plans, a capitated insurance contract stipulates as part of the contract exactly which healthcare services are covered and which ones are not.

Capitated premiums are calculated on the projected cost of providing covered services **per patient per month** or **per member per month** (PPPM or PMPM). The capitated premium for an individual member of a plan includes all the services covered by the plan, regardless of the number of services actually provided during the period or their cost. If the average member of the plan actually used more services than originally assumed in the PPPM calculation, the plan would show a loss for the period. If the average member actually used fewer services, the plan would show a profit.

The purchasers of capitated coverage (usually the member's employer) pay monthly premiums to the managed care plan. The individual enrollees usually pay part of the premium as well. The plan then compensates the providers who actually furnished the services. In some arrangements, the managed care plan accepts all the risk involved in the contract. In others, some of the risk is passed on to the PCPs who agreed to act as gatekeepers for the plan.

The capitated managed care organization may own or operate some or all of the healthcare facilities that provide care to members and directly employ clinical professionals. Staff model HMOs operate in this way. Alternatively, the capitated managed care organization may purchase services from independent physicians and facilities, as do group model HMOs. For example:

> The ABC HMO awarded a capitated contract to the XYZ Medical Center for a total compensation of $3,600,000 in the year 2004. According to the terms of the contract, the medical center agreed to provide comprehensive healthcare services to all 500 enrollees covered under the contract for twelve months. The medical center received lump-sum payments of $300,000 per month over the twelve-month period. A large, multispecialty PHO owned by the hospital acted as primary care gatekeepers and provided medical services to the enrollees. Inpatient and outpatient services were provided directly by the medical center.

Global Payment

Global payment methodology is sometimes applied to radiological and similar types of procedures that involve professional and technical components. Global payments are lump-sum payments distributed among the physicians who performed the procedure or interpreted its results and the healthcare facility that provided the equipment, supplies, and technical support required. The procedure's **professional component** is supplied by physicians (for example, radiologists), and its **technical component** (for example, radiological supplies, equipment, and support services) is supplied by a hospital or freestanding diagnostic or surgical center. For example:

> Larry Timber underwent a scheduled carotid angiogram as a hospital outpatient. He had complained of ringing in his ears and dizziness, and his physician scheduled the procedure to determine whether there was a blockage in one of Larry's carotid arteries. The procedure required a surgeon to inject radiopaque contrast material through a catheter into Larry's left carotid artery. A radiological technician then took an x-ray of Larry's neck. The technician was supervised by a radiologist, and both were employees of the hospital.

Professional component: Injection of radiopaque contrast material by the surgeon

Technical component: x-ray of the neck region

Global payment: The facility received a lump-sum payment for the procedure and paid for the services of the surgeon from that payment.

Global Surgery Payments

A single **global surgery payment** covers all the healthcare services entailed in planning and completing a specific surgical procedure. In other words, every element of the procedure from the treatment decision through normal postoperative patient care is covered by a single bundled payment. For example:

> Tammy Murdock received all the prenatal, perinatal, and postnatal care involved in the birth of her daughter from Dr. Thomas Michaels. She received one bill from the physician for a total of $2,200. The bill represented the total charges for the obstetrical services associated with her pregnancy. However, the two-day inpatient hospital stay for the normal delivery was not included in the global payment nor were the laboratory services she received during her hospital stay. Tammy received a separate bill for these services. In addition, if she had suffered a postdelivery complication (for example, a wound infection) or an unrelated medical problem, the physician and hospital services required to treat the complications would not have been covered by the global surgical payment.

Medicare Ambulatory Surgery

CMS defines an **ambulatory surgery center** (ASC) as a state-licensed, Medicare-certified supplier (not a provider) of surgical healthcare services. ASCs must **accept assignment** on Medicare claims, which means the supplier accepts as payment in full whatever Medicare reimburses. Because payments are subject to Medicare Part B deductible and coinsurance requirements, reimbursement is 80 percent of the prospectively determined rate (adjusted for regional wage variations). CMS replaced the ASC rates (which categorized approximately 2,500 surgical procedures into what were then eight payment groups) with the **ambulatory payment classification (APC) system** and the **outpatient prospective payment system** (OPPS) in 2000 for hospital-based outpatient services and procedures.

To qualify as a Medicare-certified ASC, the surgery center must be a separate entity distinguishable from any other entity or type of facility. This means that the ASC must be separate from any other organization with respect to licensure, accreditation, governance, professional supervision, administrative functions, clinical services, record keeping, financial and accounting systems, and national identifier or supplier number. The ASC can be physically located within the space of another entity and still be considered separate for Medicare payment purposes when the preceding criteria are met.

Medicare pays a prospectively determined fee for ASC services that are included on the approved list. Should the ASC perform a procedure that is not on the approved list, no reimbursement will be provided. The services that fall within the scope of ASC services include, but are not limited to, services performed by nurses and technicians, supplies, drugs and biologicals, surgical dressings, housekeeping services, and use of the facility.

The professional services of physicians and other practitioners do not fall within the scope of ASC facility services. Therefore, the ASC facility fee does not include payment for the professional services of physicians and other practitioners. ASCs should not bill for the following physicians' services: anesthesiology, surgery, or assistance at surgery services. The anesthesiologist, surgeon, and assistant surgeon submit separate claims.

CMS's ASC rates are now categorized into nine separate payment groups. (See table 7.6.) The payment groups are based on the complexity of the surgical procedures involved. CMS also updates and publishes the rate-setting methodology and establishes wage index (WI) tables for use in urban and rural areas.

Special rules apply when more than one surgical procedure is performed during the same operative session. The ASC is reimbursed at 100 percent for the procedure classified in the highest payment group, and any other procedure performed during the same session is reimbursed at 50 percent of the procedure's applicable group rate. Bilateral procedures are reimbursed at 150 percent of the applicable rate. The reimbursement of physicians for ASC-approved procedures is subject to 20 percent coinsurance and deductible provisions. Payment is made at 80 percent of the Medicare physician fee schedule, which is discussed in more detail later in this chapter. Fees for approved procedures in an ASC setting are noted on the fee schedule as a facility fee.

Table 7.6. ASC payment groups and rates, 2005

ASC Group	Reimbursement Rate
Group 1 Procedure	$333
Group 2 Procedure	$446
Group 3 Procedure	$510
Group 4 Procedure	$630
Group 5 Procedure	$717
Group 6 Procedure	$826 ($676 + $150 for intraocular lenses)
Group 7 Procedure	$995
Group 8 Procedure	$973 ($823 + $150 for intraocular lenses)
Group 9 Procedure	$1,339

Source: CMS 2005b.

Prospective Payment

In 1983, CMS implemented a PPS for inpatient hospital care provided to Medicare beneficiaries. This PPS methodology is called **diagnosis-related groups** (DRGs). The DRG system was implemented as a way to control Medicare spending. It reimburses hospitals a predetermined amount for each Medicare inpatient stay. Payments are determined by the DRG to which each case is assigned according to the patient's **principal diagnosis,** which is defined as the condition which, after study, is determined to have occasioned the admission of the patient to the hospital for care.

After DRG implementation in 1983, expenditures for Medicare post-acute care benefits quickly escalated. According to the HHS, post-acute expenditures totaled approximately $2.5 billion in 1986, but more than $30 billion in 1996. This dramatic shift in spending alarmed Medicare policy makers. In response, the BBA mandated PPS implementation for non–acute care services, including care in SNFs, outpatient services and procedures, home health care, and rehabilitation care. In addition, the act included a legislative proposal on a PPS for long-term care.

Check Your Understanding 7.6

Instructions: Select the correct term for each of the following statements.

1. ____ The type of payment system where the amount of payment is determined before the service is delivered:
   a. Fee-for-service
   b. Per diem
   c. Prospective
   d. Retrospective

2. ____ These payment arrangements are streamlined by the use of chargemasters:
   a. Fee-for-service
   b. Per diem
   c. Prospective
   d. Retrospective

3. ____ This payment is based on the amount representing reasonable compensation for the service/procedure in a specific area of the country:
   a. CFR
   b. ERA
   c. IRF
   d. UCR

4. ____ The most typical cost share ratio between insurance plans and patients is:
   a. 50:50
   b. 75:25
   c. 80:20
   d. 100:0

5. ____ The utilization control most closely associated with managed fee-for-service reimbursement:
   a. Chargemaster
   b. EOC payments
   c. Global surgery
   d. Prospective review

6. ____ Lump-sum payments to providers to compensate them for all healthcare services delivered to a patient for a specific illness and/or over a specific period of time:
   a. APC
   b. EOC
   c. MCO
   d. PPPM

7. ____ Based on per-person premiums or membership fees:
   a. Capitation
   b. Fee-for-service
   c. Managed fee-for-service
   d. UCR

8. ____ Prospective payment system implemented in 1983:
   a. APC
   b. DRG
   c. OPPS
   d. URC

9. ____ Payment system for hospital-based outpatient services and procedures:
   a. APC
   b. DRG
   c. OPPS
   d. URC

10. ____ Ambulatory surgical center rates are calculated on a:
    a. Capitation basis
    b. Fee-for-service basis
    c. Prospective basis
    d. Retrospective basis

Medicare Prospective Payment Systems

As discussed briefly in the preceding section, Congress enacted the first Medicare PPS in 1983 as a cost-control measure. Implementation of the **acute care prospective payment system** resulted in a shift of clinical services and expenditures away from the inpatient hospital setting to outpatient settings. As a result, spending on non–acute care exploded.

Congress responded by passing the **Omnibus Budget Reconciliation Act** (OBRA) of 1986, which mandated that HCFA develop a prospective system for hospital-based outpatient services provided to Medicare beneficiaries. In subsequent years, Congress mandated the development of PPSs for other healthcare providers.

Medicare Acute Care Prospective Payment System

As mentioned previously, prior to 1983, Medicare Part A payments to hospitals were determined on a traditional FFS reimbursement methodology. Payment was based on the cost of services provided, and reasonable cost and/or per-diem costs were used to determine payment.

Diagnosis-Related Groups

During the late 1960s, just a few years after the Medicare and Medicaid health programs were implemented, Congress authorized a group at Yale University to develop a system for monitoring quality of care and utilization of services. This system was known as diagnosis-related groups (DRGs). DRGs were implemented on an experimental basis by the New Jersey Department of Health in the late 1970s as a way to predetermine reimbursement for hospital inpatient stays.

At the conclusion of the New Jersey DRG experiment, Congress passed the **Tax Equity and Fiscal Responsibility Act of 1982** (TEFRA). TEFRA modified Medicare's retrospective reimbursement system for inpatient hospital stays by requiring implementation of the DRG PPS in 1983. Medicare now pays most hospitals for inpatient hospital services according to a predetermined rate for each discharge under DRGs.

At this time, several types of hospitals are excluded from Medicare acute care PPS. The following facilities are still paid on the basis of reasonable cost, subject to payment limits per discharge or under a separate PPS:

- Psychiatric and rehabilitation hospitals and psychiatric and rehabilitation units within larger medical facilities

- **Long-term care hospitals,** which are defined as hospitals with an average length of stay of twenty-five days or more

- Children's hospitals

- Cancer hospitals

- Critical access hospitals

To determine the appropriate DRG, a claim for a healthcare encounter is first classified into one of twenty-five **major diagnostic categories,** or MDCs. Most MDCs are based on body systems and include diseases and disorders relating to a particular system. However, some MDCs include disorders and diseases involving multiple organ systems (for example, burns). The number of DRGs within a particular MDC varies.

The principal diagnosis determines the MDC assignment. The principal diagnosis is the condition established after study to have resulted in the inpatient admission. Within each MDC, decision trees are used to determine the correct DRG. (See figure 7.1.) Within most MDCs, cases are divided into surgical DRGs (based on a surgical hierarchy that orders individual procedures or groups of procedures by resource intensity) and medical DRGs. Medical DRGs generally are differentiated on the basis of diagnosis and age. Some surgical and medical DRGs are further differentiated on the basis of the presence or absence of **complications** or **comorbidities.** Complications are conditions that arise during the hospitalization, for example a postoperative wound infection. Comorbidities are coexisting conditions, for example, hypertension.

Under the **acute care prospective payment system,** a predetermined rate based on the DRG (only one is assigned per case) assigned to each case is used to reimburse hospitals for inpatient care provided to Medicare beneficiaries. Hospitals determine DRGs by assigning **ICD-9-CM** codes to each patient's principal diagnosis, comorbidities, complications, **principal procedure,** and/or secondary procedures. These code numbers with other information on the patient (age, gender, and discharge status) are entered into a **DRG grouper.** A DRG grouper is a computer software program that assigns appropriate DRGs according to the information provided for each episode of care.

Reimbursement for each episode of care is based on the DRG assigned. Different diagnoses require different levels of care and expenditures of resources. Therefore,

Figure 7.1.   Portion of MDC6, Diseases and Disorders of the Digestive System

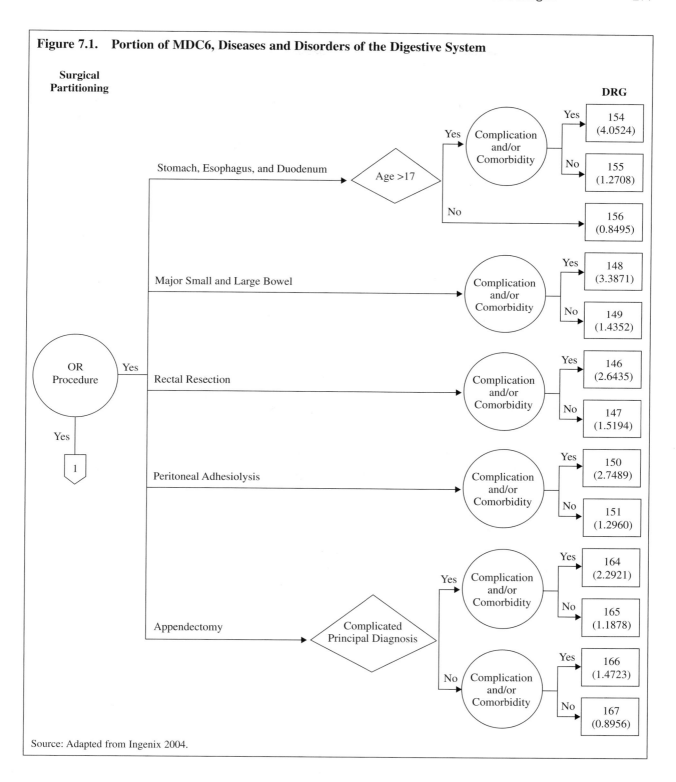

Source: Adapted from Ingenix 2004.

each DRG is assigned a different level of payment that reflects the average amount of resources required to treat a patient assigned to that DRG. Only one DRG is assigned per discharge/episode of care. Each DRG is associated with a description, a relative weight, a geometric mean length of stay (LOS), and an arithmetic mean LOS. The relative weight represents the average resources required to care for cases in that particular DRG relative to the national average of resources used to treat all Medicare patients. A DRG with a relative weight of 2.000, on average, requires twice as many resources as a DRG with a relative weight of 1.000. The geometric mean LOS is defined as the total days of service, excluding any outliers or transfers, divided by the total number of patients; the arithmetic mean LOS is defined as the total days of service divided by the total number of patients.

For example, DRG 1, organized within MDC 01, is described as SURG CRANIOTOMY AGE >17 WCC and has a relative weight of 3.3344, a geometric mean LOS of 7.5 and an arithmetic mean LOS of 10.0.

CMS adjusts the Medicare DRG list and reimbursement rates every fiscal year (October 1 through September 30). For fiscal year 2004–2005, the list includes 543 DRGs (approximately twenty of which are invalid).

In some cases, the DRG payment received by the hospital may be lower than the actual cost of providing Medicare Part A inpatient services. In such cases, the hospital must absorb the loss. In other cases, the hospital may receive a payment for more than its actual cost and, therefore, makes a profit. It is expected that, on average, hospitals will be reimbursed for their total costs in providing services to Medicare patients.

Special circumstances also can apply to inpatient cases and result in an outlier payment to the hospital. An outlier case results in exceptionally high costs when compared with other cases in the same DRG. For fiscal year (FY) 2005, to qualify for a **cost outlier,** a hospital's charges for a case (adjusted to cost) must exceed the payment rate for the DRG by $25,800. The additional payment amount is equal to 80 percent of the difference between the hospital's entire cost for the stay and the threshold amount.

Case-Mix Group Relative Weights

The DRG system creates a hospital's **case-mix index** (types or categories of patients treated by the hospital) based on the relative weights of the DRG. The case-mix index can be figured by multiplying the relative weight of each DRG by the number of discharges within that DRG. This provides the total weight for each DRG. The sum of all total weights divided by the sum of total patient discharges equals the case-mix index. A hospital may relate its case-mix index to the costs incurred for inpatient care. This information allows the hospital to make administrative decisions about services to be offered to its patient population. For example:

> The hospital's case-mix report indicated that a small population of patients was receiving obstetrical services, but that the costs associated with providing such services was disproportionately high. This report along with other data might result in the hospital's administrative decision to discontinue its obstetrical services department.

All Patient DRG

An **all patient DRG** (AP-DRG) system was developed in 1988 by 3M Health Information Systems as the basis for New York's hospital reimbursement program for non-Medicare discharges. AP-DRGs are still used in a number of states as a basis for payment of non-Medicare claims. AP-DRGs use the patient's age, sex, discharge status, and ICD-9-CM diagnoses and procedure codes to determine a DRG that, in turn, determines reimbursement.

3M also has developed **all patient refined DRGs** (APR-DRGs) as an extension of the DRG concept. APR-DRGs adjust patient data for severity of illness and risk of mortality, help to develop clinical pathways, are used as a basis for quality assurance programs, and are used in comparative profiling and setting capitation rates (3M HIS 2002).

Resource-Based Relative Value Scale (RBRVS) System

In 1992, CMS implemented the **resource-based relative value scale** (RBRVS) system for physician's services such as office visits covered under Medicare Part B. The system reimburses physicians according to a fee schedule based on predetermined values assigned to specific services.

Medicare Fee Schedule

The **Medicare fee schedule** (MFS) is the listing of allowed charges that are reimbursable to physicians under Medicare. Each year's MFS is published by CMS in the *Federal Register.*

Relative Value Units

To calculate fee schedule amounts, Medicare uses a formula that incorporates the following factors:

- **Relative value units** for physician work (RVUw)
- Practice expenses (RVUpe)
- Malpractice costs (RVUm)

Sample 2005 RVUs for selected HCPCS codes are shown in table 7.7.

Geographic Practice Cost Indices

Payment localities are adjusted according to three **geographic practice cost indices** (GPCIs):

- Physician work (GPCIw)
- Practice expenses (GPCIpe)
- Malpractice costs (GPCIm)

Table 7.7.   Sample 2005 RVUs for selected HCPCS codes

HCPCS Code	Description	Work RVU	Practice Expense RVU	Malpractice Expense RVU
99203	Office visit	1.34	.48	.09
99204	Office visit	2.00	.71	.12
10080	I&D of pilonidal cyst, simple	1.17	1.11	.11
45380	Colonoscopy with biopsy	4.43	1.73	.35
52601	TURP, complete	12.35	5.1	.87

Sample GPCIs for selected U.S. cities are shown in table 7.8.

A geographic cost index is a number used to multiply each RVU so that it better reflects a geographical area's relative costs. For example, costs of office rental prices, local taxes, average salaries, and malpractice costs are all affected by geography.

National Conversion Factor

A **national conversion factor** (CF) converts the RVUs into payments. In 2005, the CF was $37.8975.

The RBRVS fee schedule uses the following formula:

$$[(RVUw \times GPCIw) + (RVUpe \times GPCIpe) + (RVUm \times GPCIm)] \times CF = Payment$$

As an example, payment for performing a drainage of a skin abscess in Birmingham, Alabama, in 2005, can be calculated. RVU values include:

- Work RVU (RVUw) = 1.17
- Practice expense RVU (RVUpe) = 0.93
- Malpractice RVU (RVUm) = 0.12

GPCI values include:

- Work GPCI (GPCIw) = 1.00
- Practice expense GPCI (GPCIpe) = 0.858
- Malpractice GPCI (GPCIm) = 0.752
- National CF = $37.8975

The calculation is as follows:

$$(1.17 \times 1.00) + (0.93 \times 0.858) + (0.12 \times 0.752) \times \$37.8975$$

$$1.17 + 0.80 + 0.09 \times \$37.8975$$

$$2.06 \times \$37.8975$$

Fee schedule payment = $78.00

Table 7.8.   Sample GPCIs for selected U.S. cities

City	Work GPCI	Practice Expense GPCI	Malpractice Expense GPCI
St. Louis	1.000	.946	.941
Dallas	1.010	1.063	1.061
Seattle	1.010	1.115	.819
Philadelphia	1.020	1.098	1.386

Medicare Skilled Nursing Facility Prospective Payment System

The BBA mandated implementation of a **skilled nursing facility prospective payment system** (SNF PPS). The system was to cover all costs (routine, ancillary, and capital) associated with covered SNF services furnished to Medicare Part A beneficiaries. Certain educational activities were exempt from the new system.

The SNF PPS was implemented on July 1, 1998. Under the PPS, SNFs are no longer paid under a system based on reasonable costs. Instead, they are paid according to a per-diem PPS based on case mix–adjusted payment rates.

Medicare Part A covers posthospital SNF services and all items and services paid under Medicare Part B before July 1, 1998 (other than physician and certain other services specifically excluded under the BBA). Major elements of the SNF PPS include rates, coverage, transition, and consolidated billing. OBRA required CMS to develop an assessment instrument to standardize the collection of SNF patient data. That instrument is known as the **Resident Assessment Instrument** (RAI) and includes the **Minimum Data Set 2.0** (MDS). A draft of MDS 3.0 is under review.

The MDS is the minimum core of defined and categorized patient assessment questions that serves as the basis for documentation and reimbursement in a SNF. The MDS form contains a face sheet for documentation of resident identification information, demographic information, and the patient's customary routine.

Resource Utilization Groups

SNF reimbursement rates are paid according to **Resource Utilization Groups, Version III** (RUG-III) (a resident classification system) based on the MDS resident assessments.

The RUG-III classification system uses resident assessment data from the MDS collected by SNFs to assign residents to one of forty-four groups. SNFs complete MDS assessments according to a schedule specifically designed for Medicare payment (that is, on the fifth, fourteenth, thirtieth, sixtieth, and ninetieth days after admission to the SNF). For Medicare billing purposes, specific codes are associated with each of the forty-four RUG-III groups, and each assessment applies to specific days within a resident's SNF stay. SNFs that fail to perform timely assessments are paid a default payment for the days they are not in compliance with this schedule.

Resident Assessment Validation and Entry

HCFA (now called CMS) developed a computerized data-entry system for long-term care facilities that offers users the ability to collect MDS assessments in a database and transmit them in CMS-standard format to their state database. The data-entry software is entitled **Resident Assessment Validation and Entry** (RAVEN). RAVEN imports and exports data in standard MDS record format; maintains facility, resident, and employee information; enforces data integrity via rigorous edit checks; and provides comprehensive online help. It includes a data dictionary and a RUG calculator.

Consolidated Billing Provision

The BBA includes a billing provision that requires an SNF to submit consolidated Medicare bills for its residents for services covered under either Part A or Part B except for a limited number of specifically excluded services. For example, when a physician provides a diagnostic radiology service to an SNF patient, the SNF must bill for the technical component of the radiology service because this is included in the SNF consolidated billing payment. The rendering physician must develop a business relationship with the SNF in order to receive payment from the SNF for the services he or she rendered. The professional component of the physician services is excluded from SNF consolidated billing and must be billed separately to the **Medicare carrier.**

There are, of course, other exclusions to this provision, including physician assistant services, nurse practitioner services, and clinical nurse specialists when these individuals are working under the supervision of, or in collaboration with, a physician, certified midwife services, qualified psychologist services, and certified registered nurse anesthetist services. Other exclusions include hospice care, maintenance dialysis, selected services furnished on an outpatient basis such as cardiac catheterization services, CAT scans and MRIs, radiation therapy, and ambulance services. In addition, SNFs report **Healthcare Common Procedure Coding System** (HCPCS) codes on all Part B bills.

Medicare/Medicaid Outpatient Prospective Payment System

The BBA authorized implementation of a Medicare PPS for outpatient services. The OPPS, implemented in October 2001, applies to the following services:

- Services provided by hospital outpatient departments, including **partial hospitalization** services
- Certain Part B services provided to hospital inpatients who have no Part A coverage
- Partial hospitalization services provided by community mental health centers (CMHCs)
- Vaccines, splints, casts, and antigens provided by HHAs that provide medical and health-related services
- Vaccines provided by comprehensive outpatient rehabilitation facilities (CORFs)
- Splints, casts, and antigens provided to hospice patients for the treatment of non-terminal illnesses

The OPPS does not apply to critical access hospitals (CAHs) or hospitals in Maryland that are excluded because they qualify under the Social Security Act for payment under the state's payment system. In addition, IHS hospitals and hospitals located outside the fifty states, the District of Columbia, and Puerto Rico are excluded.

Implementation of the OPPS resulted in the discontinuation of the blended payment method for radiology and other diagnostic services and for ASC services provided in hospital-based outpatient departments. In addition, the following provisions are associated with the OPPS:

- Payments are established in a budget-neutral manner.
- OPPS payment weights, rates, payment adjustments and groups, and annual consultation are reviewed and updated annually by an expert provider advisory panel.
- Budget-neutral outlier adjustments are based on charges, adjusted to costs, for all OPPS services included on outpatient bills submitted before January 1, 2002, and, thereafter, based on individual services billed.

- Provisions for transitional pass-throughs are related to additional costs of new and current medical devices, drugs, and biologicals.

- Provisions are in place for OPPS payment for implantable devices, including DME, prosthetics, and implantable devices used in diagnostic testing.

The OPPS is not applicable to clinical diagnostic laboratory services, orthotics, prosthetics, and take-home surgical dressings. These services are paid on the basis of individual fee schedules. Chronic dialysis is reimbursed under the composite rate, but acute dialysis (for example, for treatment of poisonings) is paid under the OPPS. Reimbursement for screening mammographies is based on the Medicare physician fee schedule. Outpatient rehabilitation services (physical, speech-language-pathology, and occupational therapy) are reimbursed under the Medicare physician fee schedule.

Ambulatory Payment Classification Groups (APCs)

The calculation of payment for services under the OPPS is based on the categorization of outpatient services into APC groups according to **CPT**/HCPCS codes. ICD-9-CM coding is not utilized in the selection of APCs. The more than 700 APCs are categorized into significant procedure APCs, radiology and other diagnostic APCs, medical visit APCs, and a partial hospitalization APC. Services within an APC are similar, both clinically and with regard to resource consumption, and each APC is assigned a fixed payment rate for the facility fee or technical component of the outpatient visit. Payment rates then are adjusted according to the hospital's wage index. Multiple APCs may be appropriate for a single episode of care as the patient may receive various types of services such as radiology or surgical procedures.

Payment Status Indicators

Medicare has assigned **payment status indicators** (PSIs) (table 7.9) to HCPCS/CPT codes to indicate whether a service/procedure is to be reimbursed under the OPPS.

OPPS payments will be made for clinical diagnostic laboratory tests and radiology and other diagnostic services in addition to the payment for a surgical procedure or medical visit performed on the same day. However, the OPPS also incorporates the **packaging** of certain items, such as anesthesia, supplies, certain drugs, and the use of recovery and observation rooms.

Discounting applies to multiple surgical procedures furnished during the same operative session. For discounted procedures, the full APC rate is paid for the surgical procedure with the highest APC reimbursement rate and other surgical procedures performed at the same time are reimbursed at 50 percent of the APC rate. Similar discounting occurs under the physician fee schedule and the payment system for ASCs.

Surgical procedures terminated after a patient is prepared for surgery, but before induction of anesthesia, are paid for at 50 percent of the APC rate. In addition, when multiple surgical procedures are performed during the same operative session, the beneficiary's coinsurance is discounted in proportion to the APC payment.

Note: Medicare does not reimburse for services that are identified as "inpatient only" when they are provided on an outpatient basis, except in cases where the procedure is performed on an emergency basis on a patient who expires before being registered to inpatient status.

Table 7.9.	OPPS payment status indicators and description of payment under OPPS
Status Indicator	**Description of Payment under OPPS**
SI A	Services paid under some other method (such as a fee schedule): • Ambulance services • Clinical diagnostic laboratory services • Nonimplantable prosthetic and orthotic devices • EPO for ESRD patients • Physical, occupation, and speech therapy • Routine dialysis services for ESRD patients provided in a certified dialysis unit of a hospital • Diagnostic mammography • Screening mammography
SI B	Codes that are not recognized by OPPS when submitted on an outpatient hospital Part B bill type
SI C	Inpatient procedures
SI D	Discontinued codes
SI E	Items, codes, and services not covered by Medicare
SI F	Corneal tissue acquisition; certain CRNA services
SI G	Pass-through drugs, biologicals, and radiopharmaceutical agents
SI H	Pass-through device categories; brachytherapy sources
SI K	Non-pass-through drugs, biologicals, and radiopharmaceutical agents
SI L	Influenza vaccine; Pneumococcal pneumonia vaccine
SI N	Items and services packaged into APC rates
SI P	Partial hospitalization
SI S	Significant procedure, not discounted when multiple
SI T	Significant procedure, multiple reduction applies
SI V	Clinic or emergency department visit
SI Y	Nonimplantable durable medical equipment
SI X	Ancillary services

Home Health Prospective Payment System

The BBA called for the development and implementation of a **home health prospective payment system** (HH PPS) for reimbursement of services provided to Medicare beneficiaries. The PPS for HHAs was implemented on October 1, 2000.

OASIS and Home Assessment Validation and Entry

HHAs use the OASIS data set and the Home Assessment Validation and Entry (HAVEN) data-entry software to conduct all patient assessments, not just the assessments for Medicare beneficiaries. OASIS stands for **Outcome and Assessment Information Set.** It consists of data elements that (1) represent core items for the comprehensive assessment of an adult home care patient and (2) form the basis for measuring patient outcomes for the purpose of outcome-based quality improvement (OBQI). OASIS is a key component of Medicare's partnership with the home care industry to foster and monitor improved home health care outcomes. The Conditions of Participation for HHAs require that HHAs electronically report all OASIS data.

CMS also developed the OASIS data-entry system called HAVEN **(Home Assessment Validation and Entry).** HAVEN is available to HHAs at no charge through CMS's Web site or on CD-ROM. HAVEN offers users the ability to collect OASIS data in a database and transmit them in a standard format to state databases. The data-entry software imports and exports data in standard OASIS record format; maintains agency, patient, and employee information; maintains data integrity through rigorous edit checks; and provides comprehensive on-line help.

Home Health Resource Groups

Home health resource groups (HHRGs) represent the classification system established for the prospective reimbursement of covered home care services to Medicare beneficiaries during a sixty-day episode of care. Covered services include skilled nursing visits, home health aide visits, therapy services (for example, physical, occupational, and speech therapy), medical social services, and nonroutine medical supplies. DME is excluded from the episode-of-care payment and is reimbursed under the DME fee schedule.

The classification of a patient into one of eighty HHRGs is based on OASIS data, which establish the severity of clinical and functional needs and services utilized. Grouper software is used to establish the appropriate HHRG. The HHRG is a six-character alphanumeric code that represents severity levels in three domains: clinical, functional, and service utilization. (See table 7.10.) For example:

> OASIS data collected on a seventy-six-year-old male home care patient resulted in an HHRG of C3F4S3. This HHRG is interpreted as a clinical domain of high severity, a functional domain of high severity, and a service utilization domain of high utilization.

EOC reimbursements vary from $1,000 to almost $6,000 and are affected by treatment level and regional wage differentials. The initial episode is reimbursed under a 60:40 split, with 60 percent paid at the start of treatment and the remainder paid at the end of the episode. Additional episodes are paid under a 50:50 split. There is no limit to the number of sixty-day episodes of care that a patient may receive as long as Medicare coverage criteria are met.

Table 7.10.	HHRG severity levels in three domains: Clinical, functional, and service utilization		

Domain	Score	Points	Severity Level
Clinical	C0	0–7	Minimal severity
	C1	8–19	Low severity
	C2	20–40	Moderate severity
	C3	41+	High severity
Functional	F0	0–2	Minimal severity
	F1	3–15	Low severity
	F2	16–23	Moderate severity
	F3	24–29	High severity
	F4	30+	Maximum severity
Service utilization	S0	0–2	Minimum utilization
	S1	3	Low utilization
	S2	4–6	Moderate utilization
	S3	7	High utilization

Low Utilization and Outlier Payments

When a patient receives fewer than four home care visits during a sixty-day episode, an alternate (reduced) payment, or **low-utilization payment adjustment** (LUPA), is made instead of the full HHRG reimbursement rate. HHAs are eligible for a **cost outlier adjustment,** which is a payment for certain high-cost home care patients whose costs are in excess of a threshold amount for each HHRG. The threshold is the sixty-day episode payment plus a fixed-dollar loss that is constant across the HHRGs.

Ambulance Fee Schedule

A new Medicare payment system for medically necessary transports effective for services provided on or after April 1, 2002, was included as part of the BBA. The final rule established a five-year transition period during which time payment will be based on a blended amount, based in part on the ambulance fee schedule and in part on reasonable cost or reasonable charge. By year five (CY 2006), the fee schedule will be fully implemented with 100 percent of payment based on the schedule. The new payment system applies to all ambulance services, including volunteer, municipal, private, independent, and institutional providers (hospitals, critical access hospitals, SNFs, and HHAs).

Ambulance services are reported on claims using HCPCS codes that reflect the seven categories of ground service and two categories of air service. Mandatory assignment is required for all ambulance service providers.

The seven categories of ground (land and water) ambulance services include:

- Basic life support
- Basic life support—emergency
- Advanced life support, level 1
- Advanced life support, level 1—emergency
- Advanced life support, level 2

- Specialty care transport
- Paramedic intercept

The air service categories include fixed-wing air ambulance (airplane) and rotary-wing air ambulance (helicopter).

Inpatient Rehabilitation Facility (IRF) Prospective Payment System

The BBA (as amended by the **Balanced Budget Refinement Act of 1999**) authorized implementation of a per-discharge PPS for care provided to Medicare beneficiaries by inpatient rehabilitation hospitals and rehabilitation units, referred to as **inpatient rehabilitation facilities** (IRFs). The PPS for IRFs became effective on January 1, 2002.

IRFs must meet the regulatory requirements to be classified as a rehabilitation hospital or rehabilitation unit that is excluded from the PPS for inpatient acute care services.

During a most recent, consecutive, and appropriate twelve-month time period, the hospital treated an inpatient population that met or exceeded the following percentages:

- For cost-reporting periods beginning on or after July 1, 2004, and before July 1, 2005, the hospital must have served an inpatient population of whom at least 50 percent required intensive rehabilitative services for treatment of one or more of the medical conditions specified in figure 7.2.

- For cost-reporting periods beginning on or after July 1, 2005, and before July 1, 2006, the hospital must have served an inpatient population of whom at least 60 percent required intensive rehabilitative services for treatment of one or more of the medical conditions specified in figure 7.2.

- For cost-reporting periods beginning on or after July 1, 2006, and before July 1, 2007, the hospital must have served an inpatient population of whom at least 65

Figure 7.2. Medical conditions that are criteria for classification as inpatient rehabilitation facility

1. Stroke
2. Spinal cord injury
3. Congenital deformity
4. Amputation
5. Major multiple trauma
6. Fracture of femur (hip fracture)
7. Brain Injury
8. Neurological disorders including multiple sclerosis, motor neuron diseases, polyneuropathy, muscular dystrophy, and Parkinson's disease
9. Burns
10. Active, polyarticular rheumatoid arthritis, psoriatic arthritis, and seronegative arthropathies
11. Systemic vaculidities with joint inflammation
12. Severe or advanced osteoarthritis involving two or more weight-bearing joints
13. Knee or hip joint replacement or both

Source: CMS 2005a.

percent required intensive rehabilitative services for treatment of one or more of the medical conditions specified in figure 7.2.

- For cost-reporting periods beginning on or after July 1, 2007, the hospital must have served an inpatient population of whom at least 75 percent required intensive rehabilitative services for treatment of one or more of the medical conditions specified in figure 7.2.

Patient Assessment Instrument

IRFs are required to complete a patient assessment instrument (PAI) on all patients upon each patient's admission and also discharge from the facility. CMS provides facilities with IRVEN **(Inpatient Rehabilitation Validation and Entry)** system to collect the IRF-PAI in a database that can be transmitted electronically to the IRF-PAI national database. These data are used in assessing clinical characteristics of patients in rehabilitation settings. Ultimately, they can be used to provide survey agencies with a means to objectively measure and compare facility performance and quality and to allow researchers to develop improved standards of care.

The IRF PPS uses information from the IRF-PAI to classify patients into distinct groups on the basis of clinical characteristics and expected resource needs. Data used to construct these groups called **case-mix groups** (CMGs) include rehabilitation impairment categories (RICs), functional status (both motor and cognitive), age, comorbidities and other factors deemed appropriate to improve the explanatory power of the groups. There are currently 100 CMGs into which patients are classified.

CMG Relative Weight

An appropriate weight, called the **CMG relative weight,** is assigned to each case-mix group that measures the relative difference in facility resource intensity among the various groups. Separate payments are calculated for each group, including the application of case- and facility-level adjustments. Facility-level adjustments include wage-index adjustments, low-income patient adjustments, and rural facility adjustments. Case-level adjustments include transfer adjustments, interrupted-stay adjustments, and cost outlier adjustments.

Long-Term Care Hospitals (LTCHs) Prospective Payment System

The Balanced Budget Refinement Act of 1999 amended by the Benefits Improvement Act of 2000 mandated the establishment of a per discharge, DRG-based PPS for longer-term care hospitals beginning on October 1, 2002. There is a five-year transition period with full implementation by October 1, 2006. This transition period is applicable only to existing hospitals and replaces the cost-based payment system previously used. New facilities are paid 100 percent of the LTC-DRG.

LTCHs are defined as having an average inpatient LOS greater than twenty-five days.

LTC-DRGs

Patients are classified into distinct diagnosis groups based on clinical characteristics and expected resource use. These groups are based on the current inpatient DRGs. There are approximately 170 LTC-DRGs. The payment system includes the following three primary elements:

1. Patient classification into a LTC-DRG weight.
2. Relative weight of the LTC-DRG. The weights reflect the variation in cost per discharge as they take into account the utilization for each diagnosis.

3. Federal payment rate. Payment is made at a predetermined per discharge amount for each LTC-DRG.

Adjustments

The PPS does provide for case-(patient)-level adjustments such as short-stay outlier, interrupted stays, and high-cost outliers. Facility-wide adjustments include area wage index and cost of living adjustments.

A short-stay outlier is an adjustment to the payment rate for stays that are considerably shorter than the average length of stay (ALOS) for a particular LTC-DRG. A case would qualify for short-stay outlier status when the LOS is between one day and up to and including five-sixths of the ALOS for the LTC-DRG. Both the ALOS and the five-sixths of the ALOS periods are published in the *Federal Register.* Payment under the short-stay outlier is made using different payment methodologies. (See table 7.11 for examples of LTC-DRGs and the ALOS for each.)

An interrupted stay occurs when a patient is discharged from the long-term care hospital and then is readmitted to the same facility for further treatment after a specific number of days away from the facility. There are different policies if the patient is readmitted to the facility within three days (called three-day or less interrupted-stay policy) or if the patient is away from the facility greater than three days (called the greater than three-day interrupted-stay policy).

A high-cost outlier is an adjustment to the payment rate for a patient when the costs are unusually high and exceed the typical costs associated with a LTC-DRG. High-cost outlier payments reduce the facility's potential financial losses that can result from treating patients who require more costly care than is normal. A case qualifies for a high-cost outlier payment when the estimated cost of care exceeds the high-cost outlier threshold, which, for example, in 2005 was $17,864.

Table 7.11.   Examples of LTC-DRGs, relative weights, geometric ALOS, and five-sixths of the geometric ALOS

LTC-DRG	Description	Relative Weight	Geometric ALOS	Five-sixths of the Geometric ALOS
2	Craniotomy age >17 w/o CC	1.1899	28.5	23.8
3	Craniotomy age 0–17	1.1899	28.5	23.8
6	Carpal tunnel release	0.6064	21.1	17.6
26	Seizure and headache age 0–17	0.6064	21.1	17.6
30	Traumatic stupor and coma less than 1 hour age 0–17	0.8508	24.3	20.3
32	Concussion age >17 w/o CC	0.6064	21.1	17.6
36	Retinal procedures	0.4586	16.9	14.1
195	Cholecystectomy w CDE w CC	1.8658	38.6	32.2

Inpatient Psychiatric Facilities (IPFs) Prospective Payment System

The Balanced Budget Refinement Act of 1999 mandated the development of a per diem PPS for inpatient psychiatric services furnished in hospitals and exempt units. The PPS became effective on January 1, 2005, establishing a standardized per diem rate to **inpatient psychiatric facilities** (IPFs) based on the national average of operating, ancillary, and capital costs for each patient day of care in the IPF. The system uses the same DRGs as the acute care hospital inpatient system.

CMS is phasing in the PPS for existing facilities over a three-year period with full payments under the PPS beginning in the fourth year. The per diem payment is adjusted to reflect both patient and facility characteristics that cause significant cost increases.

Adjustments

Patient-level or case-level adjustments are provided for age, specified DRGs, and certain comorbidity categories. Payment adjustments are made for eight age categories beginning with age 45 at which point, statistically, costs are increased as the patient ages.

The IPF receives a DRG payment adjustment for a principal diagnosis that groups to one of fifteen psychiatric DRGs. See table 7.12. Seventeen comorbidity categories that require comparatively more costly treatment during an inpatient stay also generate a pay-

Table 7.12. Psychiatric DRGs	
DRG	**DRG Description**
424	Procedure with principal diagnosis of mental illness
425	Acute adjustment reaction
426	Depressive neurosis
427	Neurosis, except depressive
428	Disorders of personality
429	Organic disturbances
430	Psychosis
431	Childhood disorders
432	Other mental disorders
433	Alcohol/Drug use, left against medical advice
521	Alcohol/Drug use, w CC
522	Alcohol/Drug use, w/o CC
523	Alcohol/Drug use, w/o rehab
12	Degenerative nervous system disorders
23	Nontraumatic stupor and coma

ment adjustment. The list of comorbidity categories and their associated ICD-9-CM diagnosis codes can be found in table 7.13.

There also is a variable per diem adjustment to recognize higher costs in the early days of a psychiatric stay.

The IPF PPS also includes an outlier policy for those patients who require more expensive care than expected in an effort to minimize the financial risk to the IPF. Although the basis of the system is a per diem rate, outlier payments are made on a per case basis rather than on the per diem basis.

Table 7.13.   Comorbidity categories affecting IPS payment

Category	ICD-9-CM Diagnosis Codes
Developmental disabilities	317, 318.0, 318.1, 318.2, and 319
Coagulation factor deficit	286.0 through 286.4
Tracheostomy	519.00 through 519.09; V44.0
Renal failure, acute	584.5 through 584.9, 636.3, 637.3, 638.3, 639.3, 669.32, 669.34, 958.5
Renal failure, chronic	403.01, 403.11, 403.91, 404.02, 404.03, 404.12, 404.13, 404.92, 404.93, 585, 586, V45.1, V56.0, V56.1, V56.2
Oncology treatment	140.0 through 239.9 with either 99.25 or a code from 92.21 through 92.29
Uncontrolled Type I diabetes mellitus with or without complications	250.02, 250.03, 250.12, 250.13, 250.22, 250.23, 250.32, 250.33, 250.42, 250.43, 250.52, 250.53, 250.62, 250.63, 250.72,250.73, 250.82, 250.83, 250.92, 250.93
Severe protein calorie malnutrition	260 through 262
Eating and conduct disorders	307.1, 307.50, 312.03, 312.33, 312.34
Infectious diseases	010.01 through 041.10,042,045.00 through 053.19, 054.40 through 054.49,055.0 through 077.0,078.2 through 078.89, 079.50 through 079.59
Drug and/or alcohol-induced mental disorders	291.0, 292.0, 292.12, 292.2, 303.00, 304.00
Cardiac conditions	391.0, 391.1, 391.2, 402.01,404.03, 416.0, 421.0, 421.1, 421.9
Gangrene	440.24, 785.4
Chronic obstructive pulmonary disease	491.21, 494.1, 510.0, 518.83, 518.84, V46.1
Artificial openings—digestive and urinary	569.60 through 569.69, 997.5, V44.1 through V44.6
Severe musculoskeletal and connective tissue disorders	696.0, 710.0, 730.00 through 730.09, 730.10 through 730.19, 730.20 through 730.29
Poisoning	965.00 through 965.09, 965.4, 967.0 through 969.9, 977.0, 980.0 through 980.9, 983.0 through 983.9, 986, 989.0 through 989.7

The PPS also includes regulations on payments when there is an interrupted stay, meaning the patient is discharged from an IPF and returns to the same or another facility before midnight on the third consecutive day. The intent of the policy is to prevent a facility from prematurely discharging a patient after the maximum payment is received and subsequently readmitting the patient.

Facility adjustments include a wage-index adjustment, a rural location adjustment, and a teaching status adjustment.

Check Your Understanding 7. 7

Instructions: Select the best term to complete each of the following statements.

1. _____ Congress enacted the first Medicare prospective payment system in _____.
   a. 1966
   b. 1972
   c. 1983
   d. 2001

2. _____ Prior to implementation of the DRG prospective payment system, Medicare Part A payments to hospitals were based on a _____.
   a. Fee-for-service reimbursement methodology
   b. Level of care and expenditure of resources system
   c. Managed care capitated payment schedule
   d. Predetermined rate for each inpatient discharge

3. _____ The DRG prospective payment rate is based on the _____ diagnosis.
   a. Primary
   b. Principal

4. _____ The computer software program that assigns appropriate DRGs according to information provided for each episode of care is called a _____.
   a. Classification
   b. Catalog
   c. Register
   d. Grouper

5. _____ _____ hospitals are excluded from the Medicare acute care prospective payment system.
   a. Children's
   b. Small community
   c. Tertiary
   d. Trauma

6. _____ Diagnosis-related groups are organized into _____.
   a. Case-mix classifications
   b. Geographic practice cost indices
   c. Major diagnostic categories
   d. Resource-based relative values

7. _____ _____ are associated with the Medicare fee schedule.
   a. APCs
   b. DRGs
   c. RBRVS
   d. RUG-III

8. ____ ____ mandated the implementation of a skilled nursing facility prospective payment system.
    a.   BBA
    b.   COBRA
    c.   OBRA
    d.   TEFRA

9. ____ Resident assessment data are collected from the ____ to assign SNF residents to the appropriate resource utilization group.
    a.   MDS
    b.   RAP
    c.   RAVEN
    d.   RUG

10. ____ ____ are (is) associated with the outpatient prospective payment system.
    a.   APCs
    b.   DRGs
    c.   RBRVS
    d.   RUG-III

11. ____ ____ are not reimbursed according to the outpatient prospective payment system.
    a.   CMHC partial hospitalization services
    b.   Critical access hospitals
    c.   Hospital outpatient departments
    d.   Vaccines provided by CORFs

12. ____ When multiple surgical procedures are furnished during the same operative session, a concept called ____ is applied.
    a.   Bundling of services
    b.   Outlier adjustment
    c.   Pass-through payment
    d.   Discounting of procedures

13. ____ The home health prospective payment system uses the ____ data set for patient assessments.
    a.   HEDIS
    b.   OASIS
    c.   RAI
    d.   UHDDS

14. ____ A new Medicare payment system for medically necessary transports effective for services provided on or after 1/1/01 was included as part of the ____.
    a.   BBA
    b.   HH PPS
    c.   MDS-PAC
    d.   RUG-III

15. ____ A per-discharge PPS for care provided to Medicare beneficiaries by inpatient rehabilitation hospitals and rehabilitation units was phased in on ____.
    a.   October 1, 2000
    b.   January 1, 2001
    c.   April 1, 2001
    d.   October 1, 2001

Processing of Reimbursement Claims

Understanding payment mechanisms is an important foundation for accurately processing claims forms. However, it is not enough just to understand payment mechanisms.

A facility's patient accounts department is responsible for billing third-party payers, processing **accounts receivable** and verifying insurance coverage. Medicare carriers and **fiscal intermediaries** (FIs) contract with CMS to serve as the financial agent between providers and the federal government to locally administer Medicare's Part A and Part B.

Coordination of Benefits

In many instances, patients have more than one insurance policy and the determination of which policy is primary and which is secondary is necessary so that there is no duplication of benefits paid. This process is called the coordination of Benefits (COB) or the **coordination of benefits transaction.** The monies collected from third-party payers cannot be greater than the amount of the provider's charges.

Explanation of Benefits/Remittance Advice

An **Explanation of Benefits** (EOB) is a statement sent to the patient to explain services provided, amounts billed and payments made by the health plan. Medicare replaced its Explanation of Medicare Benefits (EOMB) with the **Medicare Summary Notice** (MSN). See figure 7.3 for a sample Part B MSN.

A **remittance advice** (RA) is sent to the provider to explain payments made by third-party payers. Prior to the availability of the ANSI ASC X12 835, commonly known as the **electronic remittance advice** (ERA), providers used either paper or tape transmissions to post payments to their accounts; however, tape transmissions are no longer an option. (See figure 7.4, p. 297, for a sample RA.)

Third-Party Payers

Depending on the services provided to patients, either the **CMS-1500** or the **UB-92** (CMS-1450) claim form is submitted to the third-party payer for reimbursement purposes. The CMS-1500 is used to bill third-party payers for provider services (for example, physician's office visit), and the UB-92 is submitted for inpatient, outpatient, home health care, hospice, and long-term care services. Health claims data are frequently transmitted electronically between a healthcare organization and a third-party payer using electronic data interchange (EDI), which is addressed in chapter 7.

CMS-1500
In 1958, the Health Insurance Association of America (HIAA) and the American Medical Association (AMA) originally created a standardized insurance claim form called the **Attending Physician Statement** (APS) (or COMB-1). However, some third-party payers did not accept its use. In April 1975, the AMA and CMS cochaired the Uniform Claim Form Task Force, which approved a universal claim form now known as CMS-1500. (See figure 7.5, p. 298.) CMS-1500 is used for processing both group and individual healthcare claims. It has specific form locators (FLs) that must be completed according to third-party payer guidelines. (See table 7.14, p. 299.)

Figure 7.3. Sample Medicare summary notice

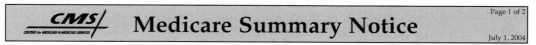

| Page 1 of 2 |
| **Medicare Summary Notice** |
| July 1, 2004 |

CUSTOMER SERVICE INFORMATION

Your Medicare Number: 111-11-1111A

If you have questions, write or call:
Medicare
555 Medicare Blvd., Suite 200
Medicare Building
Medicare, US XXXXX-XXXX

Local: (XXX) XXX-XXXX
Toll-free: 1-800-XXX-XXXX
TTY for Hearing Impaired: 1-800-XXX-XXXX

BENEFICIARY NAME
STREET ADDRESS
CITY, STATE   ZIP CODE

BE INFORMED: Beware of "free" medical services or products. If it sounds too good to be true, it probably is.

This is a summary of claims processed from 05/15/2004 through 06/10/2004.

PART A HOSPITAL INSURANCE – INPATIENT CLAIMS

Dates of Service	Benefit Days Used	Non-Covered Charges	Deductible and Coinsurance	You May Be Billed	See Notes Section
Claim Number: 12435-84956-84556-45621 **Cure Hospital, 213 Sick Lane, Dallas, TX 75555** Referred by: Paul Jones, M.D.					a
04/25/04 – 05/09/04	14 days	$0.00	$876.00	$776.00	b, c
Claim Number: 12435-84956-845556-45622 **Continued Care Hospital, 124 Sick Lane, Dallas, TX 75555** Referred by: Paul Jones, M.D.					
05/09/04 – 06/20/04	11 days	$0.00	$0.00	$0.00	

PART B MEDICAL INSURANCE – OUTPATIENT FACILITY CLAIMS

Dates of Service	Services Provided	Amount Charged	Non-Covered Charges	Deductible and Coinsurance	You May Be Billed	See Notes Section
Claim Number: 12435-8956-8458 **Medicare Hospital, 123 Medicare Lane, Dallas, TX 75209** Referred by: Paul Jones, M.D.						d
04/02/04	L.V. Therapy (Q0081)	$33.00	$0.00	$6.60	$6.60	
	Lab (3810)	1,140.50	0.00	228.10	228.10	
	Operating Room (31628)	786.50	0.00	157.30	157.30	
	Observation Room (99201)	293.00	0.00	58.60	58.60	
	Claim Total	**$2,253.00**	**$0.00**	**$450.60**	**$450.60**	
						(continued)

THIS IS NOT A BILL – Keep this notice for your records.

(Continued on next page)

Figure 7.3. *(Continued)*

Your Medicare Number: 111-11-1111A

Notes Section:

a The amount Medicare paid the provider for this claim is $XXXX.XX.

b $776.00 was applied to your inpatient deductible.

c $30.00 was applied to your blood deductible.

d The amount Medicare paid the provider for this claim is $XXXX.XX.

Deductible Information:

You have met the Part A deductible for this benefit period.

You have met the Part B deductible for 2004.

You have met the blood deductible for 2004.

General Information:

You have the right to make a request in writing for an itemized statement which details each Medicare item or service which you have received from your physician, hospital, or any other health supplier or health professional. Please contact them directly, in writing, if you would like an itemized statement.

Compare the services you receive with those that appear on your Medicare Summary Notice. If you have questions, call your doctor or provider. If you feel further investigation is needed due to possible fraud and abuse, call the phone number in the Customer Service Information Box.

Appeals Information—Part A (Inpatient) and Part B (Outpatient)

If you disagree with any claims decision on either Part A or Part B of this notice, you can request an appeal by November 1, 2004. Follow the instructions below:

1) Circle the item(s) you disagree with and explain why you disagree.

2) Send this notice or a copy, to the address in the "Customer Service Information" box on Page 1. (You may also send any additional information you may have about your appeal.)

3) Sign here _____ Phone number _____

Revised 02/04

In 1995, the Uniform Claim Form Task Force was replaced by the **National Uniform Claim Committee** (NUCC). The NUCC developed a standard data set to be used in the transmission of noninstitutional provider claims to and from third-party payers. NUCC membership includes representation from the following organizations:

- Alliance for Managed Care
- American Association of Health Plans
- AMA
- ANSI ASC X12N
- Blue Cross and Blue Shield Association
- CMS (formerly HCFA)
- Health Insurance Association of America
- **Medical Group Management Association**

Figure 7.4.   Sample single-claim remittance advice

Medicare National Standard Intermediary Remittance Advice

FPE:		07/30/04
PAID:		01/25/04
CLM#:		2
TOB:		111

PATIENT:	JOHN DOE				PCN:	235617
HIC:	123456		SVC FROM:	01/05/04	MRN:	124767
PAT STAT:	01	CLAIM STAT: 1	THRU:	01/06/04	ICN:	987654

CHARGES:		PAYMENT DATA: 140=DRG		0.000	=REIM RATE
1939.90	=REPORTED	2741.69	=DRG AMOUNT	0.00	=MSP PRIM PAYER
0.00	=NONCOVERED	2497.26	=DRG/OPER	0.00	=PROF COMPONENT
0.00	=DENIED	244.43	=DRG/CAPITAL	0.00	=ESRD AMOUNT
1939.90	=COVERED	0.00	=OUTLIER	0.00	=HCPCS AMOUNT
DAYS/VISITS:		0.00	=CAP OUTLIER	0.00	=ALLOWED AMOUNT
1	=COST REPT	768.00	=CASH DEDUCT	0.00	=G/R AMOUNT
1	=COVD/UTIL	0.00	=BLOOD DEDUCT	0.00	=INTEREST
0	=NONCOVERED	0.00	=COINSURANCE	-801.79	=CONTRACT ADJ
0	=COVD VISITS	0.00	=PAT REFUND	675.00	=PER DIEM AMT
0	=NCOV VISITS	0.00	=MSP LIAB MET	1973.69	=NET REIM AMT

ADJ REASON CODES: CO A2 –801.79
                     PR   1
                     768

REMARK CODES: MA02

Figure 7.5. CMS-1500 claim form

PLEASE DO NOT STAPLE IN THIS AREA

PICA **HEALTH INSURANCE CLAIM FORM** PICA

CARRIER

1. MEDICARE (Medicare #) MEDICAID (Medicaid #) CHAMPUS (Sponsor's SSN) CHAMPVA (VA File #) GROUP HEALTH PLAN (SSN or ID) FECA BLK LUNG (SSN) OTHER (ID)

1a. INSURED'S I.D. NUMBER (FOR PROGRAM IN ITEM 1)

2. PATIENT'S NAME (Last Name, First Name, Middle Initial)

3. PATIENT'S BIRTH DATE MM DD YY SEX M F

4. INSURED'S NAME (Last Name, First Name, Middle Initial)

5. PATIENT'S ADDRESS (No., Street)

6. PATIENT RELATIONSHIP TO INSURED Self Spouse Child Other

7. INSURED'S ADDRESS (No., Street)

CITY STATE

8. PATIENT STATUS Single Married Other

CITY STATE

ZIP CODE TELEPHONE (Include Area Code) ( )

Employed Full-Time Student Part-Time Student

ZIP CODE TELEPHONE (INCLUDE AREA CODE) ( )

9. OTHER INSURED'S NAME (Last Name, First Name, Middle Initial)

10. IS PATIENT'S CONDITION RELATED TO:

11. INSURED'S POLICY GROUP OR FECA NUMBER

a. OTHER INSURED'S POLICY OR GROUP NUMBER

a. EMPLOYMENT? (CURRENT OR PREVIOUS) YES NO

a. INSURED'S DATE OF BIRTH MM DD YY SEX M F

b. OTHER INSURED'S DATE OF BIRTH MM DD YY SEX M F

b. AUTO ACCIDENT? YES NO PLACE (State)

b. EMPLOYER'S NAME OR SCHOOL NAME

c. EMPLOYER'S NAME OR SCHOOL NAME

c. OTHER ACCIDENT? YES NO

c. INSURANCE PLAN NAME OR PROGRAM NAME

d. INSURANCE PLAN NAME OR PROGRAM NAME

10d. RESERVED FOR LOCAL USE

d. IS THERE ANOTHER HEALTH BENEFIT PLAN? YES NO *If yes*, return to and complete item 9 a-d.

READ BACK OF FORM BEFORE COMPLETING & SIGNING THIS FORM.

12. PATIENT'S OR AUTHORIZED PERSON'S SIGNATURE I authorize the release of any medical or other information necessary to process this claim. I also request payment of government benefits either to myself or to the party who accepts assignment below.

SIGNED DATE

13. INSURED'S OR AUTHORIZED PERSON'S SIGNATURE I authorize payment of medical benefits to the undersigned physician or supplier for services described below.

SIGNED

PATIENT AND INSURED INFORMATION

14. DATE OF CURRENT: MM DD YY ILLNESS (First symptom) OR INJURY (Accident) OR PREGNANCY(LMP)

15. IF PATIENT HAS HAD SAME OR SIMILAR ILLNESS. GIVE FIRST DATE MM DD YY

16. DATES PATIENT UNABLE TO WORK IN CURRENT OCCUPATION FROM MM DD YY TO MM DD YY

17. NAME OF REFERRING PHYSICIAN OR OTHER SOURCE

17a. I.D. NUMBER OF REFERRING PHYSICIAN

18. HOSPITALIZATION DATES RELATED TO CURRENT SERVICES FROM MM DD YY TO MM DD YY

19. RESERVED FOR LOCAL USE

20. OUTSIDE LAB? YES NO $ CHARGES

21. DIAGNOSIS OR NATURE OF ILLNESS OR INJURY. (RELATE ITEMS 1,2,3 OR 4 TO ITEM 24E BY LINE)

1. ___ . __ 3. ___ . __

2. ___ . __ 4. ___ . __

22. MEDICAID RESUBMISSION CODE ORIGINAL REF. NO.

23. PRIOR AUTHORIZATION NUMBER

24. A DATE(S) OF SERVICE From MM DD YY	To MM DD YY	B Place of Service	C Type of Service	D PROCEDURES, SERVICES, OR SUPPLIES (Explain Unusual Circumstances) CPT/HCPCS MODIFIER	E DIAGNOSIS CODE	F $ CHARGES	G DAYS OR UNITS	H EPSDT Family Plan	I EMG	J COB	K RESERVED FOR LOCAL USE
1											
2											
3											
4											
5											
6											

25. FEDERAL TAX I.D. NUMBER SSN EIN

26. PATIENT'S ACCOUNT NO.

27. ACCEPT ASSIGNMENT? (For govt. claims, see back) YES NO

28. TOTAL CHARGE $

29. AMOUNT PAID $

30. BALANCE DUE $

31. SIGNATURE OF PHYSICIAN OR SUPPLIER INCLUDING DEGREES OR CREDENTIALS (I certify that the statements on the reverse apply to this bill and are made a part thereof.)

SIGNED DATE

32. NAME AND ADDRESS OF FACILITY WHERE SERVICES WERE RENDERED (If other than home or office)

33. PHYSICIAN'S, SUPPLIER'S BILLING NAME, ADDRESS, ZIP CODE & PHONE #

PIN# GRP#

PHYSICIAN OR SUPPLIER INFORMATION

(APPROVED BY AMA COUNCIL ON MEDICAL SERVICE 8/88) ***PLEASE PRINT OR TYPE*** APPROVED OMB-0938-0008 FORM CMS-1500 (12-90), FORM RRB-1500, APPROVED OMB-1215-0055 FORM OWCP-1500, APPROVED OMB-0720-0001 (CHAMPUS)

Table 7.14.   CMS-1500 form locators and brief description of information to be entered into each

Form Locator	Brief Description	Form Locator	Brief Description
1	Type of insurance	17a	ID Number of referring physician
1a	Insured's ID number	18	Hospitalization dates related to current services
2	Patient's name	19	Reserved for local use
3	Patient's birth date/sex	20	Outside lab
4	Insured's name	21	Diagnosis or nature of illness or injury
5	Patient's address	22	Medicaid resubmission
6	Patient's relationship to insured	23	Prior authorization number
7	Insured's address	24A	Dates of service
8	Patient's marital status/employment status	24B	Place of service
9	Other insured's name	24C	Type of service
9a	Other insured's policy or group number	24D	Procedures, services, or supplies
9b	Other insured's date of birth/sex	24E	Diagnosis code
9c	Employer's name or school name	24F	Charges
9d	Insurance plan name or program name	24G	Days or units
10a–10c	Indicate whether patient's condition is related to a work injury, an automobile accident, or another type of accident	24H	EPSDT family plan
10d	Reserved for local use	24I	Emergency
11	Insured's policy group or FECA number	24J	Coordination of benefits
11a	Insured's date of birth/sex	24K	Reserved for local use
11b	Employer's name or school name	25	Federal tax ID number
11c	Insurance plan name or program name of insured	26	Patient's account number
11d	Indicate whether there is another health benefit plan	27	Accept assignment or not
12	Patient's or authorized person's signature	28	Total charge
13	Insured or authorized person's signature	29	Amount paid
14	Date of current illness or injury or pregnancy	30	Balance due
15	Date when patient first consulted provider for treatment of the same or similar condition	31	Signature of physician or supplier
16	Dates patient unable to work in current occupation	32	Name and address of facility where services were rendered
17	Name of referring physician or other source	33	Physician/supplier's billing name, address, ZIP code, and telephone number

- National Association of Insurance Commissioners

- National Association of Medical Equipment Services

- National Association of State Medicaid Directors

- **National Uniform Billing Committee** (NUBC)

CMS-1500 was revised in 1990 and printed in red ink to meet optical scanning guidelines. In May 1992, Medicare required that all services delivered to patients by physicians and suppliers except for ambulance services be billed on this scannable form. CMS-1500 contains 33 blocks that are completed according to third-party payer guidelines. Noninstitutional providers and suppliers submit it in accordance with these guidelines. It is important to follow payer guidelines when completing the claim form; otherwise, reimbursement will be delayed until the form is corrected.

UB-92 (CMS-1450)

Healthcare facilities, such as hospitals, currently submit the UB-92 (figure 7.6), or Uniform Bill, to third-party payers for reimbursement of patient services. The data elements and design of the UB-92 are the responsibility of the NUBC, which includes representation from the following organizations:

- American Association of Health Plans

- American Health Care Association

- American Hospital Association

- AHA's state hospital association representatives

- Alliance for Managed Care

- **American National Standards Institute Accredited Standards**

- Committee X12N-Insurance Subcommittee (ANSI ASC X12N)

- Blue Cross and Blue Shield Association

- Center for Healthcare Information Management

- Federation of American Health Systems

- CMS: Medicare

- CMS: Medicaid

- Health Insurance Association of America-National Association for Home Care

- National Association of State Medicaid Directors

- National Uniform Claim Committee

- Public Health/Health Services Research (national)

- Public Health/Health Services Research (state)

- TRICARE (CHAMPUS)

Figure 7.6.   UB-92 (CMS-1450) claim form

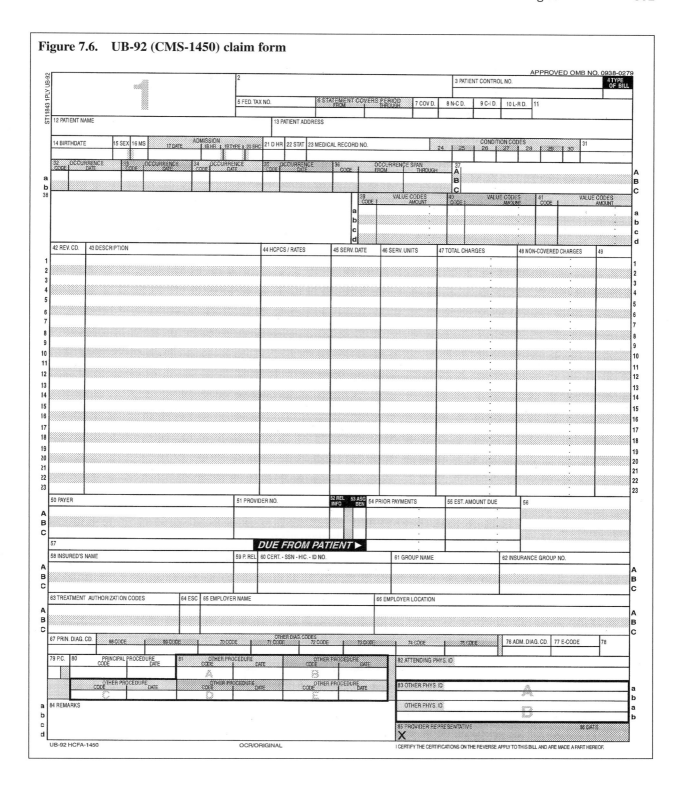

The UB-92 form and instructions are used by institutional and other selected providers to complete a Medicare, Part A, claim for submission to Medicare FIs (and other third-party payers). UB-92 contains eighty-six FLs, which are completed according to third-party payer guidelines. (See table 7.15.) FLs of particular importance are those that require entry of revenue codes, which identify services provided to patients as reported on the UB-92. The types of organizations that submit the UB-92 include:

- Ambulance companies
- Ambulatory surgery centers
- HHAs
- Hospice organizations
- Hospitals (emergency department and inpatient and outpatient services)
- Psychiatric and drug/alcohol treatment facilities (inpatient and outpatient services)
- SNFs
- Subacute facilities
- Stand-alone clinical/laboratory facilities
- Walk-in clinics

UB-04
The NUBC began work to replace the UB-92 in 2001. The intent was to make the new form more HIPAA compliant, to improve the denial rate, and to reduce the need for resubmittals. The **UB-04** data set includes a number of improvements and enhancements resulting from nearly four years of surveys and study.

One of the most significant changes is in the number of diagnosis and procedure code fields available. The newly designed form will include nine additional diagnosis fields and more fields for E codes. The anticipated UB-04 will include 80 FLs.

In addition, the UB-04 anticipates the move to ICD-10-CM with expanded code fields. It also provides a space for national provider identifiers and national health plan identifiers.

January 2007 is the targeted implementation date for the new UB-04. (See figure 7.7, p. 304.)

Medicare Carriers
Medicare carriers process Part B claims for services by physicians and medical suppliers. Examples of carriers might include a state Blue Shield plan or commercial insurance companies or other organizations under contract with Medicare. Carriers are responsible for performing the following functions:

- Determining the charges allowed by Medicare
- Maintaining the quality of performance records
- Assisting in fraud and abuse investigations
- Providing education to providers, suppliers, and beneficiaries as necessary
- Making payments to physicians and suppliers for Part B–covered services

Table 7.15.   UB-92 (CMS-1450) form locators and brief description of information to be entered into each

Form Locator	Brief Description	Form Locator	Brief Description
1	Provider's Name, Address, and Telephone Number	46	Units of Service
2	Unlabeled Field—State Use	47	Total Charges (by Revenue Code Category)
3	Patient's Control Number (Account Number)	48	Noncovered Charges
4	Type of Bill	49	Unlabeled Field—National Use
5	Federal Tax Number	50A–C	Payer Identification
6	Statement Covers Period	51A–C	Provider Number
7	Covered Days	52A–C	Release of Information Certification Indicator
8	Noncovered days	53A–C	Assignment of Benefits Certification Indicator
9	Coinsurance Days	54A–C, P	Prior Payments—Payers and Patient
10	Lifetime Reserve Days	55A–C, P	Estimated Amount Due
11	Unlabeled Field—State Use	56	DRG Number and Grouper ID
12	Patient Name	57	Unlabeled Field—National Use
13	Patient Address	58A–C	Insured's Name
14	Patient Birthdate	59A–C	Patient's Relationship to Insured
15	Patient Sex	60A–C	Health Insurance Claim Identification Number
16	Patient Marital Status	61A–C	Insured Group Name
17	Admission Date	62A–C	Insurance Group Number
18	Admission Hour	63A–C	Treatment Authorization Code
19	Type of Admission	64A–C	Employment Status Code
20	Source of Admission	65A–C	Employer Name
21	Discharge Hour	66A–C	Employer Location
22	Patient Status	67	Principal Diagnosis Code
23	Medical/Health Record Number	68–75	Other Diagnosis Codes
24–30	Condition Codes	76	Admitting Diagnosis
31	Unlabeled Field—National Use	77	External Cause of Injury Code (E-Code)
32–35a,b	Occurrence Codes and Dates	78	Not Titled
36a,b	Occurrence Span Codes and Dates	79	Procedure Coding Method Used
37	Internal Control Number (ICN)	80	Principal Procedure Code and Date
38	Responsible Party Name and Address	81A–E	Other Procedure Codes and Dates
39–41a–d	Value Codes and Amounts	82	Attending Physician ID
42	Revenue Code	83a–b	Other Physician ID
43	Revenue Description	84a–d	Remarks
44	HCPCS/Rates	85	Provider Representative Signature
45	Service Date	86	Date Bill Submitted

Figure 7.7. UB-04 (CMS-1450) claim form

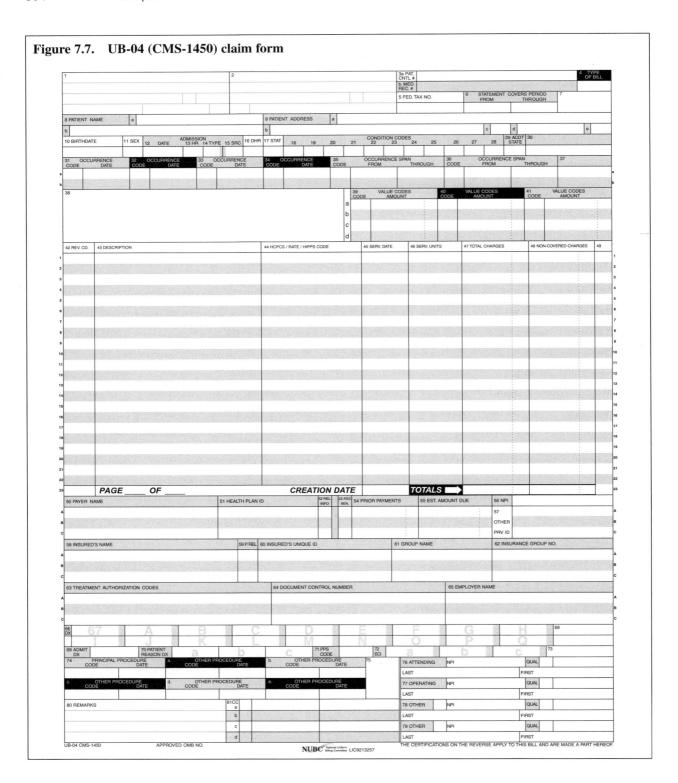

Medicare Fiscal Intermediaries

Medicare FIs process Part A claims and hospital-based Part B claims for institutional services, including inpatient hospital claims, SNFs, HHAs, and hospice services. They also process outpatient claims for supplemental medical insurance (Medicare Part B). Examples of FIs include Blue Cross and Blue Shield organizations and commercial insurance companies under contract with Medicare.

FIs are responsible for performing the following functions:

- Determining costs and reimbursement amounts

- Maintaining records

- Establishing controls

- Safeguarding against fraud and abuse or excess use

- Conducting reviews and audits

- Making payments to providers for covered services

- Providing education to facilities and beneficiaries as necessary

National Correct Coding Initiative (NCCI)

CMS implemented the **National Correct Coding Initiative** (NCCI) in 1996 to develop correct coding methodologies to improve the appropriate payment of Medicare Part B claims.

NCCI policies are based on:

- Coding conventions defined in the CPT codebooks

- National and local policies and coding edits

- Analysis of standard medical and surgical practice

- Review of current coding practices

The NCCI edits explain what procedures and services cannot be billed together on the same day of service for a patient. The mutually exclusive edit applies to improbable or impossible combinations of codes. For example, code 58940, Oophorectomy, partial or total, unilateral or bilateral, would never be used with code 58150, Total abdominal hysterectomy (corpus and cervix), with or without removal of tube(s), with or without removal of ovary(s). Modifiers may be used to indicate circumstances in which the NCCI edits should not be applied and payment should be made as requested. Modifier –59, for example, is used when circumstances require that certain procedures or services be reported together even though they usually are not.

Briefly describe comprehensive/component code matches since mutually exclusive code matches are specifically discussed.

Portions of the NCCI are incorporated into the **outpatient code editor** (OCE) against which all ambulatory claims are reviewed. The OCE also applies a set of logical rules to determine whether various combinations of codes are correct and appropriately represent services provided. Billing issues result from these CCI/OCE edits that often result in claim denials.

Physician Query Process

There are instances, however, when it is necessary to query the physician for clarification of data that may influence proper code assignment. This might include instances when there is conflicting or incomplete information in the record. Query forms have proved to be an effective means of communication with physicians. AHIMA cautions coders that these forms are used to improve documentation and understanding of the clinical situation, but not to increase reimbursement (Prophet 2001).

The facility should develop a standard form to be used in communicating with physicians. Characteristics of a good query form are noted in figure 7.8.

Electronic Data Interchange

Electronic data interchange (EDI) is the electronic transfer of information, such as health claims transmitted electronically, in a standard format between trading partners. EDI originated when a number of industries identified cost savings through the electronic transmission of business information. They were convinced that the standardization of formatted information was the most effective means of communicating with multiple trading partners.

EDI allows entities within the healthcare system to exchange medical, billing, and other information and to process transactions quickly and cost-effectively. EDI substantially reduces handling and processing time compared to paper and eliminates the risk

---

Figure 7.8.   Characteristics of a good query form

The query form should:

- Be clearly and concisely written

- Contain precise language

- Present the facts from the medical record and identify why clarification is needed

- Present the scenario and state a question that asks the physician to make a clinical interpretation of a given diagnosis or condition based on treatment, evaluation, monitoring, and/or services provided. "Open-ended" questions that allow the physician to document the specific diagnosis are preferable to multiple-choice questions or questions requiring only a "yes" or "no" response. Queries that appear to lead the physician to provide a particular response could lead to allegations of inappropriate upcoding

- Be phrased such that the physician is allowed to specify the correct diagnosis. It should not indicate the financial impact of the response to the query. The form should not be designed so that all that is required is a physician signature

- Include: patient name, admission date, medical record number, name and contact information (phone number and e-mail address) of the coding professional, specific question and rationale, place for the physician to document his or her response, place for the physician to sign and date his or her response

Source: Prophet 2001, pp. 88I–M.

of lost paper documents. It also can eliminate the inefficiencies of handling paper documents and thus can significantly reduce administrative burden, lower operating costs, and improve overall data quality.

The American National Standards Institute (ANSI) coordinates voluntary standards in the United States. Many standards developers and participants support ANSI as the central body responsible for the identification of a single consistent set of voluntary standards called American National Standards. ANSI provides an open forum for all concerned interests to identify specific business needs, plan to meet those needs, and agree on standards.

ANSI itself does not develop standards. However, its approval of standards indicates that the principles of openness and due process have been followed in the approval process and that a consensus of those participating in the approval process has been achieved.

In 1979, ANSI chartered a new committee, known as the **Accredited Standards Committee (ASC) X12, Electronic Data Interchange** (referred to as ASC X12). The charge of the committee is to develop uniform standards for the electronic interchange of business transactions. The work of ASC X12 is conducted primarily by a series of subcommittees and task forces whose major function is the development of new, and the maintenance of existing, EDI standards. The standards adopted for EDI are called ANSI ASC X12N and include:

- Professional/institutional X12N 837 Healthcare Claim Transactions, version 4010

- X12N 837 Coordination of Benefits (COB) transactions

- X12N 835 Health Care Claim (HCC) Payment/Advice (or remittance advice, RA) transactions

To implement the HIPAA administrative simplification provisions, the above transaction standards are included under part 162 of title 45 of the Code of Federal Regulations (CFR) as the standard for processing electronic healthcare claims, coordination of benefits, and **remittance advice** (RA) transmissions. All other formats for electronic healthcare claims, **coordination of benefits** (COB) **transactions,** and RA transmissions became obsolete for submission of claims data, exchange of COB data, and submission of remittance data within two years after the effective date of the publication of part 162 in the *Federal Register.* For most providers, compliance was required by October 2003 for the electronic transaction rule (and by April 2003 for the HIPAA privacy rule).

The healthcare claims transaction is the transmission of a request to obtain payment for healthcare, along with the necessary accompanying information from a healthcare provider to a health plan. If no direct claim is transmitted because the reimbursement contract is based on a mechanism other than charges or reimbursement rates for specific services (for example, managed care capitation contract), the transaction is the transmission of encounter information for the purpose of reporting healthcare. Transactions including coordination of benefits (COB), explanation of benefits (EOB), and remittance advice (RA) are discussed at the beginning of this section.

Check Your Understanding 7.8

Instructions: Indicate whether the following statements are true or false (T or F).

1. _____ Medicare carrier and fiscal intermediaries serve as the financial agent between providers and the federal government to locally administer Medicare Part A and Part B.

2. _____ The CMS-1500 is submitted to Medicare carriers to process hospital outpatient claims.

3. _____ The UB-92 is also referred to as the CMS-1500.

4. _____ The data elements and design of the CMS-1450 are the responsibility of the National Uniform Claim Committee.

5. _____ The UB-92 is submitted to Medicare fiscal intermediaries, and the CMS-1500 is submitted to Medicare carriers.

6. _____ Revenue codes are associated with the CMS-1450.

7. _____ Medicare carriers process Part A claims for providers.

8. _____ The abbreviation used to describe the electronic transfer of information (for example, electronic claim) is EDI.

9. _____ Uniform standards for the electronic interchange of business transactions are the responsibility of the ASC X12 EDI committee.

10. _____ A Medicare electronic remittance advice can be submitted on paper or tape.

Reimbursement Support Processes

Reimbursement support processes are routinely reviewed and revised by third-party payers to control payments to providers. Healthcare facilities also implement reimbursement support processes to make sure that they are receiving the level of reimbursement to which they are entitled. Third-party payers revise fee schedules, and healthcare facilities revise chargemasters, evaluate the quality of documentation and coding, conduct internal audits, and implement compliance programs.

Management of the Fee Schedules

Third-party payers that reimburse providers on a fee-for-service basis generally update fee schedules on an annual basis. A fee schedule is a list of healthcare services and procedures (usually CPT/HCPCS codes) and charges associated with each. (See table 7.16.) The fee schedule (sometimes referred to as a table of allowances) represents the approved payment levels for a given insurance plan (for example, Medicare, Medicaid, and BC/BS).

Physicians, practitioners, and suppliers must notify Medicare by December 31 of each year whether they intend to participate in the Medicare program during the coming year. Medicare participation means that the provider or supplier agrees to accept assignment for all covered services provided to Medicare patients. To accept assignment means the provider or supplier accepts, as payment in full, the allowed charge (from the fee schedule). The provider or supplier is prohibited from **balance billing,** which means the patient cannot be held responsible for charges in excess of the Medicare fee schedule.

However, participating providers may bill patients for services that are not covered by Medicare. Physicians must notify a patient that the service will not be paid for by giving the patient a Notice of Exclusions from Medicare Benefits.

Table 7.16. Sample section from a chargemaster

Charge Code	Item Description	CPT/HCPCS Code			Revenue Code	G/L Key	Activity Date
		Insurance Code A	Insurance Code B	Insurance Code C			
2110410000	ECHO ENCEPHALOGRAM	76506	76506	Y7030	320	15	12/2/2004
2110410090	F/U ECHO ENCEPHALOGRAM	76506	76506	Y7040	320	15	12/2/2004
2110413000	PORT US ECHO ENCEPHALOGRAM	76506	76506	Y7050	320	15	12/2/2004
2120411000	ULTRASOUND SPINAL CONTENTS	76800	76800	Y7060	320	15	12/2/2004
2130401000	THYROID SONOGRAM	76536	76536	Y7070	320	15	1/1/2006
2151111000	TM JOINTS BILATERAL	70330	70330	Y7080	320	15	8/12/2005
2161111000	NECK LAT ONLY	70360	70360	Y7090	320	15	10/1/2004
2162111000	LARYNX AP & LATERAL	70360	70360	Y7100	320	15	10/1/2004
2201111000	LONG BONE CHLD AP	76061	76061	Y7110	320	15	8/12/2005
2201401000	NON-VASCULAR EXTREM SONO	76880	76880	Y7120	320	15	10/1/2004
2210111000	SKULL 1 VIEW	70250	70250	Y7130	320	15	1/1/2006
2210112000	SKULL 2 VIEWS	70250	70250	Y7140	320	15	8/12/2005
2210114000	SKULL 4 VIEWS	70260	70260	Y7150	320	15	8/12/2005
2211111000	MASTOIDS	70130	70130	Y7160	320	15	1/1/2006
2212111000	MANDIBLE	70110	70110	Y7170	320	15	12/2/2004
2213111000	FACIAL BONES	70140	70140	Y7180	320	15	12/2/2004
2213114000	FACIAL BONES MIN 4	70150	70150	Y7190	320	15	12/2/2004
2214111000	NASAL BONES	70160	70160	Y7200	320	15	1/1/2006
2215111000	ORBITS	70200	70200	Y7210	320	15	1/1/2006
2217111000	PARANASAL SINUSES	70220	70220	Y7220	320	15	1/1/2006

If a provider believes that a service may be denied by Medicare because it could be considered unnecessary, he must notify the patient before the treatment begins using an **Advance Beneficiary Notice** (ABN). (See figure 7.9, p. 310.)

Nonparticipating providers (NonPAR) do not sign a participation agreement with Medicare but may or may not accept assignment. If the nonPAR physician elects to accept assignment, he or she is paid 95 percent (5% less than participating physicians) of the MFS. For example, if the MFS amount is $200, the PAR provider receives $160 (80% of $200), but the nonPAR provider receives only $152 (95% of $160).

NonPAR providers who choose not to accept assignment are subject to Medicare's limiting charge rule, which states that a physician may not charge a patient more than 115 percent of the nonparticipating fee schedule. The provider collects the full amount from the patient, and Medicare reimburses the patient. figure 7.10, p. 311, illustrates the various fee schedules by type of provider.

Management of the Chargemaster

The chargemaster (table 7.17, p. 311), also called the charge description master (CDM), contains information about healthcare services (and transactions) provided to a patient. Its primary purpose is to allow the provider to accurately charge routine services and supplies to the patient. Services, supplies, and procedures included on the chargemaster generate reimbursement for almost 75 percent of UB-92 claims submitted for outpatient services alone.

Figure 7.9.   Advance Beneficiary Notice (ABN)

Patient's Name: _____   Medicare # (HICN): _____

ADVANCE BENEFICIARY NOTICE (ABN)

NOTE: You need to make a choice about receiving these health care items or services.

We expect that Medicare will not pay for the item(s) or service(s) that are described below. Medicare does not pay for all of your health care costs. Medicare only pays for covered items and services when Medicare rules are met. The fact that Medicare may not pay for a particular item or service does not mean that you should not receive it. There may be a good reason your doctor recommended it. Right now, in your case, **Medicare probably will not pay for –**

Items or Services:

Because:

The purpose of this form is to help you make an informed choice about whether or not you want to receive these items or services, knowing that you might have to pay for them yourself. Before you make a decision about your options, you should **read this entire notice carefully.**
- x Ask us to explain, if you don't understand why Medicare probably won't pay.
- x Ask us how much these items or services will cost you (**Estimated Cost: $**_____), in case you have to pay for them yourself or through other insurance.

PLEASE CHOOSE **ONE** OPTION. CHECK **ONE** BOX.   **SIGN & DATE** YOUR CHOICE.

Option 1. YES.   I want to receive these items or services.

I understand that Medicare will not decide whether to pay unless I receive these items or services. Please submit my claim to Medicare. I understand that you may bill me for items or services and that I may have to pay the bill while Medicare is making its decision. If Medicare does pay, you will refund to me any payments I made to you that are due to me. If Medicare denies payment, I agree to be personally and fully responsible for payment. That is, I will pay personally, either out of pocket or through any other insurance that I have. I understand I can appeal Medicare's decision.

Option 2. NO.   I have decided not to receive these items or services.

I will not receive these items or services. I understand that you will not be able to submit a claim to Medicare and that I will not be able to appeal your opinion that Medicare won't pay.

_____   _____
       Date   **Signature of patient or person acting on patient's behalf**

NOTE: Your health information will be kept confidential. Any information that we collect about you on this form will be kept confidential in our offices. If a claim is submitted to Medicare, your health information on this form may be shared with Medicare. Your health information which Medicare sees will be kept confidential by Medicare.

OMB Approval No. 0938-0566   Form No. CMS-R-131-G   (June 2002)

Figure 7.10. Examples of physician reimbursement methodologies

Participating Provider
Physician's fee	$180.00
MFS	$105.00
Medicare pays 80% of MFS or	$ 84.00
Patient pays 20% of MFS or	$ 21.00
Physician write-off ($180–$105)	$ 75.00

Nonparticipating provider who accepts assignment
Physician's fee	$180.00
MFS	$105.00
Medicare nonPAR fee (95% of $105)	$ 99.75
Medicare pays 80% of nonPAR fee	$ 79.80
Patient pays 20% of nonPAR fee	$ 19.95
Physician write-off ($180–$99.75)	$ 80.25

Nonparticipating provider who does not accept assignment
Physician's normal fee	$180.00
MFS	$105.00
Medicare nonPAR fee (95% of $105)	$ 99.75
Limiting charge (115% of $99.75)	$114.71
Patient billed	$114.71
Medicare pays patient (80% of nonPAR fee)	$ 79.80
Patient out of pocket ($114.71–$79.80)	$ 34.91

Table 7.17. Partial 2005 physician fee schedule payment amounts for services covered by the Medicare physician fee schedule—Western New York State region

Carrier Number	Locality Code	CPT Code	Nonfacility Fee Schedule Amount	Facility Fee Schedule Amount
00801	99	10040	81.86	74.10
00801	99	10060	90.06	80.20
00801	99	10061	161.77	150.49
00801	99	10080	156.42	86.28
00801	99	10081	242.71	152.13
00801	99	10120	125.79	83.50
00801	99	10121	233.86	172.89

The information that makes up a chargemaster line item may vary from one facility to another. There are, however, some common elements found in a typical chargemaster (Schraffenberger 2005, pp. 135–36). These include:

- *Description of service:* Examples might be the evaluation and management visit, observation, or emergency room visit.

- *CPT/HCPCS code:* This code must correspond to the description of the service.

- *Revenue code (also called the UB-92 code):* The revenue code is a three-digit code that describes a classification of a product or service provided to the patient. These revenue or UB-92 codes are required by CMS for reporting services. (See table 7.18 for examples of revenue codes.)

- *Charge amount:* This is the amount the facility charges for the procedure or service. It is not necessarily what the facility will be reimbursed by the third-party payer.

- *Charge or service code:* The charge or service code is an internally assigned number that is unique to the facility. It identifies each procedure listed on the chargemaster and identifies the department or revenue center that initiated the charge. The charge code can be very useful for revenue tracking and budget analysis.

- *General ledger key:* The general ledger key is a two- or three-digit number that assigns a line item to a section of the general ledger in the hospital's accounting system.

- *Activity/status date:* The activity/status date indicates the most recent activity of an item.

Chargemasters may allow more than one CPT/HCPCS code per item to differentiate between payment schedules for different payers.

The CDM also can be used as a tool for collecting workload statistics that can be used to monitor production and compile budgets. (Use of the CDM for tracking productivity is not best practice.) It is often used as a decision support tool to evaluate costs related to resources and to prepare for contract negotiations with managed care organizations.

The CDM relieves coders from coding repetitive services and supplies that require little, if any, formal documentation analysis. In these circumstances, the patient is billed automatically by linking the service to the appropriate CPT/HCPCS code (referred to as **hard-coding**). The advantage of hard-coding is that the code for the procedure will be reproduced accurately each time that a test, service, or procedure is ordered. Services in the following areas are typically hard-coded: radiology, laboratory, EEG and EKG, rehabilitative services, and respiratory therapy (Schraffenberger 2005, p. 134).

Maintenance of the Chargemaster
The chargemaster must be updated routinely. Maintenance of the chargemaster is best accomplished by representatives from health information management, clinical services, finance, the business office/patient financial services, compliance, and information systems. The HIM professionals are generally consulted regarding the update of CPT codes. The CDM is updated when new CPT codes become available, when departments request a new item, and when the medical fee schedules/PPS rates are updated.

Table 7.18. Examples of UB-92 revenue codes

Revenue Code	Description
250	Pharmacy—General
251	Pharmacy—Generic Drugs
252	Pharmacy—Nongeneric Drugs
253	Pharmacy—Take-Home Drugs
260	IV Therapy—General
261	IV Therapy—Infusion Pump
262	IV Therapy—IV Therapy/Pharmacy Services
263	IV Therapy—IV Therapy/Drug/Supply Delivery
270	Medical/Surgical Supplies and Devices—General
271	Medical/Surgical Supplies and Devices—Nonsterile Supply
272	Medical/Surgical Supplies and Devices—Sterile Supply
273	Medical/Surgical Supplies and Devices—Take-Home Supplies
280	Oncology—General
289	Oncology—Other
290	DME—General
291	DME—Rental
292	DME—Purchase of New DME
293	DME—Purchase of Used DME
300	Laboratory-General
301	Laboratory—Chemistry
302	Laboratory—Immunology
303	Laboratory—Renal Patient (Home)
310	Laboratory Pathological—General
311	Laboratory Pathological—Cytology
312	Laboratory Pathological—Histology
320	Radiology—Diagnostic—General
321	Radiology—Diagnostic—Angiocardiography
322	Radiology—Diagnostic—Arthrography
360	Operating Room Services—General
361	Operating Room Services—Minor Surgery
362	Operating Room Services—Organ Transplant—Other Than Kidney
370	Anesthesia—General
371	Anesthesia—Incident to Radiology
372	Anesthesia—Incident to Other Diagnostic Services
410	Respiratory Services—General
411	Respiratory Services—Inhalation Services
412	Respiratory Services—Hyperbaric Oxygen Therapy

Some of the basic responsibilities of the CDM committee include (Rhodes 1999):

- Developing policies and procedures for the chargemaster review process

- Performing an annual chargemaster review when new CPT/HCPCS codes are available

- Reviewing key elements of the annual chargemaster review, including all CPT codes for accuracy, validity, and relationship to the CDM

- Reviewing all procedures and service descriptions for accuracy and clinical appropriateness

- Reviewing all revenue codes for accuracy and linkage to charge description numbers

- Ensuring that the usage of all HCPCS, CPT, and revenue codes is in compliance with Medicare guidelines or other existing payer contracts

- Reviewing all charge dollar amounts for appropriateness by payer

- Reviewing all charge description numbers for uniqueness and validity

- Reviewing all department code numbers for uniqueness and validity

- Performing ongoing chargemaster maintenance as the facility adds new procedures or deletes obsolete ones, updates technology, or changes services provided

- Establishing a procedure to allow clinical department directors to submit chargemaster change requests for new, deleted, or revised procedures or services

- Making sure there is no duplication of code assignment by coders and chargemaster-assigned codes in any department

- Reviewing all charge ticket and order-entry screens for accuracy against the chargemaster and appropriate mapping to CPT/HCPCS codes, when required

- Reviewing and complying with directives in Medicare bulletins, transmittals, Medicare manual updates, and official coding guidelines

- Complying with guidelines in the NCCI or other known coding or bundling edits

- Carefully considering any application that involves one charge description number "exploding" into more than one CPT/HCPCS code to prevent inadvertent **unbundling** and unearned reimbursement for services

- Reviewing and taking action on all RA denials involving HCPCS/CPT coding or CMS coding guidelines

An inaccurate chargemaster adversely affects facility reimbursement, compliance, and data quality. According to a 1999 AHIMA practice brief (Rhodes 1999), negative effects that may result from an inaccurate chargemaster include overpayment, underpayment, undercharging for delivery of healthcare services, claims rejections, and fines/penalties. Chargemaster programs are automated and involve the billing of numerous services for high volumes of patients, often without human intervention. Therefore, it is highly likely that a single error on the chargemaster could result in multiple errors before it is identified and corrected, resulting in a serious financial impact.

Management of the Revenue Cycle

Revenue cycle management involves many different processes and people, all working to make sure that the healthcare facility is properly reimbursed for the services provided. Effectively managing the revenue cycle is paramount to improving the revenues received by the facility. Delays in payment, denied claims, and other lost revenues impact tremendously on the facility's financial health.

The revenue cycle involves many functions in addition to the process of billing. According to an AHIMA practice brief (Youmans 2004), the major functions typically include:

- Admitting, patient access management
- Case management
- Charge capture
- Health information management
- Patient financial services, business office
- Finance
- Compliance
- Information technology

Revenue Cycle Management Committee

An effective method for managing the revenue cycle is through a revenue cycle management committee or team composed of individuals from all the departments involved in the revenue cycle. The HIM professional is an important player on this team. Various team members should analyze the revenue cycle indicators, which include:

- Value and volume of discharged, not final billed encounters
- Number of accounts receivable (AR) days
- Number of bill-hold days
- Percentage and amount of write-offs
- Percentage of clean claims
- Percentage of claims returned to provider
- Percentage of denials
- Percentage of accounts-missing documents
- Number of query forms
- Percentage of late charges

- Percentage of accurate registrations

- Percentage of increased point-of-service collections for elective procedures

- Percentage of increased DRG payments due to improved documentation and coding (Youmans 2004)

The HIM professional's area of expertise is varied and will be extremely useful in denials management, data analysis and presentation, write-off preparation, policy development, response to patient financial services requests, and review of OCEs and groupers.

Chapter 25 of this text also addresses revenue cycle management in relation to the financial management of the facility.

Management of Documentation and Coding Quality

According to Deborah Elder, manager of inpatient and outpatient coding services, Medical Management Plus, Inc., in Birmingham, Alabama:

> The importance of complete and accurate coding cannot be underestimated. ICD-9-CM and CPT-4 coding drives reimbursement and also presents a mechanism by which external and internal agents evaluate utilization of services, quality of care, and the hospital's patient acuity level. This numerically abbreviated medical information is only as complete as the physician documentation and is only as accurate as the coder's translation. Coders have a monumental impact on the hospital and this impact will broaden as other health care services are converted to a prospective payment method of reimbursement, including Outpatient Services, Extended Care Facilities and Home Health Agencies (Elder 2000).

The cornerstone of accurate coding is physician documentation. According to an AHIMA practice brief (Prophet 2001, pp. 88I–M), ensuring the accuracy of coded data is a shared responsibility between coding professionals and physicians. Accurate diagnostic and procedural coded data originate from collaboration between physicians, who have a clinical background, and coding professionals, who have an understanding of classification systems.

Complete, accurate, legible, and timely documentation should:

- Address the clinical significance of abnormal test results

- Support the intensity of patient evaluation and treatment and describe the thought processes and complexity of decision making

- Include all diagnostic and therapeutic procedures, treatments, and tests performed, in addition to their results

- Include any changes in the patient's condition, including psychosocial and physical symptoms

- Include all conditions that co-exist at the time of admission, that subsequently develop, or that affect the treatment received and the length of stay. This encompasses all conditions that affect patient care in terms of requiring clinical evaluation, therapeutic treatment, diagnostic procedures, extended length of hospital stay, or increased nursing care and monitoring

- Be updated as necessary to reflect all diagnoses relevant to the care or services provided

- Be consistent and discuss and reconcile any discrepancies (this reconciliation should be documented in the medical record)

- Be legible and written in ink, typewritten, or electronically signed, stored and printed (Prophet 2001)

Coding and Corporate Compliance

The federal government has initiated efforts to investigate healthcare fraud and to establish guidelines to ensure corporate compliance with the government guidelines. Part of the initiative involved providing healthcare organizations with guidelines for developing comprehensive compliance programs with specific policies and procedures.

History of Fraud and Abuse and Corporate Compliance in Healthcare

Probably the most pertinent fact in the history of corporate compliance related to healthcare organizations is that the federal government, specifically the HHS, is the largest purchaser of healthcare in the United States. Because one of the federal government's duties is to use the taxpayers' monies wisely, federal agencies must ensure that the healthcare provided to enrollees in federal healthcare programs is appropriate and is actually provided.

Several federal initiatives and pieces of legislation related to investigating, identifying, and preventing healthcare fraud and abuse have been passed. Interestingly, the basis of these initiatives and laws lies within the Civil False Claims Act, which was passed during the Civil War to prevent government contractors from overbilling for services provided. The original law was updated and reinforced in subsequent legislation and is still used to prosecute offenders.

Several government agencies are involved in detecting, prosecuting, and preventing fraud and abuse. Among them are the HHS, the Office of the Inspector General (OIG), the Department of Justice (the attorney general), the Federal Bureau of Investigation (FBI), CMS, the Drug Enforcement Agency (DEA), the Internal Revenue Service (IRS), and state attorney generals.

Many initiatives are joint efforts among the agencies. For example, Operation Restore Trust, which began in 1995, is a joint effort of HHS, OIG, CMS, and the Administration on Aging. Operation Restore Trust spent only $7.9 million in the first two years to identify $188 million in overpayments to providers. It also led to implementation of special fraud alerts notifying providers of current investigative findings and to the **Voluntary Disclosure Program.**

The federal government began to actively investigate fraud in the Medicare program in 1977 with passage of the Anti-Fraud and Abuse Amendments of 1977 to Title XIX of the Social Security Act (SSA). However, detecting, preventing, and prosecuting fraud and abuse did not reach true prominence until the Health Insurance Portability and Accountability Act of 1996 (HIPAA) established Sections 1128C and 1128D of the SSA. Sections 1128C and 1128D authorized the OIG to conduct investigations, audits, and evaluations related to healthcare fraud. The BBA focused on fraud and abuse issues specifically relating to penalties.

The BBA also required that physicians and practitioners provide diagnostic information (to show medical necessity) prior to a facility performing lab or radiology services for a patient.

As previously mentioned, HIPAA expanded the OIG's duties to include:

- Coordination of federal, state, and local enforcement efforts targeting healthcare fraud
- Provision of industry guidance concerning fraudulent healthcare practices
- Establishment of a national data bank for reporting final adverse actions against healthcare providers

Significantly, HIPAA authorizes the OIG to investigate cases of healthcare fraud that involve private healthcare plans as well as federally funded programs, although, according to information on the OIG Web site, present policies restrict the OIG's investigative focus to cases of fraud that affect federally funded programs.

A major portion of HIPAA focused on identifying medically unnecessary services, **upcoding,** unbundling, and billing for services not provided. Upcoding is the practice of assigning a diagnosis or procedure code specifically for the purpose of obtaining a higher level of payment. It is most often found when reimbursement-grouping systems are used.

Unbundling is the practice of using multiple codes that describe individual components of a procedure rather than an appropriate single code that describes all steps of the procedure performed. Unbundling is a component of the NCCI.

HIPAA also expanded sanctions related to mandatory exclusion from Medicare, length of exclusion, failure to comply with statutory obligations, and antikickback penalties (Schraffenberger 2005).

From February 1998 until the present, the OIG continues to issue **compliance program guidance** for various types of healthcare organizations. The OIG Web site (www.oig.hhs.gov) posts the documents that most healthcare organizations need to develop fraud and abuse compliance plans. The goal of compliance programs is to prevent accusations of fraud and abuse, make operations run more smoothly, improve services, and contain costs (Anderson 2000).

Elements of Corporate Compliance

In the February 23, 1998 *Federal Register* (p. 8989), the OIG outlined the following seven elements as the minimum necessary for a comprehensive compliance program:

1. The development and distribution of written standards of conduct, as well as written policies and procedures that promote the hospital's commitment to compliance and that address specific areas of potential fraud, such as claims development and submission processes, code gaming, and financial relationships with physicians and other healthcare professionals

2. The designation of a chief compliance officer and other appropriate bodies, for example, a corporate compliance committee, charged with the responsibility for operating and monitoring the compliance program, and who report directly to the CEO and the governing body

3. The development and implementation of regular, effective education and training programs for all affected employees

4. The maintenance of a process, such as a hotline, to receive complaints and the adoption of procedures to protect the anonymity of complainants and to protect whistleblowers from retaliation

5. The development of a system to respond to allegations of improper/illegal activities and the enforcement of appropriate disciplinary action against employees who have violated internal compliance policies, applicable statutes, regulations, or federal healthcare program requirements

6. The use of audits and/or other evaluation techniques to monitor compliance and assist in the reduction of identified problem areas

7. The investigation and remediation of identified systemic problems and the development of policies addressing the nonemployment or retention of sanctioned individuals

The OIG believes that a compliance program conforming to these elements above will not only "fulfill the organization's legal duty to ensure that it is not submitting false or inaccurate claims to government and private payers," but will also result in additional potential benefits, including, among others:

- Demonstration of the organization's commitment to responsible conduct toward employees and the community

- Provision of a more accurate view of behavior relating to fraud and abuse

- Identification and prevention of criminal and unethical conduct

- Improvements in the quality of patient care

In the January 31, 2005 *Federal Register,* the supplemental compliance program guidance for hospitals was published. This document supplements rather than replaces the 1998 compliance program guidance (CPG) document. The supplemental CPG contains new compliance recommendations and an expanded discussion of risk areas, current enforcement priorities, and lessons learned in the area of corporate compliance.

(For additional resources on compliance and fraud and abuse, see figure 7.11.)

Figure 7.11.   Online compliance resources

Department of Health and Human Services, Office of the Inspector General	www.oig.hhs.gov
American Health Information Management Association	www.ahima.org
Health Care Compliance Association	www.hcca-info.org
National Health Care Anti-Fraud Association	www.nhcaa.org
Centers for Medicare and Medicaid Services	www.cms.hhs.gov
CMS Fraud Page	www.medicare.gov

Relationship between Coding Practice and Corporate Compliance

Any corporate compliance program must contain references to complete and accurate coding. Many of the documented fraud and abuse convictions have centered on the coding function.

OIG Work Plan

At the beginning of each fiscal year, the OIG publishes guidance on its "special areas of concern" for the upcoming year. The OIG refers to this as its work plan. The table of contents for the 2005 Work Plan is shown in figure 7.12; the full plan can be found on the OIG web site (oig.hhs.gov).

The HIM Compliance Program

As mentioned above, one element of the corporate compliance program addresses the coding function. Because the accuracy and completeness of ICD-9-CM and CPT code assignment determine the provider payment, the reference to coding is not surprising. Thus, it is important that healthcare organizations have a strong coding compliance program. This coding compliance plan should be based on the same principles as that of the corporate-wide program. The basic elements of a coding plan should include:

- Code of conduct
- Policies and procedures
- Education and training
- Communication
- Auditing
- Corrective action
- Reporting

Code of Conduct
The HIM department should develop a code of conduct or perhaps adopt AHIMA's Standards of Ethical Coding.

Policies and Procedures
Policies and procedures that describe the facility's coding standards and functions should be documented. This should be done through a coding compliance manual. Some of the items that should be included in this manual include policies on the following: ambiguous or incomplete documentation, rebilling of problem claims, use of official coding guidelines, issues where no official guidelines exist, and clarification of new or confusing coding issues.

Education and Training
Periodic and staff-appropriate education of staff is a key factor in a successful coding compliance program. Education for coders should be provided monthly (Schraffenberger 2005).

Figure 7.12.   HHS/OIG fiscal year 2005 work plan table of contents

Medicare Hospitals
Quality Improvement Organization Mediation of Beneficiary Complaints
Medical Education Payments for Dental and Podiatry
    Residents
Nursing and Allied Health Education Payments
Graduate Medical Education Voluntary Supervision in Nonhospital
    Settings
Postacute Care Transfers
Diagnosis-Related Group Coding
Inpatient Prospective Payment System Wage Indices
Inpatient Outlier and Other Charge-Related Issues
Inpatient Rehabilitation Facilities Payments
Inpatient Rehabilitation Payments–Late Assessments
Medical Necessity of Inpatient Psychiatric Stays
Consecutive Inpatient Stays
Long-Term Care Hospital Payments
Level of Care in Long-Term Care Hospitals
Critical Access Hospitals
Organ Acquisition Costs
Rebates Paid to Hospitals
Coronary Artery Stents
Outpatient Cardiac Rehabilitation Services
Outpatient Outlier and Other Charge-Related Issues
Lifetime Reserve Days
Hospital Reporting of Restraint-Related Deaths

Medicare Home Health
Beneficiary Access to Home Health Agencies
Effect of Prospective Payment System on Quality of Home Health Care
Home Health Outlier Payments
Enhanced Payments for Home Health Therapy

Medicare Nursing Homes
Access to Skilled Nursing Facilities under the Prospective Payment System
Use of Additional Funds Provided to Skilled Nursing Facilities
Nurse Aide Registries
Nursing Home Deficiency Trends
Nursing Home Compliance with Minimum Data Set Reporting
    Requirements
Nursing Home Resident Assessment and Care Planning
Enforcement Actions against Noncompliant Nursing Homes
Nursing Home Informal Dispute Resolution
Nursing Home Residents' Rights
Skilled Nursing Facilities' Involvement in Consecutive Inpatient Stays
Imaging and Laboratory Services in Nursing Homes
Skilled Nursing Facility Rehabilitation and Infusion Therapy Services
State Compliance with Complaint Investigation
    Guidelines

Medicare Physicians and Other Health Professionals
Billing Service Companies
Medicare Payments to VA Physicians
Care Plan Oversight
Ordering Physicians Excluded from Medicare
Physician Services at Skilled Nursing Facilities
Physician Pathology Services
Cardiography and Echocardiography Services
Physical and Occupational Therapy Services
Part B Mental Health Services
Wound Care Services
Coding of Evaluation and Management Services
Use of Modifier –25
Use of Modifiers with National Correct Coding Initiative Edits
"Long Distance" Physician Claims
Provider-Based Entities

Medicare Medical Equipment and Supplies
Medical Necessity of Durable Medical Equipment
Medicare Pricing of Equipment and Supplies

Medicare Drug Reimbursement
Prescription Drug Cards
Employer Subsidies for Drug Coverage
Beneficiary Understanding of Drug Discount Card Program
Computation of Average Sales Price
Collecting and Maintaining Average Sales Price Data
Adequacy of Reimbursement Rate for Drugs under ASP
Payments for Non-End-Stage Renal Disease Epoetin Alfa

Other Medicare Services
Laboratory Services Rendered during an Inpatient Stay
Laboratory Proficiency Testing
Independent Diagnostic Testing Facilities
Therapy Services Provided by Comprehensive Outpatient Rehabilitation
    Facilities
New Payment Provisions for Ambulance Services
Air Ambulance Services
Quality of Care in Dialysis Facilities
Monitoring of Market Prices for Part B Drugs
Follow-up on Medicare Part B Payments for Ambulance Services
Follow-up on Medicare Part B Payments for Radiology Services
Emergency Health Services for Undocumented Aliens

Medicare Managed Care
Benefit Stabilization Fund
Adjusted Community Rate Proposals
Follow-up on Adjusted Community Rate Proposals
Administrative Costs
Managed Care Encounter Data
Enhanced Managed Care Payments
Enhanced Payments under the Risk Adjustment Model
Managed Care Excessive Medical Costs
Duplicate Medicare Payments to Cost-Based Plans
Prompt Payment
Marketing Practices of MCOs
Managed Care "Deeming" Organizations

Medicare Contractor Operations
Preaward Reviews of Contract Proposals
CMS Oversight of Contractor Performance
Program Safeguard Contractor Performance
Accuracy of the Provider Enrollment, Chain, and Ownership System
Handling of Beneficiary Inquiries
Carrier Medical Review: Progressive Corrective Action
Duplicate Medicare Part B Payments
Contractors' Administrative Costs
Pension Segmentation
Pension Costs Claimed
Unfunded Pension Costs
Pension Segment Closing
Postretirement Benefits and Supplemental Employee Retirement
    Plan Costs

Medicaid Hospitals
Medicaid Graduate Medical Education Payments
Hospital Outlier Payments
Medicaid Diagnosis-Related Group Payment Window
Disproportionate Share Hospital Payments
Hospital Eligibility for Disproportionate Share Hospital Payments

(Continued on next page)

Figure 7.12. *(Continued)*

Medicaid Long-Term and Community Care
Payments to Public Nursing Facilities
Community Residence Claims
Assisted Living Facilities
Medicaid Home Health Care Services
Targeted Case Management
Personal Care Services
Home- and Community-Based Services Administrative Costs
Medicaid Eligibility and the Working Disabled

Medicaid Mental Health Services
Nursing Home Residents with Mental Illness and Mental Retardation
Claims for Residents of Institutions for Mental Diseases
Medicaid Services for Mentally Disabled Persons
Rehabilitation Services for Persons with Mental Illnesses
Community Mental Health Centers
Medicaid Reimbursement for Intermediate Care Facilities
Restraint and Seclusion in Children's Psychiatric Residential Treatment
    Facilities

Medicaid/State Children's Health Insurance Program
Duplicate Claims for Medicaid and State Children's Health Insurance
    Program
Enrollment of Medicaid Eligibles in SCHIP
State Evaluations of SCHIP Programs
Detecting and Investigating Fraud and Abuse in SCHIP

Medicaid Drug Reimbursement
Average Manufacturer Price and Average Wholesale Price
Medicaid Drug Rebates–Computation of AMP and Best Price
Oversight of Drug Manufacturer Recalculations for Medicaid Drug
    Rebates
Indexing the Generic Drug Rebate
Drug Rebate Impact from Drugs Incorrectly Classified as Generic
Dispute Resolution in the Medicaid Prescription Drug Rebate
    Program
Medicaid Drug Rebate Collections
Overprescribing of OxyContin and Other Psychotropic Drugs
Accuracy of Pricing Drugs in the Federal Upper-Limit Program
Medicaid Drug Utilization Review Program

Other Medicaid Services
Family Planning Services
School-Based Health Services
Adult Rehabilitative Services
Controls over the Vaccine for Children Program
Outpatient Alcoholism Services
Claims Paid for Clinical Diagnostic Laboratory Services
Payments for Services Provided after Beneficiaries' Deaths
Marketing and Enrollment Practices by Medicaid Managed Care
    Entities
Factors Affecting the Development, Referral, and Disposition of Medicaid
    Fraud Cases: State Agency and Medicaid Fraud Control Unit
    Experiences

Medicaid Administration
Contingency Fee Payment Arrangements
Upper Payment Limits
Calculation of Upper Payment Limits for Transition States
State Match for Medicaid Upper-Payment Limit Reimbursement
Medicaid Provider Tax Issues
State-Employed Physicians and Other Practitioners
Skilled Professional Medical Personnel
Physician Assistant Reimbursement
Medicaid Claims for Excluded Providers
Administrative Costs of Other Public Agencies
Administrative Costs for Medicaid Managed Care Contracts
University-Contributed Indirect Costs
Federal Financial Participation for Medicaid Cost Allocation Plans
Medicaid Accounts Receivable
Section 1115 Demonstration Waiver
Medicaid Management Information System Expenditures
Appropriateness of Medicaid Payments
Medicaid FFS Payments for Beneficiaries Enrolled in Managed Care
CMS Oversight of Home- and Community-Based Waivers

Information Systems Controls
Security Planning for CMS Systems under Development
Accuracy of the Fraud Investigation Database
Medicaid Statistical Information System
State Controls over Medicaid Payments and Program Eligibility
Replacement State Medicaid System
Smart Card Technology
Compliance with the Health Insurance Portability and Accountability Act
    Privacy Final Rule–University Hospital
MCO's Compliance With HIPAA

General Administration
FY 2004 Medicare Error Rate Estimate
FY 2005 Medicare Error Rate Estimate
Group Purchasing Organizations
Contractual Arrangements with Suppliers
Corporate Integrity Agreements
State Medical Boards as a Source of Patient Safety Data
Payments for Services to Dually Eligible Beneficiaries
Nursing Home Quality of Care: Promising Approaches
Payments to Psychiatric Facilities Improperly Certified as Nursing
    Facilities

Investigations
Health Care Fraud
Provider Self-Disclosure

Legal Counsel
Compliance Program Guidance to the Healthcare Industry
Resolution of False Claims Act Cases and Negotiation of Corporate
    Integrity Agreements
Providers' Compliance with Corporate Integrity Agreements
Advisory Opinions and Fraud Alerts
Antikickback Safe Harbors
Patient Antidumping Statute Enforcement
Program Exclusions
Civil Monetary Penalties

Areas that could be covered at training sessions include:

- The OIG work plan
- Clinical information related to problematic body systems, diagnoses, and procedures
- Changes to the PPSs
- Changes to ICD-9-CM, HCPCS Level II, and CPT codes
- Application of the ICD-9-CM Official Guidelines for Coding and Reporting
- Issues in *Coding Clinic for ICD-9-CM*
- Issues in *CPT Assistant*

All newly hired coding personnel should receive extensive training on the facility's and HIM department's compliance programs.

Education of the medical staff on documentation is likewise important to the success of any coding compliance program. Documentation education may be provided monthly, bimonthly, or quarterly depending on the importance of the issues covered (Schraffenberger 2005).

Examples of documentation problems that may need to be addressed with physicians include:

- Inconsistent documentation
- Incomplete progress notes
- Undocumented care
- Test results not addressed in physician documentation
- Historical diagnoses being documented as current diagnoses
- Long-standing, chronic conditions that are not documented
- Lack of documentation of postoperative complications
- Illegibility
- Documentation not completed on time (Bowman 2004)

Communication

Communication between the coding supervisor and the coding professionals is vital to ensure consistency in following coding policies and issues.

Internal Audits

Ongoing evaluation is critical to successful coding and billing for third-party payer reimbursement. In the past, the goal of internal audit programs was to increase revenues for the provider. Today, the goal is to protect providers from sanctions or fines. Healthcare organizations can implement monitoring programs by conducting regular, periodic audits of (1) ICD-9-CM and CPT/HCPCS coding and (2) claims development and submission. In addition, audits should be conducted to follow up on previous reviews that resulted in the identification of problems (for example, poor coding quality or errors in claims submission).

Auditing involves the performance of internal and/or **external reviews** to identify variations from established baselines (for example, review outpatient coding as compared with CMS outpatient coding guidelines). Internal reviews are conducted by facility-based staff (for example, HIM professionals), and external reviews are conducted by either consultants hired for this purpose (for example, corporations that specialize in such reviews and independent health information consultants) or third-party payers.

The scope and frequency of audits and the size of the sample depend on the size of the organization, available resources, the number of coding professionals, the history of noncompliance, risk factors, case complexity, and the results of initial assessments (Bowman 2004).

One of the elements of the auditing process is identification of risk areas. Some major risk areas include:

- DRG coding accuracy

- Variations in case mix

- Discharge status (transfers versus discharges)

- Services provided under arrangement

- Three-day payment window, formerly called the 72-hour rule (Under this rule, diagnostic services provided within three days of admission should be included [bundled] in the DRG, whether or not they are related to the admission. Non-diagnostic services provided within three days of admission should be included in the DRG only if they are related to the admission. All nondiagnostic services that are unrelated to the admission can be billed separately.)

- Medical necessity

- Evaluation and management services

- Chargemaster description

Selecting types of cases to review also is important. Some examples of various case selection possibilities are found in figure 7.13.

The frequency of audits depends on the individual facility; daily, weekly, monthly or quarterly audits may be considered.

The results of the audits must be analyzed to determine the reason(s) for the coding errors. Focused reviews in one particular area may be necessary to review a higher volume of cases in which there were frequent errors. Certainly, focused reviews aimed at OIG target areas would be appropriate. Significant variations from baselines should prompt an investigation to determine cause(s).

Feedback on the results of audits should be presented to interested parties such as coding staff, supervisors, and physicians.

Corrective Action
Certainly, the goal of corrective action activities is the prevention of the same or a similar problem in the future. Typical corrective actions for resolving problems identified during coding audits include:

- Revisions to policies and procedures

- Development of additional policies and procedures

- Process improvements

- Education of coders, physicians, and/or other organizational staff depending on the nature of the identified problem

- Revision or addition of routine monitoring activities

- Revisions to the chargemaster

- Additions, deletions, or revisions to systems edits

- Documentation improvement strategies

- Disciplinary action (Bowman 2004, pp. 73–74)

Reporting

Documentation on coding compliance activities should be maintained and reported as stated in the policies and procedures. Adverse findings should be reviewed with the corporate compliance officer and steps taken as necessary to report these findings.

Figure 7.13.   Examples of various case selections for auditing

Simple random sample

Medical DRGs by high dollar and high volume

Surgical DRGs by high dollar and high volume

Medical DRGs without comorbid conditions or complications

Surgical DRGs without comorbid conditions or complications

Major diagnostic category by high dollar and high volume

Most common diagnosis codes

Most common procedure codes

Significant procedure APCs by high dollar and high volume

Unlisted CPT codes

"Separate procedure" CPT codes reported in conjunction with related CPT codes

Unusual modifier usage patterns

Not elsewhere classified (NEC) and not otherwise specified (NOS) codes

Highest-level evaluation and management (E/M) codes

Consultation E/M codes

Critical Care E/M codes

Chargemaster review by service

Superbill, encounter form, and charge sheet review by specialty

Check Your Understanding 7.9

Instructions: Select the best term to complete each of the following statements.

1. _____ Fee schedules are updated by third-party payers
   a. Annually
   b. Monthly
   c. Semiannually
   d. Weekly

2. _____ To accept assignment means that the
   a. Patient authorizes payment to be made directly to the provider
   b. Provider accepts as payment in full whatever the payer reimburses
   c. Balance billing is allowed on patient accounts, but at a limited rate
   d. Participating provider always receives a higher rate of reimbursement

3. _____ A fee schedule is
   a. Developed by third-party payers and includes a list of healthcare services and procedures and charges of each
   b. Developed by providers and includes a list of healthcare services provided to a patient
   c. Developed by third-party payers and includes a list of healthcare services provided to a patient
   d. Developed by providers and lists charge codes

4. _____ An inaccurately generated chargemaster affects reimbursement, resulting in
   a. Overpayments
   b. Underpayments
   c. Claims rejections
   d. Any of the above

5. _____ Correct Coding Initiative policies implemented in 1996 to develop correct coding methodologies to improve appropriate payment of Medicare Part B claims are based on
   a. Conventions defined in the CPT codebooks
   b. Guidelines developed by the American Hospital Association
   c. An analysis of standard medical and surgical practice
   d. A review of historical coding practices and coding audits

6. _____ The goal of coding compliance programs is to prevent
   a. Accusations of fraud and abuse
   b. Delays in claims processing
   c. Billing errors
   d. Inaccurate code assignments

7. _____ The practice of assigning a diagnosis or procedure code specifically for the purpose of obtaining a higher level of payment is called:
   a. Billing
   b. Unbundling
   c. Upcoding
   d. Unnecessary service

8. _____ The essential elements of a Corporate Compliance Program are defined by
   a. CMS
   b. HIPPA
   c. Medicare
   d. OIG

Real-World Case

Itemized charges on the UB-92 that are not supported by patient record documentation are unlikely to be reimbursed by a third-party payer. Examples of charges that would not be paid upon review of the patient record in comparison to the UB-92 include the following:

- Duplicate charges for services rendered one time only (for example, multiple charges for same service, such as surgery)

- Laboratory panel tests for which there should be a single charge

- Medications and diagnostic tests not prescribed by a physician

- Medications that a patient did not receive

- Tests repeated because of hospital error

- Services listed for dates after the patient was discharged from the facility

- Professional services performed by nurses or technicians (for example, equipment monitoring)

Summary

From its very beginnings, financial reimbursement for healthcare services has followed several paths. Among these are private pay, commercial insurance, employer self-insurance, and various government programs. The mixture of payment mechanisms has made healthcare reimbursement in the United States very complex.

As a consequence, the processing of medical claims can be complicated. How a claim is processed, what documentation is required, and how much reimbursement will be paid depend on the payer and the type of claim. Many attempts have been made to create a uniform healthcare claim that would accommodate all payment mechanisms. Claims processed for payment under Medicare have been consolidated into a uniform bill.

Healthcare organizations have developed several tools to help manage the billing and reimbursement process, including development of fee schedules and chargemasters. The HIM professional is frequently called on to provide expertise in the development, management, and auditing of these tools. In addition, organizations have recognized that ongoing evaluation of the entire billing process is essential to ensure accurate payment as well as to avoid fraud and abuse sanctions or fines. The HIM professional's work is likely to involve helping to develop such audit programs in addition to conducting the audits themselves.

Over the past two decades, the billing and reimbursement process has become an integral part of the job functions of many HIM professionals. The expertise brought to bear on the process to ensure accurate and timely claims submission is critical to the operations of any healthcare organization.

Payments for the delivery of healthcare services increased from $27 billion in 1960 to more than $1.1 trillion in 1998. In response, private insurers introduced managed care programs and the federal government implemented prospective payment systems to replace the costly per diem (or traditional fee-for-service) reimbursement methods. The federal government also incorporated managed care into its healthcare programs.

Health claims reimbursement processing has evolved from the submission of hand-written CMS-1500 and UB-92 forms to specially designed forms to be used for optical scanning purposes to electronic data interchange. EDI was greatly affected by HIPAA legislation passed in 1996. Of recently enacted federal legislation affecting claims reimbursement processing, the NCCI and the OIG coding compliance programs have had the most effect on HIM professionals.

References

Abraham, P.R. 2001. *Documentation and Reimbursement for Home Health and Hospice Programs.* Chicago: American Health Information Management Association.

American Medical Association. 2004. *Current Procedural Terminology,* 2005 edition. Chicago: American Medical Association.

American Nursing Association. 1997. Position Statement. *Backgorund for ANA Position Statement on Privatization and For-Profit Conversion.* Available online from: nursingworld.org/readroom/position/practice/prpvtbkg.htm.

Anderson, S. 2000. Audit outpatient bills to get all the money you deserve. *Medical Records Briefing* 15(12):6.

Averill, R.F. 1999. Honest mistake or fraud? Meeting the coding compliance challenge. *Journal of American Health Information Management Association* 70(5):16–21.

Bowman, S. 2004. *Health Information Management Compliance: A Model Program for Healthcare Organizations.* Chicago: American Health Information Management Association.

Campbell, C., H. Schmitz, and L. Waller. 1998. *Financial Management in a Managed Care Environment.* Albany, NY: Delmar Thomson Learning.

Campbell, T. Opportunities for HIM in revenue cycle management. *Journal of American Health Information Management Association* 74(10):62–63.

Centers for Medicare and Medicaid Services. 2005. IRVEN: CMS's IRF-PAI data entry software. Available online from www.cms.hhs.gov.

Centers for Medicare and Medicaid Services. 2004. Transmittal 347, Inpatient Rehabilitation Facility (IRF) Classification Requirements. October 29, 2004.

Centers for Medicare and Medicaid Services. 2002. Transmittal AB-02-131, Implementation of the Ambulance Fee Schedule. September 27, 2002.

Coder's Desk Reference. 2004. Salt Lake City: Ingenix.

Davis, J.B. 2000. *Reimbursement Manual for the Medical Office: A Comprehensive Guide to Coding, Billing and Fee Management.* Los Angeles: Practice Management Information Corporation.

Davison, J., and M. Lewis. 2000. *Working with Insurance and Managed Care Plans: A Guide for Getting Paid.* Los Angeles: Practice Management Information Corporation.

Dougherty, M. 2000. New home care PPS brings major changes. *Journal of American Health Information Management Association* 71(10):78–82.

Elder, D. 2000. Coding: The key to compliance. Birmingham, Ala.: Medical Management Plus. Available online from mmplusinc.com

Gannon, E.J. HCFA outlines new PPS for rehabilitation facilities. Available online from mxcity.com.

Green, M.A., and J.C. Rowell. 2004. *Understanding Health Insurance: A Guide to Professional Billing.* Albany, NY: Delmar Thomson Learning.

Harkins, P.D. 2000. The alphabet soup of Medicare reimbursement. *Advance for Health Information Professionals,* October 16, p. 25.

Hazelwood, A., and C. Venable. 2004. *ICD-9-CM Diagnostic Coding for Physician Services.* Chicago: American Health Information Management Association.

Health Care Financing Administration. 2000. HHS announces electronic standards to simplify health care transactions. Available online from aspe.hhs.gov/admnsimp/final/txfin00.htm.

Himmelstein, D.V., Woolhandler, S., Hellander, I., Wolfe, S.M. Quality of care in investor-owned vs not-for-profit HMOs. 1999. *JAMA* 282: 159-163.

Johnson, S.L. 2000. *Understanding Medical Coding: A Comprehensive Guide.* Albany, NY: Delmar Thomson Learning.

Jones, J., editor. 2001. *Reimbursement Methodologies for Healthcare Services.* Chicago: American Health Information Management Association.

Kim, C., D.F. Williamson, C.M. Mangione, M.M. Safford, J.V. Selby, D.G. Marrero, J.D. Curb, T.J. Thompson, K.M. Venkat Narayan, W.H. Herman. 2004. Managed care organizations and the quality of diabetes care: The translating research into action for diabetes (TRIAD) study. *Diabetes Care* (27):1529–1534.

Lewis, M. 2003. *Medicare Rules and Regulations.* Los Angeles: Practice Management Information.

Make sure that your APC claim makes it through the OCE. 2000. *Medical Records Briefing* 15(9):1.

Medicare and You. 2005. Centers for Medicare and Medicaid Services. Available online from cms.hhs.gov/partnerships/2005medandyou.asp.

Medicare Hospital Outpatient Payment System Quick Reference Guide. 2004. Available online at cms.hhs.gov.

National Committee for Quality Assurance. ncqa.org.

Newby, C. 2005. *From Patient to Payment.* New York: McGraw-Hill.

Palmer, K. 1999. A brief history: Universal health care efforts in the US: late 1800s to Medicare. Available online from pnhp.org.

Prophet, S. 2001. Practice brief: Developing a physician query process. *Journal of American Health Information Management Association* 72(9):88I–M.

Rhodes, H. 1999. Practice brief: The care and maintenance of charge masters. *Journal of American Health Information Management Association* 70(7).

Rizzo, C.D. 2000. *Uniform Billing: A Guide to Claims Processing.* Albany, NY: Delmar Thomson Learning.

Role of the physician in the home health prospective payment system. 2000. Medicare Newsroom, November 7. Available online from hgsa.com.

Schraffenberger, L.A. 2004. *Basic ICD-9-CM Coding.* Chicago: American Health Information Management Association.

Schraffenberger, L.A. 2005. *Effective Management of Coding Services.* Chicago: American Health Information Management Association.

Schneider, E.C., A.M. Zaslaksky, A.M. Epstein. 2005 (December). Quality of care in for-profit and not-for-profit health plans enrolling Medicare beneficiaries. *American Journal of Medicine* 118(12):1392–1400.

Smith, G. 2004. *Basic CPT/HCPCS Coding.* Chicago: American Health Information Management Association.

Stewart, M. 2001. *Coding and Reimbursement under the Outpatient Prospective Payment.* Chicago: American Health Information Management Association.

3M Health Information Systems. 3Mhis.com.

Valerius, J., N. Bayes, and C. Newby. 2005. *Medical Insurance: A Guide to Coding and Reimbursement.* New York: McGraw-Hill.

Kuehn, L.. 2006. *CPT/HCPCS Coding and Reimbursement for Physician Services.* Chicago: American Health Information Management Association.

Youmans, K. 2004. Practice brief: An HIM spin on the revenue cycle. *Journal of American Health Information Management Association* 75(3):32–36.

Chapter 8
Health Information Technology Functions

Jane Roberts, MS, RHIA

Learning Objectives

- To identify the typical functions performed by the health information management (HIM) department

- To understand different operational techniques for managing traditional HIM functions

- To identify techniques used in the storage and maintenance of health records

- To understand the interrelationship between the HIM department and other key departments within the healthcare organization

- To describe the purpose, development, and maintenance of registries and indexes such as the master patient index, disease index, and operation indexes

- To discuss the functions and responsibilities of common HIM support services, including cancer and trauma registries, birth certificate completion, and statistical and research services

- To understand several techniques used in the management of the HIM department, such as policy and procedure development and the budgeting process

Key Terms

Abstracting

Alphabetic filing system

Alphanumeric filing system

APC grouper

Clinical coding

Concurrent review

Deemed status

Deficiency slip

Delinquent record

Disease index

DRG grouper

Encoder

Health record number

Joint Commission on Accreditation of Healthcare Organizations (JCAHO)

Master patient index (MPI)

Medical transcription

Numeric filing system

Operation index

Outguide

Patient account number

Policies

Procedures

Purged records

Quantitative analysis

Release of information (ROI)

Requisition

Retrospective review

Serial numbering system

Serial-unit numbering system

Standard

Straight numeric filing system

Terminal-digit filing system

Unit numbering system

Introduction

Health information management (HIM) involves a wide variety of functions that are critical to the operations of the healthcare organization and the healthcare delivery process. This chapter examines the functions of the HIM department and looks at the different management and supervisory processes that HIM professionals assume in the organization. Future directions in HIM technology and how these directions will affect the role of HIM professionals also are discussed. Other chapters in this book focus on the purpose and content of patient health records, the different technologies used in obtaining and retrieving patient information, the different information systems used in healthcare organizations, the importance of maintaining data integrity and ensuring data confidentiality, and much more.

HIM functions usually involve ensuring the quality, security, and availability of health information as it follows the patient through the health system. The HIM department also monitors the quality of patient information, ensuring that the information is maintained and protected in accordance with federal, state, and local regulations and the guidelines issued by various accrediting bodies.

Among the HIM department's most important functions is that of storage and retrieval of patient information. Although computers are used widely in healthcare organizations today, many organizations still have an enormous volume of information documented on paper. As healthcare organizations make the transition to an electronic health record (EHR), paper or hybrid record systems are used to store patient information. Regardless of the type of storage system used, patient information must be stored in a manner that ensures its accessibility to authorized users whenever and wherever it is needed.

In most healthcare organizations, the HIM department also manages several critical support services. In addition to the storage and retrieval function, the HIM department also typically manages the following support services:

- Record processing
- Monitoring of record completion
- Transcription
- Release of patient information
- Clinical coding

The services managed by the HIM department vary depending on the organization. Besides the typical HIM functions, the HIM department may manage the following functions:

- Research and statistics
- Cancer and/or trauma registries
- Birth certificate completion

An interdepartmental relationship exists between the HIM department and many other departments within a healthcare organization. HIM functions support patient care, billing, and patient registration. The functions associated with patient care, billing, and patient registration also affect the processes managed by the HIM department.

Theory into Practice

The case study presented in this section demonstrates the intertwined nature of the various HIM functions described in this chapter. It is adapted from an article by Hicks et al. (2000).

Medical transcription services are critical to any healthcare organization. Because a large component of any health record consists of dictated and transcribed reports, the transcription service must be effective and efficient.

The Kirklin Clinic (TKC) is a multispecialty ambulatory practice facility within the University of Alabama health systems. The facility sees more than 500,000 patients every year. To integrate the data from all these annual visits, TKC initially considered simply upgrading its transcription services. However, based on findings from an internal study, TKC discovered that (1) only 50 percent of transcribed notes were accessible electronically, (2) patient records were not integrated across clinics, and (3) fifty-five of the clinics used more than eighty record storage sites.

As a result of these findings, TKC decided to overhaul the entire clinical access system. It wanted an integrated system that would go beyond a transcription system and support the maintenance and access of patient lists, free-form text, and structured data for all patients as dictated by caregivers. To accomplish this goal, TKC decided to develop a dictation, transcription, and clinical document access system that would give an integrated view of all documents and lists from a Web browser system.

TKC partnered with a software vendor to develop a system that resulted in accomplishment of the following objectives:

- 100 percent availability of documents transcribed for clinic physicians

- A means of constructing and maintaining patient lists by the third clinic visit

- A patient list that would operate as a composite rather than a fragmented view of the patient's care

- Improvement of transcription accuracy and the subsequent reduction and elimination of duplicate health record numbers, misfiling, and loss of information

- Increased security of patient information by eliminating the mishandling of paper records

- Improved information management by making patient information available, as appropriate, to physicians and other caregivers in a timely manner

- Information provided across the continuum of care

- Improved access, quality, and efficiency for TKC personnel

HIM Functions and Services

HIM functions are information centered. This means that they typically involve ensuring information quality, security, and availability. The medium in which the information is stored may dictate how the specific functions are carried out. For example, storage of information in paper-based records involves different types of tasks than does storage of information in electronic records.

Figure 8.1 provides a description of a fictional HIM department. The description includes many of the HIM functions discussed in this chapter. It is important to note that these are typical functions. No two HIM departments are identical in organization or in the functions they perform. Table 8.1 summarizes the typical functions of the HIM department for paper-based records and EHRs.

Figure 8.1.   HIM functions at Community Hospital Medical Center

Community Hospital Medical Center is located in the suburbs of a large southeastern city. It is a nationally recognized leader in providing specialty and primary healthcare services and in conducting groundbreaking research in the treatment of various healthcare disorders. Located on a fifty-acre campus, the facility includes:

- A 516-licensed bed facility that includes a Level I trauma center and a 50-bed neonatal intensive care unit, a 16-bed pediatric ICU, and 25 general pediatric beds

- A cancer center with facilities for research, diagnosis, and treatment

- An outpatient center that includes specialized examination and treatment rooms, a clinical laboratory, a diagnostic radiology department, and an ambulatory surgery department

The facility is affiliated with a local medical school and provides education and training for third- and fourth-year medical students as well as internships and residencies for physician training.

The HIM department is responsible for all health records for the entire facility including both inpatient and outpatient records. The medical training aspect of the facility adds another complicated dimension to the management of the health records.

The functions performed within the HIM department include:

- Record processing (concurrent and retrospective analysis and monitoring of health record content)

- Record completion

- Storage and retrieval of health records (including monitoring and tracking of health record location)

- Release of patient information

- Clinical coding of diagnoses and procedures

- Transcription of medical reports (excluding pathology and radiology reports)

- Statistical and internal report generation

- Cancer and trauma registry

The HIM department is staffed with the equivalent of sixty-three full-time employees and operates twenty-four hours a day, seven days a week. The following organizational chart shows how the operations in the department are organized.

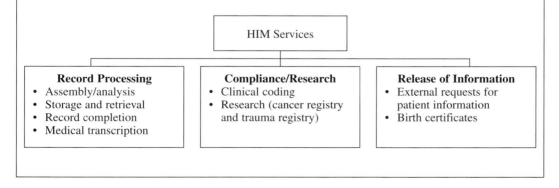

Table 8.1.	Table of common HIM functions
Function/ Service	**Description**
Storage and Retrieval	**Paper-based system:** • Records are retrieved for patient care purposes, quality improvement studies, audits, and other authorized uses. • Records are delivered to the nursing units, outpatient surgery, and the emergency room as the patient is admitted or being treated. EHR system: • Record is accessible to patient care areas via the computer. • If hospital is transitioning to the EHR, portions of the health record may be printed for use on the patient care unit.
Record Processing	**Paper-based system:** • After the patient is discharged from the hospital, the record is retrieved from the nursing unit. The record is assembled or put in an order prescribed by the facility's policy and procedure manual. For example, the face sheet is usually the first page in the paper record. • The postdischarge order is usually different from the order of the record on the nursing unit. • After the record is assembled, it is analyzed for deficiencies, such as missing reports and signatures. **EHR system:** • Portions of the record can be directly input into the EHR through computer interfaces, (transcribed reports, laboratory reports, emergency records, and so on). After the patient is discharged from the hospital, the paper record is prepared for imaging (scanning). • Records are analyzed for deficiencies either manually by the HIM staff and/or by rules built into the computer system.
Record Completion	**Paper-based system:** • Physicians visit the HIM department to complete deficiencies in records. • The record is reanalyzed after completion to ensure completeness. Deficiencies are cleared from the computer. **EHR system:** • Physicians complete the record from a computer that may be located remotely from the hospital. • If electronic signatures, computer key, and electronic completion rules are applied, the deficiency system is updated after the physician has completed his or her record.
Transcription	**Paper-based system:** • Transcription may be completed in-house or outsourced to an outside service. • Physician dictates reports into a dictation system that records the voice. The transcriptionist types (transcribes) what the physician has dictated. • The transcribed report is placed in the chart. • Reports commonly transcribed include operative reports, history and physicals, discharge summaries, radiology reports, pathology reports, and consultations. **EHR system:** • The process is basically the same as in the paper-based system, except that the transcribed reports are added electronically to the health record that resides within the computer. Speech recognition technology may be applied to the front end and back end of the transcription process to facilitate the process.

Table 8.1. (Continued)

Function/ Service	Description
Release of Information (ROI)	**Paper-based system:** • Reviews requests for health records for validity to ensure compliance with federal and state regulations • Logs and verifies validity of requests for patient information • May copy the record in response to valid requests or may provide record for an outsourced copy service to process • May go to court in response to a subpoena or court order • Must have in-depth knowledge of laws and regulations governing the release of information **EHR system:** • ROI process is basically the same as in the paper-based environment. • As the EHR evolves, there may be opportunities for the HIM professional's role to be expanded.
Clinical coding	**Paper-based system:** • Code number(s) is/are assigned to the diagnoses and procedures documented in the health record. The coder may use a coding book or enter key words into the computer using an encoder. • ICD-9-CM and CPT are the two primary coding systems used in a hospital setting. (Implementation of ICD-10-CM and ICD-10-PCS to replace ICD-9-CM is currently planned.) • Other information is abstracted from the record for reporting and reimbursement purposes. • Coding takes place on-site within the HIM department. **EHR system:** • The process is the same as the paper-based system, except that in the EHR environment, the record that is reviewed is the electronic health record. • Coding may be remote to hospital; home-based coding is possible. • As the structure of the EHR evolves, computer-assisted coding may be utilized. • Data abstracting may be reduced or eliminated as automatic data capture is implemented.[1]

Most of the above functions may be performed in a variety of healthcare settings to some degree. Therefore, an understanding of the acute care HIM functions can be applied to any healthcare setting.

[1]Tegan, Anne, et al. 2005 (May). The EHR's impact on HIM functions. *Journal of American Health Information Management Association* 76(5):56C–H.

The functions (storage and retrieval, record processing, record completion, transcription, **release of information** [ROI], **clinical coding**) discussed here might be considered the most fundamental responsibilities of most HIM departments. (The processes that support these HIM functions are discussed later in this chapter.) As mentioned earlier, in some institutions, HIM functions also include clinical quality performance activities, research and statistics, maintenance of cancer and other registries, support for medical staff committee functions, and responsibility for birth certificate submission to state departments of public health. Even though these functions may not fall within the traditional range of HIM department responsibilities, health information technicians (HITs) sometimes do perform them.

Storage and Retrieval

The storage and retrieval of patient information is one of the HIM department's most important functions. The department must ensure that health records are stored safely and that mechanisms are in place to efficiently retrieve them for patient care or other purposes. Moreover, the data contained in patient health records are confidential; thus, mechanisms must be in place to ensure that only authorized individuals have access to them.

Storage of paper-based health records has traditionally been the most common archival medium across healthcare delivery sites. In paper-based storage systems, each health record is contained in a special file folder that is filed either alphabetically or numerically, depending on the size of the organization. A small organization such as a physician's office practice may file its health records alphabetically in open-shelf files. Clinics, hospitals, long-term care facilities, and other larger facilities file their records numerically, using the patient's **health record number** as the primary identifier.

However, the in-house archival of paper-based health records is not the healthcare organization's only storage option. Health records also may be stored off-site, microfilmed, or scanned as digital images. Indeed, large HIM departments may have all these storage mechanisms in place. Many large healthcare organizations are transitioning toward or have implemented electronically stored health records. Facilities transitioning to the EHR sometimes use a hybrid health record. A hybrid health record is a combination of paper-based and electronically stored health data. The hybrid health record environment includes a combination of paper-based and EHR systems. (See table 8.1, p. 337.) The EHR is discussed in more detail in chapter 4.

Without a good storage and retrieval filing system, it would be impossible to locate and retrieve health records when they are needed. The following subsections discuss these key elements of the storage and retrieval function:

- Identification systems for paper-based health records and EHRs
- Filing systems for paper-based health records
- Storage systems
- Retrieval and tracking systems

Identification Systems for Paper-Based Health Records

The health record number (also called the medical record number) is a unique identifier and is used in numerical filing systems to locate records. Although it is typically assigned at the point of patient registration, the HIM department is usually responsible for the integrity of health record number assignment and for ensuring that no two patients receive the same number. The HIM department also ensures that the identification numbering system is such that all of an individual patient's records are stored together or can be linked together.

The health record number is important because it uniquely identifies not only the patient, but also the patient's record. Patient care documentation generated as part of the patient's episode of care is identified and physically filed or linked in an electronic system. Examples of documentation and medical reports found in health records are the history and physical, the discharge summary, operative notes, pathology reports, laboratory reports, radiology reports, and nursing notes. Thus, having a numbering system is important for efficiently storing and retrieving information about a single patient.

It is generally agreed that Social Security numbers (SSNs) should not be used as patient identifiers. The Social Security Administration is adamant in its opposition to using the SSN for purposes other than those identified by law. The American Health Information Management Association (AHIMA) is in agreement on this issue due to privacy, confidentiality, and security issues related to the use of the SSN.

The type of health record numbering system used varies from facility to facility. The three types of systems used most commonly are discussed below. An alphabetic numbering system and identification system used with EHRs are also discussed. The system used determines the procedure for assigning the health record number and the method for filing the patient record in a paper-based system.

Serial Numbering System

In the **serial numbering system,** a patient receives a unique numerical identifier for each encounter or admission to a healthcare facility. The numbering system is called serial because numbers are issued in a series. For example, Mr. Jones is admitted to the hospital at 8:00 a.m. on October 12 and given number 786544. Mrs. Wright, who registered at 8:15 a.m. on the same day, receives the next available number, 786545. Thus, in a serial numbering system each patient receives the next available number in the series.

With this system, a patient admitted to a healthcare facility on three different occasions receives three different health record numbers. The information compiled for each admission is filed with the health record for each encounter. One disadvantage to the serial numbering system is that information about the patient's care and treatment is filed in separate health records and at separate locations. This makes retrieval of all patient information less efficient and storage more costly.

In addition to retrieval inefficiencies and the costs associated with file folders, this numbering system is time-consuming in terms of documentation. Each time a patient returns to the healthcare facility, manual index cards or computer systems must be updated to reflect the addition of a new serial number and each update presents an opportunity for input error.

Unit Numbering System

The **unit numbering system** is most commonly used in large healthcare facilities. Many of the disadvantages to the serial numbering system can be addressed by using a unit number. In the unit numbering system, the patient receives a unique health record number at the time of the first encounter. For all subsequent encounters for a particular patient, the health record number that was assigned for the first encounter is used.

One advantage to this method is that all information, regardless of the number of encounters, can be filed or linked together. Having all the information related to the patient filed in one location facilitates communication among caregivers and improves operational efficiency.

For the unit numbering system to work effectively, patient demographic and health record number information must be available to all areas of the facility that process patient registrations. For example, clerks in the admitting, emergency, and clinical departments must have access to a database of previous patients and their health record numbers. Access to such information is not a problem for organizations that make the information available to the registration areas via a computer network. However, use of a manual system or an incomplete search of a computerized system increases the likelihood that duplicate numbers may be assigned to a patient. Therefore, the unit numbering system generally works best in a computerized environment.

Serial-Unit Numbering System

The **serial-unit numbering system** is an attempt to combine the strengths and minimize the weaknesses of the serial and unit numbering systems. In this system, numbers are assigned in a serial manner, just as they are in the serial numbering system. However, during each new patient encounter, the previous health records are brought forward and filed under the last assigned health record number. This creates a unit record.

The serial-unit numbering system helps alleviate the problem of access to previous patient demographic and health record number information. It also helps in addressing problems associated with retrieval and the cost of the serial system.

Alphabetic Identification and Filing System

Some small facilities and clinics use an alphabetic patient identification and filing system. In this system, the patient's last name is used as the first source of identification and his or her first name and middle initial provide further identification. The disadvantage to this system is that a given community may have several persons with the same or a similar name. In this case, the facility routinely uses date of birth as the next step in the process of identifying a patient.

There are some conveniences to alphabetic identification and filing. It is simple to locate a health record without first accessing an assigned number. However, each entry must be double-checked to verify that the correct patient record is being used.

Identification Systems for Electronic Health Records

Unit numbering is the method most commonly used as the unique identifier in the EHR environment. For search and retrieval purposes, identifiers other than the health record number can be used to locate patient records in EHRs. The **patient account number** and patient name are often used to find a patient's health record stored electronically within a computer system. Because correcting a digital record can be complex, it is very important to verify that the correct record has been accessed by checking the full name, date of birth, and other factors before making entries or using information for care. The process for checking patient records should be included in the facility's charting **policies** and **procedures.**

Filing Systems for Paper-Based Health Records

The filing system used by a healthcare facility maintaining paper-based health records refers to the procedure in which the file folders are placed on shelving units or in filing cabinets. The unique health record number assigned to a patient upon admission to a healthcare facility is the number also used to file the record in a numeric filing system. Likewise, the patient's name is used as the basis for filing in an alphabetical filing system.

Records that cannot be located and retrieved when needed serve no useful function. Thus, the HIM department must carefully consider the types of filing and storage systems it uses to ensure that they meet the needs of the organization. The three major classifications of filing systems are discussed below.

Alphabetic Filing Systems

In **alphabetic filing systems,** records are arranged in alphabetical order. This system is usually satisfactory for a very small volume of records, such as records maintained in small physician practices. The alphabetic filing system is easy to create and use. It is often called a direct filing method because it does not rely on an index or an authority file and the user can find a file by looking directly under the name of the record.

For organizations that have thousands of records, however, alphabetic filing has many disadvantages. First, it does not ensure a unique identifier. For example, a large facility may have several patients named Paula Smith. If it were relying strictly on alphabetical filing by patient last and first name, multiple health records would be labeled Paula Smith on the file shelf.

A second disadvantage is that alphabetic files do not expand evenly. Statistically, almost half the files fall under the letters *B, C, H, M, S,* and *W.* A third disadvantage to the alphabetical filing system is that it is time-consuming to purge or clean out files for inactive storage. With an alphabetical filing system, each individual record needs to be checked for the last patient encounter to determine whether it is inactive. (See figure 8.2 for the rules that apply to alphabetic filing.)

Numeric Filing Systems

In a **numeric filing system**, records are filed by using the health record number. Numeric filing is a type of indirect filing system. To use an indirect filing system, an index or authority file needs to be consulted before the user can identify a record associated with a specific patient. In healthcare, the authority file is usually the **master patient index** (MPI). The filing clerk searches the MPI by patient name. When the correct patient is located in the MPI, the clerk uses the health record number to locate the patient's health record folder within the filing system.

At first glance, the numeric filing system may seem much more work than the alphabetic system. This can be true for organizations that have a very small number of records (hundreds). However, in larger organizations, the numeric filing system actually has many advantages over an alphabetic system. Following are the most common types of numeric filing systems:

- In **straight numeric filing systems,** records are arranged consecutively in ascending numeric order. The number assigned to each file is the health record number.

Figure 8.2.   Rules for alphabetic filing

1. File each record alphabetically by the last name, followed by the first name and middle initial. For example:

   Brown, Michelle L.
   Brown, Michelle S.
   Brown, Robert A.

   When the patient has identical last and first names and middle initial, order the records by date of birth, filing the record with the earliest birth date first.

2. Last names beginning with a prefix or containing an apostrophe are filed in strict alphabetical order, ignoring any apostrophes or spaces. For example, the names Mackel, Mac Bain, and Mc Dougal would be filed as:

   Macbain
   Mackel
   Mcdougal

3. In hyphenated names such as Manasse-O'Brien, the hyphenation is ignored and the record is filed as:

   Manasseobrien

- The **terminal-digit filing system** is considered by many to be the most efficient. In this system, the last digit or group of last digits (terminal digits) is the primary unit used for filing, followed by the middle unit and the last unit of numbers. For example, 443798 could be broken down as 44-37-98, with 98 as the primary unit for filing, 37 as the secondary (middle) unit, and 44 as the tertiary unit. The record would be filed in the following arrangement: file section, 98; shelf number, 37; and folder number, 44. An example of how health records are filed using terminal-digit filing is shown in figure 8.3.

  The terminal-digit system is excellent for facilities with a heavy record volume. This is because large numbers can be divided into groups of several digits and still be easily managed for filing and retrieval purposes. In addition to ensuring that every record has a unique number, terminal-digit filing allows even file expansion, unlike an alphabetic or straight numerical filing system.

- The middle-digit filing system is very similar to the terminal-digit filing system. The primary unit is the middle unit, the secondary unit is the first unit to the left, followed by the last digits. For example, 443798 could be broken down as 37 as the primary unit, 44 as the secondary unit, and 98 as the tertiary unit. The record could be filed in the following arrangement: file section, 37, shelf number, 44; and folder number, 98.

Although the examples provided above for terminal- and middle-digit filing use a six-digit number, the number of digits in the health record number may vary depending on the healthcare facility. The length of any number and how it is divided depends on the organization. For example, one healthcare facility may have a health record number that is six digits in length. The highest number or volume of records that could be accommodated in such a numbering scheme would be 999,999 records. Another healthcare organization may have a numbering system containing seven digits. The capacity of this facility is much

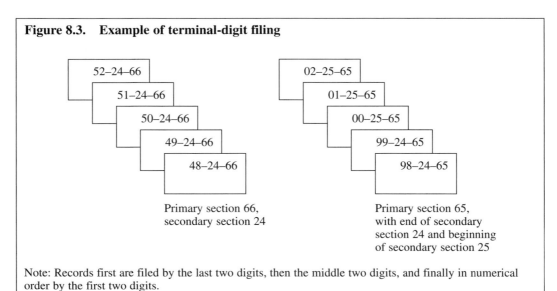

Figure 8.3.   Example of terminal-digit filing

52–24–66
51–24–66
50–24–66
49–24–66
48–24–66

Primary section 66,
secondary section 24

02–25–65
01–25–65
00–25–65
99–24–65
98–24–65

Primary section 65,
with end of secondary
section 24 and beginning
of secondary section 25

Note: Records first are filed by the last two digits, then the middle two digits, and finally in numerical order by the first two digits.

greater and can accommodate 9,999,999 records. Some facilities may have a three-digit primary unit. However, the method for filing would remain the same. The file section corresponding to the primary unit would be accessed first, followed by the secondary unit, and then the tertiary unit.

Alphanumeric Filing Systems

The **alphanumeric filing system** is the third type of system. This system uses a combination of alpha letters and numbers for identification purposes. The first two letters of the patient's last name are followed by a unique numeric identifier. The alphanumeric filing system is appropriate for small organizations. Although this system may be quicker because file clerks first file the record alphabetically, it still relies on accessing a master index or authority file to identify the unique numerical number.

Centralized Unit Filing Systems

In a centralized unit filing system, individual patient encounters are filed by the same unique identifier and in the same location. The unique identifier can be alphabetic, alphanumeric, or numeric. For example, in a small medical practice all of an individual's encounters may be filed together alphabetically by last name.

Usually, centralized unit filing is associated with the unit numbering system in which file clerks have to look in only one location for the patient's health record. In addition, the supply costs for record folders are reduced because all forms and information are filed together in one folder. Furthermore, computer or index card update issues are lessened using the unit numbering system. The patient retains the same health record number, regardless of the number of admissions or encounters.

Storage Systems

Many options are available for storing health records. Paper-based records are stored in filing cabinets or shelving units. Other storage options include microfilm, off-site storage, and imaged-based storage. As healthcare facilities transition toward and implement the EHR, imaged-based systems are increasing utilized. The choice of system depends on the needs of the facility and the amount budgeted within the department for record storage. For organizations with a high record volume, a combination of systems may be the appropriate choice. For organizations that have a very low volume of records, paper storage may be appropriate.

Storing Records in Filing Cabinets or Shelving Units

Paper-based records may be stored in vertical and lateral filing cabinets, open-shelf files, and compressible file systems. Vertical file cabinets are the traditional drawer files and come in sizes that can hold either letter or legal-sized records. The usual configuration is two or four drawers. Vertical file cabinets are appropriate for low-volume record storage. However, this type of filing equipment does not facilitate quick and easy filing and retrieval. Therefore, these file cabinets are rarely used to store health records.

Lateral filing units also have drawers. However, the drawers open laterally rather than vertically. They also include side-to-side rails for hanging files. These filing units range in size from two to five drawers and are usually thirty or thirty-six inches in width. Although easier for retrieval and filing than vertical cabinets, this type of equipment would only be used in low-volume offices.

The filing equipment of choice for housing health records is usually some configuration of shelf filing. Shelf files resemble open bookshelves. They can either be totally open or have receding doors. Shelf files are ideal for high-volume record storage. Shelving units with six shelves are usually used for record storage purposes. Moreover, shelf files save space. For example, one six-shelf unit offers file capacity equal to eight 30-inch-wide lateral file drawers.

A variation on open-shelf files is the mobile or compact file. (See figure 8.4.) Instead of having aisle space between every row of files, mobile files conserve floor space by providing only one aisle of space. This is accomplished by mounting the file shelves on tracks secured to the floor. The shelves then are moved by hand, with mechanical assistance, or electronically. This type of storage system is ideal in facilities where space is a major concern. In most situations, an organization can double or even triple storage capacity in the same floor space, even when compared to other, high-density filing systems such as open shelf.

Figure 8.4   Mobile file units

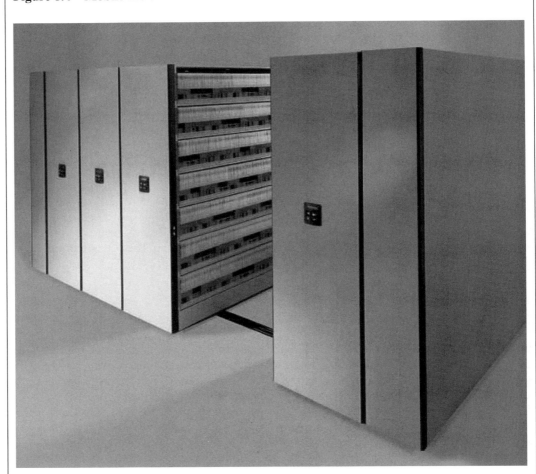

Source: Photo provided by Central Business Group, Spacesaver Corporation and Smead Software Solutions. Reprinted with permission.

A variation of mobile or compact files is the lateral mobile shelving system. This filing system consists of stationary shelving in the back and file storage shelving that slides side to side in the front. This is an inexpensive way to increase the storage capacity of existing shelving or another record storage system. However, this type of shelving is only appropriate for low-volume record filing and retrieval activity.

Variations on open-shelf files are horizontal and vertical carousel systems. The horizontal carousel contains open-shelf files that revolve around a central spine or track system. Essentially, this type of filing system brings the files to the user, thus avoiding walking through aisles of files. The vertical carousel system brings all files or records to a standing or sitting workstation and can take advantage of vertical ceiling height. Vertical carousel systems are often used to store the manual MPI.

The amount of space, volume of records, and record usage or activity must be considered when determining the type of storage system to use. When space is not sufficient to house the number of shelving units needed to hold the records for the period of time required for patient care and other purposes, older health records are purged or removed from the file area. Generally, files that have been inactive for a certain period of time (for example, three years since the patient's last visit) are removed from the active filing area. **Purged records** are often microfilmed, sent to off-site storage facilities, or scanned. How frequently paper-based records are purged from the storage system is determined by not only space availability, but also the patient readmission rate and the use of patient record data. For example, a research hospital may maintain health records in paper format for a period of time longer than other facilities because researchers may need to access information about patients who have expired or who have not been admitted to the facility for a number of years.

The volume of health records can be enormous in many organizations. For example, when an acute care facility admits fifty patients per day and treats the same number of patients in the emergency department, 100 health records are generated. Over a year, this amounts to 36,500 new records. If approximately one inch is required to store five paper records, the organization would need approximately 7,300 inches, or approximately 608 feet, of filing space.

An HIM professional often has responsibility for planning the file space and shelving units required to store paper records. He or she first must estimate the facility's storage system needs. This involves analyzing the volume indicators, such as number of discharges, size of the records, and filing inch capacity of the storage unit. For example, one could estimate the number of shelving units required by using the following information.

Shelving unit shelf width = 36 inches

Number of shelves per unit = 7 shelves

Average record thickness = $\frac{1}{2}$ inch

Average annual inpatient discharges = 8,500 patients

The following demonstrates how the HIM professional would use the information above to estimate the number of shelving units required to house one year's records:

1. Determine the linear inch capacity of each shelving unit.

    36 inches per shelf × 7 shelves per unit = 252 inches per shelving unit

2. Determine the linear filing inches needed for the volume of records.

8,500 average annual inpatient discharges $\times$ .5 average record thickness = 4,250 filing inches required to store one year of inpatient discharge records

3. Determine the number of shelving units required by dividing the required filing space by the shelving unit linear inch capacity.

$$4,250 \div 252 = 16.8 \text{ shelving units}$$

Actually, 17 shelving units would be required to store one year of inpatient records because it is impossible to purchase 16.8 shelving units.

However, most HIM departments store more than inpatient discharge records. Outpatient records also are typically stored in the HIM department, and the storage requirements for the outpatient records must be considered when estimating the record storage needs. Consider the following example:

Hospital XYZ has the following volume statistics.

Average inpatient discharges per year = 10,000

Average inpatient records thickness = 1 inch

Average outpatient visits = 22,500

Average outpatient record thickness = $1/4$ inch

Each shelving unit has 7 shelves, each 36 inches wide.

The following demonstrates how the HIM professional would estimate the number of shelving units required to house one year's records:

1. Determine the linear filing inches required to house inpatient and outpatient records.

10,000 inpatient discharges per year $\times$ 1 inch = 10,000 linear filing inches required

22,500 outpatient visits per year $\times$ $1/4$ inch = 5,625 linear filing inches required

10,000 + 5,625 = 15,625 linear filing inches needed for inpatient and outpatient records

2. Determine the linear filing inches per shelving unit.

36 inches per shelf $\times$ 7 shelves per unit = 252 inches per shelving unit

3. Divide the required filing space by the shelving unit linear inch capacity.

15,625 inches needed $\div$ 252 inches per shelving unit = 62 shelving units required to store the records

Therefore, for this example 62 shelving units would be required to store one year of records.

In an EHR environment, the HIM professional works with the software vendor and the information technology (IT) department to determine the required computer storage space and medium.

Paper-based health records that are stored on shelving units, compressible filing units or in filing cabinets are housed in filing folders. During an average inpatient encounter, a health record exceeding 100 pages is common. These various reports and documents must be sorted and stored in their own file folders. File folders come in two standard weights, eleven and fourteen point. Higher weights such as twenty point are also available. The higher weight is the most durable and would be the folder of choice for active records that receive heavy filing and retrieval activity. In addition to weight, consideration should be given to the selection of top or side tabs. Top-tabbed folders are used in vertical or lateral shelving systems. Side-tab folders, which are the usual configuration for health records, are used in all open-shelf filing systems.

Health record folders also should include some type of fastening system to hold the record documents together. Record fasteners are two pronged and can be up to two inches long. They can be placed at the top or sides of the file folder. Usually, folders are purchased with fasteners attached, although for low-volume operations self-adhesive fasteners can be used and installed by office staff. Dividers also may be placed in health records to separate clinical, inpatient, outpatient, and/or administrative documents.

Whether the facility uses an alphabetic or numeric filing system, file folders should be color coded for easy filing and retrieval. For example, in a numeric filing system, each single digit is a specific color. Therefore, one can easily locate misfiles by visually scanning a shelf for disruption of the color pattern of a particular file shelving section. Figure 8.5 demonstrates the use of color-coding on file folders. For high-volume systems, color-coding of files is done at the factory. For lower-volume systems, color-coded labels can be affixed to the file folders.

Storing Records in Microfilm-Based Storage Systems

Storage of paper-based health records consumes an enormous amount of space. There are other options for record storage that significantly reduce space needs. A traditional alternative that has been used over the past three or more decades is micrographics or microfilm. Microfilm is a good storage alternative for inactive or infrequently used health records.

Figure 8.5.   Color-coded file folders

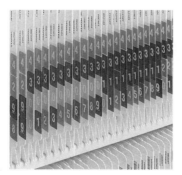

Source: Photo provided by Central Business Group, Spacesaver Corporation and Smead Software Solutions. Reprinted with permission.

Essentially, the microfilming process converts paper documents to archive-stored images by taking a picture of the original document and storing it as a very small negative. Because the images are so small, a special microfilm viewer or reader that magnifies each image must be used to read them. Microfilm comes in a variety of formats, including:

- *Roll microfilm:* This format stores each document page sequentially in a long roll. One roll of microfilm can potentially hold thousands of images and the health records of hundreds of patients. However, the fact that the roll stores document pages sequentially can be a disadvantage. For example, if the organization is using a serial numbering system, a patient's entire health record covering multiple encounters may be on separate roles of microfilm. This makes retrieval less efficient.

- *Jacket microfilm:* In this format, a roll of microfilm is cut and placed into special four-by-six-inch jackets with several sleeves to hold the images. A benefit of this option is that all the patient's records can be collected together in the same jacket or several jackets can be combined in a small paper folder. Thus, the record becomes a unit record holding all information about the patient. Jackets can be color coded with the patient's health record number and name. They are usually filed using the same type of filing system (alphabetic, straight numerical, terminal digit) used for paper files.

- *Microfiche:* This format can be a copy of a microfilm jacket or a direct copy of the source health record. It is made on Mylar film and is the same size as the microfilm jacket. When used as a copy from the source health record, the microfiche eliminates the need to cut rolls of film to fit into microfilm jackets. Sometimes organizations store their health records in microfilm jackets. These jackets are never removed from the HIM department. Instead, when the information is needed, a microfiche copy is made using a special duplicator and then provided to the requesting care areas.

One benefit of microfilm is that it is much less costly for backup than digital media. Moreover, microfilm is acceptable as courtroom evidence and provides good security because it is difficult to tamper with.

Storing Records in Off-Site Storage Systems

Because space for paper-based records has become limited and/or microfilm has become cost prohibitive, many healthcare facilities use off-site storage companies to house purged records. An off-site storage company is usually a contracted service that stores health records. The company then retrieves and delivers records requested by the healthcare facility's HIM department for a fee.

The healthcare facility should carefully evaluate the off-site storage company's capabilities for storing records securely for the entire retention period. Considerations for off-site storage include climate control, fire protection, pest and dust control, physical protection from burglary or vandalism, and cost.

Storing Records in Image-Based Storage Systems

The use of digital document imaging is increasing as healthcare facilities implement EHR or hybrid record systems. Essentially, a document imaging system scans and indexes an original source document to create a digital picture that can be retrieved via the computer.

Most document imaging solutions include production scanners that can scan hundreds or thousands of documents a day, plus a work flow or document management application that makes the scanned information available to a department or an entire enterprise. When scanned, the images are stored on electronic media, such as a magnetic or optical disk. Unlike microfilm rolls, the optical disk is a random-access device and retrieval of documents is much faster. Additionally, document images can be viewed by more than one person at one time and at different locations.

One of the greatest benefits of document imaging is increased efficiency by eliminating the requirement to move and track paper documents through work flow. Document imaging also helps solve the problem of lost or misplaced paper or microfiche documents. Moreover, it saves money by reducing the need for storage space and by decreasing the work of file clerks.

Document imaging is not necessary for information and data directly transferred into the EHR via computer interfaces. Documents commonly transmitted directly into the EHR electronically are transcribed reports, laboratory reports, and radiology reports.

Policies and procedures related to the storage and retention of paper documents that have been imaged are developed by the HIM department and take into consideration factors such as the extent of process quality assurance, cost and availability of storage space, and the organization's definition of its legal health record.

Retrieval and Tracking Systems

Tracking the location of health records removed from a paper-based storage system area is key to ensuring their accessibility to authorized persons. The **outguide** is the most common type of tracking system used to track paper-based health records. An outguide is usually made of strong colored vinyl with two plastic pockets. It is the size of a regular record folder and is placed in the record location when the record is removed from the file. Outguides normally come with either a bottom or a middle tab with the word OUT printed on it to indicate that a health record has been removed from the file shelf.

The larger of the plastic pockets is used to hold loose reports or other documents that come to the HIM department while the original record is charged out. The smaller pocket is used to house information about who checked out the health record, its current location, when it was checked out, and the expected return date. This checkout information may be either a handwritten or computerized requisition slip generated from a tracking system.

A **requisition** is a request from a clinical or other area in the organization to charge out a specific health record. The requisition may be in paper or electronic form. The information contained on a requisition usually includes patient's name, health record number, date of the request, date and time needed, name of the requestor, and location for delivery.

In a paper-based requisition system, the requisition slip has multiple copies. One copy is the routing slip that comes with the health record. Another copy goes in the outguide. A third copy may be used as a transfer notice and sent to the HIM department if the health record is subsequently transferred to another location. For example, if a record were requested from the intensive care unit (ICU), it would be transferred to the medical unit when the patient was transferred from the ICU to the medical floor.

In many institutions, the chart-tracking and requisition systems are built into their automated information system. In this case, paper requisition slips are replaced by automated requisitions sent directly to the HIM department and all pertinent data are retained in a database. Automated systems such as these are similar to a library book checkout system. With an automated system, it is easy to track how many records are charged out of the HIM department at any given time, their location, and whether they have been returned on the due dates indicated. Figure 8.6 provides an example of how the computer screen appears in a chart-tracking system. A bar code representing the health record number is often on the file folder to facilitate data entry into the computer chart-tracking system. The HIM department should create facility-wide policies and procedures for the proper use of tracking systems. Further, an audit for health records not returned in a timely manner should be performed on a regular basis.

In healthcare organizations that use hybrid or EHR systems, tools built into the systems, such as work flow automation and audit trails, can provide tracking information such as who accessed which records and for what purpose.

Record Completion

The record completion function involves making sure that information in the health record is accurate and complete. This requires that the procedures involved in maintaining the health record be performed in an organized way and that the record be monitored for quality.

Figure 8.6. Chart-tracking computer screen: History tab screen

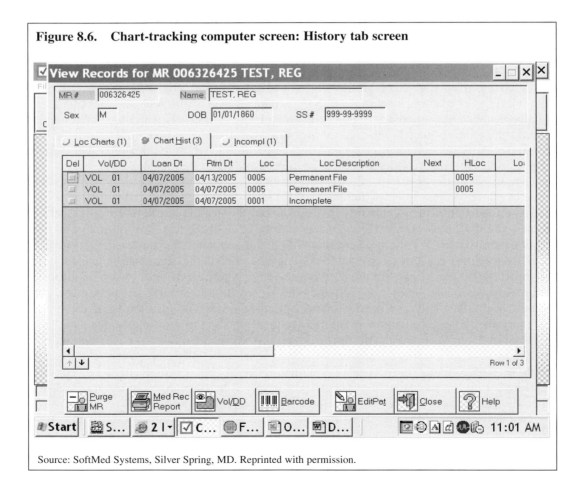

Source: SoftMed Systems, Silver Spring, MD. Reprinted with permission.

Processing the Health Record

Record processing refers to the procedures performed that support the maintenance of each individual patient record in an organized and standard manner. This function facilitates efficiency, accuracy, and completeness of the health record. The quality of patient care is adversely affected when complete and correct information is not readily available for delivery of patient care. Moreover, administrative and other functions, such as evaluating clinical quality performance, billing, and research, would be negatively affected without a complete and accurate health record.

In a paper-based system, the health record is organized or "assembled" after the patient is discharged from the hospital or other setting. *Assembly* means that each page in the patient record is organized in a pre-established order. The pre-established record order of the pages varies from facility to facility. Each page in the patient record is reviewed to ensure that it belongs to that record. After the record is assembled in the correct order, HIM professionals review or "analyze" it to make sure that there are no missing reports, forms, or required signatures and that all documents contain the patient's name and health record number. This review for deficiencies is an example of **quantitative analysis.**

The quantitative analysis or record content review process can be handled in a number of ways. Some acute care facilities conduct record review on a continuing basis during a patient's hospital stay. Using this method, personnel from the HIM department go to the nursing unit daily (or periodically) to review each patient's record. This type of process is usually referred to as a **concurrent review** because review occurs concurrently with the patient's stay in the hospital. Other acute care facilities perform the quantitative analysis the day following the patient's discharge from the hospital. This type of review is called **retrospective review** because it occurs after the patient has left the facility. In this process, the patient's health record is received in the HIM department, usually the day after discharge, and reviewed by an HIM professional.

Whether done concurrently or retrospectively, the review usually involves checking to ensure that:

- All forms and reports contain correct patient identification (name, health record number, gender, attending physician, and so on).

- All forms and reports are present. For example, when the patient is admitted for a cholecystectomy, a minimum set of operative reports, consents, and forms should be present (operative consent form, anesthesia form, operative report, recovery room report, pathology report, and so on).

- Reports requiring authentication (that is, operative, pathology, discharge summaries, history and physicals, and radiology reports) have signatures or have been appropriately authenticated.

When deficiencies are identified, the HIM professional usually completes a **deficiency slip** that indicates what reports are missing or require authentication and enters this information into a computer system that logs and tracks health record deficiencies. (See figure 8.7 for a sample paper deficiency slip.) Usually, the deficiency slip is a multipart form, one copy appended to the health record and one or more copies filed by physician name. A record with deficiencies is called an incomplete record.

Automated systems for tracking record deficiencies are commonly used to facilitate the process. An automated health record deficiency tracking system has a computer screen that looks similar to the deficiency slip to allow for data entry (see figure 8.8). If an automated deficiency system is utilized, each deficiency for a specific record is entered into the computer as is the name (or identification number) of the physician responsible for completing the deficiencies. This type of system stores the entered data into a database for later retrieval or analysis. Such systems reduce the amount of clerical work, make retrieval of deficiency information faster and easier, and provide for automatic report and statistics generation about deficiencies.

When deficiencies are identified and documented, they must be corrected. When reports or forms are missing, HIM personnel should try to locate them.

The health record content review (its requirements and how extensive it is) depends on the individual organization and its medical staff bylaws, rules, and regulations as well as

---

Figure 8.7.   Sample deficiency slip

Physician/Practitioner's Name: _____

Health Record Number: _____

Patient's Name: _____

Discharge Date: _____

Analyzed by: _____

Date: _____

Signatures Required	Dictation Required	Missing Reports
_____ History	_____ History	_____ History
_____ Physical	_____ Physical	_____ Physical
_____ Consultation	_____ Consultation	_____ Consultation
_____ Operative Report	_____ Operative Report	_____ Operative Report
_____ Discharge Summary	_____ Discharge Summary	_____ Discharge Summary
		_____ Radiology Report
Other	Other	_____ Pathology Report
_____ _____ _____	_____ _____	_____ Progress Notes
_____ _____	_____ _____	
_____ _____	_____ _____	Other
		_____ _____
		_____ _____
		_____ _____

Figure 8.8.   Chart deficiency computer screen

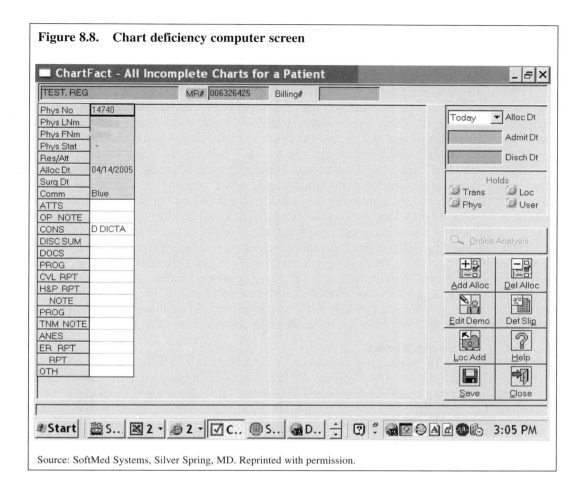

Source: SoftMed Systems, Silver Spring, MD. Reprinted with permission.

on licensing and accreditation body requirements. Other inpatient facilities, such as long-term care and rehabilitation institutions, usually follow the same processes as acute care facilities. Outpatient facilities such as clinics or physician office practices usually conduct a quantitative analysis after each patient visit or on a periodic basis.

Records are processed differently in an EHR environment than they are in a paper-based system. However, the goals of the record-processing activities in the EHR are the same as they are in the paper-based environment. The goal remains to facilitate efficiency, accuracy, and completeness of the health record.

The assembly process described above for the paper-based record is replaced by record preparation and document scanning in the EHR environment. Records are prepared for scanning by repairing torn forms, removing staples, and adding header forms to the front of the records. Additionally, checks are made to ensure that all pages are identified accurately as part of the individual patient's record. Depending on the extent to which bar-coded forms are used, the record may still need to be assembled to ensure proper order by date and type of report. The record is then scanned using high-speed scanners. After the record is scanned, the images are often reviewed to ensure that a high-quality image has been achieved. If an image is found to be unclear, the document is rescanned after adjustments are made to the computer or scanner. The amount of scanning required for the EHR depends on the amount of information directly interfaced to the EHR from computer systems.

In the EHR environment, the record also is analyzed for completeness. Automated rules may be built into the computer to identify deficiencies or HIM staff may identify deficiencies. The physician or other healthcare professional is notified electronically regarding incomplete records and the system is updated as missing or incomplete documentation is supplied.

In an EHR system where portions of the patient's records are scanned and stored in a computer, the HIM department must make certain that the scanning occurs in a timely manner and that all the forms scanned into an individual patient's record belong to that patient. Missing reports and signatures also must be identified for completion. As the EHR continues to evolve to include more structured documentation through the use of databases, the number of documents requiring scanning is likely to be reduced.

The HIM department often receives reports belonging to a health record that has already been assembled or scanned. These unprocessed reports are called "loose" reports or "loose" filing. In a paper-based system, the medical record must be located and the loose report assembled into the appropriate location within the record. In an EHR, the loose report is "indexed." Indexing is similar to filing in the paper record and ensures that documents are placed in the right location within the right record to ensure future retrievability.

Monitoring the Health Record

When deficiencies in the health record, such as reports that need to be dictated or signed by a physician or other health professional, are identified through quantitative analysis, the record is filed in a specially designated area of the HIM department, frequently called the incomplete record file. A copy of the deficiency slip also is filed, usually by the name of the responsible healthcare professional. Periodically, the HIM department notifies the appropriate individuals of the incomplete or deficient record status and requests that they come to the department to rectify it. In the EHR environment, or where electronic signatures and electronic authentication of medical records is accepted, the incomplete record file may be eliminated. Healthcare professionals can access, complete, and authenticate records using an electronic inbox, work list, or other tool. Management reports related to record completion can be generated by the system.

After the healthcare professional completes the record deficiencies, the record is reanalyzed to ensure its completeness. If no deficiencies are found, the deficiency slip is removed and/or the deficiency tracking system is updated to reflect that the health record is completed. The health record then is routed to the storage and retrieval area for filing in the permanent file.

When an incomplete record is not rectified within a specific number of days as indicated in the medical staff rules and regulations, the record is considered to be a **delinquent record.** Generally, an incomplete record is considered delinquent after it has been available to the physician for completion for fifteen to thirty days. The HIM department monitors the delinquent record rate very closely to ensure compliance with accrediting **standards.**

Medical Transcription

The medical transcription function is often included among the HIM department's responsibilities. Physicians and other clinicians use automated computer medical dictation (sometimes referred to as voice-capture) systems for dictating reports. Medical reports commonly dictated (recorded) include the clinical history, physical examination, consultation report, operative report, discharge summary, pathology reports, and radiology reports. The dictation is stored in either tape or disk format in the dictation system. Medical transcriptionists retrieve the dictated reports and type them using word-processing systems. The final typed report can be printed in paper format or stored electronically in an EHR.

Historically, the HIM department has provided medical transcription services. More recently, however, these services have been subsumed by other departments or have been centralized in a separate department. In other cases, the entire medical transcription function has been outsourced (contracted out to a vendor). In many instances, outsourcing part or all of the transcription function can provide substantial benefits, including cost reductions and relief from staffing issues that sometimes result in transcription delays.

Dictation and transcription equipment are needed to support the transcription function within the HIM department. In today's environment, particularly in a large transcription services area, dictation and transcription equipment are very closely related. In fact, many vendors supply both the dictation and the transcription components.

One of the primary issues associated with on-site transcription involves the selection of dictation and transcription equipment. Dictation equipment can be as simple as a small, single-user portable recorder or as sophisticated as a multiple-user digital desktop and recording system. Complex, multiuser dictation systems have the ability to store large amounts of voice and data material in a central area. They also offer customized programming features, such as the ability to set priority levels on reports for transcription and the ability for clinicians to listen to dictated reports prior to transcription.

More recently, large in-house transcription areas and outsourcing agencies have begun using speech recognition technology to transcribe recorded dictation. Speech recognition technology may be applied on the front end (at the point of dictation) or back end (after dictation has taken place). It enables the dictator's digitized voice recording to be processed through a computer that converts it into text. Templates or standardized documents can be used to reduce the number of errors.

The use of speech recognition will have an impact on the role of the medical transcriptionist, which is expected to become that of a medical language editor.

Release of Information (ROI)

As discussed in other chapters, protecting the security and privacy of patient information is one of the healthcare institution's top priorities. The HIM department usually has responsibility for determining appropriate access to and release of information from patient health records. For example, ROI may take the form of a patient's request to mail copies of his or her records to a healthcare provider. In this case, the HIM department usually requires the request to be in a written format, verifies the patient's signature on the ROI to the signature in the health record, and only then releases the records.

When a written request for health record information is received, information from the request is entered into a computer database. Generally, information such as patient name, date of birth, health record number, name of requester, address of requester, telephone number of requester, purpose of the request, and specific health record information requested is entered in the computer. Figure 8.9 is an example of the computer screens used for entering ROI data.

Figure 8.9.   Computer screens of ROI data

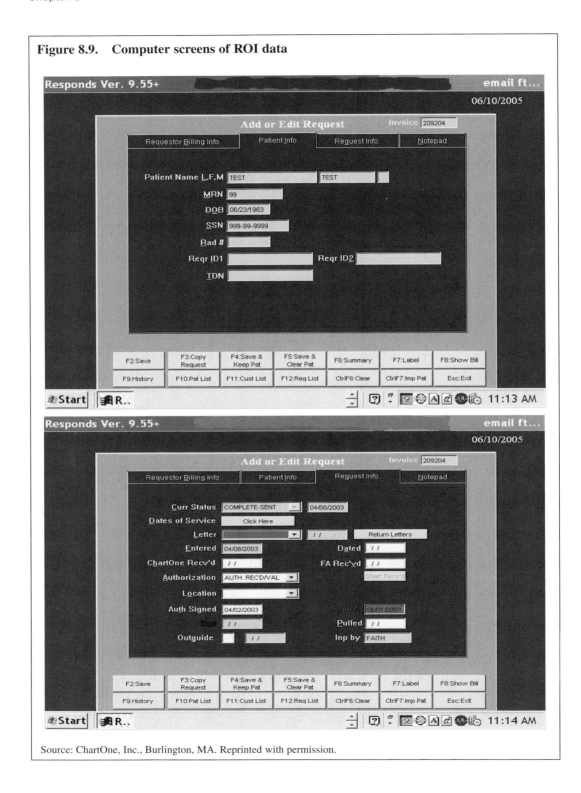

Source: ChartOne, Inc., Burlington, MA. Reprinted with permission.

Because federal regulations such as the Health Insurance Portability and Accountability Act (HIPAA) and state laws govern the release of health record information, HIM department personnel must know what information needs to be included on the authorization for it to be considered valid. If the written request or authorization is valid, the specific information is copied and sent. If the authorization is invalid, the problem with the authorization is noted in the computer and the request is returned to the sender. To comply with HIPAA standards, a healthcare facility must maintain a record that accounts for all disclosures from the health record.

In another case, ROI may take the form of a response to a subpoena *duces tecum* in a legal case. (A subpoena *duces tecum* is a judicial request for certain information or evidence.) In this instance, the HIM department verifies that the subpoena is valid and that the requested information can be released to the court in compliance with state or federal law or regulations. In such instances, a representative from the HIM department may appear in person in court or at a deposition and give sworn testimony as to the health record's authenticity.

The ROI function has grown immensely in the past decade, in part due to the HIPAA privacy standards. As a result, some HIM departments outsource this function to companies that specialize in release of medical information. Even though it has outsourced the function, the HIM department is ultimately responsible for ensuring that proper practices are followed and that all laws and regulations are adhered to.

Clinical Coding

Clinical coding is another important function usually performed by the HIM department. (The specifics of clinical coding are described in chapter 6.) Using a classification or nomenclature system such as ICD-9-CM and/or CPT, clinical coding is a method for categorizing diagnoses and procedures. (Adoption of a new coding system called ICD-10-CM and ICD-10-PCS is planned to replace ICD-9-CM in the future.) This categorization is used subsequently for billing and payment purposes as well as for research and clinical quality performance reviews.

The clinical coding function includes the processes of **abstracting** and assigning ICD-9-CM and/or CPT codes to an encounter or hospital stay. The coding professional reviews the health record and enters specific data from it into a computer database. The process of extracting data from the health record and entering them into a computer database is called abstracting. Figure 8.10 is an example, but not an exhaustive list, of data that may be abstracted and entered into the computer database. The data items included in figure 8.10 are only a partial listing of data abstracted from the health record. A hospital may abstract more than 200 data items from each record. In addition to abstracting, the coding professional also identifies the diagnoses and procedures documented in the health record. He or she assigns ICD-9-CM (or ICD-10-CM) codes to the diagnoses and procedures and CPT codes (if applicable) to procedures documented in the record. The coding function may be done manually by finding the correct codes in a coding book or done by using a computer program called an **encoder.** Encoders are software programs that help guide the coder through the various coding conventions and rules to arrive at a correct diagnosis, procedural, or service code. Other programs that are usually part of an encoding system are called DRG and APC groupers for acute care hospitals. **DRG groupers** are software programs that help coders determine the appropriate diagnosis-related group (DRG) assignment based on the logic of the system for hospital inpatients. **APC groupers** are software programs that help coders determine the appropriate ambulatory payment classification for an outpatient encounter.

In today's environment, codes for diagnoses, procedures, and services are usually entered directly into a computer system along with pertinent patient information and other demographics. Data abstracted and the clinical code(s) assigned to a health record make it possible to create automated disease, operation, and physician indexes (discussed later in this chapter). Such indexes are essential in order to retrieve data or specific health records to conduct research or clinical quality performance studies.

Like quantitative analysis, clinical coding can be either concurrent or retrospective. In some acute care and long-term care facilities, the coding of diagnoses, procedures, and services occurs during the patient's hospital stay. In this method, the HIM professional goes to the nursing unit daily or periodically, reviews the health record, and assigns appropriate

Figure 8.10.   Examples of abstracted data fields

Admit Source:
  Physician referral
  Clinic referral
  HMO referral
  Transfer from a hospital
  Transfer from a skill nursing facility
  Transfer from another healthcare facility
  Emergency room
  Court/law enforcement
  Information not available

Transfer facility

Hospital Service
  Hospice inpatient
  Psychiatric and alcohol
Inpatients/outpatients
  Skill nursing inpatients
  Surgical inpatients
  Oncology inpatients
  Obstetrics
  Trauma
  Newborn
  Cardiology
  Medicine

Discharge Disposition
  Self-care (home)
  Skilled nursing facility
  Rehabilitation facility
  Against medical advice

  Psychiatric facility
  Long term-care facility
  Intermediate care facility
  Assisted Living
  Hospice
  Home health
  Acute care facility
  Expired
  Unknown

Discharge facility

Anesthesia Type
  Conscious sedation
  General
  Monitored anesthesia care
  Regional

ASA classification

Gestation

C-section
  No previous C-section
  Previous C-section
  C-section performed for complications

VBAC (vaginal birth after cesarean section)

Apgar score (0-10)

Birth weight

**Note: This is not an exhaustive list of data items collected.

Source: Adapted from materials provided by Grant/Riverside Methodist Hospital, Columbus, Ohio.

diagnosis, procedural, and service codes. In the retrospective process, the health record is coded after patient discharge. Coding usually occurs after the health record has been assembled and analyzed for completeness.

Other HIM Functions

Research, statistical reporting, cancer registries, trauma registries, and birth certificate functions require data contained in the health record. Therefore, the HIM department often manages these functions.

Research and Statistics

Many HIM departments include a research division. The type of research assistance provided to clinicians, medical staff committees, and clinical administrative decision support varies from organization to organization. Some HIM research sections are responsible for identifying candidate health records for research projects that clinicians are conducting. An example might be that of a physician doing a study on patients diagnosed with hypertension and diabetes who are being given a specific type of medication. In this case, the research section would use disease and procedure indexes to identify and retrieve the appropriate health records. In some cases, the HIM research professionals might not only identify and retrieve the health records, but also actually review the selected records and abstract or collect data from them for the physician researchers.

In addition to research functions, many HIM departments are responsible for collecting and calculating various statistics about the operation of the healthcare facility. (See chapter 10.) Among these are ratios and percentages such as the percentage of occupancy, death and autopsy rates, and hospital census reports. Where the institution has integrated computer information systems, many of these types of statistics are generated automatically. This is particularly the case with daily hospital census reports and percentage of occupancy. However, data-entry and other errors often produce incorrect results, so it is still usually the function of the HIM department to verify the accuracy of many of the statistics calculated about institutional operations.

Cancer and Trauma Registries

The HIM department also may manage the cancer and trauma registry functions. Cancer registries use information from patient records to collect data for the study and treatment of cancer. Likewise, trauma registries use information from the patient record to collect data for the study and treatment of trauma patients. Both registries maintain large computer databases to store patient data.

Birth Certificates

Sometimes the HIM department is responsible for submitting an accurate birth certificate to the health department. A birth certificate must be completed for each newborn before the infant is discharged from the hospital. Information is gathered from the mother's and baby's medical record for completion of the birth certificate.

Check Your Understanding 8.1

Instructions: Choose the most appropriate answer for the following questions.

1. _____ The system in which a health record number is assigned at the first encounter and then used for all subsequent healthcare encounters is the _____.
   a. Serial numbering system
   b. Unit numbering system
   c. Serial–unit numbering system
   d. All of the above

2. _____ A health record number is assigned as a unique patient identifier for _____.
   a. Paper-based records
   b. Electronic health records
   c. Microfilmed records
   d. All of the above

3. _____ Consider the following sequence of numbers: 12-34-55, 13-34-55, and 14-34-54. What filing system is being used if these numbers represent the health record numbers of three records filed together within the filing system?
   a. Straight numerical filing
   b. Terminal-digit filing
   c. Middle-digit filing
   d. None of the above

4. _____ Which of the following patient identifier(s) may be used to locate an electronic health record?
   a. Patient name
   b. Health record number
   c. Patient account number
   d. All of the above

5. _____ The master patient index (MPI) is necessary to locate health records within the paper-based storage system for all the types of filing systems, except _____.
   a. Straight numerical
   b. Terminal-digit filing
   c. Middle-digit filing
   d. Alphabetical filing

6. _____ What type of paper-based storage system conserves floor space by eliminating all but one or two aisles?
   a. Open-shelf units
   b. Carousel systems
   c. Mobile filing units
   d. Filing cabinets

7. _____ What feature of the filing folder helps locate misfiles within the paper-based filing system?
   a. Fasteners
   b. Folder weight
   c. Color-coding
   d. None of the above

8. _____ In a paper-based system, individual health records are organized in a pre-established order. This process is called _____.
   a. Retrieval
   b. Assembly
   c. Analysis
   d. Reordering

9. _____ Reviewing a health record for missing signatures and missing medical reports is called _____.
   a. Assembly
   b. Indexing
   c. Analysis
   d. Coding

10. _____ Reviewing the record for deficiencies after the patient is discharged from the hospital is an example of review.
    a. Concurrent
    b. Retrospective
    c. Real–time
    d. None of the above

11. _____ Which of the following chart-processing activities does not occur in the EHR that uses scanned images?
    a. Chart preparation
    b. Scanning
    c. Assembly
    d. Quality review

12. _____ Incomplete records that are not completed by the physician within the time frame specified in the healthcare facility's policies are called _____.
    a. Suspended records
    b. Delinquent records
    c. Loose records
    d. Default records

13. _____ The function within the HIM department responsible for listening to dictated reports and typing them into a medical report format is called _____.
    a. Clinical coding
    b. Medical transcription
    c. Clerical services
    d. Release of information

14. _____ Reviewing requests for health record copies and determining if they are valid is part of the _____ function within the HIM department.
    a. Analysis function
    b. Clinical coding
    c. Storage and retrieval function
    d. Release of information function

15. _____ Assigning ICD-9-CM and CPT codes to the diagnoses and procedures documented in the medical record is called _____.
    a. Clinical coding
    b. Release of information
    c. Billing
    d. Medical transcription

HIM Interdepartmental Relationships

The HIM department (especially the clinical coding function), patient care departments, patient registration, and the billing department all interact and have an impact on the healthcare organization's revenue cycle. These departments must interact to ensure that the chargemaster data are correct and that the health record is accurately reflects the patient's condition and the services provided.

Patient Registration

Typically, the first point of data collection in any healthcare organization is patient registration. During the registration process, the patient provides the registration or admitting clerk with personal information. The patient's information is needed for the identification, treatment, and payment of healthcare services. For example, the patient provides demographic information such as name, address, telephone number, and emergency contact information. He or she also provides information about how payment should be handled (for example, insurance company name and insurance group number). For inpatient or same-day surgery admissions, other information, including attending physician, provisional diagnosis, and planned treatment, is provided by the patient's attending physician and integrated into the registration data collection and processing. For a laboratory or radiology referral, an order for a test or treatment must be accompanied by a tentative diagnosis or a reason for the order. The patient registration function essentially begins the process of documenting the patient's care and treatment.

Thus, patient registration is the area where the health record begins. Additionally, it is the area where the health record number is assigned. The accuracy of the information entered into the computer by the patient registration area has a significant impact on the HIM department, patient care areas, and billing department.

Data quality always begins at the source of the data. When data are recorded or obtained incorrectly at the start of the process, the errors follow the data throughout its use in the healthcare organization's business and patient care processes. For example, an error made in entering a patient's health insurance number in the computer system will likely cause serious problems for the billing office. An error made in recording a patient's provisional diagnosis may have adverse effects on the delivery of patient care. An error in assigning a new health record number to a patient who has previously been a patient at the facility and already has a number can cause filing and MPI problems if a unit numbering system is used. Two numbers assigned to a single patient are often referred to as "duplicate" numbers. Because the health record is filed in the storage area using the health record number, duplicate numbers result in the record having two separate locations and compromise the integrity of the MPI (discussed later in this chapter). Thus, the importance of getting information correct the first time and at the point where it is initially collected, entered, or recorded cannot be overstated.

Figure 8.11 shows the various areas where patient registration can occur in a large healthcare organization. In some organizations, responsibility for patient registration or admitting falls to the director of HIM services. In others, the admitting department reports to nursing or some other unit or is a separate department.

In smaller organizations such as freestanding clinics or long-term care facilities, patient registration usually occurs in, and is the responsibility of, only one area. In larger facilities,

Figure 8.11.   Points of patient registration in a large healthcare facility

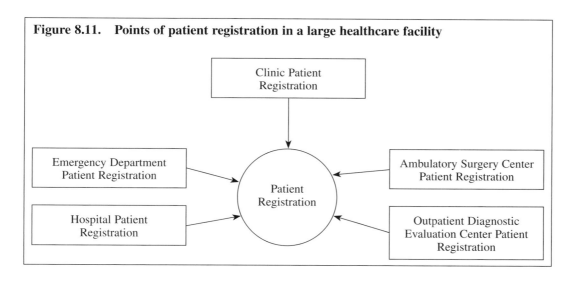

it can occur in various areas. For example, when the patient is being admitted to an acute care hospital, registration usually occurs in the patient registration or admitting department. However, when the patient comes to the emergency department for diagnosis or treatment, registration can occur in that department. Still another scenario is that the patient is being seen for the first time in one of the healthcare facility's clinics. In this case, patient registration occurs in the clinic office.

Documentation of information gathered during patient registration is handled either electronically or in paper format. Most acute care facilities now process all patient registration data using computer systems. Although patients may complete a paper form, the registration clerk usually enters their information into a computer system. In a smaller healthcare delivery unit such as a physician's office, however, registration data may still be collected and stored in a paper file.

Billing Department

The billing department also uses health record information that is entered into the computer by the HIM department. The HIM department assigns clinical codes and abstracts information from the patient's health record that is required on the patient's bill. Therefore, the patient's bill cannot be submitted for payment until the HIM department enters the required health record information into the computer.

The HIM department also affects the healthcare facility's reimbursement cycle by tracking health records where coding has been delayed and the bill has not been sent for payment. In many facilities, a report is generated weekly that identifies patient accounts that have not been billed because of missing ICD-9-CM codes and/or CPT codes. It is HIM personnel who locate the records to determine why there has been a delay in coding and initiate completion of the coding process so the bill can be submitted to the party responsible for payment of services.

The ROI function in the HIM department also can affect the billing process. Third-party payers often request additional information from the health record before payment (reimbursement for services provided) is sent to the healthcare facility.

Patient Care Departments

The HIM department also works closely with patient care departments such as nursing, laboratory, radiology, physical and occupational therapy, and so on. All patient care departments document the services they provide to patients in the health record. Therefore, they are contributors to health record content.

In a paper-based record system, the HIM department also delivers health records from previous admissions to the nursing units when the patient is readmitted to the hospital. In other healthcare settings, the HIM department pulls and delivers charts of established patients to clinics or other patient care areas. When the patient is discharged from the hospital or leaves a clinic, the HIM department retrieves records from previous admissions or visits in addition to records of the patient's recent admission/visit. The health record then is routed to the record-processing area of the HIM department.

Check Your Understanding 8.2

Instructions: Choose the most appropriate answer for the following questions.

1. ____ Where does the health record begin?
   a. Patient registration
   b. Nursing unit
   c. Billing department
   d. HIM department

2. ____ What department within the hospital uses the information abstracted and coded by the HIM department to send for payment from third-party payers?
   a. Patient registration
   b. Nursing unit
   c. Billing department
   d. Administration

3. ____ The documentation of clinical information that makes up the health record is entered into the record by ____.
   a. Patient registration
   b. Nursing
   c. Billing
   d. Administration

4. ____ In a paper-based system, the HIM department routinely delivers health records to ____?
   a. Patient registration
   b. Nursing units
   c. Billing department
   d. Administration

5. ____ The health record number is typically assigned by ____.
   a. Patient registration
   b. Nursing
   c. Billing
   d. HIM staff

Management of Health Record Content and Processes

As explained in chapter 2, the health record is the principal repository for data and information about the healthcare services provided to individual patients. Traditionally, the HIM department has been responsible for a variety of content issues. In fulfilling this role, the HIM department has worked with appropriate medical staff committees, clinical departments, and administration.

With regard to a paper-based health record, HIM usually sets standards for record content, chart order, and forms design and development to ensure that content meets accrediting, licensing, and other best practices for documentation. HIM performs many of the same functions when working with an EHR. The department helps ensure that record content and authentication (signatures) in the EHR meet accreditation and licensing requirements and also participates in user-interface design for computerized data input.

Accreditation and Licensing Documentation Requirements

Accrediting bodies such as the **Joint Commission on Accreditation of Healthcare Organizations** (JCAHO) and state licensing bodies are among the groups that have established standards for health record documentation. JCAHO is a not-for-profit organization that offers an accreditation program for hospitals and other healthcare organizations based on pre-established accreditation standards.

In addition to the JCAHO, other entities that have established documentation standards include:

- Medicare Conditions of Participation

- National Committee for Quality Assurance (NCQA)

- American Accreditation Health Care Commission/Utilization Review Accreditation Commission (AAHCC/URAC)

- American Osteopathic Association (AOA)

- Commission on Accreditation of Rehabilitation Facilities (CARF)

- Health Accreditation Program of the National League of Nursing

- College of American Pathologists (CAP)

- American Association of Blood Banks (AABB)

- American College of Surgeons (ACS)

- Accreditation Association for Ambulatory Health Care (AAAHC)

- American Medical Accreditation Program (AMAP)

Today, over 80 percent of U.S. hospitals, as well as the majority of other healthcare organizations, seek JCAHO accreditation. For several decades, JCAHO accreditation has been an indicator that the accredited hospital or healthcare facility provides high-quality care. As part of the accreditation process, the healthcare facility undergoes an on-site evaluation by a team of JCAHO surveyors. As described in *Hospital Accreditation Standards 2005* (JCAHO 2005), it is during the survey that JCAHO evaluates the quality of care provided to patients, the systems in place for ensuring caregiver and medical staff competence, and the performance of important patient functions.

In the past, the on-site survey was a scheduled event. However, "the JCAHO plans to transition to all unannounced surveys by 2006" (JCAHO 2005, APP-5). The accreditation process also includes a Periodic Performance Review (PPR) and a Priority Focus Process (PFP) that facilitates the newer continual standards compliance process. Midpoint in the accreditation process, the hospital must submit the PPR to JCAHO. The PPR is a hospital's review of standards, compliance with standards, action plans implemented to address noncompliance with standards, and measures to follow up on the success of the action plans. The PFP uses information from the PPR and other data sources to identify "priority focus areas" that are used to guide the survey process. The JCAHO survey, PPR and the PFP are used to indicate that the healthcare facility is in compliance with JCAHO standards.

Healthcare organizations accredited by JCAHO are also "deemed" to be in compliance with the Medical Conditions of Participation. This is referred to as **deemed status.** Medicare randomly selects hospitals recently surveyed by JCAHO and conducts another survey to validate the JCAHO survey results.

It is essential that HIM professionals become familiar with the JCAHO and Medicare standards and documentation requirements. An example of JCAHO standards from the 2005 manual appears in figure 8.12. "Standards are statements that define the performance expectations and/or structures or processes that must be in place for a hospital to provide safe, high quality care, treatment and services" (JCAHO 2005, HB 22). For each JCAHO standard, there are elements of performance "that detail specific performance expectations and/or structures or processes that must be in place" (JCAHO 2005, HB22). The next section of this chapter discusses the monitoring of accreditation and licensure standards.

Figure 8.12.   Examples of JCAHO Information Management Standards

Standard IM.2.10

Information privacy and confidentiality are maintained.

Standard IM 3.10

The hospital has processes in place to effectively manage information, including the capturing, reporting, processing, storing, retrieving, disseminating, and displaying of clinical/service and nonclinical data and information.

Standard IM 6.10

The hospital has a complete and accurate medical record for every individual assessed, cared for, treated, or served.

Standard IM 6.60

The hospital can provide access to all relevant information from a patient's record when needed for use in patient care, treatment, and services.

Source: © Joint Commission Resources: *Hospital Accreditation Standards 2005.* Oakbrook Terrace, IL: Joint Commission on Accreditation of Healthcare Organizations, 2005, pages IM3–IM4. Reprinted with permission.

It is important to note that each accrediting and licensing agency has its own standards, which must be followed by the healthcare facilities under their auspices.

Monitoring of Accreditation and Licensure Requirements

No program for ensuring the quality of health record content would be complete without a process for monitoring accreditation, licensure, and other state or federal agency requirements. Good documentation practices require organizations to be in compliance with regulations and standards from a variety of groups. The HIM department director should establish a mechanism that targets specific regulatory or standards groups and monitors for compliance with these standards. New standards and changes to regulations must be monitored and HIM functions revised, if necessary.

Because the HIM department is entrenched in review and analysis of the health record, several processes are typically in place to monitor the healthcare facility's compliance with JCAHO standards. Following are examples of the typical processes in place within the HIM department to monitor compliance:

- Record completion process

    —*Monitoring delinquency rates:* As part of its record completion processes, the HIM department monitors the number of delinquent records. Many facilities determine the number of delinquent records each month and notify their medical staff members of their incomplete and delinquent records. The HIM professional determines the quarterly medical record delinquency rate for the facility and determines whether the hospital is in compliance with JCAHO standard IM 6.10, which states, "The hospital has a complete and accurate medical record for every individual assessed, cared for, treated and served." The JCAHO element of performance for standard 6.10 states, "The medical record delinquency rate averaged from the last four quarterly measurements is not greater than 50% of the average monthly discharge (AMD) rate and no quarterly measurement is greater than 50% of the AMD rate" (JCAHO 2005, IM-21). If the hospital is not in compliance with JCAHO, the medical records committee, administration, and other appropriate parties are notified and corrective is action taken. There may be various consequences for physicians when they have not completed delinquent charts within a specified period of time.

    —*Monitoring timely completion of medical reports:* Other JCAHO standards specify time frames within which various medical reports (history and physicals, operative reports, autopsy reports, and so on) must be completed. The HIM department's transcription area may monitor compliance in this area. The transcriptionist can compare the date a report was dictated against the date of service or admission to determine whether the report has been completed within the time frame specified by the standards.

    —*Monitoring health record completion:* The quantitative analysis function of the HIM department monitors whether health record documents have been authenticated. Unauthenticated parts of the health record are identified for completion by either handwritten or electronic signature. If the physician does not complete the record within a timely manner, the record is counted in the delinquent record rate. JCAHO standard 6.10 also requires authentication of various medical reports. (See figure 8.12, p. 366.)

- Documentation

  —*Monitoring the use of abbreviations, acronyms and symbols:* Transcriptionists can assist with monitoring the use of abbreviations, acronyms, and symbols as they transcribe dictation. Clinical coding personnel also can identify the use of unauthorized abbreviations, acronyms, and symbols as they abstract information from health records. This is an example of the HIM professional's role in monitoring hospital compliance with JCHAO standard IM 3.10 (figure 8.12) and the element of performance, which states "abbreviations, acronyms, and symbols are standardized throughout the hospital and there is a list of abbreviations, acronyms, and symbols not to use" (JCAHO 2005, IM-16).

- Confidentiality of information

  —*Monitoring access to protected health information:* The HIM department's daily ROI activities can help ensure and monitor access to patient-specific information after discharge. HIM personnel are knowledgeable in the laws and regulations governing the release of patient information. Thus, the department's ROI function is instrumental in monitoring compliance with JCAHO standard 2.10. (See figure 8.12.)

- Access to patient records

  —*Storage and retrieval processes:* The storage and retrieval processes are managed to ensure that health information is accessible for patient care. These processes are pivotal for the compliance of JCAHO standard IM 6.60. (See figure 8.12.)

There are many additional JCAHO standards beyond those listed in the sample shown in figure 8.12. The HIM professional must consult the *Hospital Accreditation Standards Manual* published by JCAHO for a complete listing of standards and elements of performance. JCAHO also publishes accreditation manuals for specialty areas, such as long-term care and behavioral healthcare facilities. In addition to monitoring performed as part of daily HIM functions, health record reviews are often done periodically to ensure facility compliance with other standards. The health records review process is a multidisciplinary process coordinated by the HIM department.

Forms Design and Development

An important part of ensuring adequate health record content is the function of forms design and development. In a paper record system, forms make possible the capture of adequate healthcare documentation. The HIM department often participates in forms design in consultation with a forms vendor. The basic concept behind any form is that it must meet the needs of the end user. This means that the form must fulfill its intended purpose, include all the necessary data, and be easy to use.

One of the first steps in forms design is to identify the purpose, use, and potential users of the form. This basic information will drive the rest of the design process. For example, when the purpose of the form is to meet a licensing requirement, the data elements contained on it must comply with the requirement. When the form is to be used by multiple individuals, a multicopy version might be appropriate. When it is to be completed by hand, it must allow enough space for handwriting.

After the purpose, use, and potential users of the form have been identified, it is important to ensure that the new form does not duplicate one already in place. Organizations often needlessly duplicate forms because they have no mechanism for forms tracking.

Any forms design project should follow a number of guidelines. The following are common design elements for paper forms (AHIMA 1997):

- All forms should contain a unique identifying number for positive identification and easy inventory control.

- Each form should include original and revised dates for the tracking and purging of obsolete forms.

- Each form should have a concise title that clearly identifies the form's purpose.

- The facility's name and logo should appear on each page of the form.

- For clinical forms, patient identification information (name, health record number, billing number, physician name and number, date of birth, admission date, and room number) should appear on every page.

- For clinical forms, a signature line should appear at the bottom, and there should be no question about what has been authenticated. If initials are used, space also should be provided for the full name and title so that each set of initials is identified.

- Data-entry methodology should be considered when the information is to be keyed into a computer. The order of the form should mirror the data-entry order to ensure that information is entered consistently.

- Optical character reader codes and bar codes should be printed in the upper left-hand corner of the form when imaging the health record is a possibility.

- A standard of eight and a half by eleven inches is the best size for a document. Bifold and trifold documents are difficult to handle and copy in a closed chart.

- Form colors should be black ink on white paper. If color-coding is desired, a strip of color along one margin is the best option.

- Documents that contain punched holes should have a margin of at least three-quarters of an inch. All other margins should be at least three-eighths of an inch wide.

- Vertical and horizontal lines assist the user in completing and reviewing the form. Bold lines should be used to draw the reader's eye to an important field.

- Sufficient space should be provided to complete the entry (for example, one-sixteenth of an inch for typed letters and one-third inch high for handwritten entries).

- Titles for boxes and fields should be located in the top left-hand corner of the box or field.

- Paper ranging from twenty to twenty-four pounds in weight is recommended for use in copiers, scanners, and fax machines.

- Type size should be no smaller than nine points for lowercase letters and ten points for uppercase letters.

The principles of good design are critical when forms are used in document imaging systems. For example, the use of colored paper or ink other than black should be minimized or eliminated because the color can adversely affect the quality of the scanned images. Also, the use of scanned images requires forms to contain a bar code that identifies the document type, thus enabling the form to be placed in the proper location within the EHR. Forms not containing a bar code must be indexed separately when scanned into the computer.

In today's practice, computer data entry is becoming more commonplace. Good design and computer–user interface also are essential for computer views or reports generated by EHRs. The following general principles should be considered when developing user views or screens:

- Navigation design

  —All controls should be clear and placed in an intuitive location on the screen.

  —Limit choices and label commands.

  —Provide "undo" buttons to make mistakes easy to override.

  —Use consistent grammar and terminology.

  —Provide a confirmation message for any critical function (such as deleting a file).

- Input design

  —Simplify data collection.

  —Sequence data input to follow work flow.

  —Provide a title for each screen.

  —Minimize keystrokes by using pop-up menus.

  —Use text boxes to enter text.

  —Use a number box to enter numbers.

  —Use a selection box to allow the user to select a value from a predefined list:

    –Check boxes (used for multiple selections)

    –Radio buttons (used for single selections)

    –On-screen list boxes

    –Drop-down list boxes

    –Combo boxes

- Data validation

  —Perform a completeness check to ensure that all required data have been entered.

—Perform a format check to ensure that data are the right type (numeric, alphabetic, and so on).

—Perform a range check to ensure that numeric data are in the correct range.

—Perform a consistency check to ensure that combinations of data are correct.

—Perform a database check to compare data against a database or file to ensure data are correct as entered.

- Output design

—Minimize the number of "clicks" needed to reach data or a specific screen.

—Chunk data into a single organized menu to eliminate layers of screens.

Clinical Forms Committee

Every healthcare organization should have a forms or design (for EHR systems) committee. The medical records committee also may function in this capacity. This committee should provide oversight for the development, review, and control of all enterprise-wide information capture tools, including paper forms and design of computer screens. The committee should be composed of information users and include representatives from the following departments:

- Health information management

- Medical staff

- Nursing staff

- Purchasing

- Information services

- Performance improvement

- Support or ancillary departments

- Forms vendor representative

In addition, anyone directly affected by the new form or computer view should be invited to attend the forms committee meeting. For example, when a form is being redesigned for use in the intensive care unit, nurses or physicians from that clinical area should be invited to give their input.

Forms Control, Tracking, and Management

Forms control, tracking, and management are important issues. At a minimum, a good forms control program includes the following activities (Barnett 1996):

- *Establishing standards:* Written standards and guidelines are essential to ensure that good design and production practices are followed. A forms manual should be developed. Standards are fixed rules that must be followed for every form (for example, where the form title should be located). A guideline, on the other hand, provides general direction about the design of a form (for example, usual size of the font used).

- *Establishing a numbering and tracking system:* A unique numbering system should be developed to identify all organizational forms. A master form index should be established, and copies of all forms should be maintained for easy retrieval. At a minimum, information in the master form index should include form title, form number, origination date, revision dates, form purpose, and legal requirements. Ideally, the tracking system should be automated.

- *Establishing a testing and evaluation plan:* No new or revised form should be put into production or use without a field test and evaluation. Mechanisms should be in place to ensure appropriate testing of any new or revised form.

- *Checking the quality of new forms:* A mechanism should be in place to check all newly printed forms prior to distribution. This should be a quality check to ensure that the new form conforms to the original procurement order.

- *Systematizing storage, inventory, and distribution:* Processes should be in place to ensure that forms are stored appropriately. Paper forms should be stored in safe and environmentally appropriate environments. Inventory should be maintained at a cost-effective level, and distribution should be timely.

- *Establishing a forms database:* In an electronic system that supports document imaging, a forms database may be used to store and facilitate updating of forms. Such a database can provide information on utilization rates, obsolescence, and replacement of individual forms or documentation templates.

Quality Control and Monitoring for Health Record Systems

All the HIM functions discussed in this chapter must be managed appropriately to ensure the quality of health record content as well as the security, accessibility, and timeliness of the information contained in the health record. However, merely having a process for health record review does not totally ensure content quality. Further, having good forms design practices does not necessarily mean that all forms that are developed are necessary. Therefore, the organization must establish systems to help monitor and control the quality of record content and processes. The strategies discussed thus far help ensure quality control over the management of health record content.

In addition to quality monitoring performed to ensure compliance with JCAHO standards, HIM functions should be monitored for accuracy and timeliness. Below are examples of control measures that may be established to ensure that processes are being performed correctly and that systems are functioning as expected. The department should establish standards and criteria that indicate an acceptable level of performance. After quality control standards are established, it is important to establish a monitoring system to determine whether goals are being met. Corrective action should be implemented when error or accuracy rates are deemed to be at an unacceptable level.

- *Storage and retrieval:* Various standards can be set to monitor the quality of the storage and retrieval process. Filing accuracy can be checked by conducting a random audit of the storage area. To conduct a study, a section of the permanent file room can be checked for misfiles. Any misfiles found are noted, and a filing accuracy rate can be determined and compared against the established standard. For example, if the standard is that "99 percent of the health records will be filed correctly," a sample of filed records can be checked for misfiles. If 550 health records are checked and 7 misfiles are found, the error rate is 1.27 percent (7 divided by 550 multiplied by 100, which would make the accuracy rate 98.7 percent). Some organizations have a rechecking process whereby a record is filed and tagged and another employee follows up and checks the accuracy of the filing. Similarly, in a digital imaging system, indexing and quality should be checked through a defined quality assessment process to ensure the retrievability of health information.

Timeliness of the storage and retrieval processes also can be monitored. Examples of standards that may be established to determine the timeliness of HIM services are:

—An average of fifty records will be filed in an hour.

—Records for the emergency department will be retrieved within ten minutes of the request.

—Loose materials will be filed in either the record or the outguide pocket within twenty-four hours of receipt in the HIM department.

—An hourly average of 190 pages for indexing scanned records

—Scanned records will be available online within twenty-four hours of discharge.

• *Record processing:* In a paper-based health record system, physicians come to the incomplete record area to dictate and sign medical records. If records are unavailable when they arrive, the chart completion process is delayed. The availability of records can be monitored by comparing the incomplete chart lists for a sample of physicians against the charts available to the physicians when they come to the HIM department. For example, if seven physicians worked on completing charts on a particular day with a total of 210 incomplete records collectively and a total of 35 charts were not available, the nonavailable chart rate is 16.6, or 17 percent (35 divided by 210 multiplied by 100).

As discussed previously, in an EHR, imaged documents are reviewed to ensure that a quality image is achieved.

• *Medical transcription:* To monitor transcription accuracy, a sample of the transcriptionists' reports can be checked for wrong terms, misspelled words, incorrect format, and/or grammatical errors. The number of errors found is noted, and an error or accuracy rate is determined and compared against an established standard.

Transcription turnaround time also can also be monitored to determine whether reports are being transcribed within the expected time frame set in a standard. Most dictation/transcription computer management systems track the date and time reports are dictated and transcribed. A report indicating dictation and transcription time and date can be used to determine turnaround time.

- *Release of information:* The turnaround time for the ROI function also can be monitored. The date a request is received and the date the record copies are sent are entered into a computer database. This information can be used to generate a report that will determine whether the records are being sent in a timely manner.

The accuracy of the ROI function can be monitored by checking a sample of authorization forms that have been sent or that are ready to be sent to verify the validity of the authorization and to ensure compliance with federal and state regulations. The error rate or accuracy rate can be determined and compared against a set standard.

- *Clinical coding:* To monitor the clinical coding function for accuracy, a sample of records for each clinical coder can be reviewed to verify that coding rules and principles are being applied. Criteria such as correct code assignment, missing codes, extra codes, and sequencing of codes can be established. Any errors found should be noted, and an error or accuracy rate can be calculated to determine whether the quality standard is being met.

Check Your Understanding 8.3

Instructions: Choose the most appropriate answer for the following questions.

1. _____ One of the most sought after accreditation distinction by healthcare facilities is offered by the _____.
   a. American Medical Association
   b. American Hospital Association
   c. Joint Commission on Accreditation of Healthcare Organizations
   d. American Health Information Management Association

2. _____ Statements that define the performance expectations and/or structures or processes that must be in place are _____.
   a. Rules
   b. Policies
   c. Outcomes
   d. Standards

3. _____ Which of the following is *not* a part of the HIM department's monitoring function for compliance with accrediting standards?
   a. Monitoring delinquent chart rates
   b. Correcting clinical notes
   c. Monitoring the use of medical abbreviations
   d. Monitoring the completion of medical reports

4. _____ All forms should _____.
   a. Contain a unique identifier
   b. Include origination and revision dates
   c. Include the facility name and logo
   d. All of the above

5. _____ What should be done when the HIM department's error or accuracy rate is deemed unacceptable?
    a. A corrective action should be taken.
    b. The problem should be treated as an isolated incident.
    c. The formula for determining the rate may need to be adjusted.

6. _____ The forms or design committee _____.
    a. Provides oversight for the development, review, and control of forms and computer screens
    b. Is multidisciplinary
    c. Is sometimes the responsibility of the medical records committee
    d. All of the above

Indexes and Registries

As stated earlier, HIM departments often also have responsibility for maintaining indexes and registries. An index is a guide that serves as a pointer or indicator to locate something. For example, the index at the back of this book lists key terms. The page number(s) by each term indicates where in the book the reader can find information about that particular term.

Following is a brief overview of indexes and registries. More detailed information is provided in chapter 9.

Master Patient Index

Probably the most important index used by the HIM department is the master patient index (MPI). The MPI functions as the primary guide to locating pertinent demographic data about the patient and his or her health record number. Without the information contained in the MPI, it would be almost impossible to locate a patient's health record in most organizations that use a numeric filing system.

The amount of information contained on each patient in the MPI varies from facility to facility. However, the basic information usually includes:

- Patient's last, first, and middle names

- Patient's health record number(s)

- Patient's date of birth

- Patient's gender

- Dates of encounter (admission and discharge dates are usually maintained for inpatients)

Additional information such as address, telephone number, and attending physician for each encounter also may be recorded in the index.

Today, it is common practice to have an automated MPI instead of a manually maintained index. Often the patient registration system, also known at the admission, discharge, transfer (ADT) system, functions as the MPI. The benefits of an automated system include the ability to access data by more than one individual at a time. In addition, edit checks can be applied against specific fields in the database to better ensure data accuracy. An automated index also can be easily cross-referenced, for example, when a patient has used more than one name during hospital or clinic visits.

Small facilities may still use a manual MPI. In a manual MPI, index cards (usually three by five inches) are used to record patient information in typewritten format. MPI cards are usually filed in strict alphabetical order in rotary files or vertical carousel storage files described previously.

Manual MPI indexes are prone to problems. One major concern is misfiled cards. A misfiled MPI card makes it almost impossible to locate a patient's health record. At the very least, record retrieval time is increased significantly. This is why monitoring systems must be in place to ensure correct alphabetical filing of every card. Many HIM departments have established a process whereby another employee rechecks every filed MPI card for proper alphabetical location. For example, all MPI cards filed on the day shift are tagged and an employee from the evening shift rechecks the accuracy of each card's location.

Another disadvantage to the manual system is that usually only one person at a time can access the index. This definitely slows down retrieval time. Furthermore, updating, cross-referencing, and maintaining a manual system is more time-consuming than an automated system.

Disease and Operation Indexes

Compiling and maintaining **disease** and **operation indexes** has always been an important function of the HIM department. In these indexes, diagnoses and operative codes, such as those used in a classification system such as ICD-9-CM, are used as guides or pointers to the health records of patients who have had a specific disease or operation. Disease and operation indexes are essential for locating health records to conduct quality improvement and research studies, as well as for monitoring quality of care.

The minimal amount of data required for a disease or operation index usually includes:

- The principal diagnosis and relevant secondary diagnoses
- Associated procedures
- Patient's health record number
- Patient's gender, age, and race
- Attending physician's code or name
- The hospital service
- The end result of hospitalization
- Dates of encounter (including admission and discharge for inpatients)

Given this type of information, the index can be used as a guide for retrieving health records for research or other studies. For example, if the clinical quality committee wanted to see the health records for all male patients who had been diagnosed with myocardial infarction, were fifty years old or less, had been treated in the past six months, and had been discharged alive, the records could be easily identified and subsequently retrieved using the information in the index.

Today, most indexes are automated, except for those in very, very small facilities. The automated disease and operation index usually is accomplished by generating standard or ad hoc reports of data already existing in the computer. Ad hoc reporting capabilities enable the user to select the field items he or she wants in the reports. Standard reports are preexisting reports that have been programmed into the computer to include predefined data fields.

In many institutions, much of the information needed for disease and operation indexes is entered into the computer system concurrently with the diagnosis coding process. In other facilities, the data may be entered during a separate function of abstracting data from the health record and entering them into the computer system. In some cases, pertinent demographic patient information is exchanged from the automated R-ADT system and passed to the coding system. This type of data exchange helps to reduce work and data-entry redundancy and to increase data integrity and consistency.

In a manual indexing system, special index cards are used to record the pertinent data. The cards are preprinted with the pertinent categories of data to be collected. Usually, several entries (such as encounters) can be made on one card. There are various methods for filing disease and operation index cards. One common method is to enter encounters sequentially by date of discharge starting at the beginning of each year. Each card is then numbered sequentially beginning with the numeral one and filed by year.

This description illustrates how difficult it is to compile, maintain, and retrieve data from a manual index. As with any manual system, opportunities abound for data-entry error. Cross-indexing of diseases and operations is impossible without an enormous amount of data redundancy, and retrieval is very time-consuming.

Physician Index

Like the disease and operation indexes, the physician index is a guide to identifying medical cases associated with a specific physician. Often the information gathered for disease and operation indexes is sufficient for the physician index. Essentially, the data required in such an index include the physician's name or code; the health record number, diagnosis, operations, and disposition of the patients the physician treated; the dates of the patients' admission and discharge; and the patients' gender and age. In addition, certain other patient demographic information may be useful.

Registries

A registry is a chronological listing of data, or register. With regard to HIM functions, traditional registries include the patient admission and discharge register, operating room register, and birth and death registers. Most information collected today for registries is a byproduct of other automated systems. A more complete discussion of registries is provided in chapter 9.

Check Your Understanding 8.4

Instructions: Complete the following sentences.

1. _____ The primary guide to locating a record in a numerical filing system is the _____.
   a. Master patient index
   b. Admission register
   c. Discharge register
   d. Physician index

2. ____ If one needed to know the number of C-sections performed by a specific obstetrician, the ____ would be used to identify the cases.
    a. Operation index
    b. Disease index
    c. Physician index
    d. Master patient index

3. ____ The computer system that may serve as the MPI function is the ____.
    a. Patient registration system
    b. Abstract system
    c. Encoder
    d. Chart-tracking system

4. ____ A chronological listing of data is called a/an ____
    a. Index
    b. Register
    c. Abstract
    d. Record

5. ____ Most indexes and registers today ____.
    a. Are maintained on microfilm
    b. Are automated or computerized
    c. Have been eliminated
    d. Are manual

Management and Supervisory Processes

Regardless of size, all HIM departments involve a great deal of organization, management, and supervision of personnel. This section provides an overview of some of the more common supervisory responsibilities associated with the management of the HIM functions.

Policy and Procedure Development

Policies and procedures serve as the foundation for the management and supervision of employees of any department or unit. Policies are statements that describe general guidelines that direct behavior or direct and constrain decision making in the organization. Some policies apply to the entire organization; departmental policies apply only to specific business units.

Policies follow a specific format. For example, the policy statement from the University of Houston shown in figure 8.13 provides a specific format that includes a policy title, description of the scope of the policy, the expected standard, and guidelines to achieve the expected standard (University of Houston 2001). Figure 8.14 is an example of a policy that provides guidance for the assignment of overtime within the HIM department. Every policy must be dated, and if there has been a revision, the date of the revision also should appear on the policy. The format of a policy statement varies from organization to organization.

The success of policy relies on procedures. Unlike broad statements included in a policy, procedures are specific statements about how work is to be carried out. Essentially,

---

Figure 8.13.   Sample policy on computer terminal controls

Purpose: To prevent unauthorized access to University Hospital data by providing terminal controls

Scope: University Hospital's terminals

Standard: Proper physical and software control mechanisms shall be in place to control access to and use of devices connected to University Hospital's computer systems

Guidelines:

1. Hardware Terminal Locking: In areas that are not physically secured, terminals should be equipped with locking devices to prevent their use during unattended periods. The locks should be installed in addition to programmed restrictions, such as automatic disconnect after a given period of inactivity.

2. Operating System Identification of Terminal: All terminal activity should be controlled by the operating system, which should be able to identify terminals, whether they are hardwired or connected through communications lines. The operating system should inspect log-on requests to determine which application the terminal user desires. The user should identify an existing application and supply a valid user ID and password combination. If the log-on request is valid, the operating system should make a logical connection between the user and the application.

3. Limitation of Log-On Attempts: Limit system log-on attempts from remote terminal devices. More than three unsuccessful attempts should result in termination of the session, generation of a real-time security violation message to the operator and/or the ISO (and log of said message in an audit file), and purging of the input queue of messages from the terminal.

4. Time-Out Feature: Ensure that the operating system provides the timing services required to support a secure operational environment. Inactive processes or terminals (in an interactive environment) should be terminated after a predetermined period.

5. Dial-Up Control: The communications software should ensure a clean end of connection in all cases, especially in the event of abnormal disconnection.

---

they are specific instructions to help employees carry out a function or activity. Procedures provide step-by-step instructions on how to complete a specific task. Written procedures are beneficial as a training tool for new employees. They also are beneficial for providing staff with a consistent method of completing tasks.

The format of procedures varies from facility to facility. Figure 8.15 is an example of a procedure that explains the process of collecting discharge records from the nursing unit. This procedure demonstrates the detail that should be included in a written procedure. This procedure also demonstrates the interrelationship of the HIM department with the nursing units and the intra-relationship among the different functions of the HIM department.

Health information technicians have to follow both policies and procedures in their job functions. In some instances, the HIT will be involved in the development of policies and procedures as they pertain to the HIM department or information management in the organization. Figure 8.16 provides a listing of common HIM department policies and procedures. (See chapter 20 for more detailed information about policy and procedures.)

Figure 8.14.   Sample departmental policy: Overtime

HEALTH INFORMATION SERVICES STANDARD POLICY	
Title: OVERTIME	Issued:
Prepared by:	Effective:
Approved	Revised:

PURPOSE: To provide a fair, consistent guideline for assignment of overtime.

POLICY

Overtime will be assigned at the discretion of the manager/supervisor when it is deemed

- Volume of work exceeds staffing hours present
- Backlog
- Vacancy/extended absences

An Overtime Approval Form must be completed and returned to the Operations Manager/Coding Manager to obtain advanced approval of any necessary overtime.

The assignment will be based on

- past performance
- knowledge of the work area
- productivity
- availability

When overtime is deemed necessary the manager/supervisor(s) will utilize a rotating schedule of individuals trained in the area. If an individual declines an offer they will go to the end of the rotation. If the designated individual for OT fails to complete the assigned OT, it will count as an unexcused absence for the individual.

The manager/supervisor reserves the right to make the final determination in assignment of overtime based on the needs of the department.

Source: Grant Medical Center, Columbus, Ohio. Reprinted with permission.

Figure 8.15.   Sample departmental procedure: Collection of records from discharged patients

HEALTH INFORMATION SERVICES STANDARD POLICY

Title: Collection of Discharged Charts	Issued:
Prepared by:	Effective:
Approved	Revised:

PURPOSE: To provide a mechanism to follow when collecting discharged medical records from the units

PROCEDURE

The computer interface does not occur until midnight. Therefore, the discharge list will autoprint to the retrieval printer at 12:30 a.m.

I.   Separate the nursing units on the discharge list.
   A. Locate "Unit 3" on the list.
   B. Before the first "Unit 3" patient, draw a line. After the last "Unit 3," draw a line to separate "Unit 3" from the next location, "Unit 4."
   C. Do this for each unit on the list.
   D. EXCEPTIONS for the list:
     —Charts with "LD" listed as the department location will come down at a later time.

II. Making bar codes and folders from the discharge list.
   A. Make bar codes/folders for all discharges on the discharge list.

III. Picking up the charts from all floors.
   A. Pick up from all the floors.
   B. The charter is responsible for collecting any and all charts, old and new discharges, which are located in the designated collection areas on the floors.
   C. Bring all collected charts back to the Medical Record Department.

V.   Processing discharges.
   A. Separate the old charts and place them on the inbox shelf.
   B. Discharges on D/C list
     1) While placing the charts inside the folders, check each patient off by placing a small check-mark to the left of the patient's name.
     2) **Double-check the bar code information, folder information, and patient information in the chart to ensure all information matches. Check all discharge dates in computer.**
       a. Place each chart into a pile according to its next location (i.e., assembly, coding outpatient, other).
   C. Loose sheets and dictated reports may be brought down with the discharges. Some of the loose sheets and reports may belong to the collected charts. Match up the loose sheets with the discharges and place the loose sheets inside the folder. Place the loose sheets for patients that have previously been discharged in the loose sheets inbox. If the patient is still in-house, send the loose sheets or reports back up to the floor.

(Continued on next page)

Figure 8.15. *(Continued)*

    D. Uncollected charts
        1) Some charts on the discharge list may be uncollected. Track any uncollected folders to "Uncollected" in chart-tracking computer and highlight the medical record number and patient on the discharge list.
        2) Place the folder(s) in uncollected bin.
    E. Extra collections. Some charts may not be on the discharge list, but have been collected with the rest.
        1) Any collected charts that were not on the discharge list MUST be written on the discharge list with patient name and medical record number.
        2) Check the computer for the correct discharge date for the account number on the addressograph.
        3) Check the chart-tracking computer to see if the discharge date has already been tracked out to uncollected.
            a. If so, retrieve the folder from the uncollected area and track accordingly.
            b. If not, make a folder and bar code.
            c. Place the folder(s) in appropriate pile (assembly, coding outpatient, and so on).
        4) If the chart-tracking system lists a thinned part for the discharge, locate the thinned part to join the recently collected part and place in appropriate pile.
    F. Tracking charts through the computer
        1) Take the charts in the assembly pile and track them to assembly.
        2) Place the charts in assembly.
        3) Take the charts in the coding outpatient pile and track them to coding outpatient.
        4) Take the charts in the "Other" pile and decide where they need to go. Make a folder, if needed.

VI. Finishing up
    A. If, for any reason, the charter cannot finish creating, tracking, and placing the charts in the correct location, he or she must clearly label any unfinished work with what still needs to be done and let the supervisor/manager know.
    B. After all folders are created, tracked, and placed in the correct places (assembly or coding outpatient shelf), place the discharge list in the blue folder in the first shift supervisor's inbox on the office door.

VII. Monitoring discharge collection and uncollected lists
    A. The supervisor will process the discharge list daily. Statistics will be kept to report on a monthly basis to administration, nurse managers, nursing administrator, HIM director, and HIM operations manager.
    B. The supervisor will alert the appropriate nursing managers when a chart(s) is uncollected over 24 hours.
    C. If a chart is still uncollected after 48 hours, the supervisor will complete an incident report to alert risk management of the missing chart.

Source: Adapted from material provided by Grant Medical Center, Columbus, OH.

Figure 8.16.   Common HIM department policies and procedures

The following list provides an example of the types of policies and procedures that may be included in a manual for health information services. The titles and content of the policies and procedures may vary by facility or corporation. Some of the policies and procedures are listed more than once for cross-referencing purposes.

Abbreviations
Access to Automated/Computerized Records
Access to Records (Release of Information) by
        Resident and by Staff
Admission/Discharge Register
Admission Procedures
    Facility Procedures–Establishing/Closing the
        Record
    Preparing the Medical Record
    Preparing the Master Patient Index Card
    Readmission–Continued Use of Previous
        Record
    Readmission–New Record
Amendment of Clinical Records
Audit Schedule
Audit and Monitoring System
    Audit/Monitoring Schedule
    Admission/Readmission Audit
    Concurrent Audit
    Discharge Audit
    Specialized Audits (examples)
    Change in Condition
    MDS
    Nursing Assistant Flow Sheet
    Psychotropic Drug Documentation
    Pressure Sore
    Restrictive Device/Restraint
    Therapy
Certification, Medicare
Chart Removal and Chart Locator Log
Clinical Records, Definition of Records,
        and Record Service
General Policies
    Access to Records
    Automation of Records (See also
        Computerization)
    Availability
    Change in Ownership
    Coding from home
    Completion and Correction of Records
    Confidentiality
    Definition of the legal record
    Indexes
    Ownership of Records

Permanent and Capable of Being
        Photocopied
Retention
Storage of Records
Subpoena
Unit Record
Willful Falsification/Willful Omission
Closing the Record
Coding and Indexing, Disease Index
Committee Minutes Guidelines
Computerization and Security of Automated Data/
        Records
Confidentiality (See Release of Information)
Consulting Services for Clinical Records and Plan
        of Service
Content, Record *(the list provided is not all-
        inclusive and should be tailored to the
        facility/corporation)*
    General
    Advanced Directives
    Transfer Form/Discharge Plan of Care
    Discharge against Medical Advice
    Physician Consultant Reports
    Medicare Certification/Recertification
    Physician Orders/Telephone Orders
    Physician Services Guidelines and Progress
        Notes
    Physician History and Physical Exam
    Discharge Summary
    Interdisciplinary Progress Notes
Copying/Release of Records—General
Correcting Clinical Records
Data Collection/Monitoring
Definition of Clinical Records/Health Information
        Service
Delinquent Physician Visit
Denial Letters, Medicare
Destruction of Records, Log
Disaster Planning for Health Information
Discharge Procedures
    Assembly of Discharge Record
    Chart Order on Discharge

(Continued on next page)

Figure 8.16.   *(Continued)*

Completing and Filing Master Patient Index
    Card
Discharge Chart Audit
Notification of Deficiencies
Incomplete Record File
Closure of Incomplete Clinical Record
Preparation of the record, imaging of records,
    quality review
Emergency Disaster Evacuation
Establishing/Closing Record
Falsification of Records, Willful
Fax/Facsimile, Faxing
Filing Order, Discharge (Chart Order)
Filing Order, In-house (Chart Order)
Filing System
Filing System, Unit Record
Forms Management
Forms, Release of Information
Forms, Subpoena
Guide to Location of Items in the Health
    Information Department
Guidelines, Committee Minutes
Incomplete Record File
Indexes
    Disease Index and Forms for Indexing
    Master Patient Index
    Release of Information Index/Log
In-service Training Minutes/Record
Job Descriptions
    Health Information Coordinator
    Health Unit Coordinator
    Other Health Information Staff (if applicable)
Late Entries
Lost Record—Reconstruction
Master Patient Index
Medicare Documentation
    Certification and Recertification
    Medicare Denial Procedure and Letter
    Medicare Log
Numbering System
Ombudsman, Review/Access to Records
Omission, Willful
Order of Filing, Discharge
Order of Filing, In-house
Organizational Chart for Health Information
    Department
Orientation/Training of Health Information
    Department

Outguides
Physician Visit Schedule, Letters, and
    Monitoring
Physician Visits, Delinquent Visit Follow-up
Quality Assurance
    Health Information Participation
    QA Studies and Reporting
Readmission—Continued Use of Previous
    Record
Readmission—New Record
Recertification or Certification (Medicare)
Reconstruction of Lost Record
Refusal of Treatment
Release of Information
    Confidentiality
    Confidentiality Statement by Staff
    Copying/Release of Records—General
    Faxing Medical Information
    Procedure for Release—Sample Letters
        and Authorizations
    Redisclosure of Clinical Information
    Resident Access to Records
    Retrieval of Records (sign-out system)
    Subpoena
    Uses and disclosures of protected health
        information, uses and disclosures of
        de-identified documentation, business-
        associated contracts, audit trails
    Witnessing Legal Documents
Requesting Information
    From Hospitals and Other Healthcare Providers
    Request for Information Form
Retention of Records and Destruction after
    Retention Period
    Example Statement for Destruction
    Retention Guidelines
Retrieval of Records
Security of Automated Data/Electronic Medical
    Records
    General Procedures
    Back-up Procedures
    Passwords
Sign-out Logs
Storage of Records
Telephone Orders
Thinning
    In-house Records
    Maintaining Overflow Record
Unit Record System

Source: Adapted from Amatayakul 2003, and AHIMA n.d.

Budgeting Processes

A budget is a plan that converts the organization's goals and objectives into targets for revenue and spending. Essentially, it is a type of planning tool as well as an evaluation tool.

An organization's budget has many components, including:

- A *revenue budget* is a prediction of how much money an organization's activities will generate during a certain period.

- An *expense budget* is a prediction of how much expense an organization is going to generate. The expense budget includes things such as employee salaries and supplies.

- A *capital budget* is a projection or plan of what the organization intends to spend on long-lived assets such as a piece of equipment.

- A *cash budget* is the anticipated flow of cash into and out of the organization.

Most often, HITs use expense and capital budgets.

Most budgets are created for an entire year. In fact, the budgeting process may begin several months before the budget period begins. For example, department directors may be asked to submit their estimates regarding revenue and expenses to upper management in July for a budget period that actually begins the following January. After upper management receives the department director's budget projections, the director usually has to explain and justify them at a hearing before a budget committee or senior management. At or after the budget hearing, the department director is given feedback, negotiations are undertaken, and adjustments are made. Senior management makes the final budget allocations.

The HIT may be involved in helping to develop the departmental budget. This may include providing information about resource and staffing requirements that are anticipated to increase or decrease in the coming year. These types of requirements are based on considerations such as work volume, staffing needs, changes in departmental functions, and so on. For example, when senior managers predict that the volume of inpatients is going to increase in the next year, the increase may affect HIM department resources and staffing. The increased volume of patients might be reflected in the need to purchase more file folders. There will be increased dictation and thus transcription of medical reports. Additionally, there will be more health records to store and file. Such increases will have a direct impact on the HIM department's budget.

Because the budget is both an evaluation tool and a planning tool, the HIT may have to evaluate variances from the budget. A variance analysis is a report that compares actual amounts of expense and revenue to the amounts that were originally budgeted. The variance report answers the question about how far away actual expenses and revenues are from the targeted budget amounts. Budget variance reports are usually provided every month to department managers so that they can keep track of actual-versus-projected revenue and expenses and take appropriate action to try to stay within the projected budget.

Performance Review and Appraisal

An important part of any management job is conducting employee performance reviews and appraisals. This activity falls within the scope of supervision of HIM functions. To conduct employee appraisals, the HIM department must have policies, procedures, job descriptions, and work standards in place. (Chapter 11 introduces performance assessment concepts, and chapter 12 discusses various elements of performance improvement.) The combination of these domains is required for employee performance review.

Participation on Medical Staff and Organizational Committees

HIM professionals frequently serve as liaisons or support personnel on various medical staff committees. For example, the HIT may be a member of the health record, quality management, or some other medical staff committee. In a support capacity, the HIT may be responsible for taking minutes of the committee meeting, distributing the meeting agenda to committee members, and providing statistics or other required information. As a liaison, the HIT's expertise is frequently required. For example, serving on the organization's health record committee, the HIT may be asked to clarify policies, procedures, and accreditation requirements.

Future Directions in Health Information Management Technology

The role of the HIM professional continues to evolve as healthcare and technology evolve. Some of the factors influencing the evolution of the role of HIM professionals are:

- Political initiatives
- Expansion of network capabilities
- Emergence of new technologies such EHRs, natural language processing, and computer-assisted coding
- Move toward ICD-10-CM and ICD-10-PCS
- Societal and regulatory requirements for information privacy and security
- Greater demand and accountability for improved healthcare quality and patient safety that can be facilitated through the use of information technology
- Increased consumer knowledge of personal healthcare decisions and increased focus on personal health records

In his January 2004 State of the Union Address, President George W. Bush recognized the importance of moving health information into the twenty-first century. The president stated, "By computerizing health records, we can avoid dangerous medical mistakes, reduce costs, and improve care" (Bush 2004). This statement supported an initiative that the HIM profession had embraced for more than two decades. Since the State of the Union Address, many healthcare facilities have either implemented an EHR or are in the transitional stages of implementing one. Many of the EHRs today use a large amount of imaged documents. As EHRs evolve, the expanded use of database technology and direct data input will be necessary to meet industry standards and demands for information.

It has been said that we are currently in the information age. In part, this means that information is recognized as a commodity with value. As part of the information age, an explosion of information technology (IT) is transforming the workplace. Only a decade ago, the Internet as it is now known did not exist. In part, it is Internet technology that has made the EHR possible. In addition, it has made things such as electronic commerce possible. Today's intranets (private Internet systems that exist within organizations) are a direct result of the combination of IT and the need and importance of information.

The Internet and the IT explosion have transformed HIM functions and will continue to contribute to the evolution of the HIM professional's role. In addition to making EHRs possible, technology is transforming specific work tasks. The IT explosion has begun to break down the brick and mortar of the HIM department. Although the transcription function in many facilities has been possible for the past decade from the employees' home, the functionality of the process has been improved by use of the Internet. Use of the Internet allows dictation and transcribed reports to be transmitted via the Web, eliminating the need to physically transport transcribed reports to the healthcare facility for inclusion in the health record. As mentioned earlier, speech recognition technology has improved to the point that it is now being widely used at the point of transcription, changing the role of the transcriptionist.

Similarly, the Internet and its capabilities are beginning to affect the role of the clinical coder. As the EHR is implemented, more and more facilities are allowing staff to code from home. As technology and the EHR continue to evolve, it is not unrealistic to expect that natural language processing (NLP) will improve to the point that autocoding could become a reality. NLP is the process in which digital text stored on computer can be read by software and automatically coded. If or when NPL is implemented, the role of the clinical coder would most likely be reengineered and used for quality control of the automated process.

Perhaps a more immediate influence likely to affect the role of the clinical coding professional is implementation of ICD-10-CM and ICD-10-PCS. The ICD-10-CM and ICD-10-PCS coding systems have been developed to replace ICD-9-CM for coding diagnoses and procedures. Implementation of the revised or new coding systems will require that clinical coders be retrained to use them. Moreover, it will require software venders to provide new products, which could expand opportunities for HIM professionals.

Because information transcends boundaries, the HIM department may not be a department at all in the future. Instead, it may become a function that is integrated throughout the organization and exists in many departments. Thus, the HIT may be working in information functions managed by departments other than health information management.

A lot of evidence suggests that this phenomenon is already occurring as HIM professionals move into roles in data security, organizational compliance, medical staff services, and so on. AHIMA's Vision 2006 initiative, designed to move the HIM profession forward into the twenty-first century, accurately portrays a transformation of HIM roles. AHIMA outlined the following roles for the twenty-first century as those most likely to evolve in the upcoming information age:

- The *health information manager* (a line or staff manager) would have enterprise- or facility-wide responsibility for health information management. The position includes working with the chief information executive and system users to advance systems, methods, and application support and to improve data quality, access, privacy, security, and usability.

- The *clinical data specialist* would perform data management functions in a variety of application areas, including clinical coding, outcomes management, specialty registries, and research databases.

- The *patient information coordinator* would perform new service roles that help consumers manage their personal health information, including personal health history management, ROI, managed care services, and information resources.

- The *data quality manager* would perform functions involving formalized continuous quality improvement for data integrity throughout the enterprise, beginning with data dictionary and policy development and including quality monitoring and audits.

- The *data resource administrator* would be responsible for the next generation of records and data management using media such as the CPR, the data repository, and electronic warehousing for meeting current and future care needs across the continuum, providing access to the needed information, and ensuring long-term integrity and access.

- The *research and decision support analyst* would support senior management with information for decision making and strategy development using a variety of analytical tools and databases. The position would work with product and policy organizations on high-level analysis projects such as clinical trials and outcomes research.

- The security officer would manage the security of all electronically maintained information, including the promulgation of security requirements, policies and privilege systems, and performance audits.

Some HIM professionals have taken the role of security officer as the healthcare facility implements measures to comply with HIPAA. Others have assumed the role of facility/ enterprise-wide health information managers as healthcare facilities are transitioning toward the EHR. As AHIMA Vision 2006 predictions continue to become a reality, new roles for the HIM professional will continue to emerge. "New roles may include business change manager, EHR system manager, IT training specialist, business process engineer, clinical vocabulary manager, workflow and data analyst, consumer advocate, clinical alerts and reminder manager, clinical research coordinator, privacy coordinator, enterprise application specialist, and many more" (Cassidy and Hanson 2005).

Many of these positions will fall outside traditional roles and workplaces. Most will call for additional skills and education. Yet, with their unique mixture of clinical and information skills, HITs are poised for success as a profession.

As a result of the expected change in job functions, the conclusion drawn from AHIMA was that trend data indicate that employers in the twenty-first century will require flexible and multiskilled workers. Employers also will demand that employees continually add to their skill sets to meet changing needs. That is why another fundamental principle of AHIMA is the need for lifelong learning. HIM professionals must be committed to ongoing education and professional development.

Check Your Understanding 8.5

Instructions: Choose the most appropriate answer for the following questions.

1. _____ Statements that describe general guidelines that direct behavior or direct or constrain decision making are called _____.
   a. Policies
   b. Procedures
   c. Standards
   d. Criteria

2. ____ Step-by-step instructions on how to complete a specific task are called ____.
    a. Policies
    b. Procedures
    c. Standards
    d. Criteria

3. ____ The departmental budget is a ____ tool and an evaluation tool.
    a. Controlling
    b. Planning
    c. Directing
    d. Summary

4. ____ Employee salaries are part of the ____ budget.
    a. Revenue
    b. Expense
    c. Capital
    d. Cash

5. ____ The purchase of an EHR system would be planned for in the ____ budget.
    a. Revenue
    b. Expense
    c. Capital
    d. Cash

6. ____ The HIM professional may serve on which of the following committees?
    a. Health records committee
    b. Quality management committee
    c. Forms committee
    d. All of the above

7. ____ Which of the following describes the future direction of the HIM professional?
    a. The HIM professional manages the security of electronic information.
    b. The HIM professional becomes a consumer advocate.
    c. The HIM professional will increase the role of quality monitoring, especially of the EHR.
    d. All of the above

Real-World Case

Will natural language processing (NLP) replace coders? NLP is an exciting supporting information technology that may provide valuable assistance for coding diseases and operations. In fact, some say that NLP technology may even replace clinical coders. (Case study based on Warner 2000.)

Today's NLP autocoding systems promise to provide improved data management productivity and consistency without sacrificing coding accuracy. To validate whether this claim is true, a study was conducted on emergency room health records to see how well one such system measured up to the claims.

The NLP system used for the study required that the text in the emergency room records have some structure, including section headers (for example, history of present illness and physical examination). The study included 996 charts. Of these charts, the NLP system was able to assign diagnosis codes to 33 percent, or 328 cases. The remaining 67 percent of the cases either did not meet the systems formatting requirements or the system could not assign a code for other reasons.

When the 328 cases coded by the NLP system were compared with the same cases coded by expert hospital coders, there was 90 percent agreement. This means that for 90 percent of the 328 cases, the NLP system came up with the same codes as the expert coders.

Summary

The health information management department performs a variety of functions within the healthcare institution. These functions include health records storage and retrieval, monitoring record completion, clinical coding, medical transcription, and release of medical information. The department also may manage the research and statistics, cancer and trauma registry, and birth certificate completion functions. These functions vary from facility to facility. In fact, in any given HIM department, many more functions may be performed.

Probably one of the most fundamental functions of any HIM department is health record storage and maintenance. Paper systems require storage space, equipment, and a system of record identification. Most record systems use a numerical filing system. However, small organizations such as physician offices may use an alphabetic filing system. Although filing systems have been used traditionally for storage of paper records, document-imaging technologies are making it possible to scan records digitally and store them electronically. Keeping track of health records and being able to locate and retrieve them when and where they are needed is an essential HIM function. To provide high-quality retrieval services, the HIM department must have good tracking systems in place and continuously audit its filing and retrieval practices.

The record processing function performed by the HIM department is key to monitoring health record content. It includes conducting quantitative analysis of the record by checking the record content against accreditation standards, rules, and regulations internal to the organization and best practices of information handling.

Clinical coding for purposes of research, claims submission, and quality of care studies has been another foundational aspect of HIM practice. Today, various automated systems support the clinical coder, resulting in increased productivity and improved coding quality.

The HIM department has usually been the custodian of the master patient index, the key to identifying and locating any health record in a numerical filing system. Although the patient registration area assigns the health record number (the primary identifier), the HIM department is responsible for the integrity of this important index. The functions performed by the HIM department also have an impact on the billing and patient care departments and the medical staff.

Forms design and management is another critical HIM function. Accurate health information can only be developed through effective data capture methods. Thus, the role of developing good forms, whether in paper or electronic form, continues to be an important part of ensuring high-quality health record content. Associated with forms development is the entire process of tracking and managing forms. This entails development of a forms committee, establishment of forms standards, and implementation of forms numbering and tracking systems.

HIM practice will continue its evolution. Its functions are being transformed as a result of the explosion of information technologies. AHIMA's initiatives provide a picture of how functions are likely to change in the future. One thing for certain is that the HIT must become increasingly technologically savvy and remain committed to learning throughout his or her professional career.

References

Amatayakul, M. 2003 (April). Practical advice for effective policies, procedures. *Journal of American Health Information Management Association* 74(4):16A–D.

American Health Information Management Association. 2000. Practice brief: Authentication of health record entries. *Journal of American Health Information Management Association* 71(3):68A–G.

American Health Information Management Association. 1997. Practice brief: Developing information capture tools. *Journal of American Health Information Management Association* 68(3): 3-page supplement following p. 48.

American Health Information Management Association. n.d. Health Information P&P Checklist. Available online from ahima.org/infocenter/guidelines/ltcs/7.1.asp.

Barnett, R. 1996. *Managing Business Forms.* Canberra, AU: Robert Narnett and Associates.

Bush, G.W. 2004. State of the Union Address. Available online from whitehouse.gov/news/releases/2004/01/print/20040120-7.html.

Cassidy, B., and S.P. Hanson. 2005. HIM practice transformation. *Journal of American Health Information Management Association* 76(5):56A–B.

Grant Medical Center. n.d. ohiohealth.com/facilities/grant/.

Hicks, J., M. Waldrum, V. Wilson, and J. Marwill. 2000. Transcription system overhaul reaps savings, efficiency. *Journal of American Health Information Management Association* 71(10):58–63.

Joint Commission on Accreditation of Healthcare Organizations. 2005. *Hospital Accreditation Standards 2005.* Oakbrook Terrace, IL: JCAHO.

Tegan, A., et al. 2005. The EHR's impact on HIM functions. *Journal of American Health Information Management Association* 76(5):56C–H.

University of Houston. 2001. *Information Security Manual.* Available online from uh.edu/infotech/pnp/security/access.html.

Warner, H.R., Jr. 2000. Can natural language processing aid outpatient coders? *Journal of American Health Information Management Association* 71(8):78–81.

Part II
Health Statistics, Biomedical Research, and Quality Management

Chapter 9
Secondary Data Sources

Elizabeth Bowman, MPA, RHIA

Learning Objectives

- To distinguish between primary and secondary data and between patient-identifiable and aggregate data

- To identify the internal and external users of secondary data

- To compare the facility-specific indexes commonly found in hospitals

- To describe the registries used in hospitals according to purpose, methods of case definition and case finding, data collection methods, reporting and follow-up, and pertinent laws and regulations affecting registry operations

- To define the terms pertinent to each type of secondary record or database

- To discuss agencies for approval and education and certification for cancer, immunization, and trauma registries

- To distinguish among healthcare databases in terms of purpose and content

- To compare manual and automated methods of data collection and vendor systems with facility-specific systems

- To assess data quality issues in secondary records

- To recognize appropriate methods for ensuring data security and the confidentiality of secondary records

- To identify the role of the health information management professional in creating and maintaining secondary records

Key Terms

Abbreviated Injury Scale

Abstracting

Accession number

Accession registry

Activities of daily living

Agency for Healthcare Research and Quality (AHRQ)

American College of Surgeons Commission on Cancer

Audit trail

Autodialing system

Case definition

Case finding

Claim

Clinical trial

Collaborative Stage Data Set

Computer virus

Credentialing

Data confidentiality

Data security

Database

Demographic information

Disease index

Disease registry

Edit

Encryption

Facility-based registry

Facility-specific system

Food and Drug Administration (FDA)

Health services research

Healthcare Integrity and Protection Data Bank

Histocompatibility

Incidence

Index

Injury Severity Score (ISS)

Interrater reliability

Medical Literature, Analysis, and Retrieval System Online (MEDLINE)

National Practitioner Data Bank

National Vaccine Advisory Committee (NVAC)

North American Association of Central Cancer Registries (NAACCR)

Operation index

Patient-specific/identifiable data

Physician index

Population-based registry

Primary data source

Protocol

Public health

Secondary data source

Stage of the neoplasm

Traumatic injury

Unified Medical Language System (UMLS)

User groups

Vendor system

Vital Statistics

Introduction

As a rich source of data about an individual patient, the health record's primary purpose is in patient care and reimbursement for individual encounters. However, it is not easy to see trends in a population of patients by looking at individual records. For this purpose, data must be extracted from individual records and entered into **databases.** These data may be used in a facility-specific or population-based registry for research and improvement in patient care. In addition, they may be reported to the state and become part of state- and federal-level databases used to set health policy and improve healthcare.

The health information management (HIM) professional can play a variety of roles in managing secondary records and databases. He or she plays a key role in helping to set up databases. This task includes determining the content of the database and ensuring compliance with the laws, regulations, and accreditation standards that affect its content and use. All data elements included in the database or registry must be defined in a data dictionary. The HIM professional may oversee the completeness and accuracy of the data abstracted for inclusion in the database or registry.

This chapter explains the difference between primary and secondary data and their users. It also offers an in-depth look at the types of secondary databases, including indexes and registries, and their functions. Finally, the chapter discusses how secondary databases are processed and maintained.

Theory into Practice

A hospital with a level I trauma center serving a tristate area had an ongoing problem. It was required to provide care to all major trauma cases from the three states within its service area regardless of the patients' ability to pay. However, one of the states (state X) was unwilling to pay for the care provided to its indigent patients. Because trauma care can be extremely intensive and costly, the hospital was losing a lot of money.

The American College of Surgeons requires certified trauma centers to maintain a trauma registry. To demonstrate the extent of the problem, the hospital administrator asked the trauma registrar to gather data on patients from state X. The trauma registrar easily identified the patients and provided information by zip code on their location and the type and severity of their injuries. After the patients had been identified, the business office was able to calculate the cost to the hospital of providing their care. The administrator then presented this information to state X's legislature to obtain the money to pay for the care the trauma center provided to the state's indigent patients.

Differences between Primary and Secondary Data Sources and Databases

The health record is considered a **primary data source** because it contains information about a patient that has been documented by the professionals who provided care or services to that patient. Data taken from the primary health record and entered into registries and databases are considered a **secondary data source.**

Data also are categorized as either **patient-specific/identifiable data** or aggregate data. The health record consists entirely of patient-identifiable data. In other words, every fact recorded in the record relates to a particular patient identified by name. Secondary data also may be patient identifiable. In some instances, data are entered into a database along with information such as the patient's name maintained in an identifiable form. Registries are an example of patient-identifiable data on groups of patients.

More often, however, secondary data are considered aggregate data. Aggregate data include data on groups of people or patients without identifying any particular patient individually. Examples of aggregate data are statistics on the average length of stay (ALOS) for patients discharged within a particular diagnosis-related group (DRG).

Purposes and Users of Secondary Data Sources

Secondary data sources provide information that is not easily available by looking at individual health records. For example, if the HIM director doing a research study wanted to find the health records of twenty-five patients who had the principal diagnosis of myocardial infarction, he or she would have to look at numerous individual records to locate the number needed. This would be a time-consuming and laborious project.

Data taken from health records and entered into disease-oriented databases can help researchers determine the effectiveness of alternate treatment methods. They also can quickly demonstrate survival rates at different stages of diseases.

Internal Users

Internal users of secondary data are individuals located within the healthcare facility. For example, internal users include medical staff and administrative and management staff. Secondary data enable these users to identify patterns and trends that are helpful in patient care, long-range planning, budgeting, and benchmarking with other facilities.

External Users

External users of patient data are individuals and institutions outside the facility. Examples of external users are state data banks and federal agencies. States have laws that cases of patients with diseases such as tuberculosis and AIDS must be reported to the state department of health. Moreover, the federal government collects data from the states on vital events such as births and deaths.

The secondary data provided to external users is generally aggregate data and not patient-identifiable data. Thus, these data can be used as needed without risking breaches of confidentiality.

Check Your Understanding 9.1

Instructions: Indicate whether the following statements are true or false (T or F).

1. _____ A registry or database is a secondary data source.

2. _____ A patient health record contains aggregate data.

3. _____ Secondary data provide information that is not easily collected from individual health records.

4. _____ Administrative and management staff members are internal users of secondary data.

5. _____ Medical staff members are external users of secondary data.

Types of Secondary Data Sources

Secondary data sources consist of facility-specific indexes; registries, either facility or population based; or other healthcare databases.

Facility-Specific Indexes

The most long-standing secondary data sources are those that have been developed within facilities to meet their individual needs. These **indexes** enable health records to be located by diagnosis, procedure, or physician. Prior to extensive computerization in healthcare, these indexes were kept on cards. Today, most indexes are maintained as computerized reports based on data from databases routinely developed in the healthcare facility.

Master Population/Patient Index

The master population/patient index (MPI), which is sometimes called the master person index, contains patient-identifiable data such as name, address, date of birth, dates of hospitalizations or encounters, name of attending physician, and health record number. Because health records are filed numerically in most facilities, the MPI is an important source of patient health record numbers. These numbers enable the facility to quickly retrieve health information for specific patients.

Hospitals with a unit numbering system also depend on the MPI to determine whether a patient has been seen in the facility before and has an existing health record number. Having this information in the MPI avoids the duplication of record numbers. Most of the information in the MPI is entered into the facility database at the time of admission/preadmission or registration.

Disease and Operation Indexes

The **disease index** is a listing in diagnosis code number order for patients discharged from the facility during a particular time period. Each patient's diagnoses are converted from a verbal description to a numerical code, usually using the *International Classification of Diseases, Ninth Revision, Clinical Modification* (ICD-9-CM). The patient's diagnosis codes are entered into the facility's health information system as part of the discharge processing of the patient's health record. The index always includes the patient's health record number as well as the diagnosis codes so that records can be retrieved by diagnosis. Because each patient is listed with the health record number, which may be linked back to the patient's name, the disease index is considered patient-identifiable data. The disease index also may include information such as the attending physician's name and the date of discharge.

The **operation index** is similar to the disease index except that it is arranged in numerical order by the patient's procedure code(s) using ICD-9-CM or *Current Procedural Terminology* (CPT) codes. The other information listed in the operation index is generally the same as that listed in the disease index except that the surgeon may be listed in addition to, or instead of, the attending physician.

Physician Index

The **physician index** is a listing of cases in order by physician name or physician identification number. It also includes the patient's health record number and may include other information, such as date of discharge. The physician index enables users to retrieve information about a particular physician, including the number of cases seen during a particular time period.

Registries

Disease registries are collections of secondary data related to patients with a specific diagnosis, condition, or procedure. Registries are different from indexes in that they contain more extensive data. Index reports can usually be produced using data from the facility's existing databases. Registries often require more extensive entry of data from the patient record. Each registry must define the cases that are to be included in it. This process is called **case definition.** In a trauma registry, for example, the case definition might be all patients admitted with a diagnosis falling into ICD-9-CM code numbers 800–959, the trauma diagnosis codes.

After the cases to be included have been determined, the next step in data acquisition is usually **case finding.** Case finding is a method used to identify the patients who have been seen and/or treated in the facility for the particular disease or condition of interest to the registry. After cases have been identified, extensive information is abstracted from the patients' paper-based health records into the registry database or extracted from other databases and automatically entered into the registry database.

The sole purpose of some registries is to collect data from health records and to make them available for users. Other registries take further steps to enter additional information in the registry database, such as routine follow-up of patients at specified intervals. Follow-up information might include rate and duration of survival and quality of life over time.

Cancer Registries

Cancer registries have a long history in healthcare. According to the National Cancer Registrars Association (NCRA), the first hospital cancer registry was founded in 1926 at

Yale-New Haven Hospital (NCRA 2005). It has long been recognized that information is needed to improve the diagnosis and treatment of cancer. Cancer registries were developed as an organized method to collect these data. The data may be facility based (for example, within a hospital or clinic) or population based (for example, from more than one facility within a state or region).

The data from facility-based registries are used to provide information for the improved understanding of cancer, including its causes and methods of diagnosis treatment. The data collected also may provide comparisons in survival rates and quality of life for patients with different treatments and at different stages of cancer at the time of diagnosis. In **population-based registries,** emphasis is on identifying trends and changes in the **incidence** (new cases) of cancer within the area covered by the registry.

The Cancer Registries Amendment Act of 1992 provided funding for a national program of cancer registries with population-based registries in each state. According to the law, these registries were mandated to collect data such as:

- Demographic information about each case of cancer

- Information on the industrial or occupational history of the individuals with the cancers (to the extent such information is available from the same record)

- Administrative information, including date of diagnosis and source of information

- Pathological data characterizing the cancer, including site, **stage of the neoplasm,** incidence, and type of treatment

Case Definition and Case Finding in the Cancer Registry

As defined previously, case definition is the process of deciding which cases should be entered in the registry. In a cancer registry, for example, all cancer cases except skin cancer might meet the definition for the cases to be included. In addition to information on malignant neoplasms, data on benign and borderline brain/central nervous system tumors must be collected by the National Program of Cancer Registries (Ringer and Cain 2004).

In the facility-based cancer registry, the first step is case finding. One way to find cases is through the discharge process in the HIM department. During the discharge procedure, coders and/or discharge analysts can easily earmark cases of patients with cancer for inclusion in the registry. Another case-finding method is to use the facility-specific disease indexes to identify patients with diagnoses of cancer. Additional methods may include reviews of pathology reports and lists of patients receiving radiation therapy or other cancer treatments to determine cases that have not been found by other methods.

Population-based registries usually depend on hospitals, physician offices, radiation facilities, ambulatory surgery centers (ASCs), and pathology laboratories to identify and report cases to the central registry. The population-based registry has a responsibility to ensure that all cases of cancer have been identified and reported to the central registry.

Data Collection for the Cancer Registry

Data collection methods vary between facility-based registries and population-based registries. When a case is first entered in the registry, an **accession number** is assigned. This number consists of the first digits of the year the patient was first seen at the facility, and the remaining digits are assigned sequentially throughout the year. The first case in the year, for example, might be 05-0001. The accession number may be assigned manually or by the automated cancer database used by the organization. An **accession registry** of all cases can be kept manually or provided as a report by the database software. This listing of patients in accession number order provides a way to ensure that all cases have been entered into the registry.

In a facility-based registry, data are initially obtained by reviewing and collecting them from the patient's health record. In addition to **demographic information** (such as name, health record number, address), data in the registry about the patient include:

- Type and site of the cancer
- Diagnostic methodologies
- Treatment methodologies
- Stage at the time of diagnosis

The stage provides information on the size and extent of spread of the tumor throughout the body. There are currently several staging systems. The American Joint Committee on Cancer (AJCC) has worked through its Collaborative Stage Task Force with other organizations with staging systems to develop a new standardized staging system, the **Collaborative Stage Data Set.** This system uses computer algorithms to describe how far a cancer has spread (AJCC 2005). After the initial information is collected at the patient's first encounter, information in the registry is updated periodically through the follow-up process discussed below.

Frequently, the population-based registry only collects information when the patient is diagnosed. Sometimes, however, it receives follow-up information from its reporting entities. These entities usually submit information to the central registry electronically.

Reporting and Follow-up for Cancer Registry Data
Formal reporting of cancer registry data is done through an annual report. The annual report includes aggregate data on the number of cases in the past year by site and type of cancer. It also may include information on patients by gender, age, and ethnic group. Often a particular site or type of cancer is featured with more in-depth data provided.

Other reports are provided as needed. Data from the cancer registry are frequently used in the quality assessment process for a facility as well as in research.

Another activity of the cancer registry is patient follow-up. On an annual basis, the registry attempts to obtain information about each patient in the registry, including whether he or she is still alive, status of the cancer, and treatment received during the period. Various methods are used to obtain this information. For a facility-based registry, the facility's patient health records may be checked for return hospitalizations or visits for treatment. Additionally, the patient's physician may be contacted to determine whether the patient is still living and to obtain information about the cancer.

When patient status cannot be determined through these methods, an attempt may be made to contact the patient directly using information in the registry such as the patient's address and telephone number and other contacts. In addition, contact information from the patient's health record may be used to request information from the patient's relatives. Other methods used include reading newspaper obituaries for deaths and using the Internet to locate patients through sites such as the Social Security Death Index and online telephone books. The information obtained through follow-up is important to allow the registry to develop statistics on survival rates for particular cancers and different treatment methodologies.

Population-based registries do not always include follow-up information on the patients in their databases. However, those that do usually receive the information from the reporting entities such as hospitals, physician offices, and other organizations providing follow-up care.

Standards and Agencies in the Approval Processes

Several organizations have developed standards or approval processes for cancer programs. The **American College of Surgeons** (ACS) **Commission on Cancer** has an approval process for cancer programs. One of the requirements of this process is the existence of a cancer registry as part of the program. The ACS standards are published in the Cancer Program Standards (ACS COC 2005). When the ACS surveys the cancer program, part of the survey process is a review of cancer registry activities.

The **North American Association of Central Cancer Registries** (NAACCR) has a certification program for state population-based registries. Certification is based on the quality of data collected and reported by the state registry. NAACCR has developed standards for data quality and format and works with other cancer organizations to align their various standards sets.

The Centers for Disease Control and Prevention (CDC) also has national standards regarding the completeness, timeliness, and quality of cancer registry data from state registries through the National Program of Cancer Registries (NPCR). NPCR was developed as a result of the Cancer Registries Amendment Act of 1992. The CDC collects data from the NPCR state registries.

Education and Certification for Cancer Registrars

Traditionally, cancer registrars have been trained through on-the-job training and professional workshops and seminars. The National Cancer Registrars Association (NCRA) has worked with colleges to develop formal educational programs for cancer registrars. A cancer registrar may become credentialed as a certified cancer registrar (CTR) by passing an examination provided by the National Board for Certification of Registrars (NBCR). Eligibility requirements for the certification examination include a combination of experience and education (NCRA 2005).

Trauma Registries

Trauma registries maintain databases on patients with severe traumatic injuries. A **traumatic injury** is a wound or other injury caused by an external physical force such as an automobile accident, a shooting, a stabbing, or a fall. Information collected by the trauma registry may be used for performance improvement and research in the area of trauma care. Trauma registries may be facility based or may include data for a region or state.

Case Definition and Case Finding for Trauma Registries

The case definition for the trauma registry varies from registry to registry but frequently involves inclusion of cases with diagnoses from ICD-9-CM sections 800–959, the trauma diagnosis codes. To find cases with trauma diagnoses, the trauma registrar can access the disease indexes looking for cases with codes from this section of ICD-9-CM. In addition, the registrar may look at deaths in services with frequent trauma diagnoses—such as trauma, neurosurgery, orthopedics, and plastic surgery—to find additional cases.

Data Collection for Trauma Registries
After the cases have been identified, information is abstracted from the health records of the injured patients and entered into the trauma registry database. The data elements collected in the **abstracting** process vary from registry to registry but usually include:

- Demographic information on the patient

- Information on the injury

- Care the patient received before hospitalization (such as care at another transferring hospital or care from an emergency medical technician who provided care at the scene of the accident and/or in transport from the accident site to the hospital)

- Status of the patient at the time of admission

- Patient's course in the hospital

- ICD-9-CM diagnosis and procedure codes

- **Abbreviated Injury Scale** (AIS)

- **Injury Severity Score** (ISS)

The AIS reflects the nature of the injury and the threat to life of the injury by body system. It may be assigned manually by the registrar or generated as part of the database from data entered by the registrar. The ISS is an overall severity measurement calculated from the AIS scores for the three most severe injuries of the patient (Trauma.org 2005).

Reporting and Follow-up for Trauma Registries
Reporting varies among trauma registries. An annual report is often developed to show the activity of the trauma registry. Other reports may be generated as part of the performance improvement process, such as self-extubation (patients removing their own tubes) and delays in abdominal surgery or patient complications. Some hospitals report data to the National Trauma Data Bank (ACS Trauma Programs 2005).

Trauma registries may or may not do follow-up of the patients entered in the registry. When follow-up is done, emphasis is frequently on the patient's quality of life after a period of time. Unlike cancer, where physician follow-up is crucial to detect recurrence, many traumatic injuries do not require continued patient care over time. Thus, follow-up is often not given the emphasis it receives in cancer registries.

Standards and Agencies for Approval of Trauma Registries
The ACS certifies levels I, II, III, and IV trauma centers. As part of its certification requirements, the ACS states that the level I trauma center must have a trauma registry (Garthe 1997, 26).

Education and Certification of Trauma Registrars
Trauma registrars may be registered health information technicians (RHITs), registered health information administrators (RHIAs), registered nurses (RNs), licensed practical nurses (LPNs), emergency medical technicians (EMTs), or other health professionals. Training for trauma registrars is through workshops and on-the-job training. The American Trauma Society (ATS), for example, provides core and advanced workshops for trauma registrars. It also provides a certification examination for trauma registrars through its

Registrar Certification Board. Certified trauma registrars have earned the credential CSTR (certified specialist in trauma registry).

Birth Defects Registries

Birth defects registries collect information on newborns with birth defects. Often population based, these registries serve a variety of purposes. For example, they provide information on the incidence of birth defects for the study of causes and prevention of birth defects, monitor trends in birth defects to improve medical care for children with birth defects, and target interventions for preventable birth defects, such as folic acid to prevent neural tube defects.

In some cases, registries have been developed after specific events have put a spotlight on birth defects. After the Persian Gulf War, for example, some feared an increased incidence of birth defects among the children of Gulf War veterans. The Department of Defense subsequently started a birth defects registry to collect data on the children of these veterans to determine whether any pattern could be detected.

Case Definition and Case Finding for Birth Defects Registries

Birth defects registries use a variety of criteria to determine which cases to include in the registry. Some registries limit cases to those with defects found within the first year of life. Others include those with a major defect that occurred in the first year of life and was discovered within the first five years of life. Still other registries include only children who were live born or stillborn babies with discernible birth defects.

Cases may be detected in a variety of ways, including review of disease indexes, labor and delivery logs, pathology and autopsy reports, ultrasound reports, and cytogenetic reports. In addition to information from hospitals and physicians, cases may be identified from rehabilitation centers and children's hospitals and from vital records such as birth, death, and fetal death certificates.

Data Collection for Birth Defects Registries

A variety of information is abstracted for the birth defects registry, including:

- Demographic information
- Codes for diagnoses
- Birth weight
- Status at birth, including live born, stillborn, aborted
- Autopsy
- Cytogenetics results
- Whether the infant was a single or multiple birth
- Mother's use of alcohol, tobacco, or illicit drugs
- Father's use of drugs and alcohol
- Family history of birth defects

Diabetes Registries

Diabetes registries include cases of patients with diabetes for the purpose of assistance in managing care as well as for research. Patients whose diabetes is not kept under good control frequently have numerous complications. The diabetes registry can keep up with whether the patient has been seen by a physician in an effort to prevent complications.

Case Definition and Case Finding for Diabetes Registries

There are two types of diabetes mellitus: insulin-dependent diabetes (type I) and non–insulin-dependent diabetes (type II). Registries sometimes limit their cases by type of diabetes. In some instances, there may be further definition by age. Some diabetes registries, for example, only include children with diabetes.

Case finding includes the review of health records of patients with diabetes. Other case-finding methods include review of the following types of information:

- ICD-9-CM diagnostic codes
- Billing data
- Medication lists
- Physician identification
- Health Plans

Although facility-based registries for cancer and trauma are usually hospital based, facility-based diabetes registries are often found in physician offices or clinics. The office or clinic is the main location for diabetes care. Thus, data about the patient to be entered into the registry are available at these sites rather than at the hospital. The health records of diabetes patients treated in physician practices may be identified through ICD-9-CM code numbers for diabetes, billing data for diabetes-related services, medication lists for patients on diabetic medications, or identification of patients as the physician sees them.

Health plans also are interested in optimal care for their enrollees because diabetes can have serious complications when not managed correctly. The plans can provide information to the office or clinic on enrollees who are diabetics.

Data Collection for Diabetes Registries

In addition to demographic information about the cases, other data collected may include laboratory values such as HBA1c. This test is used to determine the patient's blood glucose for a period of approximately sixty days prior to the time of the test. Moreover, facility registries may track patient visits to follow up with patients who have not been seen in the past year.

Reporting and Follow-up for Diabetes Registries

A variety of reports can be developed from the diabetes registry. For facility-based registries, one report might keep up with laboratory monitoring of the patient's diabetes to allow intensive intervention with patients whose diabetes is not well controlled. Another report might concern patients who have not been tested within a year or have not had a primary care provider visit within a year.

Population-based diabetes registries might provide reporting on the incidence of diabetes for the geographic area covered by the registry. Registry data also might be used to investigate risk factors for diabetes.

Follow-up is aimed primarily at ensuring that the diabetic is seen by the physician at appropriate intervals to prevent complications.

Implant Registries

An implant is a material or substance inserted into the body, such as breast implants, heart valves, and pacemakers. Implant registries have been developed for the purpose of tracking the performance of implants, including complications, deaths, and defects resulting from implants, as well as longevity.

In the recent past, the safety of implants has been questioned in a number of highly publicized cases. In some cases, implant registries have been developed in response to such events. For example, there have been questions about the safety of silicone breast implants and temporomandibular joint implants. When such cases arise, it has often been difficult to ensure that all patients with the implants have been notified of safety questions. At one time, there was a national implant registry, but it was halted after several years because of minimal participation (Shelton 2001). It was felt that the legal implications of problem implants have prevented more interest in implant registries.

A number of federal laws have been enacted to regulate medical devices, including implants. These devices were first covered under Section 15 of the Food, Drug and Cosmetic Act. The Safe Medical Devices Act of 1990 was passed and then amended through the Medical Device Amendments of 1995. These acts required facilities to report deaths and severe complications thought to be due to a device to the manufacturer and the **Food and Drug Administration** (FDA). The 1995 Medical Device Amendments changed that requirement so that only a selected subset of user facilities would be required to report. Implant registries can help in complying with the legal requirement for reporting for the sample of facilities required to report.

Case Definition and Case Finding for Implant Registries

Implant registries sometimes include all types of implants but often are restricted to a specific type of implant such as cochlear, saline breast, or temporomandibular joint.

Data Collection for Implant Registries

Demographic data on patients receiving implant are included in the registry. The FDA requires that all reportable events involving medical devices include the following information (Center for Devices and Radiological Health 1996, 4):

- User facility report number

- Name and address of the device manufacturer

- Device brand name and common name

- Product model, catalog, serial, and lot numbers

- Brief description of the event reported to the manufacturer and/or the FDA

- Where the report was submitted (for example, to the FDA, manufacturer, or distributor)

Thus, these data items also should be included in the implant registry to facilitate reporting.

Reporting and Follow-up for Implant Registries

Data from the implant registry may be used to report to the FDA and the manufacturer when devices cause death or serious illness or injury.

Follow-up is important to track the performance of the implant. When patients are tracked, they can be easily notified of product failures, recalls, or upgrades (Shelton 2001).

Transplant Registries

Transplant registries can have varied purposes. Some organ transplant registries maintain databases of patients who need organs. When an organ becomes available, a fair way then may be used to allocate the organ to the patient with the highest priority. In other cases, the purpose of the registry is to provide a database of potential donors for transplants using live donors, such as bone marrow transplants. Posttransplant information also is kept on organ recipients and donors.

Because transplant registries are used to try to match donor organs with recipients, they are often national or even international in scope. Examples of national registries include the Scientific Registry of the United Network for Organ Sharing (UNOS) and the registry of the National Marrow Donor Program (NMDP).

Data collected in the transplant registry also may be used for research, policy analysis, and quality control.

Case Definition and Case Finding for Transplant Registries

Physicians identify patients needing transplants. Information about the patient is provided to the registry. When an organ becomes available, information about it is matched with potential donors. For donor registries, donors are solicited through community information efforts similar to those carried out by blood banks to encourage blood donations.

Data Collection for Transplant Registries

The type of information collected varies according to the type of registry. Pretransplant data about the recipient include:

- Demographic data
- Patient's diagnosis
- Patient's status codes regarding medical urgency
- Patient's functional status
- Whether the patient is on life support
- Previous transplantations
- **Histocompatibility** (compatability of donor and recipient tissues)

Information on donors varies according to whether the donor is living. For organs harvested from patients who have died, information is collected on:

- Cause and circumstances of the death
- Organ procurement and consent process
- Medications the donor was taking
- Other donor history

For a living donor, information includes:

- Relationship of the donor to the recipient (if any)
- Clinical information

- Information on organ recovery
- Histocompatibility

Reporting and Follow-up for Transplant Registries

Reporting includes information on donors and recipients as well as survival rates, length of time on the waiting list for an organ, and death rates.

Follow-up information is collected for recipients as well as living donors. For living donors, the information collected might include complications of the procedure and length of stay in the hospital. Follow-up on recipients includes information on status at the time of follow-up (for example, living, dead, lost to follow-up), functional status, graft status, and treatment, such as immunosuppressive drugs. Follow-up is carried out at intervals throughout the first year after the transplant and then annually after that.

Immunization Registries

Children are supposed to receive a large number of immunizations during the first six years of life. These immunizations are so important that the federal government has set several objectives related to immunizations in Healthy People 2010, a set of health goals for the nation. These include increasing the proportion of children and adolescents that are fully immunized (objective 14-24) and increasing the proportion of children in population-based immunization registries (objective 14-26).

Immunization registries usually have the purpose of increasing the number of infants and children who receive the required immunizations at the proper intervals. To accomplish this goal, registries collect information within a particular geographic area on children and their immunization status. They also help by maintaining a central source of information for a particular child's immunization history, even when the child has received immunizations from a variety of providers. This central location for immunization data also relieves parents of the responsibility of maintaining immunization records for their children.

Case Definition and Case Finding for Immunization Registries

All children in the population area served by the registry should be included in the registry. Some registries limit their inclusion of patients to those seen at public clinics, excluding those seen exclusively by private practitioners. Although children are usually targeted in immunization registries, some registries do include information on adults for influenza and pneumonia vaccines.

Children are often entered in the registry at birth. Registry personnel may review birth and death certificates and adoption records to determine which children to include and which children to exclude because they died after birth. In some cases, children are entered electronically through a connection with an electronic birth record system.

Data Collection for Immunization Registries

The National Immunization Program at the CDC has worked with the **National Vaccine Advisory Committee** (NVAC) to develop a core set of immunization data elements to be included in all immunization registries. These data elements include (CDC 2005a):

- Patient's name (first, middle, and last)
- Patient's birth date
- Patient's sex
- Patient's birth state/country

- Mother's name (first, middle, last, and maiden)

- Vaccine type

- Vaccine manufacturer

- Vaccination date

- Vaccine lot number

Other items may be included as needed by the individual registry.

Reporting and Follow-up for Immunization Registries
Because the purpose of the immunization registry is to increase the number of children who receive immunizations in a timely manner, reporting should emphasize immunization rates, especially changes in rates in target areas. Immunization registries also can provide automatic reporting of children's immunization to schools to check the immunization status of their students.

Follow-up is directed toward reminding parents that it is time for immunizations as well as seeing whether parents fail to bring the child in for the immunization after a reminder. Reminders may include a letter or postcard or telephone calls. **Autodialing systems** may be used to call parents and deliver a prerecorded reminder. Moreover, registries must decide how frequently to follow up with parents who do not bring their children for immunization. Maintaining up-to-date addresses and telephone numbers is an important factor in providing follow-up. Registries may allow parents to opt out of the registry if they prefer not to be reminded.

Standards and Agencies for Approval of Immunization Registries
The CDC, through its National Immunization Program, provides funding for some population-based immunization registries. It has identified twelve minimum functional standards for immunization registries (CDC 2005a), including:

- Electronically store data on all NVAC-approved core data elements.

- Establish a registry record within six weeks of birth for each newborn child born in the catchment area.

- Enable access to and retrieval of immunization information in the registry at the time of the encounter.

- Receive and process immunization information within one month of vaccine administration.

- Protect the confidentiality of healthcare information.

- Ensure the security of healthcare information.

- Exchange immunization records using Health Level Seven (HL7) standards.

- Automatically determine the routine childhood immunization(s) needed, in compliance with current ACIP (Advisory Committee on Immunization Practices) recommendations, when an individual presents for a scheduled immunization.

- Automatically identify individuals due/late for immunization(s) to enable the production of reminder/recall notifications.

- Automatically produce immunization coverage reports by providers, age groups, and geographic areas.

- Produce official immunization records.

- Promote the accuracy and completeness of registry data.

It has been proposed that the CDC develop a certification program for immunization registries.

Other Registries

Registries may be developed for any type of disease or condition. Other commonly kept types of registries are HIV/AIDS and cardiac registries.

In addition, registries may be developed for administrative purposes. The National Provider Registry is an example of an administrative registry. Data collected for healthcare administrative purposes are discussed in the next subsection.

Healthcare Databases

Databases also may be developed for a variety of purposes. For example, the federal government has developed a variety of databases to enable it to carry out surveillance, improvement, and prevention duties. HIM managers may provide information for these databases through data abstraction or from data reported by a facility to state and local entities. They also may use these data to do research or work with other researchers on issues related to reimbursement and health status.

National and State Administrative Databases

Some databases are established for administrative rather than disease-oriented reasons. For example, some are developed for **claims** data submitted on Medicare claims. Other administrative databases assist in the **credentialing** and privileging of health practitioners.

Medicare Provider Analysis and Review File

The Medicare Provider Analysis and Review (MEDPAR) file is made up of acute care hospital and skilled nursing facility (SNF) claims data for all Medicare claims. It consists of the following types of data:

- Demographic data on the patient
- Data on the provider
- Information on Medicare coverage for the claim
- Total charges
- Charges broken down by specific type of service, such as operating room, physical therapy, and pharmacy charges
- ICD-9-CM diagnosis and procedure codes
- DRGs

The MEDPAR file is frequently used for research on topics such as charges for particular types of care and DRGs. The limitation of the MEDPAR data for research purposes is that the file contains only Medicare patients.

National Practitioner Data Bank

The **National Practitioner Data Bank** (NPDB) was mandated under the Health Care Quality Improvement Act of 1986 to provide a database of medical malpractice payments, sanctions taken by boards of medical examiners, and certain professional review actions (such as denial of medical staff privileges) taken by healthcare entities such as hospitals against physicians, dentists, and other healthcare providers. The problem that the NPDB was developed to alleviate was the lack of information about malpractice decisions, denial of medical staff privileges, or loss of medical license. Because these data were not widely available, physicians who lost their license to practice in one state or facility could move to another state or another facility and begin practicing again with the current state and/or facility unaware of previous actions against the physician.

Information in the NPDB is provided through a required reporting mechanism. Entities making malpractice payments, including insurance companies, boards of medical examiners, and entities such as hospitals and professional societies, must report to the NPDB. The information to be reported includes information about the practitioner, the reporting entity, and any judgment or settlement. Information about physicians must be reported, but the reporting of information about other healthcare providers is not mandatory but will be accepted. Monetary penalties may be assessed for failure to report.

The law requires healthcare facilities to query the NPDB as part of the credentialing process when a physician initially applies for medical staff privileges and every two years thereafter.

Healthcare Integrity and Protection Data Bank

Part of the Health Insurance Portability and Accountability Act of 1996 (HIPAA) mandated the collection of information on healthcare fraud and abuse because there was no central place to obtain this information. As a result, the national **Healthcare Integrity and Protection Data Bank** (HIPDB) was developed. The types of items that must be reported to the data bank include reportable final adverse actions such as:

> Actions related to provider, supplier, and practitioner practices that are inconsistent with accepted sound fiscal, business or medical practices, directly or indirectly resulting in: (1) unnecessary costs to the program; (2) improper payment; (3) services that fail to meet professionally recognized standards of care or that are medically unnecessary; or (4) adverse patient outcomes, failure to provide covered or needed care in violation of contractual arrangements, or delays in diagnosis or treatment (OIG 1998, 58341–58342).

Reportable events include federal or state criminal convictions related to the delivery of healthcare, civil judgments related to the delivery of healthcare, exclusions from participation in federal or state healthcare programs such as Medicare and Medicaid, and other adjudicated actions or decisions. Civil judgments resulting in malpractice payments are not included because they are incorporated in the NPDB. There may be some overlap with the NPDB, so a single report is made and then sorted to the appropriate data bank.

Information to be reported includes information about the healthcare provider, supplier, or practitioner that is the subject of the final adverse action, the nature of the act, and a description of the actions on which the decision was based. Only federal and state government agencies and health plans are required to report, and access to the data bank is limited to these organizations and to practitioners, providers, and suppliers who may only query about themselves.

States also frequently have health-related administrative databases. For example, many states collect either UHDDS or UB-92 data on patients discharged from hospitals located within their area. The Statewide Planning and Research Cooperative System (SPARCS) in New York state is an example of this type of administrative database. It combines UB-92 data with data required by the state of New York.

National, State, and County Public Health Databases

Public health is the area of healthcare dealing with the health of populations in geographic areas such as states or counties. One of the duties of public health agencies is surveillance of the health status of the population within their jurisdiction.

The databases developed by public health departments provide information on the incidence and prevalence of diseases, possible high-risk populations, survival statistics, and trends over time. Data for the databases may be collected using a variety of methods, including interviews, physical examinations of individuals, and reviews of health records. Thus, the HIM manager may have input in these databases through data provided from health records. At the national level, the National Center for Health Statistics has responsibility for these databases.

National Health Care Survey

One of the major national public health surveys is the National Health Care Survey. To a large extent, it relies on data from patients' health records. It consists of a number of parts, including:

- The National Hospital Discharge Survey

- National Survey of Ambulatory Surgery

- National Employer Health Insurance Survey

- National Health Provider Inventory

- The National Ambulatory Medical Care Survey

- The National Nursing Home Survey

- The National Hospital Ambulatory Medical Care Survey

- The National Home and Hospice Care Survey

Data in the National Discharge Survey are either abstracted manually from a sample of acute care discharge records or obtained from state or other discharge databases. Items collected follow the Uniform Hospital Discharge Data Set (UHDDS), including demographic data, admission and discharge dates, and final diagnoses and procedures.

The National Ambulatory Medical Care Survey includes data collected by a sample of office-based physicians and their staffs from the health records of patients seen in a one-week reporting period. Data included are demographic data, the patients' reasons for visit, the diagnoses, diagnostic/screening services, therapeutic and preventive services, ambulatory surgical procedures, and medications/injections, in addition to information on the visit disposition and time spent with the physician.

The National Nursing Home Survey provides data on each facility, current residents, and discharged residents. Information is gathered through an interview process. The administrator or designee provides information about the facility being surveyed. For information on the residents, the nursing staff member most familiar with the resident's care is interviewed. The staff member uses the resident's health record for reference during the interview. Data collected on the facility include information on ownership, size, certification status, admissions, services, full-time equivalent employees, and basic charges. Interviews about both current and discharged residents provide demographic information on the resident as well as LOS, diagnoses, level of care received, **activities of daily living (ADL)**, and charges.

Data for the National Hospital Ambulatory Medical Care Survey are collected on patient visits to hospital-based emergency departments and outpatient clinics. Information is obtained through an abstracting process from the patient health record. Different abstracting forms are used for the emergency department records and the outpatient clinics. The emergency department abstract includes demographic data on the patient, expected source of payment, how soon the patient should be seen, the patient's complaints or reason for visit, diagnoses, diagnostic/screening services, procedures, medications/injections, providers seen, and visit disposition. The outpatient department abstract includes similar information. Facility personnel do the abstracting.

For the National Home and Hospice Care Survey, data are collected on the home health or hospice agency as well as on their current and discharged patients. For the facility, data collected include agency identifier, number of current patients, type of ownership, certification status (for example, Medicare or Medicaid), number of staff, and services available. For current and discharged patients, data include patient demographic information, current living arrangements, source of referral, diagnoses, type of care received, primary caregiver, vision and hearing status, ADL, and expected sources of payment. Facility data are obtained through an interview with the administrator or designee. Patient information is obtained from the caregiver most familiar with the patient's care. The caregiver may use the patient's health record in answering the interview questions.

Because of the bioterrorism scares in recent years, the CDC is developing the National Electronic Disease Surveillance System (NEDSS). This system will provide a national surveillance system by connecting the CDC with local and state public health partners. It would allow the CDC to monitor trends from disease reporting at the local and state levels to look for possible bioterrorism incidents.

Other national public health databases include the National Health Interview Survey and the National Immunization Survey. Table 9.1 summarizes the national databases.

State and local public health departments also develop databases, as needed, to perform their duties of health surveillance, disease prevention, and research. An example of state databases is infectious/notifiable disease databases. Each state has a list of diseases that must be reported to the state, such as AIDS, measles, and syphilis, so that containment and prevention measures can be taken to avoid large outbreaks of these diseases. As mentioned above, state and local reporting systems will be connected with the CDC through NEDSS to evaluate trends in disease outbreaks. There also may be statewide databases/registries that collect extensive information on particular diseases and conditions such as birth defects and cancer.

Database	Type of Setting	Content	Data Source	Method of Data Collection
Table 9.1. National health care databases				
National Ambulatory Medical Care Survey	Office-based physician practice	Data on the patient and the visit	State discharge databases Office-based physician records	Abstract
National Nursing Home Survey	Nursing home	Data on the facility, current and discharged residents	Administrator Nurse caregiver	Interview
National Hospital Ambulatory Medical Care Survey	Hospital emergency departments and outpatient clinics	Data on the patient, the visit, and the method of payment	Emergency department and outpatient clinic records	Abstract
National Home and Hospice Care Survey	Home health and hospice	Facility data and patient data	Administrator Caregiver	Interview
National Electronic Disease Surveillance System (NEDSS)	Public health departments	Possible bioterrorism incidents	Local and state public health departments	Electronic surveillance

Vital Statistics

Vital statistics include data on births, deaths, fetal deaths, marriages, and divorces. Responsibility for the collection of vital statistics rests with the states. The states share information with the National Center for Health Statistics (NCHS). The actual collection of the information is carried out at the local level. For example, birth certificates are completed at the facility where the birth occurred and then are sent to the state. The state serves as the official repository for the certificate and provides vital statistics information to the NCHS. From the vital statistics collected, states and the national government develop a variety of databases.

One vital statistics database at the national level is the Linked Birth and Infant Death Data Set. In this database, the information from birth certificates is compared to death certificates for infants under one year of age who die. This database provides data to conduct analyses for patterns of infant death. Other national programs that use vital statistics data include the National Maternal and Infant Health Survey, the National Mortality Followback Survey, the National Survey of Family Growth, and the National Death Index (CDC 2005b). In some of these databases, such as the National Maternal and Infant Health Survey and the National Mortality Followback Survey, additional information is collected on deaths originally identified through the vital statistics system.

Similar databases using vital statistics data as a basis are found at the state level. Birth defects registries, for example, frequently use vital records data with information on the birth defect as part of their data collection process.

Clinical Trials

A **clinical trial** is a research project in which new treatments and tests are investigated to determine whether they are safe and effective. The trial proceeds according to a **protocol,** which is the list of rules and procedures to be followed. Clinical trials databases have been developed to allow physicians and patients to find clinical trials. A patient with cancer or AIDS, for example, might be interested in participating in a clinical trial but not know how to locate one applicable to his or her type of disease. Clinical trials databases provide the data to enable patients and practitioners to determine what clinical trials are available and applicable to the patient.

The Food and Drug Administration Modernization Act of 1997 mandated that a clinical trials database be developed. The National Library of Medicine has developed the database, called ClinicalTrials.gov, which is available on the Internet for use by both patients and practitioners (NLM 2005). Information in the database includes:

- Study identification number
- Study sponsor
- Brief title
- Brief summary
- Location of trial
- Recruitment status
- Contact information
- Eligibility criteria
- Study type
- Study design
- Study phase
- Condition
- Intervention
- Data provider
- Date last modified

Each data element has been defined. For example, the study sponsor is the organization carrying out the clinical trial. The brief summary gives an overview of the treatments being studied and types of patients to be included. The location of the trial tells where the trial is being carried out so patients can select trials in convenient locations. Recruitment status indicates whether subjects are currently being entered in the trial or will be in the future or whether the trial is closed to new subjects. Eligibility criteria include information on the type of condition to be studied (in some cases, the stage of the disease) and what other treatments are allowed during the trial or must be completed before entering the trial. Age is a frequent eligibility criterion. Study types include diagnostic, genetic, monitoring, natural history, prevention, screening, supportive care, training, and treatment (McCray and Ide 2000, 316). Study design includes the research design being followed.

A clinical trial consists of four study phases. Phase I studies research the safety of the treatment in a small group of people. In phase II studies, emphasis is on determining the treatment's effectiveness and further investigating safety. Phase III studies look at effectiveness and side effects and make comparisons to other available treatments in larger populations. Phase IV studies look at the treatment after it has entered the market.

Some clinical trials databases concentrate on a particular disease. The Department of Health and Human Services, for example, has developed ACTIS, the AIDS Clinical Trials Information Service. The National Cancer Institute sponsors PDQ (Physician Data Query), a database for cancer clinical trials. These databases contain information similar to ClinicalTrials.gov.

Although ClinicalTrials.gov has been set up for use by both patients and health practitioners, some databases are more oriented toward practitioners. Moreover, some efforts have been made to develop databases of published articles and proceedings from meetings on the subject of clinical trials. The Cochrane Central Register of Controlled Trials, for example, is a bibliographic database of literature on clinical trials developed by the Cochrane Library, an electronic library.

Health Services Research Databases

Health services research is research concerning healthcare delivery systems, including organization and delivery and care effectiveness and efficiency. Within the federal government, the organization most involved in health services research is the **Agency for Healthcare Research and Quality** (AHRQ). AHRQ looks at issues related to the efficiency and effectiveness of the healthcare delivery system, disease protocols, and guidelines for improved disease outcomes.

A major initiative for AHRQ has been the Healthcare Cost and Utilization Project (HCUP). HCUP uses data collected at the state level from either claims data from the UB-92 or discharge-abstracted data, including the UHDDS items reported by individual hospitals and, in some cases, by freestanding ambulatory care centers. Which data are reported depends on the individual state. Data may be reported by the facilities to a state agency or to the state hospital association, depending on state regulations. The data then are reported from the state to AHRQ, where they become part of the HCUP databases.

HCUP consists of a set of databases, including:

- The Nationwide Inpatient Sample (NIS), which consists of inpatient discharge data from a sample of approximately a thousand hospitals throughout the United States

- The State Inpatient Database (SID), which includes data collected by states on hospital discharges

- The State Ambulatory Surgery Database (SASD), which includes information from a sample of states on hospital-affiliated ASCs and, from some states, data from freestanding surgery centers

- The Kids Inpatient Database (KID), which is made up of inpatient discharge data on children younger than nineteen years old

These databases are unique because they include data on inpatients whose care is paid for by all types of payers, including Medicare, Medicaid, private insurance, self-pay, and uninsured. Data elements include demographic information, information on diagnoses and procedures, admission and discharge status, payment sources, total charges, LOS, and information on the hospital or freestanding ambulatory surgery center. Researchers may use these databases to look at issues such as those related to the costs of treating particular diseases, the extent to which treatments are used, and differences in outcomes and cost for alternative treatments.

National Library of Medicine

The National Library of Medicine (NLM) produces two databases of special interest to the HIM manager: MEDLINE and UMLS.

Medical Literature, Analysis, and Retrieval System Online.   **Medical Literature, Analysis, and Retrieval System Online** (MEDLINE) is the best-known database from the NLM. It includes bibliographic listings for publications in the areas of medicine, dentistry, nursing, pharmacy, allied health, and veterinary medicine. HIM managers use MEDLINE to locate articles on HIM issues as well as articles on medical topics necessary to carry out quality improvement and medical research activities.

Unified Medical Language System.   The **Unified Medical Language System** (UMLS) provides a way to integrate biomedical concepts from a variety of sources to show their relationships. This process allows links to be made between different information systems for purposes such as electronic health record systems. The system is of particular interest to the HIM manager because medical vocabularies such as the *International Classification of Diseases, Ninth Revision, Clinical Modification* (ICD-9-CM), *Current Procedural Terminology* (CPT), and the *Healthcare Common Procedure Coding System* (HCPCS) are among the items included.

Check Your Understanding 9.2

Instructions: Select the best answer for each of the following questions.

1. _____ Which of the following indexes is an important source of patient health record numbers?
   a. Physician index
   b. Master patient index
   c. Operation index
   d. Disease index

2. _____ After the cases to be included in a registry have been determined, what is the next step in data acquisition?
   a. Case registration
   b. Case definition
   c. Case abstracting
   d. Case finding

3. _____ What number is assigned to a case when it is first entered in a cancer registry?
    a. Accession number
    b. Patient number
    c. Health record number
    d. Medical record number

4. _____ What are patient data such as name, age, address, and so on called?
    a. Demographic data
    b. Secondary data
    c. Aggregate data
    d. Identification data

5. _____ What type of registry maintains a database on patients injured by an external physical force?
    a. Implant registry
    b. Birth defects registry
    c. Trauma registry
    d. Transplant registry

6. _____ In addition to collecting patient data, what activities do many types of registries engage in?
    a. Abstracting and follow-up
    b. Follow-up and case finding
    c. Reporting and case finding
    d. Reporting and follow-up

7. _____ Why is the MEDPAR file limited in terms of being used for research purposes?
    a. It only provides demographic data about patients.
    b. It only contains Medicare patients.
    c. It uses ICD-9-CM diagnoses and procedure codes.
    d. It breaks charges down by specific type of service.

8. _____ Which of the following acts mandated establishment of the National Practitioner Data Bank?
    a. Health Care Quality Improvement Act of 1986
    b. Health Insurance Portability and Accountability Act of 1996
    c. Safe Medical Devices Act of 1990
    d. Food and Drug Administration Modernization Act of 1997

9. _____ Which one of the following is not part of the National Health Care Survey?
    a. The National Nursing Home Survey
    b. The National Immunization Program Survey
    c. The National Home and Hospice Care Survey
    d. The National Ambulatory Medical Care Survey

10. _____ What two databases produced by the National Library of Medicine are of special interest to HIM professionals?
    a. MEDLINE and MEDPAR
    b. UHDDS and UMLS
    c. MEDLINE and UMLS
    d. UHDDS and UMLS

Processing and Maintenance of Secondary Databases

Several issues surround the processing and maintenance of secondary databases. HIM managers are often involved in decisions concerning these issues.

Manual versus Automated Methods of Data Collection

Although registries and databases are almost universally computerized, data collection is commonly done manually. The most frequent method is abstracting. Abstracting is the process of reviewing the patient health record and entering the required data elements into the database. In some cases, the abstracting may be done initially on an abstract form. The data then would be entered into the database from the form. In many cases, it is done directly from the primary patient health record into a data collection screen in the computerized database system.

However, not all data collection is done manually. In some cases, data can be downloaded directly from other electronic systems. Birth defects registries, for example, often download information on births and birth defects from the vital records system. In some cases, providers such as hospitals and physicians send information in electronic format to the registry or database. The National Discharge Survey from the National Center for Health Statistics uses information in electronic format from state databases.

Vendor Systems versus Facility-Specific Systems

A **vendor system** is an information system developed by an outside company and sold to a variety of organizations. A **facility-specific system** is an information system developed within the facility for its own use.

One clear advantage to using vendor systems is that they have been used at a variety of sites. Thus, the vendor likely has developed expertise in the system based on past experience. When investigating possible systems, purchasers can find out about the performance of vendor systems from other users. As changes in healthcare occur, such as the recent HIPAA privacy and security regulations, it is often easier for a vendor to make the necessary changes because its entire business is related to a limited number of products. In addition, **user groups** are often developed from organizations that have purchased the system and they can be helpful in maximizing the system's performance.

One disadvantage to a vendor system is that the vendor may not be able to modify it to meet all the organization's needs. Moreover, the level of training and problem-solving support varies from vendor to vendor. In some cases, vendors are unavailable to help with system problems after the initial start-up period.

Facility-specific systems have the advantage that they can be developed to meet the specific information needs of the healthcare facility. Because the system's developers are on-site, training and problem solving are always available.

However, if the system is not well documented when it is developed, it will be difficult to sustain maintenance in the event the original developers leave the facility. Moreover, in-house developers may not have the broad experience in the type of product developed that a vendor is likely to have. The ability of facility personnel to undertake the development and maintenance of the system should be considered very carefully before deciding to develop a system in-house.

Data Quality Issues

Indexes, registries, and databases are only helpful when the data they contain are accurate. Decisions concerning new treatment methods, healthcare policy, and physician credentialing and privileging are based on these databases. Incorrect data will likely result in serious errors in decision making.

Several factors must be addressed when assessing data quality. These include data validity, reliability, completeness, and timeliness.

Validity of the Data

Validity refers to the accuracy of the data. For example, in a cancer registry, the stage of the neoplasm must be recorded accurately because statistical information on survival rates by stage is commonly reported.

Several methods may be used to ensure validity. One method is to incorporate **edits** in the database. An edit is a check on the accuracy of the data, such as setting data types. If a particular data element, such as admission date, is set up with a data type of date, the computer will not allow other types of data, such as name, to be entered in that field. Other edits may use comparisons between fields to ensure accuracy. For example, an edit might check to see that all patients with the diagnosis of prostate cancer are listed as males in the database.

Reliability of the Data

Another factor to be considered in looking at data quality is reliability. *Reliability* refers to the consistency of the data. For example, all patients in a trauma registry with the same level, severity, and site of injury should have the same Abbreviated Injury Score. Reliability is frequently checked by having more than one person abstract data for the same case. The results are then compared to identify any discrepancies. This is called an **interrater reliability** method of checking. Several different people may be used to do the checking. In a cancer registry, for example, physician members of the cancer committee may be called on to check the reliability of the data.

The use of uniform terminology is an important way to improve data reliability. This has been evident in case definition for registries. The criteria for including a patient in a registry must have a clear definition. Definitions for terms such as race, for example, must include the categories to be used in determining race. If uniform terms are not used, the data will not be consistent. Also, it will be impossible to make comparisons between systems if uniform terms have not been used for all data. A data dictionary in which all data elements are defined helps ensure that uniform data definitions are being followed.

Completeness of the Data

Completeness is another factor to be considered in data quality. Missing data may prevent the database from being useful for research or clinical decision making. To avoid missing data, some databases will not allow the user to move to the next field without making an entry in the current one, especially for fields considered crucial. Looking at a variety of sources in case finding is a way to avoid missing patients who should be included in a registry.

Timeliness of the Data

Another concept important in data quality is timeliness. Data must be available within a time frame helpful to the user. Factors that influence decisions may change over time, so it is important that the data reflect up-to-date information.

Data Security and Confidentiality Issues

Data security usually refers to efforts to control access to health information. **Data confidentiality** usually refers to efforts to guarantee the privacy of personal health information. When looking at data security and confidentiality issues, it is important to consider the HIPAA regulations for privacy and security. Under HIPAA, the data collection done by registries is considered part of "healthcare operations." Therefore, the patient does not have to sign an authorization for release of protected health information (PHI) to the registry. Reporting of notifiable diseases to the state also comes under "healthcare operations" and does not require patient authorization for release (*In Confidence* 2003, 7).

Data Security

A number of methods may be used to ensure that only authorized people have access to patient data in the facility's computer system. One common method is the use of passwords. Other methods may involve biometric identification systems that use retinal scans or fingerprints. Tokens such as identification badges also may be used.

Moreover, the facility may establish levels of access to the computer system. In this case, each user would be allowed access to only certain parts of the system. Only those parts of the system to which the users have access appear on the screen. In addition, a record of all transactions in the system, called an **audit trail,** is maintained and reviewed for instances of unauthorized access.

Loss of data is another important consideration in data security. Although data sometimes are lost as a result of unauthorized access, more often they are lost in more routine ways. For example, a computer malfunction can cause data to be erased or lost. Backing up the data on electronic media such as tapes or disks is commonly done to avoid such losses. The backup must be done frequently, and the backup media must be kept away from the site where the main system is kept. If the backup were kept on-site, it would be vulnerable to the same destruction affecting the main system from sources such as fire and flood.

Computer viruses constitute yet another threat to data security. These are computer programs that attack systems and reproduce themselves. They may alter or destroy data. Facilities must use antivirus software to combat viruses. Moreover, they must keep the antivirus software up-to-date because new viruses appear regularly.

Physical security of the system is another consideration. Computer terminals must be kept in areas that are not physically accessible to unauthorized people. Reports and printouts from the system should not be left where they can be seen. When they are no longer needed, they should be destroyed.

Finally, it may be necessary to encrypt sensitive data. **Encryption** is a method of scrambling data so that they cannot be read without first being decoded. An AIDS registry, for example, might want to use an encryption method to protect patient-identifiable information.

Data Confidentiality

Maintaining the confidentiality of health data is a traditional role of HIM professionals. Patient-specific information requires more protection than aggregate data because individual patients cannot be identified in aggregate data. Policies on who may access the data provide a basic protection for confidentiality.

The type of data maintained also may affect policies on confidentiality. For many of the government databases discussed earlier, the information is aggregate and the data are readily available to any interested users. For example, public health data are frequently published in many formats including printed reports, Internet access, and direct computer access.

Employees working with the data should receive training on confidentiality. Further, they should be required to sign a yearly statement indicating that they have received the training and understand the implications of failure to maintain the confidentiality of data.

Trends in the Collection of Secondary Data

The main trend in collecting secondary data seems to be the increased use of automated data entry. Registries and databases are more commonly using data already available in electronic form rather than manually abstracting all data. As the electronic health record becomes more common, separate databases for various diseases and conditions such as cancer, diabetes, and trauma will be unnecessary. The patient health record itself will be a database that can be queried for information currently obtained from specialized registries.

Check Your Understanding 9.3

Instructions: Indicate whether the following statements are true or false (T or F).

1. _____ Now that registries and databases are almost universally computerized, data collection is no longer done manually.

2. _____ One advantage to a vendor system is that purchasers can find out about the system's performance from other users.

3. _____ With regard to data quality, validity refers to the consistency of the data.

4. _____ The record of transactions in a computer system is called the audit security.

5. _____ Among the HIM professional's traditional roles is that of maintaining the confidentiality of health data.

Real-World Case

In an article titled "Benchmarking with National ICD-9-CM Coded Data," Carol Osborn stated that:

> As HIM professionals, we want to be assured that we are providing the highest quality data for reimbursement and research and research purposes. We can review coded data internally, but this does not give us a clear picture of the total information that is being submitted to the Health Care Financing Administration (HCFA) [now called the Centers for Medicare and Medicaid Services, CMS]. . . . Recently a new tool has come out that helps HIM professionals evaluate the quality of coded data. This tool, *DRG Resource Book: Data for Benchmarking and Analysis,* is published by the Center for Healthcare Industry Performance Studies in Columbus, OH. The book contains comparative information for the top 50 medical and the top 25 surgical DRGs for the Medicare population, so HIM professionals can compare their coded data to a national database. The source of this information is the HCFA [CMS] Medicare Provider and Review File (MEDPAR file) for the federal fiscal year 1995, which consists of data compiled from UB-92 data submitted by hospitals for inpatient Medicare discharges (1999, 59).

This resource reports DRG summary information, cost analysis information, state-specific profiles of charges per discharge and by department, utilization and quality indicators, and clinical coding analysis, all by DRG. This article [analyzes] the ICD-9-CM codes reported for the seventy-five medical and surgical DRGs.

Summary

Health records contain extensive information about individual patients but are difficult to use when attempting to perceive trends in care or quality. For that reason, secondary records were developed. One type of secondary record is the index. An index is a report from the hospital database that provides information on patients and allows retrieval by diagnosis, procedure, or physician. Health information management departments routinely produce indexes.

Disease registries are developed when extensive information is needed about specific diagnoses, procedures, or conditions. They are commonly used for research and to improve patient care and health status. From the database created through the data collection process, reports can be developed to answer questions regarding patient care or issues such as rates of immunization and birth defects. In some cases, patient follow-up is done to assess survival rates and quality of life after a disease or accident.

HIM professionals perform a variety of roles in relation to registries. In some cases, they work on setting up the registry. Moreover, they may work in data collection and management of registry functions. HIM professionals are well suited to such positions because of their background and training in management, patient health record content, regulatory and legal compliance, and medical science and terminology.

Today, organizations and institutions of all types commonly maintain databases pertaining to healthcare. At the federal level, some administrative databases provide data and information for decisions regarding claims and practitioner credentialing. Other databases focus on the public health area, using data collected at the local level and shared with states and the federal government. These databases assist in government surveillance of health status in the United States. Some databases, such as the clinical trials database, are mandated by law and help patients and providers to locate clinical trials regardless of source or location.

Registries and databases raise a number of managerial issues. Data collection is often time-consuming, so some databases now use automated entry methods. In addition, decisions must be made between vendor and facility-specific products. Finally, the quality of the data is an important issue because the decisions made based on data in registries and databases depend on the data's validity, reliability, accuracy, and timeliness.

Another important issue related to registries and databases is the security of their data. Facilities must adopt methods that will ensure controlled access to data as well as prevent the loss of data. Confidentiality is always of concern to the HIM department, and steps must be taken to protect it.

In the future, separate registries and databases may become less common with the advent of electronic health record systems. In essence a large database, the EHR can be queried directly rather than having to first abstract data from the primary record into a secondary record.

References

All Kids Count. 2005. allkidscount.org.

American College of Surgeons Commission on Cancer. 2005. Available online from facs.org/cancer/.

American College of Surgeons Trauma Programs. 2005. Available online from facs.org/trauma/index.html.

American Joint Committee on Cancer. 2005. Available online from cancerstaging.org.

Center for Devices and Radiological Health. 1996. Medical device reporting for user facilities. Available online from fda.gov/cdrh/mdruf.pdf.

Centers for Disease Control. 2005b. National Center for Health Statistics. Available online from cdc.gov/nchs/nvss.htm.

Centers for Disease Control. 2005c. National Health Care Survey. Available online from cdc.gov/nchs/nhcs.htm.

Centers for Disease Control. 2005a. National Immunization Program. Available online from cdc.gov/nip/registry/min-funct-stds2001.htm#1.

Garthe, E. 1997. Overview of trauma registries in the United States. *Journal of American Health Information Management Association* 68(7):26,28,30–31.

Handling cancer registry requests for information. 2003 (May). *In Confidence* 11(8):7.

McCray, A., and N.C. Ide. 2000. Design and implementation of a national clinical trials registry. *Journal of the American Medical Informatics Association* 7:313–23.

National Cancer Registrars Association. 2005. ncra-usa.org.

National Library of Medicine. 2005. Available online from clinicaltrials.gov.

Office of the Inspector General. 1998. Health Care Fraud and Abuse Data Collection Program: Reporting of Final Adverse Actions, Notice of Proposed Rulemaking. *Federal Register* 63(210):58341–58342.

Osborn, C.E. 1999. Benchmarking with national ICD-9-CM coded data. *Journal of American Health Information Management Association* 70(4):59–69.

Ringer, D., and W. Cain. 2004 (February 2). COC revises cancer standards, creates FORDS. *Advance for Health Information Professionals.* Available online from advanceforhim.com.

Shelton, D.L. 2001 (February 14). Retrieved implants could be a source of important data. *American Medical News.*

Trauma.org. 2005. trauma.org.

Chapter 10
Healthcare Statistics

Carol Osborn, PhD, RHIA

Learning Objectives

- To understand how statistics are used in healthcare
- To differentiate between descriptive and inferential statistics
- To define hospital-related statistical terms
- To understand how to calculate hospital-related inpatient and outpatient statistics
- To define community-based morbidity and mortality rates
- To understand how to calculate community-based morbidity and mortality rates
- To define and calculate measures of central tendency and variability
- To describe the characteristics of the normal distribution
- To identify the relationships of measures of central tendency and variation to the normal distribution
- To see how to display healthcare data using tables, charts, and graphs, as appropriate
- To locate healthcare-related online state and federal databases on the Internet
- To understand how to use healthcare data collected from online databases in comparative statistical reports

Key Terms

Average daily census

Bar chart

Bed count (complement)

Bed count day

Benchmarking

Case fatality rate

Cause-specific death rate

Census

Crude death rate

Daily inpatient census

Descriptive statistics

Fetal autopsy rate

Fetal death (stillborn)

Fetal death rate

Frequency distribution

Frequency polygon

Gross autopsy rate

Gross death rate

Histogram

Hospital-acquired infection

Hospital autopsy rate

Hospital (nosocomial) infection rate

Incidence rate

Inpatient bed occupancy rate (percentage of occupancy)

Inpatient service day

Institutional Review Board

Length of stay (LOS)

Line graph

Maternal death rate

Maternal mortality rate

Mean

Median

Mode

Net autopsy rate

Net death rate

Newborn

Newborn autopsy rate

Notifiable disease

Normal distribution

Pie chart

Postoperative infection rate

Prevalence rate

Proportion

Proportionate mortality ratio (PMR)

Range

Rate

Ratio

Standard deviation

Table

Total length of stay (discharge days)

Variance

Introduction

Complete and accurate information is at the heart of good decision making. The health information management (HIM) professional is responsible for ensuring that health record data are accurate and organized into information that is useful to healthcare decision makers.

The primary source of clinical data in the healthcare facility is the health record. The data in the health record are compiled in various ways to help in making decisions about patient care, the facility's financial status, and/or facility planning, to name a few.

This chapter discusses the descriptive rates used to describe hospital and community populations. It also introduces measures of central tendency and variability and the **normal distribution.** Finally, it includes a brief discussion of online databases.

Theory into Practice

The Department of Quality Improvement at Community Hospital asked the director of health information management to provide the hospital's Cesarean-section (C-section) rate for the previous year for benchmarking purposes. It was recommended that the C-section rate for any hospital not exceed 15 percent. For the previous year, the hospital performed 556 C-sections out of 4,233 deliveries. Its C-section rate is 13.1 percent ([556/4,233] × 100). The quality improvement coordinator is pleased that the hospital's C-section rate falls within national guidelines.

The hospital administration is evaluating the appropriateness of an expansion program. The associate administrator in charge of facility planning asks the HIM director for the bed occupancy rate for the hospital and its major services for the past five years and the number of outpatient and emergency department visits for the same time period. The director's report is displayed in table 10.1 and figure 10.1.

Table 10.1. Bed occupancy rates, Community Hospital, 2000–2004					
Hospital Service	**2000**	**2001**	**2002**	**2003**	**2004**
Total	85%	88%	90%	92%	95%
Medicine	90%	90%	92%	92%	95%
Surgery	80%	85%	85%	88%	90%
Obstetrics	65%	70%	72%	77%	79%
Pediatrics	85%	88%	88%	86%	89%

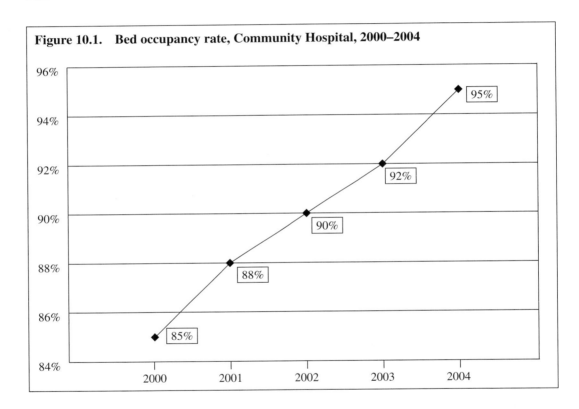

Figure 10.1.   Bed occupancy rate, Community Hospital, 2000–2004

Descriptive Statistics

Descriptive statistics are the most common type of statistics that the health information technician (HIT) will encounter or be responsible for producing. They describe populations. A population might be, for example, all the patients treated in the hospital during a certain month or an entire city or community of people. The rates reported in healthcare facilities and communities describe illnesses, births, and deaths for specific periods of time. As an example, the death rate, or mortality rate, for Community Hospital for the month of January is 2 percent. Thus, two patients died in the hospital for every 100 patients discharged during that month.

Reporting the death rate for a hospital is similar to reporting one for a community. As an example, a community's death rate for the month of January is two people for every 100,000 population. Regardless of whether hospital or community rates are being reported, the actual population of interest is the denominator in calculations of rates that describe populations. Rates for hospitals are reported as the number of cases per 100, or the percent of the hospital population. Rates for communities are reported as per 1,000, per 10,000, or per 100,000 people living in the community.

Ratios, Proportions, and Rates

Many healthcare statistics are reported in the form of a **ratio, proportion,** or **rate.** These measures are used to report morbidity (illness), mortality (death), and natality (birthrate) at the local, state, and national levels. Basically, these measures indicate the number of times something happened relative to the number of times it *could have* happened. All three measures are based on the following formula:

$$\text{Ratio, proportion, rate} = (x/y) \times 10^n$$

In this formula, x and y are the quantities being compared and x is divided by y. 10^n is 10 to the nth power. The size of 10^n may be equal to 10, 100, 1,000, 10,000, and so on, depending on the value of n:

$$10^0 = 1$$
$$10^1 = 10$$
$$10^2 = 10 \times 10 = 100$$
$$10^3 = 10 \times 10 \times 10 = 1,000$$

For example, if the hospital discharged 500 patients in January and 10 of them died, what would the hospital's death rate be for that month? The formula above can be used to compare how many times something occurred (10 deaths) to how many times something could have occurred (500 discharged patients). Therefore, in the formula, x, which is how many deaths occurred (10), is divided by y, which is how many times deaths could have occurred (500). This gives an answer of 0.02. However, as stated earlier, rates for hospitals are based on the number of cases per 100 cases. Thus, to complete the formula, it will be necessary to multiply 0.02 by 100 (or 10^2) to get an answer of 2 percent.

Ratios

In a ratio, the quantities being compared, such as patient discharge status (x = alive, y = died), may be expressed so that x and y are completely independent of each other or x can be included in y. For example, the outcome of patients discharged from Community Hospital could be compared in one of two ways:

Alive/died, or x/y

Alive/(alive + died), or $x/(x + y)$

In the first example, x is completely independent of y. The ratio represents the number of patients discharged alive compared to the number of patients who died. In the second example, x is part of the whole ($x + y$). The ratio represents the number of patients discharged alive compared to all patients discharged. Both expressions are considered ratios.

Proportions

A proportion is a type of ratio in which x is a portion of the whole $(x + y)$. In a proportion, the numerator is always included in the denominator. Figures 10.2 and 10.3 describe the procedures for calculating ratios and proportions.

Rates

Rates are often used to measure an event over a period of time. Sometimes they also are used in performance improvement studies. Like ratios and proportions, rates may be reported daily, weekly, monthly, or yearly. This allows for trend analysis and comparisons over time. The basic formula for calculating a rate is (the number above the fraction line is the numerator and the number below the line is the denominator):

$$\frac{\text{Number of cases occurring during a given time period}}{\text{Total cases or population at risk during the same time period}}$$

Figure 10.2.   Calculation of a ratio, discharge status of patients discharged in May 20xx

1. Define x and y
    x = number of patients discharged alive
    y = number of patients who died

2. Identify x and y
    $x = 235$
    $y = 22$

3. Set up the ratio x/y
    235/22

4. Reduce the fraction so that either x or y equals 1:
    10.68/1

There were 10.68 live discharges for every patient who died.

Figure 10.3.   Calculation of a proportion, discharge status of patients discharged in May 20xx

1. Define x and y
    x = number of patients discharged alive
    y = number of patients who died

2. Identify x and y
    $x = 235$
    $y = 22$

3. Set up the ratio $x/(x + y)$
    $235/(235 + 22) = 235/257$

4. Reduce the fraction so that either x or y equals 1:
    0.91/1

The proportion of patients discharged alive was 0.91.

Healthcare facilities calculate many types of morbidity and mortality rates. For example, the C-section rate is a measure of the proportion, or percentage, of C-sections performed during a given period of time. C-section rates are closely monitored because they present more risk to the mother and baby and are more expensive than vaginal deliveries.

In calculating the C-section rate, the number of C-sections performed during the specified period of time is counted and this value is placed in the numerator. The number of cases, or the population at risk, is the number of women who delivered during the same time period. This number is placed in the denominator. As mentioned above, inpatient hospital rates are reported as the rate per 100 cases ($10^n = 10^2 = 10 \times 10 = 100$) and are expressed as percentages.

Figure 10.4 shows the procedure for calculating a rate. In the example, 33 of the 263 deliveries at hospital X during the month of May were C-sections. In the formula, the numerator is the number of C-sections performed in May (given period of time) and the denominator is the total number of deliveries (the population at risk) performed in the same time frame, including C-sections. In calculating the rate, the numerator is always included in the denominator. Also, when calculating the rate, the numerator is first multiplied by 100 and then divided by the denominator.

Because hospital rates rarely result in a whole number, they usually must be rounded. The hospital should set a policy on whether rates are to be reported to one or two decimal places. The division should be carried out to at least one more decimal place than desired.

In rounding, when the last number is five or greater, the preceding number should be increased by one. In contrast, when the last number is less than five, the preceding number should remain the same. For example, when rounding 25.56 percent to one decimal place, the rate becomes 25.6 percent. When rounding 1.563 percent to two places, the rate becomes 1.56 percent. Rates of less than 1 percent are usually carried out to three decimal places and rounded to two. For rates less than 1 percent, a zero should precede the decimal to emphasize that the rate is less than 1 percent (for example, 0.56 percent).

Figure 10.4.   Calculation of a rate, C-Section rate, Community Hospital, May 20xx

During May, 263 women delivered; of these, 33 deliveries were by C-section. What is the C-section rate for May?

1. Define the numerator (number of times an event occurred) and the denominator (number of times an event could have occurred):
    Numerator = total number of C-sections performed during the time period
    Denominator = total number of deliveries, including C-sections, in the same time period

2. Identify the numerator and the denominator:
    Numerator = 33
    Denominator = 263

3. Set up the rate:
    33/263

4. Multiply the numerator by 100 and then divide by the denominator:
    ([33 $\times$ 100]/263) = 12.5%

The C-section rate for May is 12.5%.

Check Your Understanding 10.1

Instructions: Match the following statistics with the appropriate terms.

1. ____ Female discharges outnumber male discharges 3 to 1.
2. ____ Of the 100 discharges on October 1, 60 were female and 40 were male. Therefore, 0.60 of the discharges were women.
3. ____ Of the 100 patients discharged on October 1, 99 percent were discharged alive.

a. Rate
b. Ratio
c. Proportion

Measures of Central Tendency and Variability

Measures of central tendency and variability also can be used to describe populations. The measures of central tendency discussed below are the **mean,** the **median,** and the **mode.** The measures of variability discussed below are the **range,** the **variance,** and the **standard deviation.** HITs will likely be more involved in calculating means, medians, modes, and ranges than in calculating variance or standard deviations. However, this section includes a discussion of variance and standard deviation as a reference in the event the HIT's job task involves this type of statistical analysis.

Measures of Central Tendency: Mean, Median, and Mode

Before discussing the measures of central tendency that include the mean, median, and mode, it is important to understand the fundamental concept of a **frequency distribution.** This is because the mean, median, and mode are all related to a frequency distribution.

A frequency distribution shows the values that a variable can take and the number of observations associated with each value. For example, for the variable **length of stay** (LOS), five patients were discharged with the following lengths of stay:

Patient	LOS
1	2 days
2	3 days
3	4 days
4	2 days
5	3 days

The frequency distribution for LOS, in ascending order, is 2, 2, 3, 3, and 4. Examples of other variables include race, gender, height, and weight.

For instance, if Community Hospital wants to construct a frequency distribution to show the LOS for patients who were discharged on May 10, it wants to see how many of these patients were in the hospital for a particular LOS (for example, four days). The variable is the LOS, and the frequency is the number of times that LOS occurred among the patients discharged on May 10.

To construct a frequency distribution, all the values that the particular LOS can take must be listed, from the lowest-observed value to the highest. Then the number of times a discharged patient had that particular LOS is entered. Table 10.2 shows a frequency distribution for LOS on May 10. It lists all the values for LOS between the lowest and the highest, even when there are no observations for some of the values. For example, there

Table 10.2. Frequency distribution for LOS, Community Hospital

Patient Discharges, May 10	
LOS in Days	**Number of Patients (frequency)**
1	2
2	2
3	0
4	6
5	6
6	11
7	6
8	5
9	3
10	1
Total	42

are no observations of patients spending three days in the hospital. Six patients have an LOS of four days.

An understanding of a frequency distribution helps to clarify what a measure of central tendency is. Measures of central tendency are measures of location. They indicate the typical value of a frequency distribution. For example, to determine the "typical" value or LOS for a patient listed in table 10.2, it is necessary to calculate a mean, a median, or a mode, depending on the purpose of the analysis.

The Mean
The mean is the arithmetic average of a frequency distribution. Put simply, it is the sum of all the values in a frequency distribution divided by the frequency. In the preceding example with five patients, the sum of the values would be 2 + 2 + 3 + 3 + 4 = 14. To arrive at the arithmetic mean, 14 (the sum of all the values in the frequency distribution) is divided by 5 (the frequency). This gives a mean, or average, of 2.8 days.

Because the HIT will likely encounter a variety of mathematical expressions, it is important to understand some of the notations used in statistical analysis. For example, the symbol for the mean is $\overline{X}$ (pronounced X bar). The formula for calculating the mean in a frequency distribution is:

$$\overline{X} = \sum_{i}^{n} X_i / N$$

where Σ is summation, Xi is each successive observation from the first one in the frequency distribution ($i = 1$) to the last observation (n), and N is the total number of observations. To simply translate this equation, the mean ($\overline{X}$) equals the sum (Σ) of all the observations in the frequency distribution (14) divided by the total number (N) of observations (5) in the distribution.

The following is another example of working with the mathematical equation for the mean. To calculate the mean, or the average length of stay (ALOS), for the data in table 10.2, the appropriate figures could be substituted into the formula:

$$\overline{X} = \sum_{i}^{n} X_i / N$$

$$\overline{X} = \frac{\begin{array}{c} 1 + 1 + 2 + 2 + 4 + 4 + 4 + 4 + 4 + 4 + 5 + 5 + 5 + 5 + 5 + 5 \\ + 6 + 6 + 6 + 6 + 6 + 6 + 6 + 6 + 6 + 6 + 6 + 7 + 7 + 7 + 7 + 7 + 7 \\ + 8 + 8 + 8 + 8 + 8 + 9 + 9 + 9 + 10 \end{array}}{42}$$

$$\overline{X} = 245/42$$

$$\overline{X} = 5.8$$

The ALOS for patients discharged from Community Hospital on May 10 is 5.8 days (rounded).

Although the mean is a convenient measure of central tendency, there are two disadvantages to using it as the most typical value in a frequency distribution:

- In this example, the LOS for the 42 patients are integers (whole numbers). However, the ALOS is fractional (5.8), even though there is no fractional LOS. Fractional values are considered more a problem of interpretation than a result that is not meaningful. In this case, the ALOS is interpreted as, "On average, the ALOS for the patients discharged from Community Hospital on May 10 is between 5 and 6 days."

- The mean is sensitive to extreme measures. That is, it is strongly influenced by outliers. For example, if the 10-day LOS were actually a 25-day LOS, the ALOS would increase to 6.2 days.

Thus, the average or arithmetic mean may not always be the most appropriate way to summarize the most typical value of a frequency distribution. The measure of central tendency selected to describe the typical value of a frequency distribution should be based on the characteristics of that particular frequency distribution.

The Median

The median is the midpoint of a frequency distribution. It is the point at which 50 percent of observations fall above and 50 percent fall below.

If the frequency distribution has an odd number of observations, the median is the middle number. In the following distribution, the median is 13. Three observations fall above the value of 13, and three fall below it.

10 11 12 $\boxed{13}$ 14 15 16

If the frequency distribution has an even number of observations, the median is the midpoint between the two middle observations. It is found by averaging the two middle scores, $(x + y)/2$. In the following example, the median is 13.5 ($[13 + 14]/2$):

10 11 12 $\boxed{13\ 14}$ 15 16 17

When the two middle observations take on the same value, the median is that value. When determining the median, it does not matter whether there are duplicate observations in the frequency distribution. For example:

$$10\ 11\ 11\ 12\ \boxed{13\ 13}\ 14\ 15\ 16\ 17$$

In this frequency distribution, the median falls between the fifth and sixth observations. Therefore, the median is 13 ([13 + 13]/2).

Table 10.2 records LOS data for forty-two patients. In this example, the median falls between the twenty-first and twenty-second observations. Placed in order from lowest to highest, the distribution is:

$$1\ 1\ 2\ 2\ 4\ 4\ 4\ 4\ 4\ 5\ 5\ 5\ 5\ 5\ 5\ 6\ 6\ 6\ \boxed{6\ 6}\ 6\ 6\ 6\ 6\ 7\ 7\ 7\ 7\ 7\ 7\ 8\ 8\ 8\ 8\ 8\ 9\ 9\ 9\ 10$$

The median is 6 ([6 + 6]/2). The median offers the following three advantages:

- It is relatively easy to calculate.

- It is based on the whole distribution and not just a portion of it, as is the case with the mode.

- Unlike the mean, extreme values or unusual outliers in the frequency distribution do not influence the median.

The Mode

The mode is the simplest measure of central tendency. It is used to indicate the most frequent observation in a frequency distribution.

The mode has several advantages, including:

- It is easy to obtain and interpret.

- It is not sensitive to extreme observations in the frequency distribution.

- It is easy to communicate and explain to others.

However, the mode also has disadvantages, including:

- It may not be descriptive of the distribution when the most frequent observation does not occur very often, especially when there is a large number of observations.

- It may not be unique. That is, more than one mode may be in a distribution. A frequency distribution may be unimodal, bimodal, or multimodal. When each observation occurs an equal number of times, the distribution does not have a mode.

- It does not provide information about the entire distribution, only the observation that occurs most frequently.

In table 10.2, the mode is six because eleven patients had an LOS of six days.

To summarize, for the LOS data in table 10.2, the measures of central tendency are similar. The mean is 5.8 days, the median is 6 days, and the mode is 6 days.

Measures of Variability

In addition to measures of central tendency, the hospital may use measures of variability to describe frequency distributions. These measures indicate how widely the observations are spread out around the measures of central tendency, such as the mean, the median, or the mode. The measures of spread increase with greater variation in the frequency distribution. The spread is equal to zero when there is no variation (for example, when all the values in a frequency distribution are the same). This section discusses the following measures of spread: the range, the variance, and the standard deviation.

The Range

The range is the simplest measure of spread. It is the difference between the smallest and largest values in a frequency distribution:

$$\text{Range} = X_{max} - X_{min}$$

The range for the LOS data in table 10.2 is 9 (10 − 1 = 9).

One disadvantage to the range is that extreme values, or outliers, in the distribution can affect it. Also, the range varies widely from sample to sample. Only the two most extreme observations in the distribution affect its value. Thus, it is not sensitive to other observations in the distribution.

Two frequency distributions may have the same range but differ greatly in variation. For example, the range for the following frequency distributions is 9 (10 − 1 = 9):

Distribution 1: 1 2 3 4 5 6 7 8 9 10

Distribution 2: 1 1.5 3 3.5 3.7 7 8 8.26 10 10

However, when the two distributions are compared, distribution 2 has more variation than distribution 1. This is demonstrated when the variance is calculated. The variance for distribution 1 is 3.03, and the variance for distribution 2 is 3.44. To remedy the problem associated with reporting only the range of observations, another statistic can be used. This statistic is called the variance, and it does not have the shortcomings of the range.

The Variance

The calculation of variance, and also something called the standard deviation, is usually covered in a beginning statistics course. As mentioned earlier, most HITs will not have to calculate or interpret the variance or standard deviation. These sections are included here as a reference and for purposes of completion.

The variance of a frequency distribution is the average of the square deviations from the mean. The variance of a sample is symbolized by s^2. The variance of a distribution is larger when the observations are widely spread. The formula for calculating the variance is:

$$s^2 = \sum_{i}^{n} (X_i - \overline{X})^2 / N - 1$$

In the equation above, s^2 stands for variance. As explained earlier, the symbol Σ stands for summation. To calculate the deviations from the mean, it is necessary to first calculate the mean. Then, the squared deviations of the mean are calculated by subtracting the mean of the frequency distribution from each value in the distribution. The difference between the two values is squared $(X - \overline{X})^2$. The squared differences are summed and divided by $N - 1$. The calculations for the variance for the LOS data in table 10.2 are shown in table 10.3.

Table 10.3.   Calculation of the variance, LOS data

LOS	LOS − Mean (5.8) $(X - \overline{X})$	$(LOS - Mean)^2 (X - \overline{X})^2$
1	−4.8	23.04
1	−4.8	23.04
2	−3.8	14.44
2	−3.8	14.44
4	−1.8	3.24
4	−1.8	3.24
4	−1.8	3.24
4	−1.8	3.24
4	−1.8	3.24
4	−1.8	3.24
5	−1.8	3.24
5	−0.8	0.64
5	−0.8	0.64
5	−0.8	0.64
5	−0.8	0.64
5	−0.8	0.64
6	0.2	0.04
6	0.2	0.04
6	0.2	0.04
6	0.2	0.04
6	0.2	0.04
6	0.2	0.04
6	0.2	0.04
6	0.2	0.04
6	0.2	0.04
6	0.2	0.04
6	0.2	0.04
6	0.2	0.04
7	1.2	1.44
7	1.2	1.44
7	1.2	1.44
7	1.2	1.44
7	1.2	1.44
7	1.2	1.44
8	2.2	4.84
8	2.2	4.84
8	2.2	4.84
8	2.2	4.84
8	2.2	4.84
9	3.2	10.24
9	3.2	10.24
9	3.2	10.24
10	4.2	17.64
Total	0*	179.88

$$s^2 = \sum_{i}^{n} (X_i - \overline{X})^2 / N - 1$$
$$= 179.88/44$$
$$= 4.39$$

*rounded

In the calculations for the variance, the sum of $(X - \overline{X})$ is equal to zero. This is because the mean is the balance point in the distribution. When a value is less than the mean, the difference is negative ($1 - 5.8 = -4.8$). When the value is greater than the mean, the difference is positive ($6 - 5.8 = 0.2$). Therefore, the sum of the differences from the mean is equal to zero. In this example, the sum approximates zero because the actual mean of 5.8333 was rounded to 5.8.

The Standard Deviation
The variance for the LOS data is 4.39, but what does this mean? The interpretation of the variance is not meaningful at the descriptive level because the original units of measure (the LOS) are squared to arrive at the variance. By calculating the square root of the variance, the data are returned to the original units of measure. This is called the standard deviation, which is symbolized by s. The formula for the standard deviation is:

$$s = \sqrt{\sum_{i}^{n} (X_i - \overline{X})^2 / N - 1}$$

The standard deviation for the LOS data is 2.09.

The standard deviation is the most widely used measure of variability in descriptive statistics. Because it is easy to interpret, it is the preferred measure of dispersion for frequency distributions.

Check Your Understanding 10.2

Instructions: Fifteen infants were born at Community Hospital during the week of December 1. Calculate the measures of central tendency and variability for the infants' weights. The birth weights in grams are:

2,450	2,540	1,800
2,750	2,300	2,780
2,600	1,735	2,400
2,540	1,720	2,485
2,815	2,715	2,640

1. _____ Mean

2. _____ Median

3. _____ Mode

4. _____ Range

5. _____ Variance

6. _____ Standard deviation

The Normal Distribution
Another important concept associated with measures of central tendency and variation is the concept of normal distribution. Measures of central tendency and variation are interpreted as they relate to the normal distribution. The normal distribution is actually a theoretical family of distributions that may have any mean or any standard deviation.

Sometimes the normal distribution is called a bell-shaped curve. The normal distribution is bell-shaped and symmetrical about the mean. Because it is symmetrical, 50 percent of observations fall above the mean and 50 percent fall below it. In a normal distribution, the mean, median, and mode are equal. The values of the normal distribution range from minus infinity ($-\infty$) to plus infinity ($+\infty$).

In the normal distribution, the standard deviation indicates how many observations fall within a certain range of the mean. Typically, 68 percent of observations fall within one standard deviation of the mean, 95 percent fall within two standard deviations, and 99.7 percent fall within three standard deviations.

Figure 10.5 shows an example of a normal distribution superimposed on a **histogram.** The center of the distribution, or mean, is 6. (The median and the mode also are 6.) The standard deviation is 2.45. This means that 68 percent of the observations in the frequency distribution fall within 2.45 standard deviations of 6(6 ± 2.45). Thus, 68 percent fall between 3.55 and 8.45; 95 percent fall between 1.1 and 10.9; and 99.7 percent fall between −1.35 and 13.35.

As shown in the figure, a characteristic of the normal distribution is that each tail of the curve approaches the x-axis but never touches it, no matter how far from center the line is.

A histogram of the frequency distribution for the LOS data in table 10.2 is shown in figure 10.6. The distribution is kurtotic. *Kurtosis* is the vertical stretching of a distribution. The distribution is more peaked than the normal distribution and thus is considered kurtotic.

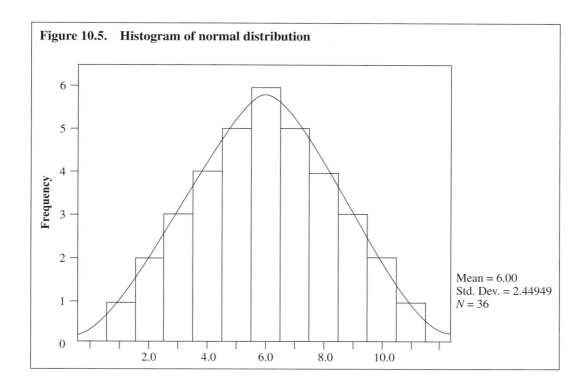

Figure 10.5.   Histogram of normal distribution

Mean = 6.00
Std. Dev. = 2.44949
N = 36

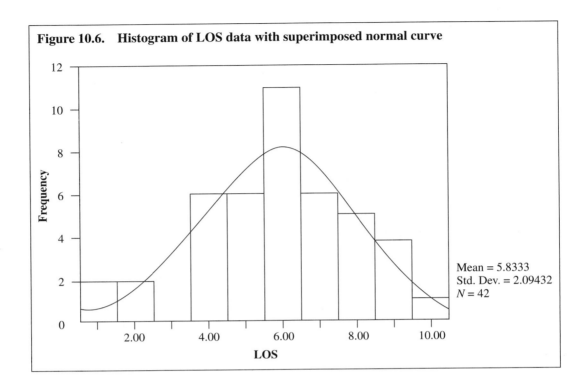

Figure 10.6.   Histogram of LOS data with superimposed normal curve

Mean = 5.8333
Std. Dev. = 2.09432
N = 42

A skewed distribution is asymmetrical. *Skewness* is the horizontal stretching of a frequency distribution to one side or the other so that one tail is longer than the other. The longer tail has more observations. Because the mean is sensitive to extreme observations, it moves in the direction of the long tail when a distribution is skewed. When the direction of the tail is off to the right, the distribution is positively skewed, or skewed to the right. When the direction of the tail is off to the left, the distribution is negatively skewed, or skewed to the left. When the mean and the median approximate one another (as with the LOS data), the distribution is not significantly skewed.

The measures of central tendency and variation discussed above may be calculated using a handheld calculator. Also, statistical packages such as SPSS are available for performing these and other descriptive and inferential statistics. The histograms were prepared using SPSS. The SPSS output for the LOS data appears in figure 10.7. The slight differences between the handheld calculator results and the SPSS results in the mean, variance, and standard deviation are because of rounding.

Graphic Display of Data

After data have been summarized in aggregate form, it is often useful to display them in graphic form. Graphic forms are effective ways of presenting large quantities of information. The purpose of **tables,** charts, and graphs is to communicate information about the data to the user of the data.

Whatever type of graphic form is used, it should:

- Display the data
- Allow the user to think about the meaning of the data

Figure 10.7.   SPSS output for LOS data

LOS

N	Valid	42
	Missing	0
Mean		5.8333
Median		6.0000
Mode		6.00
Std. Deviation		2.09432
Variance		4.386
Range		9.00
Minimum		1.00
Maximum		10.00
Sum		245.00

- Avoid distortion of the data
- Encourage the user to make comparisons
- Reveal data at several levels, from a broad overview to the fine detail

Tables

A table is an orderly arrangement of values that groups data into rows and columns. Almost any type of quantitative information can be organized into tables. Tables are useful for demonstrating patterns and other kinds of relationships. They also may serve as the basis for more visual displays of data, such as charts and graphs, where some of the detail may be lost. However, because tables are not very interesting, they should be used sparingly.

A useful first step is to prepare a table shell that shows how the data will be organized and displayed. A table shell is the outline of a table with everything in place except for the data. (See figure 10.8.)

A table should contain all the information the user needs to understand the data in it. It should have the following characteristics:

- It should be a logical unit.
- It should be self-explanatory. It should be able to stand on its own when it is photocopied and/or removed from its context.
- All sources should be specified.
- Headings for columns and rows should be specific and understandable.
- Row and column totals should have been checked for accuracy.
- Blank cells should not be left empty. When no information is available for a particular cell, the cell should contain a zero or a dash.
- Categories should be mutually exclusive and exhaustive.

Figure 10.8.   Table shell

TITLE							
		Sex				Total	
		Male		Female			
Box Head	**Age**	**Number**	**%**	**Number**	**%**	**Number**	**%**
Stub	Row Variable	→→→	→→→	→→→	→→→	→→→	→→→
	<45			Column Variable			
↓	45–54			↓			
↓	55–64			↓			
↓	65–74			↓			
↓	75+			↓			

Data contained in tables should be aligned. Guidelines for aligning text and numbers include:

- Text in the table should be aligned at left, although text that serves as a column heading may be centered.

- Numeric values should be aligned at right.

- When the numeric values contain decimals, the decimals should be aligned.

The essential components of a table are summarized in figure 10.9.

Tables contain information on one or more variables. Tables 10.4 and 10.5 are examples of one- and two-variable tables.

Charts and Graphs

Charts and graphs of various types are the best means for presenting data for quick visualization of relationships. They emphasize the main points and analyze and clarify relationships among variables.

Several principles are involved in the construction of charts and graphs. When constructing charts and graphs, the following points should be considered:

- *Distortion:* To avoid distorting the data, the representation of the numbers should be proportional to the numerical quantities represented.

- *Proportion and scale:* Graphs should emphasize the horizontal. It is easier for the eye to read along the horizontal axis from left to right. Also, graphs should be greater in length than height. A useful guideline is to follow the three-quarter-high rule. This rule states that the height (*y*-axis) of the graph should be three-fourths the length (*x*-axis) of the graph.

Figure 10.9.   Essential components of tables

Title	The title should be as complete as possible and should clearly relate to the content of the table. It should answer the following questions: • What are the data (e.g., counts, percentages)? • Who (e.g., white females with breast cancer; black males with lung cancer)? • Where are the data from (e.g., hospital, state, community)? • When (e.g., year, month)? A sample title might be: Site Distribution by Age and Sex of Cancer Patients upon First Admission to Community Hospital, 2000–2004
Box Head	The box head contains the captions or column headings. The heading of each column should contain as few words as possible but should explain exactly what the data in the column represent.
Stub	The row captions are known as the stub. Items in the stub should be grouped to make it easy to interpret the data (for example, ages grouped into five-year intervals).
Cell	The cell is the box formed by the intersection of a column and a row.
Optional Items:	
Note	Notes are used to explain anything in the table that the reader cannot understand from the title, box head, or stub. They contain numbers, preliminary or revised numbers, or explanations of any unusual numbers. Definitions, abbreviations, and/or qualifications for captions or cell names should be footnoted. A note usually applies to a specific cell(s) within the table, and a symbol (e.g., ** or #) may be used to key the cell to the note. If several notes are used, it is better to use small letters than symbols or numbers. Note any numbers that may be confused with the numbers within the table.
Source	If data are used from a source outside your research, the exact reference to the source should be given. The source lends authenticity to the data and allows the reader to locate the original information if he or she needs it.

Source: Adapted from *Self-Instructional Manual for Cancer Registries, Book 7: Statistics and Epidemiology for Cancer Registries.* Department of Health and Human Services, Public Health Services, NIH Publication No. 94-3766, 1994.

Table 10.4.   One-variable table, Community Hospital admissions by gender, 2004

Gender	Number	%
Male	3,141	46.0%
Female	3,683	54.0%
Total	6,824	100.0%

Table 10.5.   Two-variable table, Community Hospital admissions by race and gender, 2004

Race	Gender		Total
	Male	**Female**	
White	2,607	2,946	5,553
Non-White	534	737	1,271
Total	3,141	3,683	6,824

- *Abbreviations:* Any abbreviations should be spelled out in explanatory notes.

- *Color:* Colors can be used to highlight groupings that appear in the graph.

- *Print:* Both uppercase and lowercase letters should be used in titles. The use of all-capital letters can be difficult to read.

Bar Charts

Bar charts are used to display data from one or more variables. The bars may be drawn vertically or horizontally. The simplest bar chart is the one-variable bar chart. In this type of chart, one bar represents each category of the variable. For example, if the data in table 10.4 were displayed in a bar chart, sex would be the variable and male and female would be the variable categories. Figure 10.10 displays the data from table 10.4 as a bar chart. The length or height of each bar is proportional to the number of males and females discharged. Presentation of the data in a bar chart makes it easy to see that more females than males were admitted to Community Hospital in 1999.

Figure 10.11 displays the two-variable data from table 10.5 as a two-variable or grouped-variable bar chart in a three-dimensional format. Computer software makes it easy to present data in this way. However, presenting data in a three-dimensional format can be tricky. The reader may not always be able to estimate the true height of the bar. In a three-dimensional bar chart, the back edges of the bar appear higher than the front edge, as shown in figure 10.11. To make sure the reader correctly interprets the chart, the bars should include the actual values for each category.

Figure 10.12 shows guidelines for constructing bar charts.

Pie Charts

A **pie chart** is an easily understood chart in which the sizes of the slices of the pie show the proportional contribution of each part. Pie charts can be used to show the component parts of a single group or variable.

To calculate the size of each slice of the pie, first determine the proportion that each slice is to represent. Multiplying the proportion by 360 (the total number of degrees in a circle) will give the size of each slice of the pie in degrees.

Figure 10.13 shows data collected on admissions to Community Hospital by payer. The summary data for one year show that managed care was the payer for 40.1 percent of the patients, Medicare was the payer for 30.5 percent, Medicaid was the payer for 16.5 per-

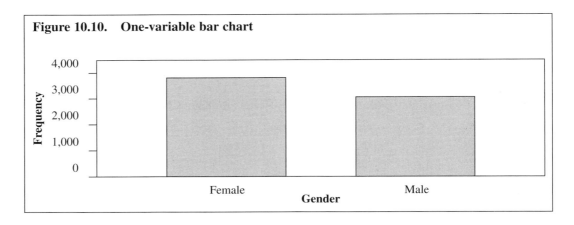

Figure 10.10.   One-variable bar chart

cent, and government managed care was the payer for 8.1 percent. The remaining patients (4.9 percent) had commercial insurance.

With 40.1 percent of the pie chart, the managed care category equals approximately 144° (360° × 0.401 = 144°), the Medicare category equals 30.5° (360° × 0.305 = 110°), the Medicaid category equals 59.4° (360° × 0.165 = 59.4°), the government managed care category equals approximately 29° (360° × 0.081 = 29°), and commercial insurance equals 17.6° (360° × 0.049 = 17.6°). Taken together, the slices equal 360° [(144 + 110 + 59.4 + 29 + 17.6) = 360].

The slices of the pie should be arranged in some logical order. By convention, the largest slices begin at twelve o'clock. Computer software is available to make the construction of pie charts easy. The pie chart in figure 10.13 was prepared using SPSS™. (Numbers may not total 100 exactly because of rounding.)

Figure 10.11.   Two-variable bar chart, Community Hospital admissions by race and sex, 2004

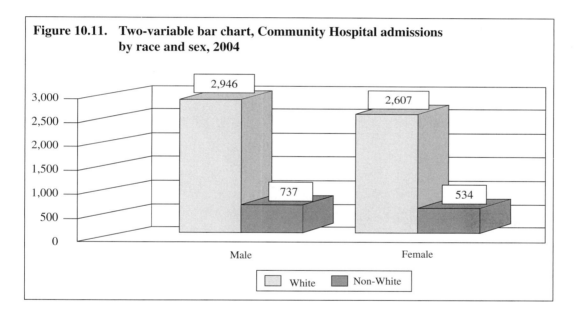

Figure 10.12.   Guidelines for constructing a bar chart

When constructing a bar chart, keep the following points in mind:

- Arrange the bar categories in a natural order, such as alphabetical order, order by increasing age, or an order that will produce increasing or decreasing bar lengths.
- The bars may be positioned vertically or horizontally.
- The length of the bars should be proportional to the frequency of the event.
- Avoid using more than three bars (categories) within a group of bars.
- Leave a space between adjacent groups of bars, but not between bars within a group.
- Code different categories of variables by differences in bar color, shading, and/or cross-hatching. Include a legend that explains the coding system.

Source: Department of Health and Human Services, Public Health Services. *Principles of Epidemiology: An Introduction to Applied Epidemiology and Biostatistics.* Atlanta: HHS, 1992, 251.

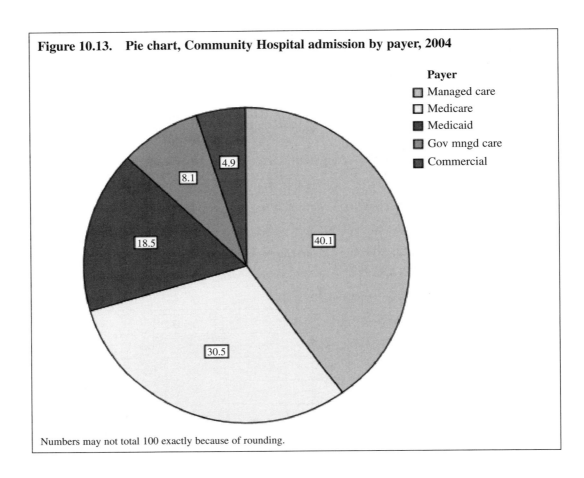

Figure 10.13.   Pie chart, Community Hospital admission by payer, 2004

Payer
- Managed care
- Medicare
- Medicaid
- Gov mngd care
- Commercial

4.9

8.1

40.1

18.5

30.5

Numbers may not total 100 exactly because of rounding.

Line Graphs

A **line graph** may be used to display time trends. The *x*-axis shows the unit of time from left to right, and the *y*-axis measures the values of the variable being plotted. A line graph does not represent a frequency distribution.

A line graph consists of a line connecting a series of points. Like all graphs, it should be constructed so that it is easy to read. The selection of the proper scale, a complete and accurate title, and an informative legend is important. When a graph is too long and narrow, either vertically or horizontally, it has an awkward appearance and may exaggerate one aspect of the data.

A line graph is especially useful for plotting a large number of observations. It also allows several sets of data to be presented on one graph.

Either actual numbers or percentages may be used on the *y*-axis. Percentages should be placed on the *y*-axis when more than one distribution is to be shown. A percentage distribution allows comparisons among groups where the actual totals are different.

When more than one set of data is plotted on the same graph, the lines should be made different (for example, solid or broken) for each set. However, the number of lines should be kept to a minimum to avoid confusion. Each line then should be identified in a legend placed on the graph itself.

There are two kinds of time-trend data: point data and period data. Point data reflect an instant in time. Figure 10.14 displays point data, the total number of admissions for each year represented in the graph. Period data are averages or totals over a specified period of time, such as a five-year time frame. Table 10.6 summarizes period data for survival rates of patients diagnosed with kidney cancer. Figure 10.15 displays these period data in a line graph.

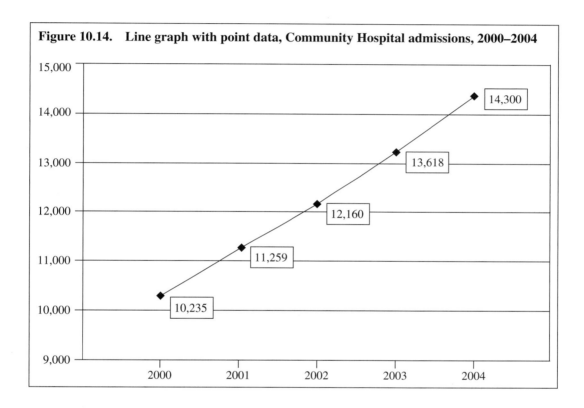

Figure 10.14. Line graph with point data, Community Hospital admissions, 2000–2004

Table 10.6. Sample five-year survival rates for kidney cancer by stage for patients diagnosed between 1996 and 2004

Year of Diagnosis	Midpoint of Interval	Survival Rate (%)		
		Localized	Regional	Distant
1996–1998	1997	80	71	28
1999–2001	2000	84	71	29
2002–2004	2003	85	74	31

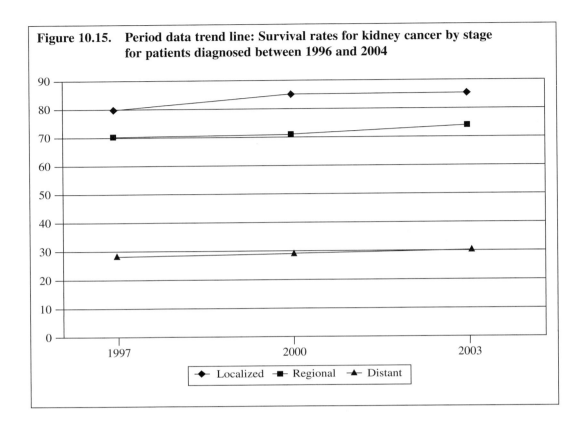

Figure 10.15.   Period data trend line: Survival rates for kidney cancer by stage for patients diagnosed between 1996 and 2004

Histograms

As mentioned earlier, a histogram is used to display a frequency distribution. It is different from a bar graph in that a bar graph is used to display data that fall into groups or categories. The categories are noncontinuous, or discrete. In a bar chart, the bars representing the different categories are separated. (See figures 10.10 and 10.11, pp. 446–47.) On the other hand, histograms are used to illustrate frequency distributions of continuous variables, such as age or LOS. A continuous variable can take on a fractional value (for example, 75.345° F). With continuous variables, there are no gaps between values because the values progress fractionally.

In a histogram, the frequency distribution may be displayed as a number or a percentage. The histogram consists of a series of bars. Each bar has one class interval as its base and the number (frequency) or percentage of cases in that class interval as its height. A class interval is a type of category. It can represent one value in a frequency distribution (for example, three years of age) or a group of values (for example, ages three to five).

In histograms, there are no spaces between the bars unless there are gaps in the data. (See figure 10.16.) The lack of spaces between bars depicts the continuous nature of the

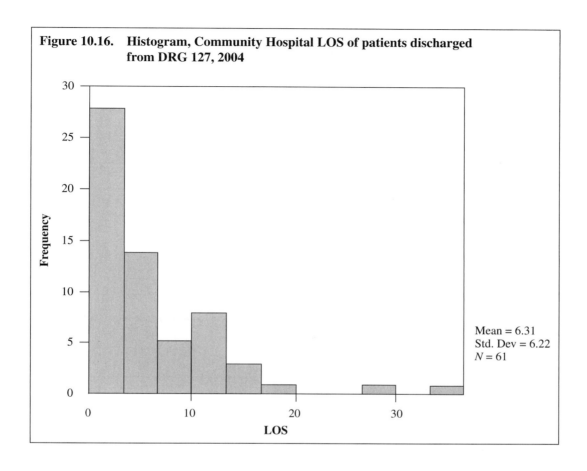

Figure 10.16.   Histogram, Community Hospital LOS of patients discharged
from DRG 127, 2004

Mean = 6.31
Std. Dev = 6.22
N = 61

distribution. The sum of the heights of the bars represents the total number, or 100 percent, of the cases. Histograms should be used when the distribution of the data needs to be
emphasized more than the values of the distribution.

Frequency Polygons
A **frequency polygon** is an alternative to a histogram. Like a histogram, it is a graph of a
frequency distribution, but in line form rather than bar form. The advantage to frequency
polygons is that several of them can be placed on the same graph to make comparisons.
Another advantage is that frequency polygons are easy to interpret.

When constructing a frequency polygon, the x-axis should be made longer than the
y-axis to avoid distorting the data. The frequency of observations is always placed on
the y-axis and the scale of the variable on the x-axis. The frequency polygon in figure
10.17 plots the same data that appear in the histogram in figure 10.16. Because the x-axis
represents the entire frequency distribution, the line starts at zero cases and ends with
zero cases.

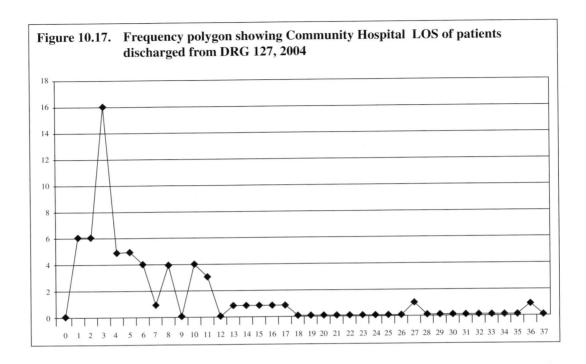

Figure 10.17.   Frequency polygon showing Community Hospital LOS of patients discharged from DRG 127, 2004

Check Your Understanding 10.3

Instructions: Match the correct word with its description.

1. _____ Data presented in rows and columns
2. _____ Graphic display technique used to display the contributions of the parts of a whole
3. _____ Graphic display technique used to show trends over time
4. _____ Graphic display technique used to display categories of a variable
5. _____ Graphic display technique that may be used to show the age distribution of a population

a.   Histogram
b.   Line graph
c.   Bar chart
d.   Table
e.   Pie chart

Hospital Statistics

Hospitals collect data about both inpatients and outpatients on a daily basis. They use these statistics to monitor the volume of patients treated daily, weekly, monthly, or within some other specified time frame. The statistics give healthcare decision makers the information they need to plan facilities and to monitor inpatient and outpatient revenue streams. For these reasons, health information management (HIM) professionals must be well versed in data collection and reporting methods.

Standard definitions have been developed to ensure that all healthcare providers collect and report data in a consistent manner. HIM professionals should be familiar with the following basic terms:

- *Hospital inpatient:* A person who is provided room, board, and continuous general nursing service in an area of the hospital where patients generally stay at least overnight.

- *Hospital newborn inpatient:* An infant born in the hospital at the beginning of the current inpatient hospitalization. **Newborns** are usually counted separately because their care is so different from that of other patients. Infants born on the way to the hospital or at home are considered hospital inpatients, not hospital newborn inpatients.

- *Inpatient hospitalization:* The period in a person's life when he or she is an inpatient in a single hospital without interruption except by possible intervening leaves of absence.

- *Inpatient admission:* The formal acceptance by a hospital of a patient who is to be provided with room, board, and continuous nursing services in an area of the hospital where patients generally stay overnight.

- *Inpatient discharge:* The termination of a period of inpatient hospitalization through the formal release of the inpatient by the hospital. The designation includes patients who are discharged alive (by physician order), who are discharged against medical advice, or who died while hospitalized. Unless otherwise indicated, inpatient discharges include deaths.

- *Hospital outpatient:* A hospital patient who receives services in one or more of the outpatient facilities when not currently an inpatient or home care patient. An outpatient may be classified as either an emergency outpatient or a clinic outpatient. An emergency outpatient is admitted to the hospital's emergency department for diagnosis and treatment of a condition that requires immediate medical, dental, or other type of emergency services. A clinic outpatient is admitted to a clinical service of the clinic or hospital for diagnosis and treatment on an ambulatory basis.

Inpatient Census Data

Even though much of the data collection process has been automated, an ongoing responsibility of the HIM professional is to verify the **census** data that are collected daily. The census reports patient activity for a twenty-four-hour reporting period. Included in the census report are the number of inpatients admitted and discharged for the previous twenty-four-hour period and the number of intrahospital transfers. An intrahospital transfer is a patient who is moved from one patient care unit (for example, the intensive care unit) to another (for example, the surgical unit). The usual twenty-four-hour reporting period begins at 12:01 a.m. and ends at 12:00 p.m. (midnight). In the census count, adults and children are reported separately from newborns.

Before compiling census data, however, it is important to understand the related terminology. The census refers to the number of hospital inpatients present at any one time. For example, the census in a 300-bed hospital may be 250 patients at 2:00 p.m. on May 1, but 245 an hour later. Because the census may change throughout the day as admissions and discharges occur, hospitals designate an official census-taking time. In most facilities, the official count takes place at midnight.

The result of the official count taken at midnight is the **daily inpatient census.** This refers to the number of inpatients present at the official census-taking time each day. Also included in the daily inpatient census are any patients who were admitted and discharged the same day. For example, if a patient was admitted to the cardiac care unit at 1:00 p.m. on May 1 and died at 4:00 p.m. on May 1, he would be counted as a patient who was both admitted and discharged the same day.

Because patients admitted and discharged the same day are not present at census-taking time, the hospital must account for them separately. If it did not, it would lose credit for the services it provided to these patients. The daily inpatient census reflects the total number of patients treated during the twenty-four-hour period. Figure 10.18 displays a sample daily inpatient census report.

A unit of measure that reflects the services received by one inpatient during a twenty-four-hour period is an **inpatient service day.** The number of inpatient service days for a twenty-four-hour period is equal to the daily inpatient census minus one service day for each patient treated. In figure 10.18, the total number of inpatient service days for May 2 is 230.

Inpatient service days are compiled daily, weekly, monthly, and annually. They reflect the volume of services provided by the healthcare facility. When the volume of services is greater, the healthcare facility receives greater revenue. Daily reporting of the number of inpatient service days is an indicator of the hospital's financial condition.

As mentioned earlier, the daily inpatient census is equal to the number of inpatient service days provided for a single day. The total number of inpatient service days for a week, a month, or some other period of time can be divided by the total number of days in the period to get the average daily inpatient census.

Figure 10.18. Sample daily inpatient census report, adults and children

May 2

Number of patients in hospital at midnight, May 1	230
+ Number of patients admitted May 2	+35
− Number of patients discharged, including deaths, May 2	−40
Number of patients in hospital at midnight, May 2	225
+ Number of patients both admitted and discharged, including deaths	+5
Daily inpatient census at midnight, May 2	230
Total inpatient service days, May 2	230

For example, a hospital might have a daily inpatient census of 240 for day one, 253 for day two, and 237 for day three. The total number of inpatient service days for the three-day period would be 730. When that total is divided by three days, the **average daily census** is 243.3. The average daily census is the average number of inpatients treated during a given period of time. The general formula for calculating the average daily census is:

$$\frac{\text{Total number of inpatient service days for a given period}}{\text{Total number of days in the same period}}$$

In calculating the average daily census, adults and children (A&C) are reported separately from newborns (NBs). This is because the intensity of services provided to A&C is greater than it is for NBs. To calculate the average daily census for A&C, the general formula is modified as follows:

$$\frac{\text{Total number of inpatient service days for A\&C for a given period}}{\text{Total number of days for the same period}}$$

The formula for the average daily census for NBs is:

$$\frac{\text{Total number of inpatient service days for NBs for a given period}}{\text{Total number of days for the same period}}$$

For example, the total number of inpatient service days provided to A&C for the week of May 1 is 1,729, and the total for NBs is 119. Using the preceding formulas, the average daily census is 247 (1,729/7) for A&C and 17 (119/7) for NBs. The average daily census for all hospital inpatients for the week of May 1 is 264 ([1,729 + 119]/7). Table 10.7 presents the various formulas for calculating the average daily census.

Table 10.7. Average daily census statistics

Indicator	Numerator (x)	Denominator (y)
Average daily inpatient census	Total number of inpatient service days for a given period	Total number of days for the same period
Average daily inpatient census for adults and children (A&C)	Total number of inpatient service days for A&C for a given period	Total number of days for the same period
Average daily inpatient census for newborns (NBs)	Total number of inpatient service days for NBs for a given period	Total number of days for the same period

---

Check Your Understanding 10.4

Instructions for questions 1 and 2: Using the information given, answer the following questions.

1. The inpatient census for Community Hospital at midnight on August 1 was 268, and the daily inpatient census for August 1 was 270. On August 2, sixteen patients were admitted, nine were discharged, and two were admitted and discharged on the same day. What were the following statistics for August 2?

    a. _____ Inpatient census

    b. _____ Daily inpatient census

    c. _____ Inpatient service days

    d. _____ Total inpatient service days for August 1 and 2

2. Nine patients were in the intensive care unit (ICU) at midnight on August 1. On August 2, two patients were admitted, two were admitted and then died, one was transferred from 3N to ICU, one was transferred from ICU to cardiology service, and one died after having been in ICU for several days. What were the statistics for the ICU on August 2?

    a. _____ Inpatient census

    b. _____ Daily inpatient census

Instructions for questions 3 through 5: Review the data in the table below and answer the questions that follow.

Summary Statistics for August
Urology, ENT, and Orthopedics Patient Care Units

	Urology	ENT	Orthopedics
Bed count	18	16	24
Census at midnight, July 31	15	12	20
Admissions	62	51	89
Live discharges	59	48	86
Deaths	1	0	1
Total inpatient service days	501	418	617

3. What is the census at midnight, August 31, for each clinical unit?

    a. _____ Urology

    b. _____ ENT

    c. _____ Orthopedics

4. _____ What is the total number of inpatient service days for all three units for the month of August?

5. What is the average daily census for each unit for the month of August?

    a. _____ Urology

    b. _____ ENT

    c. _____ Orthopedics

Inpatient Bed Occupancy Rate

Another indicator of the hospital's financial position is the **inpatient bed occupancy rate,** also called the **percentage of occupancy.** The inpatient bed occupancy rate is the percentage of official beds occupied by hospital inpatients for a given period of time. In general, the greater the occupancy rate, the greater the revenues to the hospital. For a bed to be included in the official count, it must be set up, staffed, equipped, and available for patient care. The total number of inpatient service days is used in the numerator because it is equal to the daily inpatient census or the number of patients treated daily.

The occupancy rate compares the number of patients treated over a given period of time to the total number of beds available for the same period of time. For example, if 200 patients occupied 280 beds on May 2, the inpatient bed occupancy rate would be 71.4 percent. If the rate were for two or more days, the number of beds would be multiplied by the number of days in that particular time frame. For example, if 1,729 inpatient service days were provided during the week of May 1, the number of beds (280) would be multiplied by the number of days (7), and the inpatient bed occupancy rate for that week would be 88.2 percent.

The denominator in this formula is actually the total possible number of inpatient service days. That is, if every available bed in the hospital were occupied every single day, this would be the maximum number of inpatient service days that could be provided. This is an important concept, especially when the official **bed count** changes for a given reporting period. For example, if the bed count changes from 280 beds to 300, the bed occupancy rate must reflect the change. The total number of inpatient beds times the total number of days in the period is called the total number of **bed count days.**

The general formula for the inpatient bed occupancy rate is:

$$\frac{\text{Total number of inpatient service days for a given period}}{\text{Total number of inpatient bed count days for the same period}} \times 100$$

For example, in May the total number of inpatient service days provided was 7,582. The bed count for the month of May changed from 280 beds to 300 on May 20. To calculate the inpatient bed occupancy rate for May, it is necessary to determine the total number of bed count days. May has thirty-one days, so the total number of bed count days is calculated as:

$$\text{Number of beds, May 1–May 19} = 280 \times 19 \text{ days} = 5,320 \text{ bed count days}$$

$$\text{Number of beds, May 20–May 31} = 300 \times 12 \text{ days} = 3,600 \text{ bed count days}$$

$$5,320 + 3,600 = 8,920 \text{ bed count days}$$

The inpatient bed occupancy rate for the month of May is 85 percent ([7,582/8,920] × 100).

As with the average daily census, the inpatient bed occupancy rate for adults and children is reported separately from that of newborns. To calculate the total number of bed count days for newborns, the official count for newborn bassinets is used. Table 10.8 reviews how to calculate inpatient bed occupancy rates.

It is possible for the inpatient bed occupancy to be greater than 100 percent. This occurs when the hospital faces an epidemic or disaster. In this type of situation, hospitals set up

Table 10.8.   Calculation of inpatient bed occupancy rates

Rate	Numerator	Denominator
Inpatient bed occupancy rate	Total number of inpatient service days for a given period × 100	Total number of inpatient bed count days for the same period
Inpatient bed occupancy rate for adults and children (A&C)	Total number of inpatient service days for A&C for a given period × 100	Total number of inpatient bed count days for A&C for the same period
Inpatient bed occupancy rate for newborns (NBs)	Total number of NB inpatient service days for a given period × 100	Total number of bassinet bed count days for the same period

temporary beds that are not normally included in the official bed count. As an example, Community Hospital experienced an excessive number of admissions in January because of an outbreak of influenza. In January, the official bed count was 150 beds. On January 5, the daily inpatient census was 156. Therefore, the inpatient bed occupancy rate for January 5 was 104 percent ([156 × 150]/100).

Check Your Understanding 10.5

Instructions: Using the information provided, answer the following questions.

1.   What are the inpatient bed occupancy ratios for the following patient care units for the month of August, given the statistics provided in the table?

Unit	Inpatient Service Days	Bed Count
Medical	2,850	100
Surgical	988	34
Pediatrics	422	15
Orthopedics	502	18
Obstetrics	544	20
Newborn	524	18

   a.   ____% Medical

   b.   ____% Surgical

   c.   ____% Pediatrics

   d.   ____% Orthopedics

   e.   ____% Obstetrics

   f.   ____% Newborn

   g.   ____% Total occupancy

2.   In 20xx, Community Hospital had 67,120 inpatient service days for adults and children and 4,850 inpatient service days for newborns. The bed count for adults and children was 220, and the bed count for newborn bassinets was 22.

   a.   ____   What was the average daily inpatient census for adults and children?

   b.   ____   What was the average daily inpatient census for newborns?

   c.   ____   What was the inpatient bed occupancy rate for adults and children?

   d.   ____   What was the inpatient bed occupancy rate for newborns?

Length of Stay Data

LOS is calculated for each patient after he or she is discharged from the hospital. It refers to the number of calendar days from the day of patient admission to the day of discharge. When the patient is admitted and discharged in the same month, the LOS is determined by subtracting the date of admission from the date of discharge. For example, the LOS for a patient admitted on May 12 and discharged on May 17 is five days (17 − 12 = 5).

When the patient is admitted in one month and discharged in another, the calculations must be adjusted. One way to calculate the LOS in this case is to subtract the date of admission from the total number of days in the month the patient was admitted and then to add the total number of hospitalized days for the month in which the patient was discharged. For example, the LOS for a patient admitted on May 28 and discharged on June 6 is nine days ([May 31 − May 28] + June 6).

When a patient is admitted and discharged on the same day, the LOS is one day. A partial day's stay is never reported as a fraction of a day. The LOS for a patient discharged the day after admission also is one day. Thus, the LOS for a patient who was admitted to the ICU on May 10 at 9:00 a.m. and died at 3:00 p.m. the same day is one day. Likewise, the LOS for a patient admitted on May 12 and discharged on May 13 is one day.

When the LOS for all patients discharged for a given period of time is summed, the result is the **total length of stay.** As an example, five patients were discharged from the pediatric unit on May 9. The LOS for each patient was as follows:

Patient	LOS
1	5
2	3
3	1
4	8
5	10
Total length of stay	27

In the preceding example, the total LOS is 27 days (5 + 3 + 1 + 8 + 10). The total LOS is also referred to as the number of days of care provided to patients discharged or died, or the discharge days.

The total LOS divided by the number of patients discharged is the average length of stay (ALOS). Using the data in the above example, the ALOS for the five patients discharged from the pediatric unit is 5.4 days (27/5). The general formula for calculating ALOS is:

$$\frac{\text{Total length of stay for a given period}}{\text{Total number of discharges, including deaths, for the same period}}$$

As with the other measures already discussed, the ALOS for adults and children is reported separately from the ALOS for newborns. Table 10.9 reviews the formulas for ALOS.

Figure 10.19 displays an example of a hospital statistical summary prepared by the HIM department on the basis of census and discharge data.

Table 10.9.   Calculation of LOS statistics

Indicator	Numerator	Denominator
Average LOS	Total length of stay (discharge days) for a given period	Total number of discharges, including deaths, for the same period
Average LOS for adults and children (A&C)	Total length of stay for A&C (discharge days) for a given period	Total number discharges, including deaths, for A&C for the same period
Average LOS for newborns (NBs)	Total length of stay for all NB discharges and deaths (discharge days) for a given period	Total number of NB discharges, including deaths, for the same period

Check Your Understanding 10.6

Instructions: Complete the following exercises using the statistics provided.

1. Use the statistics from the following table to calculate the total LOS and the ALOS for all patients discharged.

Number of Patients Discharged	Length of Stay
10	2
7	3
2	4
1	7
1	9
1	10
1	16

a. _____ Total LOS

b. _____ ALOS

2. Calculate the LOS for the following six patients discharged from the psychiatric unit at Community Hospital.

Patient	Admission Date	Discharge Date
Patient one	March 1	June 6
Patient two	February 28	March 31
Patient three	January 4	July 10
Patient four	April 16	May 16
Patient five	October 1	October 1
Patient six	October 1	October 2

a. _____ What is the LOS for patient one?

b. _____ What is the LOS for patient two?

c. _____ What is the LOS for patient three?

d. _____ What is the LOS for patient four?

e. _____ What is the LOS for patient five?

f. _____ What is the LOS for patient six?

g. _____ What is the total LOS for the entire group of patients?

h. _____ What is the ALOS for the entire group of patients?

Figure 10.19.   Statistical summary, Community Hospital for period ending July 20xx

Admissions	July 20xx		Year-to-Date	
	Actual	Budget	Actual	Budget
Medical	728	769	5,075	5,082
Surgical	578	583	3,964	3,964
OB/GYN	402	440	2,839	3,027
Psychiatry	113	99	818	711
Physical Medicine & Rehab	48	57	380	384
Other Adult	191	178	1,209	1,212
Total Adult	2,060	2,126	14,285	14,380
Newborn	294	312	2,143	2,195
Total Admissions	2,354	2,438	16,428	16,575

Average Length of Stay	July 20xx		Year-to-Date	
	Actual	Budget	Actual	Budget
Medical	6.1	6.4	6.0	6.1
Surgical	7.0	7.2	7.7	7.7
OB/GYN	2.9	3.2	3.5	3.1
Psychiatry	10.8	11.6	10.4	11.6
Physical Medicine & Rehab	27.5	23.0	28.1	24.3
Other Adult	3.6	3.9	4.0	4.1
Total Adult	6.3	6.4	6.7	6.5
Newborn	5.6	5.0	5.6	5.0
Total ALOS	6.2	6.3	6.5	6.3

Patient Days	July 20xx		Year-to-Date	
	Actual	Budget	Actual	Budget
Medical	4,436	4,915	30,654	30,762
Surgical	4,036	4,215	30,381	30,331
OB/GYN	1,170	1,417	10,051	9,442
Psychiatry	1,223	1,144	8,524	8,242
Physical Medicine & Rehab	1,318	1,310	10,672	9,338
Other Adult	688	699	4,858	4,921
Total Adult	12,871	13,700	95,140	93,036
Newborn	1,633	1,552	12,015	10,963
Total Patient Days	14,504	15,252	107,155	103,999

Other Key Statistics	July 20xx		Year-to-Date	
	Actual	Budget	Actual	Budget
Average Daily Census	485	482	498	486
Average Beds Available	677	660	677	660
Clinic Visits	21,621	18,975	144,271	136,513
Emergency Visits	3,822	3,688	26,262	25,604
Inpatient Surgery Patients	657	583	4,546	4,093
Outpatient Surgery Patients	603	554	4,457	3,987

Hospital Death (Mortality) Rates

The death rate is based on the number of patients discharged, alive and dead, from the facility. Deaths are considered discharges because they are the end point of a period of hospitalization. In contrast to the rates discussed in the preceding section, newborns (NBs) are not counted separately from adults and children (A&C).

Gross Death Rate

The **gross death rate** is the proportion of all hospital discharges that resulted in death. It is the basic indicator of mortality in a healthcare facility. The gross death rate is calculated by dividing the total number of deaths occurring in a given time period by the total number of discharges, including deaths, for the same time period. The formula for calculating the gross death rate is:

$$\frac{\text{Total number of inpatient deaths (including NBs) for a given period}}{\text{Total number of discharges, including A\&C and NB deaths, for the same period}} \times 100$$

For example, Community Hospital experienced twenty-one deaths (A&C and NB) during the month of May. There were 633 total discharges, including deaths. The gross death rate is 3.3 percent ([21/633] × 100).

Net Death Rate

The **net death rate** is an adjusted death rate. It is calculated in the belief that certain deaths should not "count against the hospital." It is an adjusted rate because patients who die within 48 hours of admission are not included in the net death rate. The reason for excluding them is that 48 hours is not enough time to positively affect patient outcome. In other words, the patient was not admitted to the hospital in a manner timely enough for treatment to have an effect on his or her outcome. However, in view of currently available technology, some people believe that the net death rate is no longer a meaningful indicator. The formula for calculating the net death rate is:

$$\frac{\substack{\text{Total number of inpatient deaths (including NBs)} \\ \text{minus deaths} < 48 \text{ hours for a given period}}}{\substack{\text{Total number of discharges (including A\&C and NB deaths)} \\ \text{minus deaths} < 48 \text{ hours for the same period}}} \times 100$$

Continuing with the preceding example, three of the twenty-one deaths at Community Hospital occurred within 48 hours of admission. Therefore, the net death rate is 2.9 percent ([18/630] × 100) The fact that the net death rate is less than the gross death rate is favorable to the hospital because lower death rates may be an indicator of better care.

Newborn Death Rate

Even though newborn deaths are included in the hospital's gross and net death rates, the newborn death rate can be calculated separately. Newborns include only infants born alive in the hospital. The newborn death rate is the number of newborns that died in comparison to the total number of newborns discharged, alive and dead. To qualify as a newborn death, the newborn must have been delivered alive. A stillborn infant is not included in either the newborn death rate or the gross or net death rates. The formula for calculating the newborn death rate is:

$$\frac{\text{Total number of NB deaths for a given period}}{\text{Total number of NB discharges (including deaths) for the same period}} \times 100$$

Fetal Death Rate

Stillborn deaths are called fetal deaths. A **fetal death** is a death that occurs prior to the fetus's complete expulsion or extraction from the mother in a hospital facility, regardless of the length of the pregnancy. Thus, stillborns are neither admitted nor discharged from the hospital. A fetal death occurs when the fetus fails to breathe or show any other evidence of life, such as beating of the heart, pulsation of the umbilical cord, or movement of the voluntary muscles.

Fetal deaths also are classified into categories based on the fetus's length of gestation or weight:

- *Early fetal death:* Less than 20 weeks' gestation or a weight of 500 grams or less

- *Intermediate fetal death:* At least 20 but less than 28 weeks' gestation or a weight of between 501 and 1,000 grams

- *Late fetal death:* 28 weeks' gestation or a weight of more than 1,000 grams

To calculate the **fetal death rate,** the total number of intermediate and late fetal deaths for the period should be divided by the total number of live births and intermediate and late fetal deaths for the same period. The formula for calculating the fetal death rate is:

$$\frac{\text{Total number of intermediate and late fetal deaths for a given period}}{\substack{\text{Total number of live births plus total number of intermediate and late fetal deaths} \\ \text{for the same period}}} \times 100$$

For example, during the month of May, Community Hospital experienced 269 live births and 13 intermediate and late fetal deaths. The fetal death rate is 4.6 percent ([13/282] $\times$ 100).

Maternal Death Rate (Hospital Inpatient)

Hospitals also calculate the **maternal death rate.** A maternal death is the death of any woman from any cause related to, or aggravated by, pregnancy or its management, regardless of the duration or site of the pregnancy. Maternal deaths resulting from accidental or incidental causes are not included in the maternal death rate.

Maternal deaths are classified as direct or indirect. A *direct maternal death* is the death of a woman resulting from obstetrical (OB) complications of the pregnancy, labor, or puerperium (the period lasting from birth until six weeks after delivery). Direct maternal deaths are included in the maternal death rate. An *indirect maternal death* is the death of a woman from a previously existing disease or a disease that developed during pregnancy, labor, or the puerperium that was not due to obstetric causes, although the physiologic effects of pregnancy were partially responsible for the death.

The maternal death rate may be an indicator of the availability of prenatal care in a community. The hospital also may use it to help identify conditions that could lead to a maternal death.

The formula for calculating the maternal death rate is:

$$\frac{\text{Total number of direct maternal deaths for a given period}}{\text{Total number of maternal discharges, including deaths, for the same period}} \times 100$$

For example, during the month of May, Community Hospital experienced 275 maternal discharges. Two of these patients died. The maternal death rate for May is 0.73 percent ([2/275] × 100). Table 10.10 summarizes hospital-based mortality rates.

Check Your Understanding 10.7

Instructions: Use the data provided on deaths and discharges at Community Hospital for the past calendar year to answer the following questions.

Total discharges, including deaths (A&C)	754
Total deaths (A&C)	14
Deaths < 48 hours (A&C)	6
Fetal deaths	3
Live births	140
Newborn deaths	3
Newborn deaths, including discharges	122
Maternal deaths (direct)	2
Obstetric discharges, including deaths	133

1. _____ What is the gross death rate for adults and children?

2. _____ What is the net death rate for adults and children?

3. _____ What is the fetal death rate?

4. _____ What is the newborn death rate?

5. _____ What is the gross death rate for adults and children and newborns combined?

6. _____ What is the maternal death rate (direct)?

Autopsy Rates

An autopsy is an examination of a dead body to determine the cause of death. Autopsies are very useful in the education of medical students and residents. In addition, they can alert family members to conditions or diseases for which they may be at risk.

Autopsies are of two types:

- *Hospital inpatient autopsy:* An examination of the body of a patient who died while being treated in the hospital. The patient's death marks the end of his or her stay in the hospital. A pathologist or some other physician on the medical staff who has been given responsibility performs this type of autopsy in the facility.

- *Hospital autopsy:* An examination of the body of an individual who at some time in the past had been a hospital patient but was not an inpatient at the time of

Table 10.10. Calculation of hospital-based mortality rates		
Rate	**Numerator (x)**	**Denominator (y)**
Gross death rate	Total number of inpatient deaths, including NBs, for a given period $\times$ 100	Total number of discharges, including A&C and NB deaths, for the same period
Net death rate (Institutional death rate)	Total number of inpatient deaths, including NBs, minus deaths <48 hours for a given period $\times$ 100	Total number of discharges, including A&C and NB deaths, minus deaths < 48 hours for the same period
Newborn death rate	Total number of NB deaths for a given period $\times$ 100	Total number of NB discharges, including deaths, for the same period
Fetal death rate	Total number of intermediate and late fetal deaths for a given period $\times$ 100	Total number of live births plus total number of intermediate and late fetal deaths for the same period
Maternal death rate	Total number of direct maternal deaths for a given period $\times$ 100	Total number of maternal (obstetric) discharges, including deaths, for the same period

death. A pathologist or some other physician on the medical staff who has been given responsibility performs this type of autopsy.

The following sections describe the different types of autopsy rates.

Gross Autopsy Rate

A **gross autopsy rate** is the proportion or percentage of deaths that are followed by the performance of autopsy. The formula for calculating the gross autopsy rate is:

$$\frac{\text{Total inpatient autopsies for a given period}}{\text{Total number of inpatient deaths for the same period}} \times 100$$

For example, during the month of May, Community Hospital experienced twenty-one deaths. Autopsies were performed on four of these patients. The gross autopsy rate is 19.0 percent ([4/21] $\times$ 100).

Net Autopsy Rate

The bodies of patients who have died are not always available for autopsy. For example, a coroner or medical examiner may claim a body for an autopsy for legal reasons. In these situations, the hospital calculates a **net autopsy rate.** In calculating the net autopsy rate, bodies that have been removed by the coroner or medical examiner are excluded from the denominator. The formula for calculating the net autopsy rate is:

$$\frac{\text{Total number of autopsies on inpatient deaths for a period}}{\text{Total number of inpatient deaths minus unautopsied coroners' or medical examiners' cases for the same period}} \times 100$$

Continuing with the example in the preceding section, the medical examiner claimed three of the four patients scheduled for autopsy. The numerator remains the same because four autopsies were performed. However, because three of the deaths were identified as medical examiner's cases and removed from the hospital, they are subtracted from the total of twenty-one deaths. Thus, the net autopsy rate is 22.2 percent ([4/18] × 100).

Hospital Autopsy Rate

A **hospital autopsy rate** is an adjusted rate that includes autopsies on anyone who once may have been a hospital patient. The formula for calculating the hospital autopsy rate is:

$$\frac{\text{Total number of hospital autopsies for a given period}}{\text{Total number of deaths of hospital patients whose bodies are available for hospital autopsy for the same period}} \times 100$$

The hospital autopsy rate can include either or both of the following:

- Inpatients who died in the hospital, except those removed by the coroner or medical examiner. When the hospital pathologist or another designated physician acts as an agent in the performance of an autopsy on an inpatient, the death and the autopsy are included in the percentage.

- Other hospital patients, including ambulatory care patients, hospital home care patients, and former hospital patients who died elsewhere, but whose bodies were made available for autopsy by the hospital pathologist or other designated physician. These autopsies and deaths are included when the percentage is computed.

Generally, it is impossible to determine the number of bodies of former hospital patients who may have died during a given time period. In the formula, the phrase "available for hospital autopsy" involves several conditions, including:

- The autopsy must be performed by the hospital pathologist or a designated physician on the body of a patient treated at some time in the hospital.

- The report of the autopsy must be filed in the patient's health record and with the hospital laboratory or pathology department.

- The tissue specimens must be maintained in the hospital laboratory.

Figure 10.20 explains how to calculate the hospital autopsy rate.

Newborn Autopsy Rate

Autopsy rates usually include autopsies performed on newborn infants unless a separate rate is requested. The formula for calculating the **newborn autopsy rate** is:

$$\frac{\text{Total number of autopsies on NB deaths for a given period}}{\text{Total number of NB deaths for the same period}} \times 100$$

Fetal Autopsy Rate

Hospitals also sometimes calculate the **fetal autopsy rate.** Fetal autopsies are performed on stillborn infants who have been classified as either intermediate or late fetal deaths. This is the proportion or percentage of autopsies done on intermediate or late fetal deaths out of the total number of intermediate or late fetal deaths. The formula for calculating the fetal autopsy rate is:

$$\frac{\text{Total number of autopsies on intermediate and late fetal deaths for a given period}}{\text{Total number of intermediate and late fetal deaths for the same period}} \times 100$$

Table 10.11 summarizes the different autopsy rates.

Figure 10.20.   Calculation of hospital autopsy rate

In June, 33 inpatient deaths occurred. Three of them were medical examiner's cases. Two of the bodies were removed from the hospital and so were not available for hospital autopsy. One of the medical examiner's cases was autopsied by the hospital pathologist. Fourteen other autopsies were performed on hospital inpatients who died during the month of June. In addition, autopsies were performed in the hospital on:

- A child with congenital heart disease who died in the emergency department

- A former hospital inpatient who died in an extended care facility and whose body was brought to the hospital for autopsy

- A former hospital inpatient who died at home and whose body was brought to the hospital for autopsy

- A hospital outpatient who died while receiving chemotherapy for cancer

- A hospital home care patient whose body was brought to the hospital for autopsy

- A former hospital inpatient who died in an emergency vehicle on the way to the hospital

Calculation of total hospital autopsies:

$$\begin{array}{rl} & 1 \text{ autopsy on medical examiner's case} \\ + & 14 \text{ autopsies on hospital inpatients} \\ + & 6 \text{ autopsies on hospital patients whose bodies were available for autopsy} \\ \hline & 21 \text{ autopsies performed by the hospital pathologist} \end{array}$$

Calculation of number of deaths of hospital patients whose bodies were available for autopsy:

$$\begin{array}{l} 33 \text{ inpatient deaths} \\ - 2 \text{ medical examiner's cases} \\ + 6 \text{ deaths of hospital patients} \\ \hline 37 \text{ bodies available for autopsy} \end{array}$$

Calculation of hospital autopsy rate:

$$\frac{\text{Total number of hospital autopsies for the period} \times 100}{\substack{\text{Total number of deaths of hospital patients with bodies available} \\ \text{for hospital autopsy for the period}}}$$

$$(21 \times 100)/37 = 56.8\%$$

Rate	Numerator	Denominator
Gross autopsy rate	Total number of autopsies on inpatient deaths for a given period × 100	Total number of inpatient deaths for the same period
Net autopsy rate	Total number of autopsies on inpatient deaths for a given period × 100	Total number of inpatient deaths minus unautopsied coroner or medical examiner cases for the same period
Hospital autopsy rate	Total number of autopsies on inpatient deaths for a given period × 100	Total number of deaths of hospital patients whose bodies are available for hospital autopsy for the same period
Newborn (NB) autopsy rate	Total number of autopsies on NB deaths for a given period × 100	Total number of NB deaths for the same period
Fetal autopsy rate	Total number of autopsies on intermediate and late fetal deaths for a given period × 100	Total number of intermediate and late fetal deaths for the same period

Table 10.11.   Calculation of hospital autopsy rates

Check Your Understanding 10.8

Instructions: Read the scenario below and answer the questions that follow.

In October, Community Hospital experienced forty-four deaths. Three of them were coroner's cases, and one was autopsied by the hospital pathologist. Twenty-one autopsies were performed on the remaining deaths.

1. _____ What is the gross autopsy rate for Community Hospital for the month of October?

2. _____ What is the net autopsy rate for Community Hospital for the month of October?

Hospital Infection Rates

The most common morbidity rates calculated for hospitals are related to **hospital-acquired infections,**. The hospital must monitor the number of infections that occur in its various patient care units continuously. Infection can adversely affect the course of a patient's treatment and possibly result in death. The Joint Commission on Accreditation of Healthcare Organizations (JCAHO) requires hospitals to follow written guidelines for reporting all types of infections. Examples of the different types of infections are respiratory, gastrointestinal, surgical wound, skin, urinary tract, septicemias, and infections related to intravascular catheters.

Hospital (nosocomial) infection rates may be calculated for the entire hospital or for a specific unit in the hospital. They also may be calculated for the specific types of infections. Ideally, the hospital should strive for an infection rate of 0.0 percent. The formula for calculating the nosocomial infection rate is:

$$\frac{\text{Total number of hospital infections for a given period}}{\text{Total number of discharges, including deaths, for the same period}} \times 100$$

For example, Community Hospital discharged 725 patients during the month of June. Thirty-two of these patients had hospital-acquired infections. The infection rate is 4.4 percent ([32/725] × 100).

Postoperative Infection Rate

Hospitals often track their postoperative infection rate. The **postoperative infection rate** is the proportion or percentage of infections in clean surgical cases out of the total number of surgical operations performed. A clean surgical case is one in which no infection existed prior to surgery. The postoperative infection rate may be an indicator of a problem in the hospital environment or of some type of surgical contamination.

The person calculating the postoperative infection rate must know the difference between a surgical procedure and a surgical operation. A *surgical procedure* is any separate, systematic process on or within the body that can be complete in itself. A physician, dentist, or some other licensed practitioner performs a surgical procedure, with or without instruments, for the following reasons:

- To restore disunited or deficient parts
- To remove diseased or injured tissues
- To extract foreign matter
- To assist in obstetrical delivery
- To aid in diagnosis

A *surgical operation* involves one or more surgical procedures performed on one patient at one time using one approach to achieve a common purpose. An example of a surgical operation is the resection of a portion of both the intestine and the liver in a cancer patient. This involves two procedures (removal of a portion of the liver and removal of a portion of the colon) but is considered only one operation because it involves only one approach or incision. In contrast, an esophagogastroduodenoscopy (EGD) and a colonoscopy performed at the same time would be an example of two procedures with two different approaches. In the former, the approach is the upper gastrointestinal tract; in the latter, the approach is the lower gastrointestinal tract. In this case, the two procedures do not have common approach or purpose.

The formula for calculating the postoperative infection rate is:

$$\frac{\text{Number of infections in clean surgical cases for a given period}}{\text{Total number of surgical operations for the same period}} \times 100$$

Consultation Rate

A consultation occurs when two or more physicians collaborate on a particular patient's diagnosis or treatment. The attending physician requests the consultation and explains his or her reason for doing so. The consultant then examines the patient and the health record and makes recommendations in a written report. The formula for calculating the consultation rate is:

$$\frac{\text{Total number of patients receiving consultations for a given period}}{\text{Total number of discharges and deaths for the same period}}$$

Check Your Understanding 10.9

Instructions: Use the appropriate formula to determine the rates requested below.

1. ____ Thirty patients were discharged from the Surgical Intensive Care Unit (SICU) during the week of July 1. Eight of these patients had a hospital-acquired infection. What is the hospital-acquired infection rate for the SICU for the week of July 1?

2. ____ During the month of April, 822 patients were discharged from Community Hospital. Of these, 122 patients had consults from specialty physicians. What is the consultation rate for the month of April?

National Vital Statistics System

The National Vital Statistics System (NVSS) is responsible for the official vital statistics of the United States. The term *vital statistics* refers to crucial events in life: births, deaths, marriages, divorces, fetal deaths, and induced terminations of pregnancy. Vital statistics are provided to the federal government by state-operated registration systems. NVSS is housed in the National Center for Health Statistics (NCHS) of the Centers for Disease Control (CDC).

To facilitate data collection, standard forms and model procedures for the uniform registration of events are developed and recommended for state use through cooperative activities of the individual states and NCHS. The standard certificates represent the minimum basic data set necessary for the collection and publication of comparable national, state, and local vital statistics data. The standard forms are revised about every ten years, and the last revision took place in 2003. To effectively implement these new certificates, NCHS is working with its state partners to improve the timeliness, quality, and sustainability of the vital statistics system, along with collection of the revised and new content of the 2003 certificates. These revisions can be viewed on line at cdc.gov.

The certificate of live birth is used for registration purposes and is composed of two parts. The first part contains information related to the child and parents; the second part is used to collect data on the mother's pregnancy. This part is used for the collection of aggregate data only. No identification information appears on this portion of the certificate, and it never appears on the "official" certificate of birth. Pregnancy-related information includes complications of pregnancy, concurrent illnesses or conditions affecting pregnancy, and abnormal conditions and/or congenital anomalies of the newborn. Information on lifestyle factors, such as alcohol and tobacco use, also is collected. Thus, the birth certificate is the major source of maternal and natality (birthrate) statistics. A listing of pregnancy-related information appears in figure 10.21.

A report of fetal death is completed when a pregnancy results in a stillbirth. This report contains information on the parents, the history of the pregnancy, and the cause of the fetal death. Information collected on the pregnancy is the same as that recorded on the birth certificate. To assess environmental exposures on the fetus, the parents' occupational data are collected. Data items related to the fetus include:

- The cause of fetal death (whether fetal or maternal)
- Other significant conditions of the fetus or mother
- When fetus died (before labor, during labor or delivery, or unknown)

Data collected from death certificates are used to compile causes of death in the United States. The certificate of death contains information on the decedent, place of death information, medical certification, and disposition information. Beginning in 1999, the United States implemented ICD-10 for the coding of causes of death. Examples of the content that appears in death certificates are shown in figure 10.22.

The report of induced termination of pregnancy records information on the place of the induced termination, the procedure, and the patient. Sample content of this report appears in figure 10.23.

Figure 10.21.   Content of U.S. certificate of live birth, 2003

Child's Information
Child's name
Time of birth
Sex
Date of birth
Facility (hospital) name (if not an institution, give
   street address)
City
County

Mother's Information
Current legal name
Date of birth
Mother's name prior to first marriage
Birthplace
Residence (state)
County
City
Street Number
Zip Code
Inside city limits?
Mother married?
If no, has paternity acknowledgment been signed
   in the hospital?'
Social Security number (SSN) requested for child?
Mother's SSN
Father's SSN
Education
Hispanic origin?
Race

Father
Current legal name
Date of birth
Birthplace
Education
Hispanic origin?
Race

Pregnancy History
Date of first prenatal care visit
Date of last prenatal care visit
Total number of prenatal visits for this pregnancy
Number of previous live births
Mother's height
Mother's pregnancy weight
Mother's weight at delivery
Did mother get WIC food for herself during this
   pregnancy?
Number of previous live births
Number of other pregnancy outcomes
Cigarette smoking before and during pregnancy
Principal source of payment for this delivery
Date of last live birth
Date of last other pregnancy outcome
Date last normal menses began
Risk factors in this pregnancy
Infections present and/or treated during this
   pregnancy
Obstetric procedures
Onset of labor
Characteristics of labor and delivery
Method of delivery
Maternal mortality

Newborn Information
Birthweight
Obstetric estimate of gestation
Apgar score (1 and 5 minutes)
Plurality
If not born first (born first, second, third, etc.)
Abnormal conditions of newborn
Congenital anomalies of the newborn
Was infant transferred within 24 hours of delivery?
Is infant living at time of report?
Is infant being breastfed at discharge?

Source: Department of Health and Human Services. National Center for Health Statistics. National Vital Statistics System. Available online from www.cdc.gov/nchs/nvss.htm.

Figure 10.22.   Content of U.S. certificate of death, 2003

Decedent Information
Name
Sex
Social Security number
Age
Date of birth
Birthplace
Residence (state)
County
City or town
Street and number
Zip code
Inside city limits?
Ever in U.S. armed forces?
Marital status at time of death
Surviving spouse's name (If wife, give name prior to first marriage)
Father's name
Mother's name (prior to first marriage)
Decedent's education
Hispanic origin?
Race
Informant's name
Relationship to decedent
Mailing address

Disposition Information
Method of disposition
Place of disposition (cemetery, crematory, other)
Location
Name and address of funeral facility

Place of Death Information
Place of death
  If hospital, indicate inpatient, emergency room/outpatient, dead on arrival
  If somewhere other than hospital, indicate hospice, nursing home/long-term care facility, decedent's home, other
Facility name
City, state, zip code
County

Medical Certification
Date pronounced dead
Time pronounced dead
Signature of person pronouncing death
Date signed
Actual or presumed date of death
Actual or presumed time of death
Was medical examiner contacted?
Immediate cause of death
  Due to _____
  Due to _____
  Due to _____
Other significant conditions contributing to death
Was an autopsy performed?
Were autopsy findings available to complete the cause of death?
Did tobacco use contribute to death?
If female, indicate pregnancy status
Manner of death
For deaths due to injury:
  Date of injury
  Time of injury
  Place of injury
  Injury at work?
  Location of injury
  Describe how injury occurred
  If transportation injury, specify if driver/operator, passenger, pedestrian, other

Source: Department of Health and Human Services. National Center for Health Statistics. National Vital Statistics System. Available online from www.cdc.gov/nchs/nvss.htm.

Figure 10.23. Content of U.S. standard report of induced termination of pregnancy, 1997

Place of Induced Termination
Facility name
Address (city, town, state, county)

Patient Information
Patient identification
Age at last birthday
Marital status
Date or pregnancy termination
Residence (city, town, state, county)
Inside city limits?

Zip code
Hispanic origin?
Race
Education
Date last normal menses began
Clinical estimate of gestation
Previous pregnancies
  Live births
  Other terminations
Type of termination procedure

Source: Department of Health and Human Services. National Center for Health Statistics. National Vital Statistics System. Available online from www.cdc.gov/nchs/nvss.htm.

A tool for monitoring and exploring the interrelationships between infant death and risk factors at birth is the linked birth and infant death data set. This is a service provided by NCHS. In this data set, the information from the death certificate is linked to the information in the birth certificate for each infant who dies in the United States, Puerto Rico, the Virgin Islands, and Guam. The purpose of the data set is to use the many additional variables available from the birth certificate to conduct a detailed analysis of infant mortality patterns. The files contain information from the birth certificate (such as age, race or Hispanic origin of the parents, birth weight, period of gestation, plurality, prenatal care usage, maternal education, live birth order, marital status, and maternal smoking) linked to information from the death certificate (such as age and death and underlying and multiple causes of death).

The birth, death, fetal death, and termination of pregnancy certificates provide vital information for use in medical research, epidemiological studies, and other public health programs. In addition, they are the source of data for compiling morbidity, birth, and mortality rates that describe the health of a given population at the local, state, and national levels. Because of their many uses, the data on these certificates must be complete and accurate.

Community-Based Birth and Infant Death (Mortality) Rates

Two community-based rates that are commonly used to describe a community's health are the crude birth rate and measures of infant mortality. The official international definition of a *live birth* is the delivery of a product or conception that shows any sign of life after complete removal from the mother. A sign of life may consist of a breath or cry, any spontaneous movement, a pulse or heartbeat, or pulsation of the umbilical cord. The crude birth rate is the number of live births divided by the population at risk. The formula for calculating the crude birth rate is:

$$\frac{\text{Number of live births for a given community for a specified time period}}{\text{Estimated population for the same community and the same time period}} \times 1{,}000$$

As the formula shows, community rates are calculated using the multiplier 1,000, 10,000, or 100,000. The purpose is to bring the rate to a whole number as discussed earlier in this chapter. The result of the formula would be stated as the number of live births per 1,000 population. As an example, in 1999, there were 7,532 live births in a community of 600,000. The crude birth rate is 12.6 per 1,000 population ([7,532/600,000] × 1,000).

Rates that describe infant mortality are based on age. Thus, the definitions for the various age groups must be strictly followed. The following subsections discuss the three infant mortality rates.

Neonatal Mortality Rate

The neonatal period is the period from birth up to, but not including, 28 days of age. In the formula, the numerator is the number of deaths under 28 days of age during a given time period and the denominator is the total number of live births during the same period. The neonatal mortality rate may be used as an indirect measure of the quality of prenatal care and/or the mother's prenatal behavior (for example, alcohol, drug, or tobacco use).

Postneonatal Mortality Rate

The postneonatal period is the time from 28 days of age up to, but not including, one year. In the formula, the numerator is the number of deaths among children from age 28 days up to, but not including, one year during a given time period. The denominator is the total number of live births minus the number of neonatal deaths during the same period. The postneonatal mortality rate is often used as an indicator of the quality of the infant's home or community environment.

Infant Mortality Rate

The infant mortality rate is a summary of the neonatal and postneonatal mortality rates. In the formula, the numerator is the number of deaths among children under one year of age and the denominator is the number of live births during the same period. The infant mortality rate is the most commonly used measure for comparing health status among nations. All the rates are expressed in terms of the number of deaths per 1,000. Table 10.12 summarizes the community-based birth and infant mortality rates.

Table 10.12.	Calculation of community-based birth and infant death (mortality) rates		
Measure	**Numerator (x)**	**Denominator (y)**	10^n
Crude birth rate	Number of live births for a given community for a specified time period	Estimated population for the same community and the same time period	1,000
Neonatal death rate	Number of deaths under 28 days during a given time period	Number of live births during the same time period	1,000
Postneonatal death rate	Number of deaths from 28 days up to, but not including, one year of age during a given time period	Number of live births during the same time period less neonatal deaths	1,000
Infant death rate	Number of deaths under one year of age during a given time frame	Number of live births during the same time period	1,000

Other Community-Based Death (Mortality) Rates

Other measures of mortality with which the HIM professional should be familiar include the **crude death rate,** the **cause-specific death rate,** the **proportionate mortality ratio,** the **case fatality rate,** and the **maternal mortality rate.** Table 10.13 summarizes these rates.

Crude Death Rate

The crude death rate is a measure of the actual or observed mortality in a given population. Crude death rates apply to a population without regard to characteristics (for example, age, race, or gender). They measure the proportion of the population that has died during a given period of time (usually one year) or the number of deaths in a community per 1,000 for a given period of time. The formula for calculating the crude death rate is:

$$\frac{\text{Total number of deaths for a population during a specified time period}}{\text{Estimated population for the same time period}} \times 10^n$$

Cause-Specific Death Rate

As its name indicates, the cause-specific death rate is the death rate due to a specified cause. It may be calculated for an entire population or for any age, gender, or race. In the formula, the numerator is the number of deaths due to a specified cause for a given time period and the denominator is the estimated population for the same time period.

Table 10.14 displays cause-specific death rates for men and women due to pneumonia for the year 1995. The cause-specific death rates for each age group are consistently higher for men than for women. This information could lead to an investigation of why men are more susceptible to death from pneumonia than women.

Table 10.13.   Other community-based death (mortality) rates

Rate	Numerator (x)	Denominator (y)	10^n
Crude death rate	Total number of deaths for a population during a specified time period	Estimated population for the same time period	1,000 or 10,000 or 100,000
Cause-specific death rate	Total number of deaths due to a specific cause during a specified time period	Estimated population for the same time period	100,000
Case fatality rate	Total number of deaths due to a specific disease during a specified time period	Total number of cases due to a specific disease during the same time period	100
Proportionate mortality ratio	Total number of deaths due to a specific cause during a specified time period	Total number of deaths from all causes during the same time period	NA
Maternal mortality rate	Total number of deaths due to a pregnancy-related conditions during a specified time frame	Total number of live births during the same time period	100,000

	Women			Men		
Age Group	**Population**	**Deaths**	**Rate/100,000**	**Population**	**Deaths**	**Rate/100,000**
45–54	19,971,971	702	3.51	19,256,395	1,009	5.71
55–64	13,160,005	1,117	8.49	12,155,918	1,587	13.06
65–74	10,020,545	2,918	29.12	8,301,935	3,732	44.95
75–84	7,585,929	9,383	123.69	4,996,556	9,294	148.44
85+	3,127,729	19,689	6229.50	1,320,580	10,502	795.26
Total	53,866,179	33,809	62.76	46,031,384	26,124	60.08

Table 10.14.   Cause-specific mortality rates, by sex, due to influenza and pneumonia (ICD-10 Codes J10–J18.9), age 45+, U.S., 2001

Source: Centers for Disease Control and Prevention. CDC Wonder Data Base. Available online from wonder.cdc.gov.

Case Fatality Rate

The case fatality rate measures the probability of death among the diagnosed cases of a disease (most often, acute illness). In the formula, the numerator is the number of deaths due to a specific disease that occurred during a specific time period and the denominator is the number of diagnosed cases during the same time period. The higher the case fatality rate, the more virulent the infection.

Proportionate Mortality Ratio

The proportionate mortality ratio (PMR) is a measure of mortality due to a specific cause for a specific time period. In the formula, the numerator is the number of deaths due to a specific disease for a specific time period and the denominator is the number of deaths from all causes for the same time period. Table 10.15 displays the PMRs for pneumonia in the United States in 1995.

Maternal Mortality Rate

The maternal mortality rate measures deaths associated with pregnancy for a community. It is calculated only for deaths related to the pregnancy. In the formula, the numerator is the number of deaths assigned to causes related to pregnancy during a specific time period for a given community and the denominator is the number of live births reported during the same time period for the same community. Because the maternal mortality rate tends to be very small, it is usually expressed as the number of deaths per 100,000 live births.

Check Your Understanding 10.10

Instructions: Review the mortality data in table 10.16 and answer the questions below.

1. ____ What is the AIDS crude death rate per 100,000 for men?
2. ____ What is the AIDS crude death rate per 100,000 for women?
3. ____ What is the AIDS crude death rate per 100,000 for the entire group?
4. ____ What is the AIDS crude death rate for men per 10,000 ages 35–44?
5. ____ What is the AIDS crude death rate for women per 10,000 ages 35-44?

Table 10.15.   Proportionate mortality ratios for influenza and pneumonia (ICD-10 Codes J10–J18.9), age 45+, U.S., 2001

Age Group	Influenza and Pneumonia Deaths	Total Deaths	PMR/100
0–4	411	32,675	1.26
5–9	46	3,093	1.49
10–14	46	4,002	1.15
15–19	66	13,555	0.49
20–24	115	18,697	0.62
25–34	339	41,683	0.81
35–44	983	91,674	1.07
45–54	1,801	168,065	1.07
55–64	2,704	244,139	1.11
65–74	6,650	430,960	1.54
75–84	18,677	701,929	2.66
85+	30,191	665,531	4.54

Source: Centers for Disease Control and Prevention. CDC Wonder Data Base. Available online from wonder.cdc.gov.

Table 10.16.   Deaths due to AIDS (ICD-10 Codes B20–B24) by age and sex United States, 2002

Age Group	Male	Total Population	Female	Total Population
< 20 Years	36	41,503,211	39	39,507,380
20–34 Years	1,263	30,552,917	716	29,589,019
35–44 Years	4,198	22,366,506	1,509	22,550,100
45–54 Years	3,485	19,676,321	989	20,407,616
55–64 Years	1,083	12,784,311	264	13,817,415
65–74 Years	323	8,301,005	78	9,973,210
75–84 Years	71	5,081,056	25	7,653,577
85+ Years	5	1,389,808	7	3,203,261
	10,464	141,655,135	3,627	146,701,578

Source: Centers for Disease Control and Prevention, CDC Wonder Data Base, wonder.cdc.gov.

Frequently Used Measures of Morbidity

Two measures commonly used to describe the presence of disease in a community or specific location (for example, a nursing home) are incidence and prevalence rates. Disease is defined as any illness, injury, or disability. Incidence and prevalence measures can be broken down by race, sex, age, or some other characteristic of a population.

Incidence Rate

An **incidence rate** is used to compare the frequency of disease in different populations. Populations are compared using rates instead of raw numbers because rates adjust for differences in population size. The incidence rate is the probability or risk of illness in a population over a period of time. The formula for calculating the incidence rate is:

$$\frac{\text{Total number of new cases of a specific disease during a given time period}}{\text{Total population at risk during the same time period}} \times 10^n$$

The denominator represents the population from which the case in the numerator arose, such as a nursing home, school, or organization. For 10^n, a value is selected so that the smallest rate calculated results in a whole number.

Prevalence Rate

The **prevalence rate** is the proportion of persons in a population who have a particular disease at a specific point in time or over a specified period of time. The formula for calculating the prevalence rate is:

$$\frac{\text{All new and preexisting cases of a specific disease during a given time period}}{\text{Total population during the same time period}} \times 10^n$$

The prevalence rate describes the magnitude of an epidemic. It can be an indicator of the medical resources needed in a community for the duration of the epidemic.

It is easy to confuse incidence and prevalence rates. The distinction is in the numerators of their formulas. The numerator in the formula for the incidence rate is the number of new cases occurring in a given time period. The numerator in the formula for the prevalence rate is *all* cases present during a given time period. In addition, the incidence rate includes only patients whose illness began during a specified time period. The prevalence rate includes all patients from a specified cause regardless of when the illness began. Moreover, the prevalence rate includes a patient until he or she recovers.

National Notifiable Diseases

In 1878, Congress authorized the U.S. Marine Hospital Service to collect morbidity reports on cholera, smallpox, plague, and yellow fever from U.S. consuls overseas. This information was used to implement quarantine measures to prevent the spread of these diseases to the United States. In 1879, Congress provided for the weekly collection and publication of reports of these diseases. In 1893, Congress expanded the scope to include weekly reporting from states and municipalities. To provide for more uniformity in data collection, Congress enacted a law in 1902 that directed the surgeon general to provide standard forms for the collection, compilation, and publication of reports at the national level. In 1912, the states and U.S. territories recommended that infectious disease be immediately reported by telegraph. By 1928, all states, the District of Columbia, Hawaii, and Puerto Rico were participating in the national reporting of twenty-nine specified diseases. In 1961, the CDC assumed responsibility for the collection and publication of data concerning nationally notifiable diseases.

A **notifiable disease** is one for which regular, frequent, and timely information on individual cases is considered necessary to prevent and control disease. The list of notifiable diseases varies over time and by state. The Council of State and Territorial Epidemiologists (CSTE) collaborates with the CDC to determine which diseases should be reported. State reporting to the CDC is voluntary, but all states generally report the internationally quarantinable diseases in accordance with the World Health Organization's International Health Regulations. Completeness of reporting varies by state and type of disease and may be influenced by any of the following factors:

- The type and severity of the illness
- Whether treatment in a healthcare facility was sought
- The diagnosis of an illness
- The availability of diagnostic services
- The disease-control measures in effect
- The public's awareness of the disease
- The resources, priorities, and interests of state and local public health officials

Information that is reported includes date, county, age, sex, race/ethnicity, and disease-specific epidemiologic information; personal identifiers are not included. A strict CSTE Data Release Policy regulates dissemination of the data. A list of nationally notifiable infectious diseases appears in figure 10.24. The list is updated annually.

National morbidity data are reported weekly. Public health managers and providers use the reports to rapidly identify disease epidemics and to understand patterns of disease occurrence. Case-specific information is included in the reports. Changes in age, sex, race/ethnicity, and geographic distributions can be monitored and investigated as necessary.

Check Your Understanding 10.11

Instructions: Complete the following exercises.

1. _____ Define incidence and prevalence.

2. Review the data in the table and answer the questions below:

Incidence of Cancer of the Breast, in Situ, 2001, State of Ohio

	White	Black	Total
Number of Cases	1,595	179	1,774
Total Population	5,035,239	720,544	5,755,783

Source: Center for Disease Control, National Center for Chronic Disease Prevention and Health Promotion. Cancer prevention and control. //apps.nccd.cdc.gov

    a. _____ What is the incidence rate for cancer of the breast, in situ, per 10,000 for white women? for black women?

    b. _____ What is the incidence rate, per 10,000, for the entire group for 2001 in the state of Ohio?

Figure 10.24.   Nationally notifiable infectious diseases, U.S., 2005

Acquired Immunodeficiency Syndrome (AIDS)
Anthrax
Arboviral neuroinvasive and non-neuroinvasive
   diseases
  California serogroup virus disease
  Eastern equine encephalitis virus disease
  Powassan virus disease
  St. Louis encephalitis virus disease
  West Nile virus disease
  Western equine encephalitis virus disease
Botulism
Brucellosis
Chancroid
Chlamydia trachomatis, genital
Cholera
Coccidioidomycosis
Cryptosporidiosis
Cyclosporiasis
Diphtheria
Ehrlichiosis
Enterohemorrhagic *Escherichia coli*
Giardiasis
Gonorrhea
Haemophilus influenzae, invasive disease
Hansen disease
Hantavirus pulmonary syndrome
Hemolytic uremic syndrome, post-diarrheal
Hepatitis, viral, acute
  Hepatitis A, acute
  Hepatitis B, acute
  Hepatitis B virus, perinatal infection
  Hepatitis C, acute
Hepatitis, viral, chronic
  Chronic Hepatitis B
  Hepatitis C Virus Infection (past or present)
HIV infection
Influenza-associated pediatric mortality
Legionellosis
Listeriosis
Lyme disease
Malaria
Measles
Meningococcal disease
Mumps

Pertussis
Plague
Poliomyelitis, paralytic
Psittacosis
Q fever
Rabies (animal and human)
Rocky Mountain spotted fever
Rubella
Rubella, congenital syndrome
Salmonellosis
Severe Acute Respiratory Syndrome– associated
   Coronavirus (SARS-CoV) disease
Shigellosis
Smallpox
Streptococcal disease, invasive, Group A
Streptococcal toxic-shock syndrome
Streptococcus pneumoniae, drug resistant, invasive
  disease
Streptococcus pneumoniae, invasive in children
  < 5 years
Syphilis
  Syphilis, primary
  Syphilis, secondary
  Syphilis, latent
  Syphilis, late latent
  Syphilis, latent unknown duration
  Neurosyphilis
  Syphilis, late, non-neurological
Syphilis, congenital
  Syphilitic stillbirth
Tetanus
Toxic-shock syndrome
Trichinellosis (Trichinosis)
Tuberculosis
Tularemia
Typhoid fever
Vancomycin–intermediate *Staphylococcus aureus*
  (VISA)
Vancomycin–resistant *Staphylococcus aureus*
  (VRSA)
Varicella (morbidity)
Varicella (deaths only)
Yellow fever

Source: Centers for Disease Control, Division of Public Health Surveillance and Informatics. Nationally Notifiable
Infectious Disease, United States, 2005. Available online from www.cdc.gov/epo/dphsi/infdis2005.htm.

External Sources of Healthcare Data

The HIM manager is often called on to compare organizational data with external data for benchmarking purposes. **Benchmarking** is the process of comparing an organization to a standard, a peer group, or another organization. For example, a hospital might want to compare its average length of stay with the ALOS for all hospitals nationwide. Many state and federal agencies maintain online databases that can provide comparative data. Indeed, several of the federal databases have links to the various states' departments of public health.

The following sections discuss three major sources of healthcare data: the Centers for Disease Control and Prevention, the National Center for Health Statistics, and the Agency for Healthcare Research and Quality.

Centers for Disease Control and Prevention

Located in Atlanta, the CDC is an agency of the Department of Health and Human Services (HHS). Its mission is to promote health and quality of life by preventing and controlling disease, injury, and disability.

The CDC includes many resources on its Web site that are useful to the HIM professional. One prominent feature is the CDC Wonder Data Sets. Some data sets that may prove useful include:

- *SEER (Cancer Surveillance, Epidemiology, and End Results):* SEER has counts and rates of new cases of cancer that can be sorted by a single variable. The user may seek cancer information by age, gender, race, year, state, county, or ICD-9-CM code. This data set is the responsibility of the Division of Cancer Prevention and Control, National Cancer Institute.

- *FARS (Fatal Accident Reporting):* FARS gathers data on traffic crashes that result in the loss of human life. The system was designed by the National Center for Statistics and Analysis (NCSA) to provide an overall measure of highway safety, to identify traffic safety problems, and to provide an objective basis for evaluating motor vehicle safety and highway safety programs.

- *DATA2010 . . . the Healthy People 2010 Database:* DATA2010 contains national baseline and monitoring data for each Healthy People 2010 objective. Users can browse tables and graphs of the twenty-eight health focus areas and leading health indicators. This data set is maintained by the National Center for Health Statistics, Office of Analysis, Epidemiology, and Health Promotion, Division of Health Promotion and Statistics.

- *Injury Mortality Data:* This interactive system contains the frequencies and rates of death due to injury by state, age, sex, and category of injury. It is maintained by the National Center for Injury Prevention and Control, CDC.

- *Leading Causes of Death:* This system can be queried to determine the number of injury-related deaths relative to the number of other leading causes of death in the United States or individual states. It is maintained by the National Center for Injury Prevention and Control, CDC.

- *Mortality:* This system contains counts and rates of death by age, race, gender, year, state, county of residence, and underlying cause of death (four-digit ICD-9-CM codes). The source of this data set is the Office of Analysis and Epidemiology, National Center for Health Statistics, CDC.

- *Natality:* This data set has counts of births in the United States. The data in this data set can be used in the creation of tables, graphs, and maps.

The CDC also has links to various state and local health departments. Its home page address is cdc.gov.

The National Center for Health Statistics

NCHS is part of the CDC. It is the federal government's principal vital and health statistics agency. Its mission is to provide statistical information that will guide actions and policies to improve the health of the American public. The agency houses data on vital events as well as on health status, lifestyle and exposure to unhealthy influences, the onset and diagnosis of illness and disability, and the use of healthcare services.

The National Vital Statistics System includes the following types of data:

- *Birth data:* This data set is a federally mandated national collection of births and other vital data. This information is collected in cooperation with the states.

- *Mortality data:* This is a federally mandated vital statistics collection system. Data are collected in cooperation with the states. Mortality data are a fundamental source of demographic, geographic, and cause-of-death information. The data are used to describe the characteristics of individuals dying in the United States, to determine life expectancy, and to compare mortality trends with other countries.

- *Linked births/infant deaths:* This data file contains linked birth and death data. The information from the death certificate is linked to the information for each infant under one year of age who dies in the United States, Puerto Rico, the Virgin Islands, and Guam. The linkage provides more information for the analysis of infant mortality patterns.

The National Health Care Survey contains a family of healthcare provider surveys. The survey obtains information about facilities that provide care, services rendered, and types of patients served. Data are collected directly from the facility and/or medical records rather than patients. Data are collected on hospitalizations, surgeries, and long-term stays. Policymakers, planners, researchers, and others use the information to monitor changes in the use of healthcare resources, to monitor specific diseases, and to examine the impact of new medical technologies. This family of surveys includes:

- *National Ambulatory Medical Care Survey (NAMCS):* The NAMCS was designed to meet the need for objective, reliable information about the provision and use of ambulatory services in the U.S. Findings are based on a sample of visits to non-federally employed office-based physicians who provide direct care to patients. Physicians in anesthesiology, pathology, and radiology are excluded from the survey. The survey has been conducted annually since 1989.

- *National Hospital Ambulatory Medical Care Survey (NHAMCS):* The NHAMCS was designed to collect data on the utilization and provision of ambulatory care services in hospital emergency and outpatient departments. Federal, military, and Veterans Administration hospitals are not included in the sample. Data are collected on demographic characteristics of patients, expected source of payment, patient complaints, physician diagnoses, diagnostic/screening services, procedures, medication therapy, disposition, types of healthcare professionals seen, causes of injury (where applicable), and certain characteristics of the hospital such as type of ownership. Data have been collected annually since 1992. The abstract used for data collection appears in figure 10.25.

- *National Hospital Discharge Survey (NHDS):* The NHDS has been conducted since 1965. It is a national probability survey of inpatients discharged from nonfederal, short-stay hospitals in the U.S. Only hospitals with an ALOS of less than 30 days are included. Data abstracted include elements on the patient's age, sex, race, ethnicity, marital status, and expected source of payment. Administrative data also are collected, including admission and discharge dates, and discharge status. Medical information on patient diagnoses and procedures is coded in ICD-9-CM.

- *National Survey of Ambulatory Surgery (NSAS):* The NSAS was initiated in 1994 and conducted through 1996. It is a national survey of surgical and nonsurgical procedures performed on an ambulatory (outpatient) basis. The procedures may take place in a hospital or freestanding center's general operating room, dedicated ambulatory surgery rooms, and other specialized rooms such as endoscopy units and cardiac catheterization labs. The data set includes diagnosis and procedure codes in ICD-9-CM.

- *National Home and Hospice Care Survey (NHHCS):* The NHHCS is a continuing series of surveys of home and hospice care agencies in the U.S. It includes all types of agencies regardless of Medicare certification or state license. Data are collected on referral and length of service, diagnoses, number of visits, patient charges, health status, reason for discharge, and types of services provided.

- *National Nursing Home Survey (NNHS):* The NNHS is a continuing survey of nursing homes and their residents and staff. Nursing home surveys were conducted in 1973–1974, 1977, 1985, 1995, 1997, and 1999. The database provides information from two perspectives: provider and recipient. Data on facilities include characteristics such as size, ownership, Medicare/Medicaid certification, occupancy rate, days of care provided, and expenses. For recipients, data are obtained on demographic characteristics, health status, and services received.

- *National Employer Health Insurance Survey (NEHIS):* The NEHIS was developed to produce estimates on employer-sponsored health insurance data in the U.S. This is the first federal survey designed to obtain information on all health plans offered to employees by their employer. Data were collected from approximately 39,000 employers, with nearly 47,000 health plans, in all 50 states and the District of Columbia.

The Web site address for the NCHS is cdc.gov/nchs.

Figure 10.25. NHAMCS-100 form used for data collection

Form Approved OMB No. 0920-0278 Exp. Date 05/31/2007 CDC 64.135

FORM **NHAMCS-100(ED)** (8-19-2004)

U.S. DEPARTMENT OF COMMERCE
Economics and Statistics Administration
U.S. CENSUS BUREAU
ACTING AS DATA COLLECTION AGENT FOR THE
U.S. Department of Health and Human Services
Centers for Disease Control and Prevention
National Center for Health Statistics

PATIENT RECORD NO.:

PATIENT'S NAME:

NATIONAL HOSPITAL AMBULATORY MEDICAL CARE SURVEY
2005 EMERGENCY DEPARTMENT PATIENT RECORD

Assurance of confidentiality –All information which would permit identification of an individual, a practice, or an establishment will be held confidential, will be used only by persons engaged in and for the purpose of the survey and will not be disclosed or released to other persons or used for any other purpose without consent of the individual or the establishment in accordance with section 308(d) of the Public Health Service Act (42 USC 242m).

NHAMCS-100(ED) (8-19-2004)

1. PATIENT INFORMATION

a. Date of visit Month / Day / Year 2 0 0

b. ZIP code

c. Date of birth Month / Day / Year

d. Time of day
(1) Arrival ☐ AM ☐ PM ☐ Military
(2) Time seen by physician ☐ AM ☐ PM ☐ Military
☐ Not seen by physician
(3) ED discharge ☐ AM ☐ PM ☐ Military
Mark (X) if ED discharge is more than 24 hours from arrival. ☐

e. Patient residence
1 ☐ Private residence
2 ☐ Nursing home
3 ☐ Other institution
4 ☐ Other residence
5 ☐ Homeless
6 ☐ Unknown

f. Mode of arrival – *Mark (X) one.*
1 ☐ Ambulance (air/ground)
2 ☐ Public service (nonambulance, e.g., police, social services)
3 ☐ Walk-in
4 ☐ Unknown

g. Sex
1 ☐ Female
2 ☐ Male

h. Ethnicity
1 ☐ Hispanic or Latino
2 ☐ Not Hispanic or Latino

i. Race – *Mark (X) one or more.*
1 ☐ White
2 ☐ Black/ African American
3 ☐ Asian
4 ☐ Native Hawaiian/ Other Pacific Islander
5 ☐ American Indian/ Alaska Native

j. Expected source(s) of payment for this visit – *Mark (X) all that apply.*
1 ☐ Private insurance
2 ☐ Medicare
3 ☐ Medicaid/SCHIP
4 ☐ Worker's compensation
5 ☐ Self-pay
6 ☐ No charge/Charity
7 ☐ Other
8 ☐ Unknown

2. TRIAGE

a. Initial vital signs
(1) Temperature ☐ °C ☐ °F
(2) Pulse ___ beats per minute
(3) Blood pressure ___ / ___
(4) Oriented X 3 1 ☐ Yes 2 ☐ No 3 ☐ Unknown

b. Immediacy with which patient should be seen
1 ☐ Immediate
2 ☐ 1-14 minutes
3 ☐ 15-60 minutes
4 ☐ >1 hour-2 hours
5 ☐ >2 hours-24 hours
6 ☐ No triage
7 ☐ Unknown

c. Presenting level of pain
1 ☐ None
2 ☐ Mild
3 ☐ Moderate
4 ☐ Severe
5 ☐ Unknown

3. PREVIOUS CARE

Has patient been:

a. Seen in this ED within the last 72 hours?
1 ☐ Yes
2 ☐ No
3 ☐ Unknown

b. Discharged from any hospital within the last 7 days?
1 ☐ Yes
2 ☐ No
3 ☐ Unknown

4. REASON FOR VISIT

a. Patient's complaint(s), symptom(s), or other reason(s) for this visit *Use patient's own words.*
(1) Most important:
(2) Other:
(3) Other:

b. Is this visit work related?
1 ☐ Yes
2 ☐ No
3 ☐ Unknown

5. INJURY/POISONING/ADVERSE EFFECT

a. Is this visit related to an injury, poisoning, or adverse effect of medical treatment?
1 ☐ Yes
2 ☐ No – *SKIP to item 6.*

b. Is this injury/ poisoning intentional?
1 ☐ Yes, self inflicted
2 ☐ Yes, assault
3 ☐ No, unintentional
4 ☐ Unknown

c. Cause of injury, poisoning, or adverse effect – *Describe the place and events that preceded the injury, poisoning, or adverse effect (e.g., allergy to penicillin, bee sting, pedestrian hit by car driven by drunk driver, spouse beaten with fists by spouse, heroin overdose, infected shunt, etc.).*

6. PHYSICIAN'S DIAGNOSIS FOR THIS VISIT

As specifically as possible, list diagnoses related to this visit including chronic conditions.
(1) Primary diagnosis:
(2) Other:
(3) Other:

7. DIAGNOSTIC/SCREENING SERVICES

*Mark (X) all **ordered** or **provided** at this visit.*
1 ☐ NONE

Blood tests:
2 ☐ CBC (complete blood count)
3 ☐ BUN/Creatinine
4 ☐ Cardiac enzymes
5 ☐ Electrolytes
6 ☐ Glucose
7 ☐ Liver function tests
8 ☐ Arterial blood gases
9 ☐ BAC (blood alcohol)
10 ☐ HIV serology
11 ☐ Other blood test

Other tests:
12 ☐ EKG/ECG
13 ☐ Cardiac monitor
14 ☐ Pulse oximetry
15 ☐ Pregnancy test
16 ☐ Urinalysis (UA)
17 ☐ Other test/service

Imaging:
18 ☐ X-ray
19 ☐ Ultrasound
20 ☐ MRI
21 ☐ CT scan
22 ☐ Other imaging

8. PROCEDURES

*Mark (X) all **provided** at this visit. Exclude medications.*
1 ☐ NONE
2 ☐ Bladder catheter
3 ☐ CPR
4 ☐ Endotracheal intubation
5 ☐ IV fluids
6 ☐ Nebulizer therapy
7 ☐ NG tube/gastric suction
8 ☐ OB/GYN care
9 ☐ Orthopedic care
10 ☐ Thrombolytic therapy
11 ☐ Wound care
12 ☐ Other

9. MEDICATIONS & IMMUNIZATIONS

List up to 8 drugs given at this visit or prescribed at ED discharge. Include Rx and OTC drugs, immunizations, and anesthetics.

☐ NONE

	Given in ED	Rx at discharge
(1)	1 ☐	2 ☐
(2)	1 ☐	2 ☐
(3)	1 ☐	2 ☐
(4)	1 ☐	2 ☐
(5)	1 ☐	2 ☐
(6)	1 ☐	2 ☐
(7)	1 ☐	2 ☐
(8)	1 ☐	2 ☐

10. PROVIDERS

Mark (X) all providers seen at this visit.
1 ☐ ED attending physician
2 ☐ ED resident/intern
3 ☐ On call attending physician/Fellow
4 ☐ RN/LPN
5 ☐ Nurse practitioner
6 ☐ Physician assistant
7 ☐ EMT
8 ☐ Other

11. VISIT DISPOSITION

Mark (X) all that apply.
1 ☐ No follow-up planned
2 ☐ Return if needed, PRN/ appointment
3 ☐ Return/Refer to physician/clinic for FU
4 ☐ Refer to social services
5 ☐ Left AMA
6 ☐ Left without being seen
7 ☐ DOA/died in ED
8 ☐ Transfer to different hospital - *Reason*
9 ☐ Admit to observation unit
10 ☐ **Admit to hospital**
11 ☐ Other

If "Admit to hospital" was marked, then please continue with Item 12 - HOSPITAL ADMISSION on the reverse side.

2005 ED

Figure 10.25. *(Continued)*

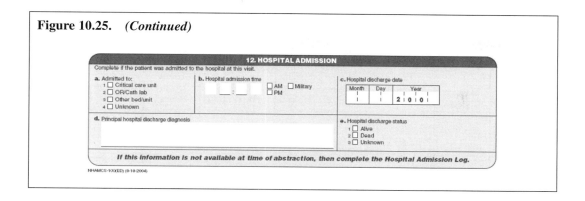

12. HOSPITAL ADMISSION

Complete if the patient was admitted to the hospital at this visit.

a. Admitted to:
1 ☐ Critical care unit
2 ☐ OR/Cath lab
3 ☐ Other bed/unit
4 ☐ Unknown

b. Hospital admission time
____ : ____   ☐ AM   ☐ Military
                        ☐ PM

c. Hospital discharge date

Month	Day	Year
		2 0 0 1

d. Principal hospital discharge diagnosis

e. Hospital discharge status
1 ☐ Alive
2 ☐ Dead
3 ☐ Unknown

If this information is not available at time of abstraction, then complete the Hospital Admission Log.

NHAMCS-100(ED) (9-18-2004)

Agency for Healthcare Research and Quality

The Agency for Healthcare Research and Quality (AHRC) is an agency of the HHS. It was created in 1989 as the Agency for Health Care Policy and Research and renamed in 1999. Its mission is as follows:

- To improve the outcomes and quality of healthcare

- To strengthen quality measurement and improvement

- To reduce the cost of healthcare

- To address patient safety and medical errors

- To broaden access to effective services

- To advance the use of information technology for coordinating patient care and conducting quality and outcomes research

This site can provide the most up-to-date information for professionals working in clinical quality improvement. Relevant topics include:

- Evidence-based practice

- Outcomes and effectiveness

- Technology assessment

- Preventive services

- Clinical practice guidelines

The Healthcare Cost and Utilization Project (HCUP), a database supported by AHRQ, can provide a wealth of information for benchmarking purposes. This interactive database allows researchers to identify, track, analyze, and compare hospital statistics at the regional, state, and national levels. Table 10.17 displays a sample report.

The Web site address for the AHRQ is ahrq.gov.

Table 10.17.   HCUP query: Outcomes by patient characteristics for DRG 416, Septicemia, age >17, 2002

Age Group	Total Number of Discharges	ALOS	Average Charges	Discharge Status						
				In-Hospital Deaths	Routine Discharge	Short Term Hospital	Other Institution	Home Health Care	Against Medical Advice	Missing Discharge Status
Total	299,479	7.3	$25,996	55,657 (18.6%)	107,531 (35.9%)	9,442 (3.2%)	93,435 (31.2%)	30,650 (10.2%)	1,658 (0.6%)	849 (0.3%)
18–44	26,210	6.9	$26,610	2,019 (7.7%)	15,731 (60.0%)	1,282 (4.9%)	3,341 (12.7%)	2,961 (11.3%)	802 (3.1%)	
45–64	63,372	7.4	$29,356	8,803 (13.9%)	31,905 (50.3%)	2,906 (4.6%)	11,898 (18.8%)	7,109 (11.2%)	571 (0.9%)	
65–84	148,087	7.5	$26,322	28,334 (19.1%)	48,879 (33.0%)	4,413 (3.0%)	50,139 (33.9%)	15,502 (10.5%)	220 (0.1%)	460 (0.3%)
85+	61,801	6.9	$21,556	16,501 (26.7%)	11,006 (17.8%)	841 (1.4%)	28,057 (45.4%)	5,078 (8.2%)	*	173 (0.3%)

Internal Use of Statistics and Patient Data for Research

The translation of data into information is part of daily life within healthcare organizations. Data are collected and reported to answer a variety of clinical and administrative research questions. Typical questions might be:

- What is the medical record delinquency rate?

- How many patients diagnosed with an acute myocardial infarction were given aspirin within one hour of arrival in the emergency department?

- How many newborns experienced a brachial plexus injury during delivery?

- What are the top 10 DRGs for inpatients discharged from our facility? How does this compare with national data?

- What is the infection rate on the Bone Marrow Transplant Unit?

- What proportion of hospital discharges are covered by Medicare?

- What is the ALOS for DRG 127, Heart Failure and Shock? How does this compare with the organization's peer group?

The list of research questions is endless. Many data queries are used to demonstrate compliance with JCAHO standards, to meet state licensure requirements, to evaluate performance of healthcare providers, and to improve organizational performance.

Check Your Understanding 10.12

Instructions: Find the appropriate information on the HCUP Web site and answer the following questions.

1. Go to the HCUPnet Web site at ahcpr.gov/hcupnet. Read the description of the information available at the Web site. Click the "new HCUPnet" link. Scroll down to "quick statistics," which contains data from the National Inpatient Sample (NIS). Click "2003" and then "overall statistics for hospital stays."

    a.   ____ What is the total number of inpatient discharges for 2003?

    b.   ____ What is the mean charge for 2003?

    c.   ____ What is the ALOS for 2003?

    d.   ____ What percentage of hospital inpatients died in 2003?

    e.   ____ What is the average age of hospital inpatients for 2003?

    f.   ____ What was the total national health bill for 2003?

Introduction to Institutional Review Boards

Healthcare organizations that conduct research on human subjects are required to have an **Institutional Review Board** (IRB). The IRB is a committee whose primary responsibility is to protect the rights and welfare of research subjects. Professionals who serve on IRBs have extensive education and experience in clinical research. Most of these individuals have medical and/or doctoral or other advanced degrees.

The IRB functions as a kind of ethics committee that focuses on what is right or wrong and what is undesirable. Because human subjects are involved, researchers are required to follow certain ethical principles that guide researcher behavior, morality, and character traits. Research ethics provide:

- A structure for analysis and decision making

- Support and reminders for researchers to protect human subjects

- Workable definitions of benefits and risks

Risk versus benefit is critical in weighing the advantages of biomedical research. A benefit may be specific to the individual subject or to others that may result from the research.

Risks are concerned with the probability or extent of harm to the research subject. Probability of harm may be stated as 1 in 100 patients may experience a certain risk. Extent of harm may be a statement that indicates minor problems such as itchiness as a result of the treatment, or it may be a major effect of treatment such as liver failure that may result in death.

In most cases, biomedical research requires that subjects be given informed consent. Informed consent is a person's voluntary agreement to participate in research or to undergo a diagnostic, therapeutic, or preventive procedure. It is based on adequate knowledge and an understanding of relevant information provided by the investigators. In giving informed consent, subjects do not waive any of their legal rights nor do they release the investigator, sponsor, or institution from liability for negligence. Federal regulations require that certain information be provided each human subject, including:

- A statement that the study involves research, the purpose of the research, the expected time frame of subject participation, a description of the procedures to be followed, and the identification of procedures that are experimental.

- A description of reasonably foreseeable risks or discomforts. The description must be accurate and reasonable, and subjects must be informed of previously reported adverse events.

- A description of the benefits to the subject or others who may reasonably benefit from the research.

- A disclosure of any appropriate alternative procedures or courses of treatment that might be available. When appropriate, a statement that supportive care with no additional disease-specific treatment is an alternative.

- A statement describing the extent to which confidentiality of records identifying the subject will be maintained. The statement should include full disclosure and description of approved agencies, such as the FDA, that may have access to the records.

- For research involving more than minimal risk, an explanation as to whether any compensation or medical treatments are available if injury occurs, and, if so, what they consist of or where further information may be obtained.

- An explanation of whom to contact for answers to pertinent questions about the research and whom to contact in the event of a research-related injury.

- A statement that participation is voluntary, that refusal to participate will involve no penalty or loss of benefits, and that the subject may discontinue participation at any time.

Federal regulations also require that informed consent be in a language that is understandable to the subject. The consent form must be translated into that language. Subjects who are not literate in their language must have an interpreter present to explain the study and to translate questions and answers between subject and investigator. A model consent form appears in figure 10.26.

Privacy Considerations in Clinical and Biomedical Research

In response to a congressional mandate in the Health Insurance Portability and Accountability Act (HIPAA), HHS issued regulations entitled Standards for Privacy of Individually Identifiable Health Information. Known as the Privacy Rule, it protects medical records and other individually identifiable health information from being used or disclosed in any form. The rule became effective on April 14, 2001, and organizations covered (covered entities) by the rule were expected to be in compliance by April 14, 2003. HIPAA privacy standards are discussed in detail in chapter 15.

Figure 10.26.   Template for informed consent for research involving human subjects

Consent to Investigational Treatment or Procedure

I, _____ , hereby authorize or direct _____ or associates of his/her choosing to perform the following treatment or procedure (describe in general terms), upon _____ (myself).

The experimental (research) portion of the treatment or procedure is:

1. Purpose of the procedure or treatment

2. Possible appropriate alternative procedure or treatment (not to participate in the study is always an option)

3. Discomforts and risks reasonably to be expected

4. Possible benefits for subjects/society

5. Anticipated duration of subject's participation (including number of visits)

I hereby acknowledge that _____ has provided information about the procedure described above, about my rights as a subject, and he/she answered all questions to my satisfaction. I understand that I may contact him/her at phone number _____ should I have additional questions. He/she has explained the risks described above, and I understand them; he/she has also offered to explain all possible risks or complications.

I understand that, where appropriate, the U.S. Food and Drug Administration may inspect records pertaining to this study. I understand further that records obtained during my participation in this study that may contain my name or other personal identifiers may be made available to the sponsor of this study. Beyond this, I understand that my participation will remain confidential.

I understand that I am free to withdraw my consent and participation in this project at any time after notifying the project director without prejudicing future care. No guarantee has been given to me concerning this treatment or procedure.

I understand that in signing this form, beyond giving consent, I am not waiving any legal rights that I might have and I am not releasing the investigator, the sponsor, or institution or its agents from any legal liability for damages that they might otherwise have.

In the event of injury resulting from participation in this study, I also understand that immediate medical treatment is available at _____ and that the costs of such treatment will be at my expense; financial compensation beyond that required by law is not available. Questions about this should be directed to the Office of Research Risks _____.

I have read and fully understand the consent form. I sign it freely and voluntarily. A copy has been given to me.

The Privacy Rule establishes a category of protected health information (PHI), which may be used or disclosed only in certain circumstances or under certain conditions. PHI is a subset of what is called individually identifiable health information. It includes what healthcare professionals typically regard as a patient's PHI, such as information in the patient's medial records as well as billing information for services rendered. PHI also includes identifiable health information about subjects of clinical research. Patient information considered "protected" is listed in figure 10.27.

The Privacy Rule defines the means by which human research subjects are informed of how their personal medical information will be used or disclosed. It also outlines their rights to access the information. Further, it protects the privacy of individually identifiable information while ensuring that researchers continue to have access to the medical information they need to conduct their research. Investigators are permitted to use and disclose PHI for research with individual authorization or without individual authorization under limited circumstances.

A valid Privacy Rule authorization is an individual's signed permission allowing a covered entity to use or disclose the patient's PHI for the purpose(s) and to the recipient(s) stated in the authorization. When an authorization is obtained for biomedical research purposes, the Privacy Rule requires that it pertain only to a specific research study, not to future unspecified projects. The core elements of the Privacy Rule authorization are:

- A description of the PHI to be used or disclosed, identifying the information in a specific and meaningful manner

- The names or other specific identification of the person or persons authorized to make the requested use or disclosure

- The names or other specific identification of the person or persons to whom the covered entity may make the requested use or disclosure

- A description of each purpose of the requested use or disclosure

- An authorization expiration date or expiration event that relates to the individual or to the purpose of the use or disclosure

- The signature of the individual and the date (If the individual's legally authorized representative signs the authorization, a description of his or her authority to act for the individual also must be provided.)

In addition, the authorization must include statements indicating:

- That the individual has the right to revoke the authorization at any time and must be provided with the procedure for doing so

- Whether treatment, payment, enrollment, or eligibility of benefits can be contingent upon authorization, including research-related treatment and consequences of refusing to sign the authorization, if applicable

- Any potential risk that the PHI will be redisclosed by the recipient and no longer protected by the Privacy Rule

Figure 10.27.   Examples of protected health information

The Privacy Rule allows covered entities to de-identify data by removing the following 18 elements that may be used to identify the individual or the individual's relatives, employers, or household members.

1. Names

2. All geographic subdivisions smaller than a state, including street address, city, county, precinct, ZIP code, except for the initial three digits of a ZIP code if, according to the current publicly available data from the Bureau of the Census:

    a. The geographic unit formed by combining all ZIP codes with the same three initial digits contains more than 20,000 people.

    b. The initial three digits of a ZIP code for all such geographic units containing 20,000 or fewer people are changed to 000.

3. All elements of dates (except year) for dates directly related to an individual, including birth date, admission date, discharge date, date of death; and all ages over 89 and all elements of dates (including year) indicative of such age, except that such ages and elements may be aggregated into a single category of age 90 or older

4. Telephone numbers

5. Facsimile numbers

6. Electronic mail addresses

7. Social Security numbers

8. Medical record numbers

9. Health plan beneficiary numbers

10. Account numbers

11. Certificate/license numbers

12. Vehicle identifiers and serial numbers, including license plate numbers

13. Device identifiers and serial numbers

14. Web universal resource locators (URLs)

15. Internet protocol (IP) address numbers

16. Biometric identifiers, including fingerprints and voiceprints

17. Full-face photographic images and any comparable images

18. Any other unique identifying number, characteristic, or code, unless permitted by the Privacy Rule for re-identification

Finally, the authorization must be written in plain language and a copy provided to the individual. A model HIPAA consent appears in figure 10.28; optional elements that may be included in the HIPAA consent are listed in figure 10.29.

Check Your Understanding 10.13

Instructions: Indicate whether the following statements are true or false (T or F).

1. ____ In signing an informed consent, a subject releases the research sponsor from any liability or negligence.

2. ____ Medical records of subjects in a research study may be released without patient authorization.

3. ____ A subject may withdraw from a research study at any time.

4. ____ Individuals who participate in clinical trials and biomedical research must sign the HIPAA consent form.

5. ____ A patient's medical record number is considered protected health information.

Figure 10.28.   Model HIPAA consent: Required elements

**Authorization to Use or Disclose (Release) Health Information
That Identifies You for a Research Study**

If you sign this document, you give permission to ___(name of healthcare providers)___ at

___(name of covered entity)___ to use or disclose (release) your health information that identifies

you for the research study described here:

(provide a description of the research study, such as title and purpose)

The health information that we may use or disclose (release) for this research includes:

The health information listed above may be used by and/or disclosed (released) to:

___(Name of covered entity)___ is required by law to protect your health information. By signing this

document, you authorize ___(name of covered entity)___ to use and/or disclose (release) your information for this research. Those persons who receive your health information may not be required by federal privacy laws (such as the Privacy Rule) to protect it and may share your information with others without your permission, if permitted by laws governing them.

Please note that (include the appropriate statement):

• You do not have to sign this Authorization, but if you do not, you may not receive research-related treatment

   (When the research involves treatment and is conducted by the covered entity or when the covered entity provides healthcare solely for the purpose of creating protected health information to disclose to a researcher)

• (Name of covered entity) may not condition (withhold or refuse) treating you on whether you sign this authorization.

   (When the research does not involve research-related treatment by the covered entity or when the covered entity is not providing healthcare solely for the purpose of creating protected health information to disclose to a researcher)

Please note that (include the appropriate statement):

• You may change your mind and revoke (take back) this authorization at any time, except to the extent that (name of covered entity) has already acted based on this authorization. To revoke this authorization, you mist write to (name of covered entity and contact information).

   (Where the research study is conducted by an entity other than the covered entity)

• You may change your mind and revoke (take back) this authorization at any time. Even if you revoke this authorization, (name of persons at the covered entity involved in the research) may still use or disclose health information they already have obtained about you as necessary to maintain the integrity or reliability of the current research. To revoke this authorization, you mist write to (name of covered entity and contact information).

This authorization does not have an expiration date.

Figure 10.29.   Model HIPAA consent: Optional elements

**Authorization to Use or Disclose (Release) Health Information
That Identifies You for a Research Study**

- Your health information will be used or disclosed when required by law.

- Your health information may be shared with a public health authority that is authorized by law to collect or receive such information for the purpose of preventing or controlling disease, injury, or disability, and conducting public health surveillance, investigations, or interventions.

- No publication or public presentation about the research described above will reveal your identity without another authorization from you.

- All information that does or can identify you is removed from your health information; the remaining information will no longer be subject to this authorization and may be used or disclosed for other purposes.

- **When the research for which the use or disclosure is made involves treatment and is conducted by a covered entity:** To maintain the integrity of this research study, you generally will not have access to your personal health information related to this research until the study is complete. At the conclusion of the research and at your request, you generally will have access to your health information that (name of covered entity) maintains in a designated record set that includes medical information or billing records used in whole or in part by your doctors or other healthcare providers at (name of covered entity) to make decisions about individuals. Access to your health information in a designated record set is described in the Notice of Privacy Practices provided to you by (name of covered entity). If it is necessary for your care, your health information will be provided to you or your physician.

- If you revoke this authorization, you may no longer be allowed to participate in the research described in this authorization.

Real-World Case

A community hospital's quality improvement committee wants to study cases of kidney and urinary tract infection among patients older than seventeen who experienced complications or had comorbidities. The committee is concerned about the wide variation in lengths of stay and total charges for this group of cases. To study the cases, the committee has asked you to prepare a profile of patients discharged from DRG 320 during the past twelve months. You create a summary report based on information from the hospital's online database. This summary appears in table 10.18.

Summary

Rates, ratios, and proportions and statistics are commonly used to describe community and hospital populations. These computations are considered descriptive statistics because they portray the characteristics of a group or population. Public health officials use community-based rates, ratios, and proportions to evaluate the general health status of a community. Morbidity and morality rates are used as an indicator of access and availability of healthcare services in a community.

Table 10.18.   Community Hospital, discharges DRG 320

Case	Principal DX	Principal Procedure	Age	LOS	Discharge Destination	Charges	Payor
1	599.0	38.93	53.5	4	HOMEIV	$8,851	MEDICAID
2	599.0	45.13	28.2	7	HOMEHEALTH	$18,966	MEDICARE
3	590.8		45.5	3	HOME	$4,370	MANAGED CARE
4	590.8	86.27	27.9	3	HOMEHEALTH	$7,121	GOV MNGD CARE
5	590.8		38.8	3	HOME	$13,350	MEDICAID
6	590.8	45.23	67.1	4	HOME	$15,854	MANAGED CARE
7	599.0	39.95	88.5	6	SNF	$22,373	MEDICARE
8	599.0		27.8	6	HOMEHEALTH	$11,381	GOV MNGD CARE
9	590.1		52.6	2	HOME	$4,082	MEDICAID
10	599.0		81.9	6	HOMEHEALTH	$17,025	MEDICARE
11	590.8		23.3	3	HOME	$5,039	MEDICAID
12	599.0	43.11	90.1	5	HOMEHEALTH	$17,411	MEDICARE
13	599.0	99.6	91.3	1	UNKNOWN	$5,302	MEDICARE
14	599.0	88.72	73.1	4	HOME	$11,091	MEDICARE
15	599.0		81.3	12	SNF	$23,341	MEDICARE
16	590.8	45.16	74.7	4	HOMEHEALTH	$16,277	MEDICARE
17	599.0		71.2	5	HOMEHEALTH	$9,239	MEDICARE
18	599.0		79.3	7	SNF	$21,050	MEDICARE
19	590.1		31.3	4	HOME	$7,085	GOV MNGD CARE
20	590.8	38.93	74.1	13	ACUTECARE	$49,487	MEDICAID
21	599.0		65.7	2	HOMEHEALTH	$8,980	MEDICARE
22	599.0	86.27	83.1	5	SNF	$11,651	MEDICARE
23	599.0		77.0	5	SNF	$12,295	MEDICARE
24	599.0	99.04	81.2	7	HOMEHEALTH	$23,745	MEDICARE
25	599.0		43.3	10	HOMEHEALTH	$25,130	MEDICARE
26	599.0		81.5	3	SNF	$10,092	MEDICARE
27	599.0	38.93	25.6	3	HOMEIV	$8,722	MEDICAID
28	599.0		61.4	2	SNF	$6,670	MEDICAID
29	599.0	45.13	76.0	8	SNF	$17,741	GOV MNGD CARE
30	590.1		44.4	4	HOME	$10,800	MANAGED CARE
31	590.8		44.8	2	HOME	$10,916	MEDICAID
32	599.0	45.13	61.2	8	SNF	$32,796	MEDICARE

Hospital-based rates are used for a variety of purposes. First, they describe the general characteristics of the patients treated at the facility. Hospital administrators use the data to monitor the volume of patients treated monthly, weekly, or within some other specified time frame. The statistics give healthcare decision makers the information they need to plan facilities and monitor inpatient and outpatient revenue streams.

Data may be presented using a variety of graphic techniques, including charts, graphs, and/or tables. Graphic forms help to summarize and clarify data for the user and are effective ways of presenting large quantities of information.

The health information management (HIM) professional is in a position to serve as a data broker for the healthcare organization. To do this, he or she must fully understand the clinical data that are collected and their application to the decision-making process. In addition, the HIM professional must know what information is needed and how to provide it in a timely manner. With this knowledge, the HIM professional can become an invaluable member of the healthcare team.

References

Agency for Health Care Policy and Research. 2005. *HCUPnet, Healthcare Cost and Utilization Project.* Rockville, MD: AHCPR. Available online from ahcpr.gov/data/hcup/hcupnet.htm.

Agency for Healthcare Research and Quality. 2000. *AHRQ Profile: Quality Research for Quality Healthcare* (AHRQ Publication No. 00-P005). Rockville, MD: AHRQ. Available online from ahrq.gov/about/provile.htm.

Amdur, R.J. 2003 *The Institutional Review Board Member Handbook.* Boston: Jones and Bartlett Publishers.

Centers for Disease Control and Prevention. CDC Wonder Data Base. Available online from wonder.cdc.gov.

Department of Health and Human Services. 2004. *Clinical Research and the HIPAA Privacy Rule.* NIH Publication Number 04-5495. Washington, DC: HHS.

Department of Health and Human Services. 2004. *HIPAA Authorization for Research.* NIH Publication Number 04-5529. Washington, DC: HHS.

Department of Health and Human Services. 2003. *Protecting Personal Health Information in Research: HIPAA Privacy Rule.* NIH Publication Number 03-5388. Washington, DC: HHS.

Horton, L. 2004. *Calculating and Reporting Healthcare Statistics.* Chicago: American Health Information Management Association.

National Center for Health Statistics. Centers for Disease Control and Prevention. 2000. *Specifications for Collecting and Editing the United States Standard Certificates of Birth and Death, 2003 Revision.* Available online from cdc.gov/nchs.

Osborn, C.E. 2005. *Statistical Applications for Health Information Management.* Boston: Jones and Bartlett Publishers.

Chapter 11
Clinical Quality Management

Susan B. Willner, RHIA

Learning Objectives

- To understand the concept of quality and its importance in healthcare

- To be aware of the increased importance of patient safety and new national patient safety goals to high-quality healthcare and clinical quality management

- To define the terms *clinical quality assessment, infection control, utilization management, case management,* and *risk management* and to differentiate among them

- To recognize the elements of a quality assessment (QA) program

- To identify the major organizations that publish clinical quality standards and guidelines

- To identify and discuss the government regulations and accreditation standards related to clinical quality management

- To explain the various ways that healthcare organizations manage the prevention and occurrence of infections

- To understand the Medicare requirements for utilization management (UM)

- To describe the organization of a hospital UM program

- To list the basic procedures in the utilization review (UR) process

- To understand the clinical and administrative use of UM information

- To identify the utilization-related activities conducted by quality improvement organizations

- To understand the use of severity-of-illness/intensity-of-service screening criteria

- To define the key elements of a risk management plan

- To identify recent national initiatives designed to manage and improve the quality and safety of patient care

Key Terms

Accreditation standards

Admission utilization review

Agency for Healthcare Research and Quality (AHRQ)

American Association of Health Plans (AAHP)

American Society for Healthcare Risk Management (ASHRM)

Case management

Claims management

Clinical pathway

Clinical practice guideline

Clinical protocol

Clinical quality assessment

Community-acquired infection

Computerized physician order entry or computerized provider order entry (CPOE)

Concurrent utilization review

Continued-stay utilization review

Corporate negligence

Critical pathway

Discharge abstract system

Discharge utilization review

Discovery process

Facilities management

Health Care Quality Improvement Program (HCQIP)

Health Plan Employer Data and Information Set (HEDIS)

Incident report

Infection control

Institute of Medicine (IOM)

Intensity-of-service screening criteria

Liability

National Guideline Clearinghouse (NGC)

National patient safety goals (NPSGs)

Occurrence screening

Office of the National Coordinator for Health Information Technology (ONC)

Outcome measure

Patient advocacy

Patient safety

Potentially compensable event

Preadmission utilization review

Professional standards review organization (PSRO)

Prospective utilization review

Quality

Quality indicator

Retrospective utilization review

Risk management

Safety management

Security management

Sentinel event

Severity-of-illness screening criteria

Tracer methodology

Universal precautions

Utilization management (UM)

Utilization review (UR)

Introduction

Within the context of healthcare services, the word *quality* is difficult to define because no single definition can adequately describe all its characteristics. Healthcare quality has a number of dimensions, each meaning something different to the people involved in providing and receiving healthcare products and services.

Quality must be considered in light of the healthcare organization's different customers. For example, when the customer is a patient, quality is tied to the end result of treatment, the personal consideration received from caregivers, and the respect demonstrated for patient privacy, confidentiality, and security. When the customer is a physician, quality means that the facility has state-of-the-art equipment, an adequate number of staff members, and an efficient scheduling system. When the customer is a third-party payer, quality depends on the benefit achieved in relation to the cost of the healthcare service.

Clinical quality management usually includes three related processes: **clinical quality assessment, utilization management** (UM), and **risk management.** Clinical quality assessment is the process of determining whether the services provided to patients meet predetermined standards of care. This chapter presents an overview of how healthcare standards are developed and who develops and disseminates them and gives examples of how healthcare organizations implement a clinical quality assessment program.

The chapter also introduces utilization management and risk management. *Utilization management* may be described as a group of processes used to measure how efficiently healthcare organizations use their resources. When applied to hospital care, for example, UM is used to determine whether a patient meets preestablished criteria for admission or continued stay. *Risk management* is the process of overseeing the medical, legal, and administrative operations within a healthcare organization. Its goal is to minimize the organization's exposure to **liability** claims. Risk management includes processes that minimize the organization's risk of being subject to clinical malpractice suits and also involves overseeing the safety of the organization's physical plant.

Further, this chapter discusses implementation of programs for clinical quality assessment, utilization management, and risk management. Quality and performance improvement is discussed in detail in chapter 12.

Finally, the chapter describes the more recent approaches and processes that, hopefully, will contribute to the successful assessment and management of clinical quality in the twenty-first century. These include implementation of electronic health record systems, development of regional health information organizations (RHIOs), development of a national healthcare information network (NHIN) and pay for performance programs.

Theory into Practice

Physicians and surgeons as well as nurses and quality managers continuously assess the quality of the clinical services they provide in healthcare organizations. They also continuously search for ways to improve it. The data collected during the process of providing patient services are the best source of information on the effectiveness of care.

One cardiovascular surgery department at a large Midwestern university hospital identified a potential problem with its program. The department's medical staff noted that many of the patients who had undergone percutaneous transluminal coronary angioplasty (PTCA) in the facility subsequently needed emergency open-heart surgery. Over a period of five years, the hospital's rate of post-PTCA coronary artery bypass graft (CABG) surgery was significantly higher than the national average.

An interdisciplinary team was convened to study the problem. Its members searched the clinical literature on the subject. Based their research, the team decided to investigate the following factors in relation to the long-term success rate for PTCAs:

- Whether a stent had been placed during the original PTCA procedure

- The patient's age, gender, and comorbidities (unstable angina, severe angina, past myocardial infarction, left ventricular function, number of vessels involved, and diabetes)

- The surgeon's age and gender

- The number of PTCAs performed each year by each surgeon

The study team wanted to perform a biostatistical analysis of these key factors to determine the root causes of the facility's high rate of emergency surgery after PTCA procedures. The team's leader contacted the director of the health information management (HIM) department and asked for information from the department's databases and the health records of former patients. In addition, the team leader asked the hospital's risk manager to compile information on the surgeons who had performed PTCAs in the facility over the past five years.

The study team was able to answer some of its questions by looking at relevant coded data abstracted from the patient's medical record and input into the hospital's **discharge**

abstract system. The team also obtained some interesting insights by analyzing the documentation in the health records of all the patients who had undergone a PTCA in the facility over the past five years or had undergone a PTCA and subsequent emergency CABG surgery. In addition, the HIM director was able to direct the study team to additional sources of clinical guidelines and protocols for PTCA and CABG procedures.

By analyzing and comparing all this information, the study team determined that most of the variance from national success rates was based on a higher-than-average level of comorbidity in the hospital's patient base. However, the team also found that the PTCA success rate was affected by the surgeon's level of experience. The surgeons who performed the most PTCA procedures had the highest success rates.

Definition of Quality

Many definitions have been proposed for quality. Meisenheimer (1997, 702) offered several definitions in her text. She reported that quality is:

> [The] distinguishing characteristics that determine the value, rank, or degree of excellence or expectation, the totality of features and characteristics of a healthcare process that bear on its ability to satisfy stated or implied needs . . . a process or outcome that consistently conforms to requirements, meets expectations, and maximizes value or utility for the customer.

The **Institute of Medicine** (IOM) has defined healthcare quality as "the degree to which health care services for individuals and populations increase the likelihood of desired health outcomes and are consistent with professional knowledge" (Genovich-Richards 1997, 85). An even simpler definition was proposed by the Hospital Corporation of America (HCA) when it suggested that quality is meeting or exceeding customer expectations.

IOM jolted the healthcare industry when it issued its 1999 report, *To Err Is Human: Building a Safer Health System,* which suggested that approximately 98,000 Americans die each year from preventable medical errors in hospitals (Kohn et al. 1999). In 2001, IOM followed with another report, *Crossing the Quality Chasm: New Health System for the 21st Century,* that criticized the American healthcare delivery system for a serious quality gap. In introducing the report, Dr. William Richardson stated:

> The U.S. healthcare system is in need of fundamental change. Americans ought to be able to count on receiving care that is safe and uses the best scientific knowledge. But there is strong evidence that this is not the case. Healthcare today harms too frequently, and fails to deliver its potential benefits routinely. As medical science and technology have advanced at a rapid pace, the health care delivery system has foundered. Between the care we have and the care we could have lies not just a gap, but a wide chasm.

These IOM reports spurred many of the key players in the American healthcare system to action. In 2003, for example, the Joint Commission on Accreditation of Healthcare Organizations (JCAHO) identified **patient safety** as its top priority and revamped its priorities and methodology for accrediting healthcare organizations to reflect the importance of patient safety to high-quality care. Patient safety now has become a critical issue in the national discussion of what constitutes high-quality healthcare.

Although an organization or individual may find it difficult to define quality or consistently meet any or all of its definitions, it certainly is worth striving toward. But how does a healthcare organization know if it is managing and achieving clinical quality, and what are the methodologies and motivations for doing so? This chapter presents an overview of traditional as well as relatively new clinical quality management processes and initiatives.

Clinical Quality Assessment

Caregivers have been concerned about the quality of care they provide to patients since ancient times. In 500 BC, for example, the Greek physician Hippocrates advised young physicians to "First, do no harm." That directive is still part of the physician's oath today.

As early as the 1860s, healthcare providers were interested in improving the outcomes of patient care. Florence Nightingale is considered to have been the founder of modern nursing. She advocated the use of a uniform method of collecting and evaluating statistics that compared mortality rates among hospitals. The results of her efforts showed wide variation among hospitals in the quality of patient care. She also implemented sanitary procedures such as simple hand-washing that greatly improved the outcomes of hospital care.

Fifty years later, Dr. Abraham Flexner conducted a survey of the medical schools then in operation in the United States. His report, published in 1910, described the poor quality of medical education. Flexner's recommendations eventually led to higher academic standards. Shortly thereafter, Dr. Ernest Avery Codman studied outcomes of care and called for the regular review of medical practice. Many of the issues he addressed in 1916 are still relevant today:

- Licensure and/or certification of healthcare professionals

- Accreditation of healthcare organizations

- Determinations of severity or stage of disease

- Consideration of comorbid conditions

- Influence of the patient's behavior on individual health

- Access or barriers to care

The American College of Surgeons (ACS) was established in 1913. One aspect of its mission was to improve patient care in hospitals. The ACS started its Hospital Standardization Program in 1918. The ACS's first survey identified severe quality problems in hospitals. Only 90 (about 13 percent) of the 692 hospitals surveyed were approved according the minimal requirements of the first survey. Through the efforts of ASC and other healthcare reformers, nearly 95 percent of hospitals met the program's **accreditation standards** just thirty years later.

Eventually, the hospital accreditation process grew to a point that ASC was no longer able to administer it. The Joint Commission on Accreditation of Hospitals (JCAH) was organized in 1952 to carry out the hospital accreditation program and encourage voluntary compliance with predefined standards of care. The standards covered every area of the hospital, including nursing, radiology, and pharmacy services.

In 1965, a major court case emphasized the importance of quality of care for healthcare organizations. The ruling in *Darling v. Charleston Memorial Hospital* held that hospitals are legally obligated to oversee the quality of the professional services provided in their facilities. In this case, a young man had broken his leg during a college football game. He was treated in a hospital emergency room by the physician on call, who had received little orthopedic training. The physician reduced the fracture and applied a toe-to-groin cast. However, the cast was applied incorrectly, and it cut off circulation to the patient's leg. The patient was admitted to the hospital for pain management. No orthopedic consult was ordered, and the patient continued to complain of pain.

After two weeks, the patient was transferred to another hospital. At the second hospital, an orthopedic surgeon discovered gangrenous (dead) tissue under the cast. Eventually, a below-the-knee amputation was performed to save the patient's life. The patient's father sued the first hospital for negligence. The court, and subsequent appeals courts, found the hospital legally responsible for the inadequate care rendered to the patient. The patient was awarded $100,000.

This case was significant because it established a new legal precedent for cases involving healthcare organizations. In earlier court cases involving hospitals organized as charitable corporations, the hospital's liability had been limited to the amount of liability insurance it carried. In *Darling v. Charleston Memorial Hospital,* the charitable hospital was held fully liable due to **corporate negligence** (McWay 1997, 47–48, 157).

Standards of Clinical Quality

A number of private and government entities develop and maintain standards of clinical quality. These entities include agencies and departments of the federal government, accreditation organizations, private for-profit organizations, and not-for-profit organizations such as medical societies and organizations dedicated to research on a specific disease. Standards of clinical quality include descriptive statements called by a number of names, including standards of care, quality of care standards, performance standards, and practice standards.

A standard is a written description of the expected features, characteristics, or outcomes of a healthcare-related service. Standards are generally based on a minimum level of performance. In other words, standards represent the level of performance expected of every healthcare provider. A current standard issued by one of the main accreditors of managed care organizations in the U.S. requires that 85 percent of women between ages 50 and 80 receive annual mammograms.

Four types of standards are relevant within the context of clinical quality assessment:

- *Clinical practice guidelines* and *clinical protocols:* Detailed step-by-step guides used by healthcare practitioners to make knowledge-based clinical decisions directly related to patient care

- *Accreditation standards:* Predefined statements of the criteria against which the performance of participating healthcare organizations will be assessed during the voluntary accreditation process

- *Government regulations:* Detailed descriptions of the compulsory requirements for participation in the federal Medicare and Medicaid programs

- *Licensure requirements:* Detailed descriptions of the criteria healthcare organizations must fulfill in order to obtain and maintain state licenses to provide specific healthcare services

Clinical Practice Guidelines and Protocols

Standards of clinical quality include both clinical practice guidelines and clinical protocols. According to the **Agency for Healthcare Research and Quality,** clinical practice guidelines are "systematically developed statements used to assist provider and patient decisions about appropriate health care for specific clinical circumstances" (AHRQ 2005). Clinical practice guidelines are developed with the goal of standardizing clinical decision making. As the word *guideline* suggests, clinical practice guidelines are not meant to be inflexible and do not apply in every case.

Every year, for example, the American Diabetes Association (ADA) issues a series of updated clinical practice recommendations to help healthcare providers treat people with diabetes. These guidelines usually reflect the results of recent research studies. In 2004, the organization recommended that statins be considered for people with diabetes over the age of 40 who have a total cholesterol level greater than or equal to 135 and that there be a blood pressure goal of less than 130/80 mmHg for people with diabetes (diabetes.org). Figure 11.1 shows the American Cancer Society's most updated (2003) clinical practice guideline for breast cancer screening. More than 1,000 other clinical guidelines are available at guideline.gov.

In contrast to clinical practice guidelines, clinical protocols are treatment recommendations that are often based on guidelines. They describe "generally accepted procedure[s] with clinical steps explicitly recommended by an authoritative body, such as the medical staff" (Larsen-Denning et al. 1997, 575). One example of a clinical protocol is the step-by-step description of the accepted procedure for preparing intravenous solutions at a specific acute care hospital. Another example is described in figure 11.2.

Clinical pathways are structured plans of care that help organizations implement clinical guidelines and protocols. Sometimes known as critical paths, care paths, and/or care maps, they are widely used by institutions hoping to reduce costs and improve quality through decreased variation in practices. **Critical pathways** display goals for patients and provide the corresponding ideal sequence and timing of staff actions to achieve those goals with optimal efficiency (Pearson, Goulart-Fisher, and Lee 1995). They have a multidisciplinary focus that emphasizes the coordination of clinical services. Figure 11.3 contains an example of a pathway for unstable angina.

Despite these specific definitions for clinical guidelines, protocols, and pathways, clinicians and researchers often use the terms interchangeably to describe current recommendations for patient care.

Agency for Healthcare Research and Quality

The **Agency for Healthcare Research and Quality** (AHRQ) is an agency within the Department of Health and Human Services (HHS). It was founded in 1989 as the Agency for Health Care Policy and Research. AHRQ's mission is to improve the quality, safety, efficiency, and effectiveness of healthcare for all Americans. In its 2001 *Crossing the Quality Chasm* report, the IOM directed HHS and AHRQ to implement select monitoring activities to track healthcare quality improvements. More recently, AHRQ has funded such research projects as the role of **computerized physician order-entry** (CPOE) systems in preventing medical errors. In June 2005, AHRQ awarded more than $8 million in grants to "help health care institutions implement safe practice interventions that show evidence of eliminating or reducing risks, hazards, and harms associated with the process of care."

Figure 11.1.   American Cancer Society guidelines for breast cancer screening

Guideline Status

This is the current release of the guideline.

This guideline updates a previous version: Leitch AM, Dodd GD, Costanza M, Linver M, Pressman P, McGinnis L, Smith RA. American Cancer Society guidelines for the early detection of breast cancer: update 1997. CA Cancer J Clin 1997 May–Jun;47(3):150–3.

Each year the American Cancer Society publishes a summary of existing recommendations for early cancer detection, including updates, and/or emerging issues that are relevant to screening for cancer.

Major Recommendations

Summary Recommendation

The American Cancer Society recommendations for breast cancer screening are presented below in abbreviated form. Readers should refer to the original full text guideline document to see the complete recommendations, along with the rationale and summary of the evidence. See http://www.guideline.gov/.

Women at Average Risk

Begin mammography at age 40.

For women in their 20s and 30s, it is recommended that clinical breast examination (CBE) be part of a periodic health examination, preferably at least every three years. Asymptomatic women aged 40 and over should continue to receive a clinical breast examination as part of a periodic health examination, preferably annually.

Beginning in their 20s, women should be told about the benefits and limitations of breast self-examination (BSE). The importance of prompt reporting of any new breast symptoms to a health professional should be emphasized. Women who choose to do BSE should receive instruction and have their technique reviewed on the occasion of a periodic health examination. It is acceptable for women to choose not to do BSE or to do BSE irregularly.

Women should have an opportunity to become informed about the benefits, limitations, and potential harms associated with regular screening.

Older Women

Screening decisions in older women should be individualized by considering the potential benefits and risks of mammography in the context of current health status and estimated life expectancy. As long as a woman is in reasonably good health and would be a candidate for treatment, she should continue to be screened with mammography.

Women at Increased Risk

Women at increased risk of breast cancer might benefit from additional screening strategies beyond those offered to women of average risk, such as earlier initiation of screening, shorter screening intervals, or the addition of screening modalities other than mammography and physical examination, such as ultrasound or magnetic resonance imaging. However, the evidence currently available is insufficient to justify recommendations for any of these screening approaches.

Type Of Evidence Supporting The Recommendations

The primary evidence supporting the recommendation for periodic screening for breast cancer with mammography derives from seven randomized controlled trials (RCTs).

Bibliographic Source(s)

• Smith RA, Saslow D, Sawyer KA, Burke W, Costanza ME, Evans WP 3rd, Foster RS Jr, Hendrick E, Eyre HJ, Sener S. American Cancer Society guidelines for breast cancer screening: update 2003. CA Cancer J Clin 2003 May–Jun;53(3):141–69. [184 references] PubMed

Date Released

1997 (revised 2003)

Guideline Developer(s)

American Cancer Society—Disease Specific Society

Source(s) of Funding

American Cancer Society

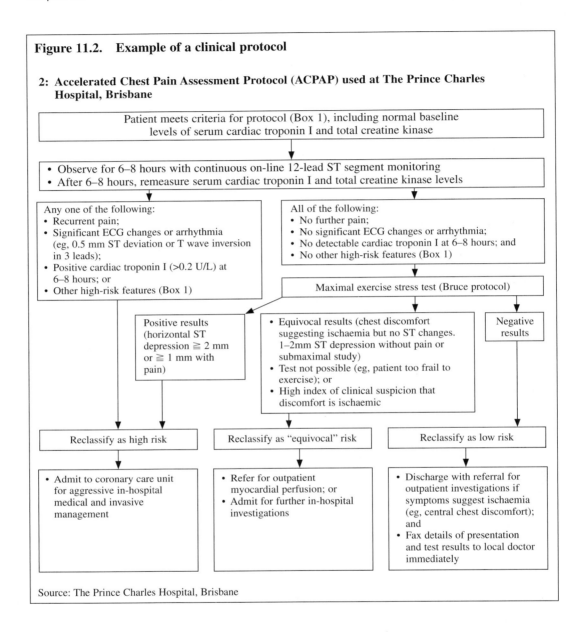

Figure 11.2.   Example of a clinical protocol

2: Accelerated Chest Pain Assessment Protocol (ACPAP) used at The Prince Charles Hospital, Brisbane

Patient meets criteria for protocol (Box 1), including normal baseline levels of serum cardiac troponin I and total creatine kinase

- Observe for 6–8 hours with continuous on-line 12-lead ST segment monitoring
- After 6–8 hours, remeasure serum cardiac troponin I and total creatine kinase levels

Any one of the following:
- Recurrent pain;
- Significant ECG changes or arrhythmia (eg, 0.5 mm ST deviation or T wave inversion in 3 leads);
- Positive cardiac troponin I (>0.2 U/L) at 6–8 hours; or
- Other high-risk features (Box 1)

All of the following:
- No further pain;
- No significant ECG changes or arrhythmia;
- No detectable cardiac troponin I at 6–8 hours; and
- No other high-risk features (Box 1)

Maximal exercise stress test (Bruce protocol)

Positive results (horizontal ST depression ≧ 2 mm or ≧ 1 mm with pain)

- Equivocal results (chest discomfort suggesting ischaemia but no ST changes. 1–2mm ST depression without pain or submaximal study)
- Test not possible (eg, patient too frail to exercise); or
- High index of clinical suspicion that discomfort is ischaemic

Negative results

Reclassify as high risk

Reclassify as "equivocal" risk

Reclassify as low risk

- Admit to coronary care unit for aggressive in-hospital medical and invasive management

- Refer for outpatient myocardial perfusion; or
- Admit for further in-hospital investigations

- Discharge with referral for outpatient investigations if symptoms suggest ischaemia (eg, central chest discomfort); and
- Fax details of presentation and test results to local doctor immediately

Source: The Prince Charles Hospital, Brisbane

The agency also works with healthcare practitioners and healthcare consumers to develop and test clinical practice guidelines. The process is based on precise methodologies that ensure the validity of the treatment protocols. AHQR publishes clinical practice guidelines for a number of diagnoses in the form of decision-making algorithms (step-by-step procedures for solving problems). The agency's goal is to develop a national database of evidence-based clinical practice information. With this goal in mind, AHQR encourages the developers of clinical practice guidelines to submit them to the **National Guideline Clearinghouse** (NGC).

Figure 11.3.   Example of a pathway for unstable angina

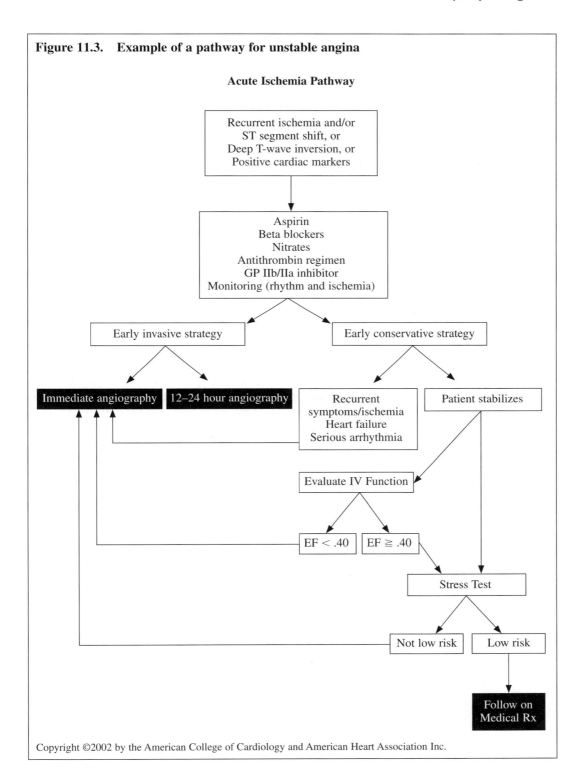

Acute Ischemia Pathway

Recurrent ischemia and/or ST segment shift, or Deep T-wave inversion, or Positive cardiac markers

Aspirin
Beta blockers
Nitrates
Antithrombin regimen
GP IIb/IIa inhibitor
Monitoring (rhythm and ischemia)

Early invasive strategy   Early conservative strategy

Immediate angiography   12–24 hour angiography

Recurrent symptoms/ischemia
Heart failure
Serious arrhythmia

Patient stabilizes

Evaluate IV Function

EF < .40   EF ≧ .40

Stress Test

Not low risk   Low risk

Follow on Medical Rx

National Guideline Clearinghouse

NGC is an Internet Web site that serves as a public resource for clinical guidelines developed by other respected organizations (guideline.gov). It represents a partnership of AHRQ, the American Medical Association (AMA), and the **American Association of Health Plans** (AAHP) that ensures that each guideline meets minimally acceptable criteria but does not judge the accuracy of the content of the guidelines themselves. The guidelines available online apply to topics such as acute pain management, benign prostate hyperplasia, cardiac rehabilitation, depression, mammography, otitis media, pressure ulcers, and sickle-cell disease.

Accreditation Standards

In the United States today, many different organizations monitor the quality of healthcare services and offer accreditation programs for healthcare organizations. All the programs base accreditation on a data collection and submission process followed by a comprehensive survey process. The survey involves measurement of a healthcare facility's performance in comparison to preestablished accreditation standards. Participation in accreditation programs is voluntary. Most accreditation standards are provided to participating healthcare organizations in the form of manuals, such as JCAHO's *Comprehensive Accreditation Manual for Hospitals.*

Joint Commission on Accreditation of Healthcare Organizations

Since its beginning in 1952, the Joint Commission Accreditation of Hospitals has continually evolved to meet the changing needs of healthcare organizations. The organization changed its name to the Joint Commission on Accreditation of Healthcare Organizations (JCAHO) in the late 1980s in recognition of changes in the U.S. health delivery system. Today, JCAHO is the largest healthcare standards-setting body in the world. It conducts accreditation surveys in more than 15,000 healthcare organizations and programs in the U.S., including more than 8,200 hospitals and home care organizations and more than 6,800 other healthcare organizations that provide long-term care, assisted living, behavioral healthcare, and laboratory and ambulatory care services (JCAHO 2005a).

In the late 1990s, JCAHO moved away from traditional quality assessment processes and began emphasizing performance and quality improvement. The ORYX initiative reflected the new approach. The goal of the ORYX initiative was to incorporate the ongoing collection of quality and performance data into the accreditation process. (The ORYX initiative is discussed in detail in chapter 5.)

Today, JCAHO's standards give organizations substantial leeway in selecting performance measures and improvement projects. Under the ORYX system, required since 1998, all hospitals and long-term care facilities must report outcome measures on at least 20 percent of their patients. **Outcome measures** document the results of care for individual patients as well as for specific types of patients grouped by diagnostic category. For example, an acute care hospital's overall rate of postsurgical infection would be considered an outcome measure. The outcome measures must be reported to JCAHO via software from vendors that have been approved by JCAHO for this purpose. (Performance improvement is discussed in more detail in chapter 12.)

In 2003–2004, JCAHO again changed its accreditation standards and its accreditation survey process. The changes, in response to IOM's 1999 and 2001 reports on the status of healthcare in America, were dramatic and extensive. Effective January 2004, JCAHO implemented a new philosophy called continuous survey readiness, a new approach to on-site surveying called **tracer methodology,** and new standards that integrated patient safety into all aspects of patient care.

At the same time, JCAHO also began issuing and scoring healthcare organizations on compliance with specific **national patient safety goals** (NPSGs). An expert advisory group composed of physicians, nurses, risk managers, and other professionals developed these NPSGs. One JCAHO safety goal, for example, requires healthcare organizations to eliminate wrong-site, wrong-patient, and wrong-procedure surgery. To accomplish this, organizations must create and use a preoperative verification process, such as a checklist, to confirm that appropriate documents (for example, medical records, imaging studies) are available. They also must implement a process to mark the surgical site and involve the patient in the marking process.

Another JCAHO safety goal requires healthcare organizations to improve the effectiveness of communication among their caregivers. To accomplish this, organizations must standardize a list of unacceptable abbreviations, acronyms, and symbols and implement rigorous standards for verbal communications related to physician orders and the reporting of critical test results. Verbal or oral orders can only be given in emergencies and therefore written orders are required for nonurgent care. Only nurses (within the scope of their state's law), respiratory therapists, nurse practitioners, and physician assistants may take oral orders, and questions need to be brought up immediately with the physician. Furthermore, when a verbal or telephone order or the reporting of critical test results takes places, the person receiving the order or test result must verify what is heard by "reading back" the complete order or test result.

JCAHO's safety goals continue to evolve and are expected to keep changing as some goals are achieved, some are difficult to attain, and new ones are identified. In 2004, for example, six goals from 2003 were carried over because organizations were struggling to comply, plus one extra was added to make seven. In 2006, two of the original goals—improving the safety of using infusion pumps and effectiveness of clinical alarm systems—were retired and new subcategories were added to several of the original ones. NPSGs are available at jcaho.org.

JCAHO also began to require a comprehensive presurvey data collection and submission process that focuses on the following fourteen priority areas:

- Assessment and care services

- Organizational structure

- Communication

- Orientation and training

- Credentialed practitioners

- Physical environment

- Equipment use

- Quality improvement expertise and activity

- Infection control

- Patient safety

- Information management
- Rights and ethics
- Medication management
- Staffing

The data collected are used to help focus the accreditation survey on patient safety and high-quality patient care and to select specific patients to "trace" during the on-site survey. This approach, first implemented in 2004, known as tracer methodology, consists of following (tracing) a few patients through their entire stay at the hospital in order to identify quality and patient safety issues that might indicate quality problems and/or patterns of less than optimum care. According to JCAHO, "tracer methodology is an evaluation method in which surveyors select a patient, resident or client and use that individual's record as a roadmap to move through an organization to assess and evaluate the organization's compliance with selected standards and the organization's systems of providing care and services" (JCAHO 2005a). A trace of a surgical patient, for example, might reveal a missing updated history and physical (H&P) on the patient's medical record within twenty-four hours before surgery. Following this lead, the surveyor might discover that the organization is having an ongoing problem with H&Ps in general, a problem with obtaining the required updated H&P within twenty-four hours before surgery, or perhaps a problem with just one particular physician.

National Committee for Quality Assurance

The National Committee for Quality Assurance (NCQA) is a private, not-for profit organization dedicated to improving the quality of healthcare. NCQA began accrediting managed care organizations in 1991 and quickly became one of the leading organizations that assess and report on the quality of the nation's managed care plans. Since then, its activities have become wider in scope. NCQA now also accredits managed behavioral health, preferred provider, and disease management organizations as well as certifying credentials verification, UM, and physician organizations.

NCQA actually has two separate arms. One focuses on the accreditation and certification processes and the other, the **Health Plan Employer Data and Information Set** (HEDIS), is used to help NCQA perform its assessments. Together, HEDIS data and NCQA accreditation give employers a way to select healthcare plans on the basis of demonstrated value in addition to cost.

HEDIS consists of more than sixty different quality and performance measures related to significant public health issues. In HEDIS, NCQA focuses on the development of performance standards in key areas such as access to services, effectiveness of care, and satisfaction with the experience of care. A list of NCQA's HEDIS measures can be viewed under the HEDIS Program at ncqa.org.

HEDIS measures are updated and revised constantly as new research and technology identify best clinical practices. In its 2006 edition of HEDIS, for example, NCQA added new measures that look at the overuse of antibiotics, proper follow-up for children and seniors taking certain medications, and diagnosis of chronic obstructive pulmonary disease (COPD).

NCQA's accreditation program for health plans measures how well they are performing on a number of basic functions. Audits of health plans include, but are not limited to, examination of their processes and databases in the following major categories:

- Quality improvement

- Quality of provider network (credentialing)

- Processes for reviewing and authorizing medical care (UM)

- Member rights and responsibilities

- Preventive health activities

The accreditation status of individual plans is reported publicly. This allows employers to determine which health plans to include in their employee benefit programs.

In addition to HEDIS and its accreditation and certification programs, NCQA issues public reports on the status of healthcare quality in America based on the data it collects. In 2004, for example, NCQA attributed widespread variation in rates of care between the best performers among health plans that collect and report data and the national rate of failure to consistently apply principles of evidence-based medicine. According to NCQA, the gap between the top 10 percent of health plans and the national average was significant in every clinical area studied. The disparity between the care most Americans receive and the care delivered through the nation's best plans results in from 42,000 to 79,000 premature deaths each year.

American Osteopathic Association

Accreditation of healthcare organizations became the focus of the American Osteopathic Association (AOA) in 1945. Osteopathic medicine emphasizes the interrelationship of the body's nerves, muscles, bones, and organs, and thus doctors of osteopathic medicine apply the philosophy of treating the whole person to the prevention, diagnosis, and treatment of illness, disease, and injury (osteopathic.org/).

Initially, AOA's primary objective was to ensure that osteopathic students received their training through rotating internships and residencies in facilities that provided effective patient care. AOA has since developed accreditation standards for hospitals, ambulatory care facilities, ambulatory surgery centers, behavioral health facilities, substance abuse treatment facilities, and physical rehabilitation facilities.

Commission on Accreditation of Rehabilitation Facilities

The Commission on Accreditation of Rehabilitation Facilities (CARF) was established in 1966. CARF is a private, not-for-profit organization that develops and maintains practical, customer-focused standards for behavioral healthcare and medical rehabilitation programs. It accredits programs and services in adult day services, assisted living, behavioral health, employment and community services, and medical rehabilitation. CARF accreditation means that the organization has made a commitment to continuously enhance the quality of its services and programs (carf.org).

Government Regulations and Licensure Requirements

Various agencies and departments of the federal, state, and local governments also review the quality of services provided in healthcare organizations. However, government regulations and licensure requirements are compulsory rather than voluntary.

Medicare Conditions of Participation

To participate in the Medicare program, healthcare providers must comply with federal regulations known as the Conditions of Participation. The Conditions of Participation are distributed by the Centers for Medicare and Medicaid Services (CMS). CMS administers the Medicare program as well as the federal portion of the Medicaid program. Participation in the Medicare program is critical to the success of many healthcare organizations because a high percentage of healthcare services is delivered to elderly Medicare beneficiaries.

In 1992, CMS and peer review organizations (PROs) working under contract with CMS instituted the **Health Care Quality Improvement Program** (HCQIP). Originally, the mission of HCQIP was to promote the quality, effectiveness, and efficiency of services to Medicare beneficiaries by strengthening the community of those committed to improving quality. HCQIP was to monitor and improve quality of care; communicate with beneficiaries, healthcare providers and practitioners; promote informed health choices; and protect beneficiaries from poor care. Today, HCQIP's approach to improving the health of Medicare beneficiaries involves the analysis of patterns of care to promote changes in the healthcare delivery system.

In 2002, CMS changed the name of the PROs to quality improvement organizations (QIOs). CMS and the QIOs collaborate with practitioners, beneficiaries, providers, plans, and other purchasers of healthcare services to achieve the following goals:

- Developing **quality indicators** that are firmly based in science
- Identifying opportunities for healthcare improvements through careful measurement of patterns of care
- Communicating with professional and provider communities about patterns of care
- Intervening to foster quality improvement through system improvements
- Conducting follow-up studies to evaluate success and redirect efforts

HCQIP began work in 1992 with a national quality improvement (QI) project on acute myocardial infarction, the Cooperative Cardiovascular Project. Since then, CMS has expanded its national QI activities and now focuses on six clinical priority areas:

- Acute myocardial infarction
- Breast cancer
- Diabetes
- Heart failure
- Pneumonia
- Stroke

Table 11.1 presents the quality indicators and data sources for each of these clinical topics. CMS selected these priorities because of their importance to public health. In addition, performance in these areas was measurable and there appeared to be a real possibility of improving quality. All are important causes of morbidity and mortality in the U.S. population as a whole and account for large numbers of hospitalizations as well as healthcare expenditures.

Table 11.1.   Quality indicators: Medicare's Health Care Quality Improvement Program

Clinical Topic	Quality Indicators	Data Sources
Acute myocardial infarction	1. Early administration of aspirin 2. Early administration of beta blocker 3. Timely reperfusion 4. Aspirin at discharge 5. Beta blocker at discharge 6. Angiotensin-converting enzyme inhibitor (ACEI) at discharge for low left ventricular ejection fraction 7. Smoking cessation counseling during hospitalization	Hospital health records for acute myocardial infarction patients
Breast cancer	8. Biennial mammography screening	Medicare claims (bills) for all female beneficiaries
Diabetes	9. Biennial retinal exam by an eye professional 10. Annual hemoglobin (HbA1c) testing 11. Biennial lipid profile	Medicare claims (bills) for all diabetic beneficiaries
Heart failure	12. Appropriate use/nonuse of ACEI at discharge [excluding discharges on angiotensin-II receptor blocker (ARB)]	Hospital health records for heart failure patients
Pneumonia	13. Influenza vaccinations 14. Pneumococcal vaccinations 15. Blood culture before antibiotics are administered 16. Appropriate initial empiric antibiotic selection 17. Initial antibiotic dose within 8 hours of hospital arrival 18. Influenza vaccination or appropriate screening 19. Pneumococcal vaccination or appropriate screening	13–14: Centers for Disease Control and Prevention Behavioral Risk Factor Surveillance System data 15–19: Hospital health records for pneumonia patients
Stroke	20. Discharged on antithrombotic [acute stroke or transient ischemic attack (TIA)] 21. Discharged on warfarin (atrial fibrillation) 22. Avoidance of sublingual nifedipine (acute stroke)	Hospital health records for stroke, TIA, and chronic atrial fibrillation patients

Source: Originally published as part of CMS publication number 10156.

CMS's seventh national priority is the reduction of disparities in the healthcare services provided to Medicare beneficiaries. For example, compared to the population overall, African-American Medicare beneficiaries receive fewer preventive services, such as influenza vaccinations. Under CMS's direction, the QIOs are analyzing these disparities in order to implement programs aimed at narrowing the gaps in service.

QIOs use medical peer review, data analysis, and other tools to identify patterns of care and outcomes that need improvement. They then work cooperatively with facilities and individual physicians to improve care. CMS established a comprehensive program in which QIOs use a data-driven approach to monitoring care and outcomes and a shared approach to working with the healthcare community to improve care. In this effort, QIOs also will pursue other types of HCQIP projects, such as important state or local issues, care provided in nonacute hospital settings, and managed care.

CMS requires QIOs to offer technical assistance and collaboration on QI projects to every Medicare+Choice plan in their state. QIOs can provide clinical and biostatistical expertise. Further, they can design and conduct quality projects, review and analyze project findings, recommend interventions, and provide advice on data collection (CMS 2005).

In April 2004, President George W. Bush established the Office of the National Coordinator for Health Information Technology to help further widespread adoption of electronic health records (EHRs) within ten years. To lend support to this endeavor, the QIOs have been contracted to help hospitals, physician practices, and home health agencies implement increased use of technology, including EHRs.

In July 2005, Medicare announced that it planned to offer physicians free software to computerize their medical practices. Believing that the EHR will improve healthcare and stating that only 20 to 25 percent of the nation's 650,000 licensed physicians outside the military and Department of Veterans Affairs (VA) are currently using electronic patient records, Medicare will offer the VA's VistA software to physicians free of charge. As part of the three-year 8th Scope of Work beginning August 2005, QIOs will assist physician practices interested in adopting EHRs with the assessment and redesign of office work flow and care processes as well as with actual implementation.

State and Local Licensure Requirements

Every state government has required the licensure of hospitals and other types of healthcare organizations since the early twentieth century. Some city and county governments also regulate healthcare facilities that operate within local boundaries. The individual states issue licenses that permit facilities to operate within a defined scope of operation. For example, a long-term care organization would be licensed to perform long-term care services, but not acute care services.

To maintain its licensed status, each facility must adhere to the state regulations that govern issues related to staffing, physical facilities, services, documentation requirements, and quality of care. Each facility's performance is usually evaluated annually by survey teams from the state department of health. Healthcare facilities that lose their licenses are no longer allowed to operate in the state.

Planning and Implementation of Clinical Quality Assessment Programs

The organizational structures and processes that constitute a quality management program must be integrated across the entire healthcare organization. To be effective, the department responsible for quality management must be able to communicate with other areas of the organization and foster interdisciplinary cooperation.

The basic responsibilities of the quality management department include:

- Helping departments or groups of departments with similar issues to identify potential clinical quality problems

- Determining the method for studying potential problems (for example, survey, chart review, or interview with staff)

- Participating in regular departmental meetings across the organization, as appropriate

In addition, the quality management department tracks progress on specific quality studies; distributes study results and recommendations to the appropriate bodies (departments, committees, administration, board of directors or trustees); facilitates implementation of educational or structural changes that flow from the recommendations; and ensures that follow-up studies are performed in a timely manner (Longo 1990). Recently, many quality management departments began to assume leadership in the assessing and tracking of organizational compliance with JCAHO standards, focus areas, and national patient safety goals.

In hospitals and other large healthcare organizations, the board of directors has ultimate responsibility for ensuring the quality of the medical care provided in the organization. In addition, the board is responsible for the organization's fiscal (financial) stability. If the board is to perform its role, it must be provided regular updates on the organization's clinical quality assessment processes and special projects (Spath 2001). A summary report of the status of quality studies performed during the year 2005 at a fictional medical center is presented in figure 11.4.

Quality management is best implemented as a cross-functional program. Staff training is critical to success, and new employee orientation should include training in quality management. A permanent multidisciplinary committee should be created to coordinate the program and ensure the consistency of clinical quality assessment processes throughout the organization. The committee should include representatives of the medical staff, nursing staff, and infection control team. Depending on the issue under study, representatives from other areas may be consulted and/or included on a particular assessment. For example, maintenance personnel, safety committee representatives, or departmental supervisors may be included on an issue concerning physical security. In some organizations, specific teams are brought together under the auspices of the quality assessment committee to study a specific issue.

Medical Staff

JCAHO requires that the medical staff organization provide oversight over the quality of patient care and have mechanisms in place for evaluating the medical staff and the quality of care they provide. Although no specific organizational structure except for the medical staff executive committee is required, the functions of the medical staff include ensuring that all members are qualified for their positions through a rigorous credentialing and privilege delineation process.

Credentialed practitioners are, in fact, a major focus of JCAHO's accreditation process. JCAHO requires that an organization's process for granting, renewing, and revising clinical privileges be outlined in the medical staff bylaws. The medical staff must evaluate practitioners (including medical staff and non-physician clinical personnel) at the time of renewal of privileges, and the organization must have a process that outlines when the medical staff may conduct a focused review of a practitioner's performance.

In addition, JCAHO requires that the medical staff be involved in QI activities. Thus, it is important that medical staff representatives serve on the organization's quality assessment committees and that the executive committee receive reports and recommendations.

Nursing Staff

Representatives from the nursing staff are essential to any quality assessment program because nursing personnel deliver the most direct patient care. Like the requirements for the medical staff, the nursing service must participate in quality assessment activities.

Figure 11.4. Excerpt from quality assessment summary report for JC Medical Center

Dept.	Subject	Dimensions of Performance	Patient Rights/Ethics	Patient Assessment	Care of Patients	Education	Continuity of Care	Performance Improvement	Leadership	Environment of Care	Human Resources	Information Management	Infection Control	Governance	Management	Medical Staff	Nursing	Outcomes
Outpatient Surgery	Postoperative Outpatient Satisfaction	Appropriate Effectiveness Continuity Respect & Caring	4	4	4		4	4										9/04: 45 pts contacted. All report pain adequately controlled; f/u in 6–9 months. 5/15/2005 89 pts: 74% = no pain, 15% = twinges, 10% = uncomfortable but tolerable. 98%: experience was positive and would return/recommend. 98% D/C instructions useful. 11/2005: 33 pts: 93% = no pain, 7% = Rx for pain ineffective. 73%: excellent experience, would return. 91%: D/C instructions useful.
2N	Restraint Audit	Effectiveness Respect & Caring Appropriateness Timeliness	4		4			4									4	Revised policy 10/04 according to HCFA regs. Audit tool revised to focus on patient outcome. 2005: Monthly chart reviews. Aggregate data compiled 10/2005. No untoward or sentinel events resulting from restraints. Goal: FY2006: reevaluate restraint competency of staff.

Figure 11.4. *(Continued)*

Dept.	Subject	Dimensions of Performance	Patient Rights/Ethics	Patient Assessment	Care of Patients	Education	Continuity of Care	Performance Improvement	Leadership	Environment of Care	Human Resources	Information Management	Infection Control	Governance	Management	Medical Staff	Nursing	Outcomes
JCMC	Pain Management	Efficacy, Appropriateness, Timeliness, Effectiveness, Respect & Caring	4	4	4	4	4	4								4	4	8/04: ER benchmark study conducted. 7/2005 Rural Connection format used to survey OB, Post Op, & Ortho patients. 9/2005: New pain protocol developed facilitywide. New pain management policy. IV standard completed. Circulating anesthesia policy completed. Patient survey begun Fall 2005, to be completed 5/2006.
Home Health Care	Physician Satisfaction Survey	Efficacy, Availability, Timeliness, Effectiveness	4	4	4		4	4										Input from physicians regarding overall care of home health patients. Satisfaction rates: 7/04 = 68%, 1/05 = 69%, 6/05 = 69%, 11/05 = 63% Modify survey to ask for recommendations to improve and resurvey in 2006
Radiology CT Contrast	Limit IV Starts in CT Contrast Scans	Effectiveness, Safety, Respect & Caring	4	4	4			4					4					12/03: Goal 88%. First time stick rate = 83%. 4/04: Goal 85%. First IV stick rate = 79%. Additional training scheduled for techs. 9/05: 87% success of first IV stick GOAL SURPASSED: CELEBRATION
Nutrition	Risk Evaluation	Appropriateness, Efficiency, Timeliness, Continuity	4	4		4		4										Timely Risk Evaluation: Goal is 100% 10/04 = 92%; 1/05 = 95%; 3/05 = 93%; 6/05 = 92%; 9/05 = 90%; 12/05 = 91%

Infection Control

In developed countries, government agencies maintain national standards for disease prevention and treatment. In the United States, the Centers for Disease Control and Prevention (CDC), part of HHS located in Atlanta, performs this function. In addition, professional groups such as the American Public Health Association and the Association for Professionals in Infection Control and Epidemiology (APIC) train communicable disease specialists. Such professional groups also establish standards of care for infectious diseases.

Healthcare accreditation and licensing organizations also require healthcare providers to meet specific **infection control** (IC) standards. Different types of healthcare organizations require different types of IC programs, depending on the type of services each organization offers. Acute care hospitals need the most stringent systems to prevent the spread of disease-causing organisms among patients, visitors, caregivers, and employees.

Caregivers in all healthcare settings are required to apply **universal precautions** to prevent exposure to disease-causing agents. Universal precautions may be defined as the application of a set of procedures specifically designed to minimize or eliminate the passage of infectious disease agents from one individual to another during the provision of healthcare services (Shaw et al. 2003, 112). Basically, universal precautions require that caregivers wash their hands between patients and wear protective gloves when they examine or treat patients. Moreover, caregivers must wear additional protection (masks, gowns, and eye protection as well as gloves) whenever they perform procedures that may bring them in contact with blood or other bodily fluids. The precautions are termed universal because they must be applied to every patient and every situation whether or not the patient or caregiver is known to be carrying an infectious disease.

Hospital IC programs are based on ongoing infection surveillance procedures. In hospitals, infections are categorized according to origin. When a patient gets an infection as the result of an exposure that occurred while he or she was hospitalized, the resulting infection is categorized as a nosocomial infection. When a patient is exposed to an infectious agent before being admitted to the hospital, the resulting infection is said to be a **community-acquired infection.** Hospital infection surveillance programs track both types of infection.

The rate of nosocomial infection is an important quality indicator. Nosocomial infections are more prevalent in intensive care units and postsurgical care units. Infection also is more prevalent among very young (newborn) and very old patients. Patients who undergo certain procedures also are prone to infection. One such infection-prone procedure is the use of an indwelling urinary catheter. Patients in long-term care facilities are especially prone to developing skin infections called decubitus ulcers.

Despite considerable attention and resources expended on infection control nationally, the CDC has estimated that as many as two million infections are acquired in hospitals each year, resulting in 90,000 deaths. One third of these were probably preventable. In response, JCAHO has identified infection control as a critical component of safe, high-quality healthcare. A seventh NPSG was added to the six 2003 goals, and new IC standards were implemented. As of January 1, 2004, all JCAHO-accredited organizations must be in compliance with the CDC's hand-washing guidelines and all unanticipated deaths associated with organization-acquired infections now must be managed as **sentinel events.** As indicated later in this chapter, a sentinel event is an infrequently occurring undesirable outcome reportable to JCAHO.

JCAHO also has identified infection control as one of its fourteen focus areas. An organization must take actions to reduce the risk of hospital-acquired infections considered epidemiologically and demographically relevant. One or more qualified individuals must manage the IC process. Furthermore, the IC standards require healthcare organizations to:

- Hold their leaders responsible for the effectiveness of their IC programs
- Allocate sufficient resources to support the IC program (for example, having an adequate number of competent IC practitioners)
- Ensure adequate staff training in infection control
- Communicate and ensure engagement of all the parties in the organization who have a role in infection control
- Coordinate efforts with the health department and other community agencies
- Intervene in a timely manner when problems arise

An effective IC program is a critical component of patient safety and high-quality care. Improved patient outcomes, decreased patient length of stay and corresponding costs, compliance with national recommendations and standards of practice, defense against litigation, and enhanced teamwork and collaboration among departments are all recognized advantages of a rigorous IC program.

Employee health is another area of concern in IC programs. In addition, sanitary conditions throughout the facility must be maintained, especially in food preparation areas.

In large healthcare organizations, permanent committees are charged with managing the IC program. Regardless of organization size, however, ongoing training is critical to the prevention of infectious disease. Because of the importance of infection control, representatives from this area must be included on all the organization's quality assessment committees.

Check Your Understanding 11.1

Instructions: Choose the answer that best completes each of the following statements.

1. _____ Federal regulations regarding the Medicare program are promulgated by _____.
   a. CMS
   b. JCAHO
   c. NCQA
   d. QIOs

2. _____ The Agency for Healthcare Research and Quality _____.
   a. Is an agency within the federal Department of Health and Human Services
   b. Works with healthcare practitioners and consumers to develop and test clinical practice guidelines
   c. Funds research projects on the effectiveness of healthcare services
   d. All of the above
   e. None of the above

3. _____ The *Darling v. Charleston Memorial Hospital* case resulted in _____.
   a. A nursing staff strike
   b. A hospital being found liable for corporate negligence
   c. No penalty for the hospital
   d. Mandatory consultations for orthopedic injuries

4. _____ Quality improvement organizations _____.
   a. Take over responsibility for all quality assessment in all hospitals
   b. Work alone to make rules about quality of care
   c. Develop protocols for care
   d. Contract with CMS to carry out the HCQIP and other projects and functions assigned in Scopes of Work

5. _____ HCQIP is _____.
   a. One of JCAHO's national patient safety goals
   b. Another name for the CMS Conditions of Participation
   c. A nonprofit agency that evaluates and accredits managed care health plans
   d. A quality initiative under CMS and its contracted QI organizations to collaborate on clinical QI projects

6. _____ Guidelines for clinical practice can be found on the Internet through provisions made by _____.
   a. CMS
   b. AHIMA
   c. AARP
   d. National Guideline Clearinghouse

7. _____ NCQA directs its evaluations of quality to the services performed under the auspices of _____.
   a. Managed care plans
   b. Medicare
   c. Skilled nursing facilities
   d. Acute care inpatient hospitals

8. _____ JCAHO requires hospitals and long-term care facilities to report outcomes for 20 percent of patients through a mechanism known as _____.
   a. LION
   b. ORYX
   c. TIGER
   d. CLAM

9. _____ Ultimate responsibility for ensuring the quality of care provided in a hospital lies with the _____.
   a. Medical staff
   b. Quality assessment department
   c. Nursing staff
   d. Board of directors

10. _____ Accreditation by JCAHO means that the healthcare organization _____.
    a. Is considered to have met the Medicare Conditions of Participation
    b. Can charge more for its services
    c. Will be paid more under DRG reimbursement
    d. Does not have to perform any further quality assessment studies

Utilization Management

UM is a set of processes used to determine the appropriateness of medical services provided during specific episodes of care. Whether the services are determined to be appropriate is based on the patient's diagnosis, the site of care, the length of stay (LOS), and other clinical factors. UM processes evaluate the level of care each patient requires. At the same time, they move services to the most appropriate healthcare setting, evaluate alternative healthcare options, manage over- and underutilization of services, and eliminate inefficient scheduling of services.

Basically, UM provides information on how efficiently and cost-effectively the healthcare organization provides the services its customers need. Medicare Conditions of Participation and JCAHO accreditation standards require acute care hospitals to institute UM programs. In addition, managed care plans such as health maintenance organizations usually conduct rigorous UM processes to control the use of expensive diagnostic, specialty, and hospital care.

Many hospitals have established alternative services to meet the cost-control demands of government payers and managed care plans. Observation beds, same-day surgery services, skilled nursing services, swing beds, and home care services all have decreased inpatient hospital care.

Hospitals can use UM information during contract negotiations with managed care plans to ensure that they are adequately reimbursed for the services they provide. UM information also can be used to evaluate the performance of individual members of the medical staff during the credentialing process.

Functions of Utilization Management

In most hospitals, UM programs perform three important functions: utilization review, **case management,** and discharge planning.

Utilization Review

Utilization review (UR) is the process of determining whether the medical care provided to a specific patient is necessary. Preestablished objective screening criteria are used as the basis of UR, which is performed according to time frames specified in the organization's UM plan.

During the UR process, information about the patient and his or her condition is provided by the patient's physician(s). That information is compared to the organization's screening criteria to determine whether an inpatient admission and/or a clinical service is appropriate and medically necessary. UR can be performed *prospectively,* before care is provided; *concurrently,* while care is being provided; or *retrospectively,* after the episode of care is complete.

Screening Criteria

UR is based on preestablished screening criteria for inpatient care. **Intensity-of-service screening criteria** determine whether the patient's needed services could be fulfilled most efficiently in an inpatient hospital setting or safely provided on an outpatient basis. For example, if the patient requires invasive surgery that involves a long recovery period, inpatient care would be appropriate. If, however, the procedure could be performed in an ambulatory surgery center, inpatient care would be inappropriate. **Severity-of-illness screening criteria** determine whether the patient's level of physical impairment requires inpatient care.

The hospital may choose whether to develop its own criteria for utilization review or to use criteria established by other sources. Regardless of the criteria selected or developed, the hospital's medical staff should review them periodically and document their formal approval. Screening criteria also are developed and applied by professional review organizations (QIOs) as well as by other third-party payers to establish medical necessity.

Timing

For hospital services, UR is usually performed before the patient is admitted for inpatient care or at the time of admission. Most health insurance and managed care plans require preadmission certification at or before admission to a hospital. Precertification is the process of collecting information to be used for advance eligibility verification, determination of insurance coverage, communication with the physician and/or insured, and initiation of preservice discharge planning and specialized programs such as disease or case management.

Preadmission utilization review is conducted to determine whether the planned service (intensity of service) or the patient's condition (severity of illness) warrants care in an inpatient setting. The purpose of preadmission (or **prospective**) utilization review is to identify patients who do not qualify for inpatient benefits before they are actually admitted. In this way, patients can be referred to the appropriate healthcare setting in a timely manner.

UR also can be conducted at the time of admission, for example, when a patient is admitted to a hospital through its emergency department. The purpose of **admission utilization review** is the same as the purpose of preadmission UR, that is, to identify patients who not require inpatient care and to direct them to the appropriate healthcare provider.

Continued-stay (or **concurrent**) **utilization review** is conducted to determine whether the patient continues to require inpatient care. The purpose of continued-stay review is to ensure that the patient's LOS is not being unnecessarily prolonged and that the hospital's resources are being used efficiently. Some third-party payers require continued stay UR at specified points during an inpatient stay.

Similar to continued-stay review, **discharge utilization review** is performed to determine whether the patient meets discharge screening criteria and no longer requires services available only in an acute care setting.

Retrospective utilization review is conducted after the patient has been discharged. Retrospective review examines the medical necessity of the services provided to the patient. It may be conducted by a peer review organization or a hospital committee. The purpose of retrospective review is to evaluate quality issues, cost issues, and LOS factors, as well as the appropriateness of the patient's admission and the utilization of hospital resources.

Utilization Review Process

Most hospitals follow a two-step UR process. Nonphysician staff members perform the initial review using information provided by the admitting physician(s). The documentation provided by the physician(s) is compared to the predetermined screening criteria for inpatient admission or continued inpatient stay. When the staff reviewer finds that the screening criteria have not been met, he or she may ask the attending physician(s) to provide additional information. Alternatively, the staff reviewer may refer the case to a member of the medical staff for peer review.

When the reviewing physician determines that the case does not meet the criteria for admission or continued stay, a written notification of denial is prepared. The notification is sent to the attending physician(s), the patient, the business office, and the peer review organization. The patient and the attending physician(s) have the right to request that the decision be reconsidered.

Case Management

Case management is the ongoing review of clinical care to ensure the necessity and effectiveness of the services being provided to the patient. It is conducted concurrently with the patient's stay and is performed by clinical professionals (usually registered nurses) employed by acute care hospitals.

The primary role of the case manager is to coordinate and facilitate care. The care-planning process extends beyond the acute care setting to ensure that the patient receives appropriate follow-up services. Many healthcare insurers and managed care organizations also employ case managers to coordinate medical care and ensure the medical necessity of the services provided to beneficiaries.

According to the Center for Case Management (2001), the process of case management is performed to meet the following goals:

- To coordinate multidisciplinary and/or multisetting patient care

- To ensure positive outcomes of care

- To manage the patient's LOS in the acute care facility

- To ensure that the healthcare organization's resources are used efficiently

The need for case management is illustrated by a June 2005 report issued by the Office of Inspector General (OIG). According to the report, which studied patients with three or more stays at an inpatient facility where the admission date for each stay was within one day of the discharge date for the previous stay, 20 percent of the consecutive inpatient stay sequences involved poor-quality care and/or unnecessary fragmentation of care. The report states that the 20 percent was the result of failure to treat patients in a timely manner, inadequate monitoring and treatment of patients, and inadequate care planning (OIG 2005).

Discharge Planning

The purpose of discharge planning is to ensure that patients are released from acute care hospitals when they no longer need inpatient care. Discharge planning is usually managed by the patient's case manager or nurse or by a clinical professional who coordinates discharge planning for the facility. The discharge planner works with the patient and his or her physician(s) and family and/or caregivers to ensure that arrangements have been made to address his or her needs after discharge from the hospital.

Careful discharge planning ensures that the patient can leave the hospital safely and receive the follow-up medical and nursing care he or she needs. For example, a stroke patient who suffered residual hemiplegia might no longer require acute care services and yet still be unable to care for herself at home. She might need continued inpatient care at a rehabilitation facility. Early discharge planning and careful assessment of her medical stability would ensure that she could be transferred safely to the other facility and that the rehabilitation facility would have a room for her after she was discharged from the acute care hospital.

Regulatory and Accreditation Requirements for Utilization Management in Acute Care Hospitals

CMS and JCAHO both require hospitals to conduct UM programs. Before implementation of the prospective payment system for acute care in 1983, UR was required as a cost-containing measure for hospital services provided to Medicare and Medicaid patients. In contrast, the current focus of UM programs is on preventing both the under- and overutilization of healthcare services.

Federal Regulatory Requirements

The original Medicare legislation passed in 1965 required hospitals and extended-care facilities to establish a plan for utilization review. The legislation also required facilities to develop UR committees. The law encouraged physicians to perform UR but gave fiscal intermediaries the power to deny payment for unnecessary medical services. Subsequent changes in the Medicare/Medicaid reimbursement system legislated in 1982 changed the focus of UM in the Medicare and Medicaid programs.

The Medicare Conditions of Participation require hospitals to maintain written UM plans. The plans must outline the hospitals' UM activities and spell out the norms and standards to be followed in the UM process.

History of Peer Review

In 1972, Public Law 92-603 instituted concurrent UR for Medicare and Medicaid patients. To accomplish concurrent review, the law established the **professional standards review organization** (PSRO) program. The function of the nonprofit PSROs was to review the hospital admissions of beneficiaries in the Medicare, Medicaid, and Maternal and Child Health programs. The PSROs evaluated patient care services for medical necessity, quality, and cost-effectiveness.

The law also required the PSROs to conduct extended-stay reviews. Physicians' review committees established the standards and criteria used to evaluate the necessity of admissions and extended hospital stays. However, UR proved to be ineffective in controlling Medicare and Medicaid spending and the PSROs were disbanded in the early 1980s.

Quality Improvement Organizations

Peer review is still an important component of UM. Federal legislation passed in 1982 created the peer review organization (PRO) program. The program's components were renamed in 2002 to reflect changes in the healthcare industry and now are called quality improvement organizations (QIOs). Nonprofit QIOs work under contract with CMS. They review the reimbursement claims of Medicare and Medicaid inpatients for medical necessity, appropriateness of care, and quality of care.

QIOs perform a number of utilization-related activities. They review the appropriateness of hospital admissions, discharges, and transfers and the completeness and quality of the care provided. Moreover, they determine whether additional payments are warranted for cases that fall outside the standard diagnosis-related groups.

QIO physician reviewers look at both utilization and quality. Utilization factors include the appropriateness of the level of care provided to the patient, specifically, whether services provided in the inpatient setting could have been performed more efficiently on an outpatient basis. Other utilization concerns include LOS and medical necessity. Quality concerns include the completeness and adequacy of care compared to professionally recognized standards of care. Possible cases of fraud and abuse also are assessed.

Reimbursement may be denied for cases that fail to meet the review criteria. Medical facilities and providers may appeal QIO decisions and request reconsideration. The beneficiaries also are notified of medical necessity denial and may request reconsideration (Watkins 1999).

Recently, CMS and its contracted QIOS have been criticized for not identifying serious quality and patient safety issues that later surface in hospitals they have reviewed. Critics also complain that the contracts between CMS and the QIOs do not allow for the release of data that could help consumers make wiser and more informed healthcare decisions and that physicians are rarely sanctioned for substandard care. Given the increased attention to quality of care and patient safety, it is likely that CMS will be reevaluating the QIOs and their procedures for reviewing the care given to Medicare beneficiaries.

Accreditation Requirements for Utilization Management

JCAHO's accreditation standards have required hospitals to conduct utilization review (UR) since the early 1970s. At that time, physicians were required to periodically review the utilization of hospital beds and other hospital resources, such as nursing, therapeutic, and diagnostic services. They determined whether these resources were made available to all patients in accordance with their medical needs.

In 1980, JCAHO separated the UR requirements from the standards covering the overall quality of professional services rendered. At that time, the UR standard required hospitals to demonstrate that they were allocating their resources appropriately through an effective UR program. JCAHO's emphasis on UR paralleled the emphasis of the Medicare program and other third-party payers on decreasing inappropriate hospital utilization. Earlier utilization requirements focused only on Medicare beneficiaries. JCAHO's requirements expanded the UR process to all hospital patients, regardless of payment source.

Today, JCAHO's *Accreditation Manual for Hospitals* incorporates UR standards into its leadership, information management, and organizational performance improvement sections. Hospitals that have earned JCAHO accreditation are deemed to have met the Conditions of Participation for Medicare and so are not required to undergo a separate validation survey. It is not unusual, however, for Medicare to conduct a postsurvey to validate the findings of JCAHO's survey team.

NCQA has extremely rigorous UM standards. Managed care plans must monitor the medical care delivered by their practitioners to detect possible over- and underuse of services. To gain NCQA accreditation, health plans must have a written UM program that is evaluated and approved annually. There must be clearly documented and consistently applied clinical criteria and procedures for approving or denying care. UM staff must be accessible to practitioners and members to discuss UM issues, and appropriate practitioners must review any denial of care based on medical necessity. Furthermore, the plan must demonstrate that decisions regarding coverage are made in a timely manner and likewise communicated to the member in acceptable time frames. As required by the national Employee Retirement Income Security Act (ERISA), the appeals process for denials is stringent in order to ensure the member's right to a fair and expedited decision.

Planning and Implementation of a UM Program

Implementation of many prospective payment systems and changes in the healthcare delivery system over the past two decades have created a competitive environment. In response, a number of healthcare organizations have undergone mergers and acquisitions. The internal incentives for utilization management are more important today than they have ever been.

Hospital UM programs are based on a UM plan. The plan should include the following components:

- A statement of the program's purpose
- A description of the lines of authority
- A description of the UM committee's structure, responsibilities, and functions
- A description of the program's reporting mechanisms
- A description of the administrative support required for the program
- A description of the relationship between UM and performance improvement activities
- A description of the procedure to be followed in reviewing and updating the UM plan on a regular basis

Administrative support for the UM program may be assigned to the quality management department or the HIM department. Regardless of the facility's organizational structure, the HIM practitioner's expertise in data collection and data analysis is critical to the operation of an efficient UM program. The program's data requirements must be integrated with other data requirements to ensure that data quality is maintained and that each data element is collected only once (Watkins 1999).

Check Your Understanding 11.2

Instructions: Match each term to the appropriate definition.

1. ____ Utilization management
2. ____ Screening criteria
3. ____ Discharge utilization review
4. ____ Preadmission utilization review
5. ____ Concurrent utilization review
6. ____ Conditions of Participation
7. ____ Admission utilization review
8. ____ Retrospective utilization review
9. ____ Prospective utilization review
10. ____ Continued-stay utilization review

a. Review of a planned admission to determine whether the services are medically necessary and whether the patient qualifies for inpatient benefits
b. Assessment of a patient's readiness to leave the hospital
c. Periodic review during a current admission to determine whether the patient still needs acute care services

d. Review of the patient's need for care and of the care provided at the time services are rendered
e. Review of the appropriateness of the care setting and resources used to treat a patient
f. Review of records some time following the patient's discharge to determine any of several issues, including the quality or appropriateness of the care provided
g. Standards that, if met, allow a hospital to receive reimbursement for care provided to Medicare beneficiaries
h. Severity-of-illness or intensity-of-service standards used to determine the most appropriate care setting
i. Review prior to a hospital admission to determine whether the planned services are medically necessary and require treatment in an acute care setting
j. Review at the time of admission to determine medical necessity and appropriateness of care in an acute care setting

Risk Management

In healthcare, risk can be defined as any occurrence or circumstance that might result in a loss. Losses include any damage to an entity's person, property, or rights, including physical injury, cognitive injury, emotional injury, wrongful death, and financial loss. Risk management, therefore, can be defined as a set of policies, processes, and procedures that identify potential operational and financial losses, prevent losses whenever possible, and lessen the effects of losses that cannot be prevented.

The purpose of the risk management program should be to link risk management functions to the related processes of quality assessment and performance improvement. The aims of the program are to (1) help provide high-quality patient care while also enhancing a safe environment for patients, employees, and visitors and (2) minimize financial loss by reducing risk through prevention and evaluation.

According to the **American Society for Healthcare Risk Management** (ASHRM), most losses in healthcare organizations fall into one or more of the following types (Hope 1997, 31):

- *Property losses:* For example, the owners of a clinic that was damaged by fire would suffer a property loss.

- *Net income losses:* For example, the owners of the clinic that was damaged by fire would suffer a net income loss during the period when the clinic was not in operation.

- *Liability losses:* For example, a patient injured during the fire in the clinic might file a lawsuit against the owners of the clinic, claiming that they should have taken steps to prevent the fire. The owners would suffer a liability loss that included legal costs as well as possible damage awards.

- *Personnel losses:* For example, the death of an employee during the fire would represent a personnel loss for the organization. Any time a situation or event resulted in the death, disability, retirement, resignation, or unemployment of a key employee, the organization would suffer a personnel loss.

As the preceding examples show, the same incident can result in a variety of losses for the healthcare organization.

The development of formal risk management programs in hospitals and other types of healthcare organizations followed the 1965 court decision in *Darling vs. Charleston Community Memorial Hospital.* Without the protection of charitable immunity from damage awards, hospitals soon faced an avalanche of medical malpractice lawsuits. When the number of malpractice claims increased dramatically in the 1970s, the liability insurance premiums of healthcare organizations and physicians skyrocketed. At about the same time, JCAHO also began to require that hospitals develop risk management plans (McWay 1997, 157).

The 1999 IOM report, *To Err is Human: Building a Safer Health System,* significantly influenced all organizations involved with risk management. JCAHO now defines patient safety as "the degree to which the risk of an intervention (for example, use of a drug or procedure) and risk in the care environment are reduced for a patient and for other persons, including healthcare practitioners" (JCAHO 2005a). ASHRM began to emphasize its commitment to a vision of safe and trusted healthcare and on the fifth anniversary of the report commented that "the IOM report was a clarion call to managers of risk who have been at the forefront of creating safe and trusted health care since ASHRM was founded in 1980" (ASHRM 2005).

Functions of Risk Management

The basic functions of healthcare risk management programs are similar for most organizations and include (Sedwick 1997, 18–26):

- Risk identification and analysis
- Loss prevention and reduction
- **Claims management**

Risk Identification and Analysis

The role of the risk manager is to collect and analyze information on actual losses and potential risks and to design systems that lessen potential losses in the future. Risk managers use information from a variety of sources to identify areas of risk exposure within the organization. Sources of risk management information include:

- **Incident reports** (sometimes called occurrence reports or occurrence screens)
- Current and past liability claims against the organization
- Performance improvement reports
- Internal inspections of the organization's physical plant and medical equipment
- Reviews conducted by the organization's insurance carriers
- Survey reports from state and local licensing agencies
- Survey reports from accreditation organizations

- Reports of complaints from patients, visitors, medical staff, and employees
- Results of patient satisfaction surveys

An incident report is a structured tool used to collect data and information about any event not consistent with routine operational procedures. In the language of risk management, this event is referred to as a **potentially compensable event.** A potentially compensable event is an event, such as an accident or medical error, that results in a personal injury or loss of property.

Incident reports are prepared to help healthcare facilities identify and correct problem areas and to prepare for legal defense. They are considered extremely confidential documents that are never filed in the patient record and should not be photocopied or prepared in duplicate.

The risk manager analyzes every potential risk identified. Practice standards published by professional medical associations such as the American College of Emergency Physicians help the risk manager to determine whether the organization's level of risk exposure in a particular service area is acceptable. When the level of risk falls outside the parameters set by the organization's safety standards and/or external practice standards, the risk manager communicates this information to the organization's administration and/or the appropriate department manager.

Loss Prevention and Reduction

The risk manager is responsible for developing systems to prevent injuries and other losses within the organization. Performance improvement actions are often initiated in response to suggestions offered by the risk manager. Education also is an invaluable tool in risk management and sometimes is the only activity required to prevent potential safety problems.

Risk managers in many healthcare organizations also are responsible for developing policies and procedures aimed at preventing accidents and injuries and reducing the organizations' risk exposure. In addition, risk managers are involved in the organization's **safety management** program, **security management** program, medication management, **facilities management** program, and infection control program.

Safety and Security Management

To fulfill their goal of loss prevention and reduction, risk management programs are concerned with environmental safety measures and security management. For example, the risk manager collects and analyzes data to promote a safe environment. This may include analyzing patient, staff, visitor, and volunteer unexpected events, such as falls and injuries. Moreover, the risk manager is involved in conducting or reviewing results of evaluations or audits that have been performed with regard to safety and security management. This also may include evaluations of facilities and technologies used by the organization.

Claims Management

Healthcare organizations can be held legally responsible for injuries that occur in their facilities or on the surrounding property they own or manage (parking garages, campus parks, and so on). Injuries can result from substandard clinical care (malpractice), medical errors, falls, equipment malfunctions, and other adverse occurrences. Every year, thousands of patients and other individuals file claims for compensatory damages (compensation for pain and harm suffered) against healthcare organizations as well as clinical professionals (physicians, nurses, and others). Some areas of healthcare delivery are considered to carry significantly higher levels of risk, including obstetrics, psychiatry, anesthesia, and surgery.

Claims management is the process of managing the legal and administrative aspects of the healthcare organization's response to injury claims. It is handled differently by different sizes and types of organizations. Accordingly, the role of the risk manager in managing claims varies (Barton 1997, 385). Many organizations place the entire process in the hands of their liability insurance vendors. In such cases, the risk manager may act as the organization's liaison with the insurance company. However, some organizations are self-insured, meaning that they establish a dedicated fund for financing future liability settlements. In such cases, the risk manager may manage the entire claims management process.

In most healthcare organizations, the claims management process involves the following general steps (Barton 1997, 385–430):

1. *Reporting of claims:* Written claims for damages and/or formal legal notifications of the intent to seek compensation for injuries are given to the person responsible for risk management in the organization. The risk manager then notifies the organization's administration and its insurance vendor and/or corporate counsel. The risk manager also reports and investigates potentially compensable events for which no claims have been filed.

2. *Initial investigation of claims:* The risk manager gathers all the information relevant to the claim or the potentially compensable event, including information about the injured parties or claimants; information about the departments and/or caregivers involved in the incident; information about the individuals named as defendants in lawsuits; dates; insurance information; extent of injuries; current status of case; summary of the claimant's allegations; summary of health record information; summaries of interviews with witnesses and participants; copies of relevant policies, procedures, clinical protocols, practice standards, and equipment maintenance records.

3. *Protection of primary and secondary health records:* The health records of patients involved in potentially compensable events and claims should be completed as soon as possible after the patients are discharged. The primary and secondary records should then be copied for use by the risk manager and the originals secured in a locked storage place. Any written incident reports, investigative reports, peer review records, and credentialing files relevant to the case also should be protected. State laws and findings in past legal cases dictate what kinds of information must be provided to the parties in a lawsuit, and risk managers should maintain the confidentiality of sensitive documents until it is determined exactly what kinds of information must be turned over to the injured party's representatives. (Information that must be turned over to the parties in a lawsuit is termed *discoverable* and is provided to the parties in a **discovery process.**) Patients and their legal representatives have automatic access to the

patients' health records, and so copies of internal incident reports must not be placed in health records.

4. *Negotiation of settlements:* Many claims for compensatory damages are settled out of court. After the healthcare organization has determined whether it is at fault in a case, the organization's risk manager, insurance representative, administration, and/or legal counsel decide whether to offer a monetary settlement or to go forward with a formal trial. Most organizations attempt to avoid going to trial when they are at fault because defending against lawsuits is extremely expensive and may damage their reputation. If the organization and the injured party agree on a settlement, the case is brought to a close before trial.

5. *Management of litigation:* Preparation for trial involves selecting legal defense counsel and providing information to legal counsel. Legal counsel then conducts expert medical and technical reviews of the evidence, manages the discovery process, interviews (deposes) witnesses, and negotiates pretrial settlements. When a pretrial settlement cannot be negotiated successfully, the legal counsel conducts the trial and various witnesses and medical experts give testimony. After testimony is complete, a jury examines the evidence and decides whether the defendant(s) is responsible in whole or in part for the injury. When the defendant(s) is found to be liable, the jury and/or the trial judge determines the size of the damage award.

6. *Use of information on claim's resolution in performance improvement activities:* The outcomes of settlements and lawsuits are used as information in the organization's performance improvement processes. The problems that resulted in the injury are examined and solutions are implemented. Performance improvements center on the need for more staff training, changes in the credentialing process, changes in equipment maintenance procedures, and so on. (Chapter 13 discusses performance improvement in detail.)

Patient Advocacy

Many large healthcare organizations such as acute care hospitals have instituted **patient advocacy** programs. In such programs, a patient representative (sometimes called an ombudsperson) responds personally to complaints from patients and their families. Many times, patients and their families are looking for nothing more than an explanation of an adverse occurrence or an apology for a mistake or misunderstanding. Patient representatives are trained to handle minor complaints and to seek remedies on behalf of patients. They also are trained to recognize serious problems that need to be forwarded to performance improvement and/or risk management personnel.

According to the healthcare ombudsperson model, all parties benefit because the ombudsperson (Houk 2004):

- Intervenes at the earliest possible opportunity at the lowest possible level

- Maintains informality, confidentiality, and independence

- Resolves potentially compensable events through timely communication

- Is a trained professional in communicating adverse outcomes and mediation skills

- Has the time built into his job to spend with patients and providers

- Is sanctioned by top leadership to move fluidly horizontally and vertically within the existing organizational structure

Process of Risk Management

According to the ASHRM, the first two functions of risk management (risk identification and analysis, and loss prevention and reduction) can best be achieved by adopting a process that ensures the continuous improvement of the organization's risk management plan (Hope 1997, 30–33). The continuous improvement process includes five basic steps:

1. Identify and analyze potential losses.

2. Examine the feasibility of alternative risk management techniques.

3. Select the best risk management technique or combination of techniques for the organization.

4. Implement the technique(s) selected.

5. Monitor and improve the organization's risk management activities.

Most healthcare organizations use a variety of techniques for managing risk. These techniques can be categorized as follows (Hagg-Rickert 1997, 44–45):

- *Risk acceptance:* Many areas of medical care are inherently risky (for example, obstetrics). Risk acceptance involves planning for losses by setting up special self-insurance funds. In addition, some risks inherently involve acceptable levels of financial loss (for example, misplacement of a patient's personal possessions).

- *Risk avoidance:* Many healthcare organizations avoid potential losses by discontinuing especially risky services (for example, high-risk obstetrics).

- *Risk reduction or minimization:* Most healthcare organizations use the risk reduction technique when they develop safety policies and procedures (for example, requiring the use of bed rails for patients with a high risk of falling) and conduct educational programs for staff.

- *Risk transfer:* Risk transfer involves purchasing liability insurance protection against potential losses.

Regulatory and Accreditation Requirements for Risk Management in Acute Care Hospitals

Risk management activities are built into virtually every healthcare regulation and accreditation program. Some requirements pertain to the development of formal risk management programs; others are meant to guarantee safe and effective patient care.

As a result of the renewed attention to patient safety and to JCAHO's recently rewritten accreditation standards, the entire area of risk management has undergone a significant change. Anything that undermines patient safety is a risk issue. All hospital activities must be evaluated as to the potential risk to the patient or to the organization. Leadership is responsible for ensuring adequate resources for patient safety.

Federal, State, and Local Regulatory Requirements

Federal and state governments have established a number of mandatory regulations that pertain to risk management activities in healthcare organizations.

Federal Regulations

The following pieces of federal legislation have direct relevance for risk management programs in healthcare organizations (Scully 1997, 125–38):

- *Food, Drug and Cosmetic Act of 1938:* This legislation requires the manufacturers of food, drug, and cosmetic products to provide package labeling that provides information on the product's content and safety.

- *Occupational Safety and Health Act of 1971:* This legislation requires employers to provide safe working environments for their employees. It also established the Occupational Safety and Health Administration.

- *Employee Retirement Income Security Act of 1974:* This legislation standardized the administrative functions of employee benefit plans across the fifty states.

- *Emergency Medical Treatment and Active Labor Act of 1985:* This legislation (sometimes called "antidumping legislation") prohibits hospital emergency departments from transferring medically unstable patients to other facilities simply because they have no health insurance coverage.

- *Health Care Quality Improvement Act of 1986:* This legislation established the National Practitioner Data Bank (NPDB). The act requires insurance companies, self-insured trusts, and state licensing boards to report information on medical malpractice and adverse actions against healthcare practitioners to the NPDB. Further, it requires hospitals to request information from the NPDB before granting clinical privileges to new practitioners (including physicians, dentists, nurse practitioners, and others).

- *Patient Self-Determination Act of 1990:* This legislation requires hospitals and skilled nursing facilities to advise patients of their right to execute advance directives (statements of the patients' wishes concerning future medical treatment).

- *Americans with Disabilities Act of 1990:* This legislation established the equal opportunity rights of people with physical and mental disabilities. It had far-reaching effects on equal access to employment, transportation, housing, and public services.

- *Safe Medical Devices Act of 1993:* This legislation requires most healthcare organizations (except physicians' offices) to report adverse events (accidents and injuries) involving medical equipment to the Food and Drug Administration.

- *Health Insurance Portability and Accountability Act of 1996:* This complex legislation requires the implementation of sweeping changes in the area of privacy protection and healthcare information security. (Both these topics are covered in depth in chapters 14 and 15.)

In addition, several federal agencies have been granted authority to monitor and regulate the safety of healthcare facilities, including:

- *Centers for Disease Control and Prevention (CDC):* The CDC is responsible for national programs concerned with communicable diseases and environmental health.

- *Centers for Medicare and Medicaid Services (CMS):* CMS administers the financial aspects of the Medicare program and the federal portion of the Medicaid program. It also publishes the Medicare Conditions of Participation for healthcare providers and professionals who provide services to Medicare beneficiaries.

- *Environmental Protection Agency (EPA):* The EPA is responsible for protecting human health and the natural environment. It regulates indoor and outdoor air quality, the safety of the water supply, and waste management.

- *Equal Employment Opportunity Commission (EEOC):* The EEOC enforces federal laws prohibiting job discrimination based on gender, race, religion, or national origin.

- *Food and Drug Administration (FDA):* The FDA is responsible for the protection of human research subjects; the safety of food, drugs, and cosmetics; the safe use of equipment that emits ionizing radiation; the safe use of medical equipment and devices; and the proper labeling of consumable products.

- *Nuclear Regulatory Commission (NRC):* The NRC licenses qualified healthcare organizations to use, handle, and store radioactive substances.

- *Occupational Safety and Health Administration (OSHA):* OSHA enforces federal laws related to safety in the workplace. Figure 11.5 lists healthcare-related areas for which OSHA administers safety standards guidelines.

- *Office of Civil Rights (OCR):* The OCR is charged with investigating complaints and enforcing the privacy provisions of the federal HIPAA legislation.

State and Local Laws

Risk management programs also are affected by regulations in their geographic locations. State laws generally regulate the following areas of healthcare:

- Malpractice and liability insurance providers
- Liability claims, including statutes of limitations and caps on damage awards
- Professional practice acts, including the licensing of physicians, nurses, and other clinical practitioners
- Licensing of healthcare organizations such as hospitals and skilled nursing facilities
- Public health departments

```
Figure 11.5.   Healthcare-related areas for OSHA safety standards guidelines

Asbestos and lead exposure in building          Communication of information on potential
   construction                                    hazards to employees
Exposure to blood-borne pathogens               Hazardous waste operations and emergency response
Exposure to airborne pathogens                  Infectious waste handling and disposal
Use of hazardous drugs                          Use of lasers
Use of hazardous substances in laboratories     Use and maintenance of hazardous equipment
Use of radioactive substances                   Use of hazardous solvents
Use of hazardous substances in sterilization    Indoor air quality
   equipment                                    Noise pollution
Use of hazardous substances in treatment        Use of personal protective equipment
   modalities                                    Use of respiratory protection
```

Moreover, city and county ordinances may be relevant in some locales. For example, local health departments may require the reporting of specific infectious diseases. Many state and local governments also enforce regulations on air and water quality, hazardous and medical waste disposal, and use of below- and above-ground storage tanks.

Accreditation Requirements for Risk Management

JCAHO's voluntary accreditation standards for hospitals require the integration of risk management activities with all clinical and operational activities. JCAHO requires healthcare organizations to conduct in-depth investigations of occurrences that resulted—or could have resulted—in life-threatening injuries to patients, medical staff, visitors, and employees. JCAHO uses the term *sentinel event* for such occurrences.

A sentinel event, therefore, describes an infrequently occurring undesirable outcome. According to JCAHO, it is:

- An unexpected occurrence involving death or serious physical or psychological injury, or the risk thereof. Serious injury specifically includes loss of limb or function. The phrase "or the risk thereof" includes any process variation for which a recurrence would carry a significant chance of a serious adverse outcome.

- An outcome of such magnitude that each event requires an investigation and response.

Examples of sentinel events include medical errors, explosions and fires, and acts of violence. When these occur, the healthcare organization is required to prepare a detailed report of its investigation to explain the root cause of the event so that similar events can be averted in the future. JCAHO issues sentinel event alerts when it detects a pattern of similar events reported by the healthcare organizations it accredits. JCAHO uses its sentinel events data as a basis for its NPSGs.

JCAHO and other accreditation organizations such as the National Committee for Quality Assurance also have standards related to the prevention of injuries in healthcare organizations. Most of the standards share common activities, such as staff training and education and monitoring and evaluation processes. These related standards fall into the following categories (West 1997, 181–83):

- *Safety management:* JCAHO standards require healthcare facilities to eliminate hazards that could cause life-threatening injuries to patients and others who visit or work in the facility. An individual must be identified who will be responsible for developing, implementing, and monitoring the safety management program as well as intervening when there are threatening conditions.

- *Security management:* JCAHO standards address physical security concerns such as traffic control, access control, and identification systems. An individual must be designated to be specifically responsible for security.

- *Hazardous materials management:* JCAHO standards require healthcare organizations to manage the use and disposal of hazardous materials and the disposal of hazardous and infectious waste. Organizations are expected to comply with all related OSHA regulations.

- *Life safety management:* JCAHO standards require healthcare organizations to implement a written management plan for fire safety that addresses the process for the regular inspection, testing, and maintenance of fire safety equipment.

- *Emergency preparedness:* JCAHO standards require healthcare organizations to plan for natural and man-made disasters within and outside the facility. Vulnerabilities must be identified and responses to all types of emergencies developed and understood by all staff.

- *Equipment management:* JCAHO standards require healthcare organizations to have a systematic program for selecting, evaluating, testing, and maintaining medical equipment.

- *Utilities management:* JCAHO standards require healthcare organizations to have a program for preventing system failures and a plan in place for managing utility risks.

- *Social environment management:* JCAHO standards emphasize meeting the patient's space requirements and need for privacy within the healthcare facility.

Role of the Health Record in Risk Management

Complete and accurate health record documentation is the foundation of effective risk management. As chapter 6 explained, the health record represents legal documentation of the services provided to patients. It is accepted as legal evidence of what happened during a specific episode of clinical care. The health record is the best source of information for determining whether caregivers met relevant standards of care. Therefore, the documentation in the health record can defend healthcare providers against malpractice charges or support the patient's claim of negligence.

Thorough documentation of the patient's condition in the health record also can prevent injuries by alerting caregivers to potential problems. The negative effects of medical errors such as medication mistakes can be better controlled when caregivers have an accurate account of the name and amount of the medication administered and the time it was given. Using information from health records, external reviewers sometimes can identify systematic shortcomings in the services offered in specific clinical departments of a healthcare organization before patients are adversely affected.

An effective risk management technique is **occurrence screening.** In this process, the risk manager carefully reviews the health records of current and discharged patients with the goal of identifying potentially compensable events. Occurrences that can result in injuries to patients and future lawsuits include instances when a wrong surgery was performed, a contraindicated medication was ordered, or an informed consent for a medical procedure was not obtained. The documentation in health records also may draw the risk manager's attention to a higher-than-average rate of nosocomial infection in one unit of the hospital. Similarly, a large number of cases of decubitus ulcers often would be the first sign of quality problems in a long-term care facility.

Figure 11.6 presents AHIMA's guidelines for health record documentation in acute care facilities. Other care settings have similar documentation guidelines for the services they provide. Complete, accurate, and legible health record documentation is fundamental

---

Figure 11.6.   General documentation guidelines

- Every healthcare facility should have policies that ensure the uniformity of the content and format of the health record. The policies should be based on applicable accreditation standards, federal and state regulations, reimbursement requirements, and professional practice standards.

- The health record should be organized systematically to facilitate data retrieval and compilation.

- Only persons authorized by the facility's policies should author documentation in the health record.

- The healthcare facility's rules and regulations should specify who may receive and transcribe physicians' verbal orders.

- Health record entries should be documented at the time the treatment they describe is rendered, and every entry should be signed and dated.

- The authors of all entries should be clearly identifiable.

- Only preapproved abbreviations and symbols should be used in the health record.

- All entries in the health records should be permanent.

- Errors should be corrected as follows: Draw a single line in ink through the incorrect entry. Then print the word error at the top of the entry. Authenticate the entry with a legal signature or initials, date, time, title, reason for change, and professional discipline of the person making the correction. Errors must never be blocked out or erased. The existing entry should be left intact. Corrections should be entered in chronological order. Late entries should be labeled as such.

- In the event the patient wishes to amend information in the record, it should be done as an addendum, without a change to the original entry. It also should be clearly identified as an additional document appended to the original health record at the direction of the patient. The patient is responsible for explaining the addendum in the future.

Source: Adapted from Smith and Dougherty 2001.

to achieving positive health outcomes in every setting, just as incomplete documentation can result in medical errors, treatment delays, and patient injuries.

In court proceedings, the health record is the only record of care that matters. If care is not recorded in the health record, it did not happen. The health record should represent a complete, chronological account of the care provided to the patient. One of the most embarrassing and damning ploys a plaintiff's attorney can use during a trial for malpractice is to show that a physician, nurse, or therapist cannot understand his or her own health record entries.

The following list provides examples of the consequences of unclear or incomplete health record documentation:

- Improperly entered medication orders can result in claims of negligence. For example, a patient who received 25 milligrams rather than 2.5 milligrams of a medication might suffer a serious drug reaction and brain damage.

- Illegible physician orders can result in serious harm or injury to a patient. A scrawled order by a physician for one medication can be erroneously interpreted and administered as another medication by a different provider or caregiver carrying out the order.

- Incorrect abbreviations of medical terminology or medications can result in serious harm or injury. The Latin abbreviations of Q.D. for "once daily" and Q.O.D. for "every other day" are easily mistaken for each other. The period after *Q* can be mistaken for *I* and *O* can be mistaken for *I*.

- Inconsistent entries make the entire health record suspect. For example, an admitting note dated 6/24 and a progress note dated 6/22 clearly indicate that something is wrong. Similarly, the diagnostic information for an emergency department patient would be questionable if the physician's note mentioned a fractured right leg, but the x-ray noted a fractured left leg.

- Time gaps in the record can cause serious problems. For example, in an actual case, a patient was brought to the emergency department at 10:00 p.m. The record noted that, upon examination, an immediate surgical consult was requested. The entry that mentioned the consult was not made until 7:00 a.m. the next morning even though the consult actually took place an hour after it was requested. Surgery was performed in the morning but resulted in only limited success. When a malpractice case went to trial four years later, no witnesses were available and the nine-hour delay evidenced in the record stood as proof of negligence.

- Contradictions and accusations of improper actions in health record entries can be deadly. For example, a nurse's note might read, "Patient going into shock. Could not get Dr. Jones to come. We never can!"

The following types of documentation must be included in the health record:

- *Justification of diagnostic procedures:* This refers to documentation showing the medical necessity of performing diagnostic procedures.

- *Abnormal results of diagnostic procedures:* In addition, any actions taken or treatment decisions made on the basis of abnormal test results should be documented. If the ramifications of abnormal test results are not mentioned in the health record, subsequent reviewers may conclude that the patient's physician ignored the test results.

- *Achievement of treatment goals:* Such notations indicate to future reviewers of the record that the patient's progress was being monitored adequately, appropriate care was being provided, and the course of treatment was concluded successfully.

- *Discontinued treatment:* The clinical indications that led to the decision that treatment was either successful and thus no longer necessary, ineffective and thus wasteful, harmful to the patient, or replaced by other therapies should be readily apparent to those reviewing the record for evidence of appropriate clinical care.

- *Discharge planning for inpatients:* In addition, the patient's medical stability at the time of discharge and the plan for follow-up care must be documented. CMS includes the documentation of adequate discharge planning among the generic quality screens that QIOs use in reviewing the records of hospital patients. In addition, the record must include a complete summary of the patient's history, current status, and future care needs to ensure appropriate continuity of care when the patient is transferred to another healthcare delivery setting.

Planning and Implementation of a Risk Management Program

Different kinds of healthcare organizations need different kinds of risk management programs. In an acute care hospital, the program's size and complexity depend on the hospital's size and service mix. Large medical centers usually have dedicated risk management departments. Small community hospitals often assign risk management to a single employee who usually has other functions to perform. Ambulatory care organizations such as physician offices and freestanding surgical centers may assign the risk management function to an office manager. Many small healthcare organizations retain outside counsel to handle risk management activities such as claims management. A dedicated department at the corporate level might handle the risk management function in a multifacility healthcare system or integrated delivery network (Sedwick 1997, 18–26).

Risk management records should be created and maintained in strict accordance with legal guidelines to prevent discoverability in future court cases. Risk management information is used administratively to accomplish several objectives: to improve operational processes, to maximize patient and employee satisfaction and clinical outcomes, and to decrease risk factors. Aggregate data are generated through organization-wide monitoring and evaluation activities, hazard surveillance, infection control, and other medical staff review activities.

Each organization's risk management plan should include the following components: the plan's objectives, key elements, responsibilities, methods, and areas of focus for the current year. (See the sample plan in figure 11.7.)

Figure 11.7.   Sample risk management plan

Objective: The objective of the JC Medical Center (JCMC) risk management plan is to control and minimize loss in order to protect the assets of the facility and the safety of all staff, patients, and visitors.

Key Elements: Risk management involves several key elements. The methods for implementing these elements are displayed later in this document. The key elements are: *identification* of risk issues, *evaluation* of areas of risk, *communication* of risk information, *education* of organizational personnel and others, and *reduction* of risk.

Responsibilities: The risk manager will be responsible for managing JCMC's risk management activities. These activities include coordinating insurance coverage, managing claims against the facility, interfacing with legal counsel, administering the risk management plan, managing and analyzing risk management data, conducting risk management educational programs, and managing the facility's compliance with the standards of JCAHO and other accrediting organizations or regulatory agencies. Although the risk manager has oversight responsibility for this plan, risk cannot be reduced without education of, and participation by, all team members at JCMC. Team members include (1) staff, (2) managers, (3) administration, and (4) medical staff. All team members are expected to report events. In addition, their respective specific responsibilities are to: (1) follow standards of practice; (2) oversee standards of practice, identify risk events, and contribute to solutions; (3) guide the organizational mission, implement systems to reduce risks, and budget monies to solve problems; and (4) participate in solving problems for areas amenable to risk reduction.

The risk manager will be available to consult with any department or manager to assist in a risk assessment of the environment or system. A professional exchange of ideas, observations, and systems will identify potential problems. The risk manager will then assist in creating a plan to reduce that risk and to enhance care for the patients.

The risk manager also will research issues and gather additional data to assist decision makers in the search for solutions. This research may include local, state, or national data. The risk manager will consult on interpretation of data and contribute information about possible laws that may contribute to and impact the outcome of the problem-solving activities.

Methods for Carrying Out Key Elements:

Identification: There are several methods for identifying risk issues. These methods of identification include, but are not limited to, incident reports, medical device reports, customer comment tracking forms, attorneys' health record requests, security reports, performance improvement referrals, medical staff/peer review reports (when appropriate), safety hazard reports, supervisor reports, documentation by staff and/or phone conversations with individuals who feel a need to speak about a risk issue, and visual inspection of all areas of the organization in order to identify potential risk situations.

Committee membership and participation are essential for risk identification. The risk manager will attend, when possible, any committee meeting that requests risk management to be present. The risk manager will assist in the credentialing process whenever there is a request or need to do so. The risk manager will research the appropriate databases and assist in obtaining profiles concerning procedures as needed or required by the medical staff bylaws.

Risk management will identify high-risk areas due to trends in practice, advanced changes in technology, and national data suggesting risk at JCMC. The high-risk areas at JCMC are the emergency department, obstetrics, surgery, anesthesia, critical care, and pediatrics. These areas have the potential for creating situations that can have a significant economic and emotional impact on the organization.

Figure 11.7. *(Continued)*

The organization has other vested interests that risk management will include when evaluating risk exposure. Risk management will monitor the off-campus sites by receiving notification of any incidents that occur off-campus, as well as through periodic visits by the risk manager to each site.

As the organization transitions into larger networks, risk management will monitor changing trends in healthcare delivery and keep the medical community apprised of these changes. Such trends may include clinical pathways, joint ventures, mergers, and community projects that promote wellness.

Maintaining information is and always will be the foundation of risk management. Most information will be maintained on the computer system for ease of data retrieval, to keep paper to a minimum, and to make record transfers easier and more timely.

Regulatory agencies are constantly changing guidelines, regulations, and statutes. The risk manager will monitor changing regulations and assist team members in implementing practice changes pertinent to the regulations. Agencies that may affect the organization are the JCAHO, HCFA, state licensing boards, state and federal legislative bodies, professional organizations (e.g., AORN, NIOSH), and others.

Evaluation: A major role of the risk management department is to continuously evaluate data, systems, processes, events, documents, and departments or areas for risk. This can be done through committee participation, reporting mechanisms such as patient satisfaction data and incident reports, and data trends such as needle sticks and reported medication errors, among others.

Risk will be classified as sentinel events; very high-risk, problem-prone occurrences; frequent occurrences with an impact on outcome; infrequent occurrences with an impact on outcome; trends in data that identify the potential for risk; and frequent occurrences with little effect or no change in outcome.

The risk management department will complete an investigation of any occurrence and rate the risk of the event. A further investigation will then occur, with priority given to all events that alter an outcome for a patient, a staff member, or a practitioner. The method of investigation will be determined by the event itself but could include data collection and review; health record review; committee participation; incident report investigation; making rounds in the area; consulting with specialists to assist in the investigation, including other managers, educators, insurance carriers, attorneys, and law enforcement; and, finally, processes such as root-cause analysis, case study, or peer review to determine what occurred.

Risk management will analyze those events that have altered outcomes and share the results with the appropriate leadership staff or committee, depending on the risk and confidentiality of the analysis. The leadership staff in the organization will then be responsible for changing processes or improving systems to reduce future occurrences and risk. The risk analysis will also be reported periodically to the board of directors for its overall direction. The risk management department will maintain confidential records of the analysis, including the progress taken to evaluate processes that may be causing increased risk and the suggested actions for improvement.

After the analysis is complete, the action steps will be implemented to solve problems or to improve the outcome for the parties involved. These action steps may be implemented by a variety of team members. The risk management department will track progress against those action steps and report to senior leadership the outcome results of the changes made. After changes have been made, a periodic evaluation of the success of the change will occur, and the evaluation will also be reported to senior leadership.

(Continued on next page)

Figure 11.7. *(Continued)*

Communication:

Communication of risk management functions, information, data collection, and risk assessment is an important function within the risk management plan. The priority for communication is to inform and educate employees, physicians and other providers, customers, and others of risk issues and problem-solving processes.

Although communication is a key component of risk management, the need to keep discrete information confidential is critical. Confidential information will be shared only on a need-to-know basis without exception. Risk management will determine the confidentiality of certain communication links for direct and discrete information. Communication may be directed to any or all of the following groups, as deemed appropriate: administration, medical staff, employees, patients, the board of directors, and employees.

Communication to the board of directors will be done on a quarterly basis. This communication mechanism will also include performance improvement activities related to the risk management plan.

Education:

Education regarding risk management activities, risk reduction opportunities, and other ways to improve the organization is a key element of the risk management plan. Education will occur at least quarterly and may be done in the form of: general orientation, root-cause analysis sessions, special education programs, conferences, medical staff meetings, employee staff meetings or employee forums, newsletter articles, e-mail announcements, printed media, board reports, department rounds, and informal discussions.

Risk management will actively work with all managers, learning resource center personnel, clinical educators, community members, physicians, and administrators to plan and provide appropriate educational opportunities. Risk management will be prepared to assist the organization in national regulatory changes that influence how our work is done. Educational opportunities will be sought out in the employee environment to reinforce the principles of risk reduction.

Reduction:

The outcome of any effective risk management plan is reduced risk. The problem-solving process of identification, evaluation, education, and communication will be the mechanism for reducing risk. This reduction of the risk will provide a safer environment for patients, staff, providers, and visitors. Each of the activities will identify action steps and personnel required to resolve issues. Problem-solving activities and their outcomes will be shared through appropriate activities. The medical center will also participate and collaborate with the parent organization's national risk management program through involvement in the Risk Management Incentive Program. Proven measures of risk reduction may result in lowered liability premium rates.

Areas of Focus in Fiscal Year 2001:

1. Timely incident reporting

2. Reduction of medication errors

3. Implementation of workplace violence program

4. Data trending of resuscitation outcomes

Check Your Understanding 11.3

Instructions: Choose the answer that best completes each of the following statements.

1. _____ In healthcare, risk includes _____.
   a. Only the things for which a hospital can be sued
   b. Any occurrence or circumstance that might result in a loss
   c. Only losses due to physical injuries to a patient
   d. The process used to determine whether the medical care provided to a specific patient was medically necessary

2. _____ The main functions of a risk management program are _____.
   a. Risk identification and analysis
   b. Loss prevention and reduction
   c. Claims management
   d. All of the above
   e. None of the above

3. _____ Health record documentation must include _____.
   a. The date of the entry
   b. The time of the entry
   c. The date and time of the entry
   d. None of the above

4. _____ Incident reports _____.
   a. Must be filed in the patient's health record
   b. Must be filed in duplicate in the patient's health record
   c. Should never be filed in the patient's health record
   d. Are copied and both copies are filed in the patient's health record

5. _____ Sentinel events _____.
   a. Are only reported to JCAHO when a patient has been injured
   b. Must be reported to JCAHO along with a root-cause analysis
   c. Usually describe a frequently occurring undesirable outcome
   d. Are the same as a national patient safety goal

6. _____ Patient advocacy is usually _____.
   a. Part of the quality assessment process
   b. Part of the utilization management process
   c. Part of the risk management process
   d. None of the above

7. _____ Occurrence screening _____.
   a. Is a technique used in risk management
   b. Involves reviewing health records of current and discharged patients
   c. Is performed to identify compensable events
   d. All of the above
   e. None of the above

8. _____ When treatment is discontinued, _____.
   a. No documentation of that fact needs to be recorded in the patient's health record.
   b. The physician can choose to document it or not.
   c. There must be documentation of the clinical indicators that led to the decision to cease the treatment.
   d. A verbal order is accepted in lieu of documentation.

9. ____ Patient safety must be integrated into a healthcare organization's ____.
   a. Quality assessment activities
   b. Utilization management activities
   c. Risk management activities
   d. Infection control activities
   e. All of the above

10. ____ JCAHO's National Patient Safety Goals ____.
   a. Are part of ORYX
   b. Are based on their own sentinel alerts
   c. Require a root-cause analysis
   d. Require an incident report

Recent Clinical Quality Management Initiatives

New initiatives and processes that seek to ensure high-quality care and patient safety characterize the beginning of the twenty-first century. Stemming from the IOM 1999 and 2001 reports on the quality of healthcare in America, a consensus developed around the need to use information technology as both a methodology and a pathway for managing and improving healthcare quality.

In 2001, the National Committee on Vital and Health Statistics (NCVHS) first sparked dialogue on how to exchange national health information electronically in a secure fashion. The feasibility of a national health information infrastructure (NHII) was considered as a solution for increasing patient safety and reducing medical errors in addition to increasing efficiency and containing costs.

In 2005, President Bush called for the rapid transition to the EHR. HHS compared this mission to the linking of the nation's railroads in the nineteenth century. According to HHS Secretary Mike Leavitt, standardizing, digitizing, and connecting all health records would transform the U.S. healthcare system by reducing medical errors, minimizing paperwork hassles, lowering costs, and improving quality of care (CMS 2005).

At the same time, the new **Office of the National Coordinator for Health Information Technology** (ONC) was created and the goals of widespread adoption of EHRs and health information exchange quickly identified. The resulting discussion changed NHII, an infrastructure that did not actually exist, to a more accessible and possible national health information network (NHIN). The NHIN could be created and implemented by a group of organizations within smaller geographical areas. Called regional health information organizations (RHIOs), their purpose was to "support access of near real-time information for routine and emergency care, monitor disease outbreaks and bioweapon attacks, and research and quality improvement" (Mon 2005). Other organizational models within this rapidly evolving field include local health information networks (LHINs) and sub-network organizations (SNOs).

In recent years, interest in CPOE systems has intensified. With CPOEs, physicians or hospital staffs enter medication orders directly into a computer linked to prescribing error prevention software. CPOEs make important information available at the time of physician ordering. Patient allergies, possible drug reactions and interactions, and calculations of dosages based on patient weight and age help physicians make optimal and safe ordering decisions. According to some studies, CPOEs may reduce serious medication prescribing errors in hospitals by more than 50 percent, which is significant because medication errors are believed to account for a large majority of adverse hospital events.

To date, physician resistance to CPOEs has had a negative impact on their widespread implementation. Furthermore, some researchers have expressed concern that poor computer screen design and downtimes in early CPOE systems might actually facilitate patient care errors. Despite these problems, however, it is expected that CPOEs will become a part of the overall package of technical improvements in healthcare in the coming years as more sophisticated systems replace earlier versions.

The beginning of the twenty-first century also has witnessed attempts to link clinical quality to reimbursement for health services. Recent pay-for-performance initiatives by the federal government, JCAHO, and private payers are rewarding organizations for quality outcomes. It is hoped that these funds will encourage healthcare providers to invest in technology that will improve patient care and safety.

In recent years, CMS has become an advocate for pay for performance within the Medicare Program. One of its efforts requires hospitals participating in the Medicare program to collect and report on ten proven hospital quality measures in three clinical areas to qualify for full inpatient prospective payment. Those that do not report their data on acute myocardial infarction, heart failure, and pneumonia face a four percent penalty per case. Medicare expects hospitals to compare their own data to national regional averages in order to identify areas for quality improvement. (See figure 11.8 for the ten clinical quality measures.)

In July 2005, CMS announced that it was developing further pay-for-performance guidelines for the Medicare program. Similarly, NCQA has suggested that systems be implemented to recognize and reward physicians and hospitals that demonstrate positive patient outcomes.

This type of activity began with the nation's largest employers, who early in the twenty-first century began directing their employees to highly rated healthcare organizations. They hoped that this would promote the health of their workforces while simultaneously lowering company expenses for healthcare. Boeing Company, for example, paid a higher percent of healthcare fees (after deductible) for employees who use hospitals that meet certain predefined standards than employees who choose to go elsewhere. Another program, Bridges to Excellence, was launched in 2003 by GE in partnership with other large employers to connect physician compensation and incentive payments to high levels of diabetes and cardiac care.

Finally, the early part of the twenty-first century has witnessed new and creative efforts to encourage medical error reporting. Federal legislation enacted in 2005 allows for the voluntary reporting of medical errors, serious adverse events, and their underlying causes. According to JCAHO President Dennis O'Leary, the Patient Safety and Quality Improvement Act "is a breakthrough in the blame and punishment culture that has literally held a death grip on health care. When caregivers feel safe to report errors, patients will be safer because we can learn from these events and put proven solutions into place" (JCAHO 2005b).

Figure 11.8.   Ten clinical quality measures

To receive full reimbursement from Medicare under the inpatient prospective payment system (IPPS), hospitals must report data for the following 10 quality measures to CMS:

Acute myocardial infarction

1. Acute myocardial infarction (AMI) patients without aspirin contraindications who received aspirin within 24 hours before or after hospital arrival

2. AMI patients without aspirin contraindications who are prescribed aspirin at hospital discharge

3. AMI patients with left ventricular systolic dysfunction (LVSD) and without angiotensin converting enzyme inhibitor (ACEI) contraindications who are prescribed ACEI at hospital discharge

4. AMI patients without beta blocker contraindications who received a beta blocker within 24 hours after hospital arrival

5. AMI patients without beta blocker contraindications who are prescribed a beta blocker at hospital discharge

Heart failure

6. Heart failure patients with documentation in the hospital record that left ventricular function was assessed before arrival, during hospitalization, or is planned for after discharge

7. Heart failure patients with LVSD and without ACEI contraindications who are prescribed an ACEI at hospital discharge

Pneumonia

8. Pneumonia patients who receive their first dose of antibiotics within four hours after arrival at the hospital

9. Pneumonia patients age 65 and older who were screened for pneumococcal vaccine status and were administered the vaccine prior to discharge, if indicated.

10. Pneumonia patients who had an assessment of arterial oxygenation by arterial blood gas measurement or pulse oximetry within 24 hours prior to or after arrival at the hospital.

Source: Adapted from CMS 2005.

Real-World Case

A client scheduled for a routine visit to the Maternity Care Center brought her daughter with her. The patient was taken to an exam room for a test, and the child stayed in the waiting area to watch a video. The child wandered in and out of the exam room without anyone paying much attention. A staff member who later went into the exam room to check on the patient realized that the child was missing and initiated a search of the clinic. The local police subsequently found the child at a nearby Seven-Eleven store.

Summary

Clinical quality management has traditionally included three related processes: clinical quality assessment, utilization management, and risk management. More recently, additional processes for managing clinical quality have focused on using information technology to manage and ensure patient safety. All are related in that the accurate and complete documentation of care-related information is crucial.

Communication among the staff members responsible for clinical quality management functions is especially important. Health information management staff involvement is critical in maintaining clinical databases, developing study parameters, retrieving data, and producing quality reports for review by various study teams.

Standards of clinical quality are developed and maintained by a number of organizations, including federal, state, and local government agencies; accreditation organizations; and professional medical associations. Meeting the standards published in the Medicare Conditions of Participation is especially important for acute care hospitals because they depend on reimbursement from the Medicare program for about half the services they provide. Healthcare organizations as well as individual healthcare professionals must meet state licensure and certification requirements.

Effective utilization management (UM) is critical for hospitals. It ensures that organizations use their resources efficiently and to the greatest benefit for all patients. The UM process is based on screening performed before, during, and after episodes of care. Preestablished screening criteria are used to assess the patient's severity of illness and the intensity of services the patient requires to meet his or her medical needs. Case management and discharge planning are vital tools in effective UM.

Risk management involves policies, processes, and procedures that identify potential operational and financial losses, prevent losses whenever possible, and lessen the effects of losses that cannot be prevented. Specifically, risk management involves three steps: identifying and analyzing potential risks; preventing and reducing the effects of accidents, medical errors, and other injuries and losses; and managing damage claims when losses occur. Programs related to risk management include safety management, security management, technology management, facility management, and infection control.

Several federal, state, and local laws and regulations are relevant to the practice of risk management in healthcare organizations. Examples include the Occupational Safety and Health Act, the Health Care Quality Improvement Act, the Safe Medical Devices Act, and the Health Insurance Portability and Accountability Act. State laws generally regulate the licensing of hospitals and skilled nursing facilities, the licensing of physicians and nurses, and the handling of malpractice claims. Accreditation standards also address risk management in healthcare organizations.

Risk management, clinical quality assessment, and UM all require accurate, complete, and timely health record documentation. The health record represents legal documentation of the services provided to the patient. It is one of the most important tools that clinicians and healthcare organizations have for assessing and ensuring the quality of care they provide to their patients.

Many creative and innovative attempts have been made in recent years to assess, manage, and improve the quality of care. The use of information technology to collect, integrate, and make health information available when needed for patient care is promising. Pay for better clinical performance and voluntary reporting of medical errors and adverse events are being tested and may prove effective.

References

Abdelhak, M., et al., eds. 2000. *Health Information: Management of a Strategic Resource,* 2nd ed. Philadelphia: W.B. Saunders.

Agency for Healthcare Research and Quality. 2005. National Guideline Clearinghouse. Available online from guideline.gov.

Agency for Healthcare Research and Quality. 2005. Clinical Practice Guidelines. Available online from ahrq.gov/clinic.

American Osteopathic Association. 2005. osteopathic.org.

American Society for Healthcare Risk Management. 2005. ashrm.org

Barton, E.J. 1997. Claims and litigation. In *Risk Management Handbook for Health Care Organizations,* 2nd ed., edited by R. Carroll. Chicago: American Hospital Publishing.

Bryant, J.M. 1997. Development of the risk management program. In *Risk Management Handbook for Health Care Organizations,* 2nd ed., edited by R. Carroll. Chicago: American Hospital Publishing.

Bryant, S.W. 2004. *Understanding JCAHO's Priority Focus Areas.* Marblehead, MA: HCPro.

Carroll, R., ed. 1997. *Risk Management Handbook for Health Care Organizations,* 2nd ed. Chicago: American Hospital Publishing.

Center for Case Management. 2001. cfcm.com.

Centers for Medicare and Medicaid Services. 2005. cms.gov.

Commission on Accreditation of Rehabilitation Facilities. 2005. carf.org.

Department of Health and Human Services. Available online from oig.hhs.gov/oei/reports/oei-03-01-00430.pdf.

Genovich-Richards, J. 1997. Selecting quality initiatives and methodologies. In *Improving Quality: A Guide to Effective Programs,* 2nd ed., edited by C. G. Meisenheimer. Gaithersburg, MD: Aspen Publishers.

Graham, N. 1990. *Quality Assurance in Hospitals: Strategies for Assessment and Implementation.* Rockville, MD: Aspen Publishers.

Hagg-Rickert, S.R. 1997. Elements of a risk management program. In *Risk Management Handbook for Health Care Organizations,* 2nd ed., edited by Roberta Carroll. Chicago: American Hospital Publishing.

Health Plan Employer Data and Information Set (HEDIS). ncqa.org.

Hope, W.T. 1997. The risk management process. In *Risk Management Handbook for Health Care Organizations,* 2nd ed., edited by R. Carroll. Chicago: American Hospital Publishing.

Horn, S., ed. 1994. *Clinical Practice Improvement: A New Technology for Developing Cost-Effective Quality Health Care,* Vol. 1. Washington, DC: Faulkner & Gray.

Houk, C. 2003 (Sept 4–5). From dispute resolution to conflict management. Presentation at NADRAC 2004 Conference, Sydney, AU. Available online from ag.gov.au.

Institute of Medicine. 2005. iom.edu.

Institute of Medicine. 2001. *Crossing the Quality Chasm: New Health System for the 21st Century.* Washington, DC: National Academy Press.

Joint Commission on Accreditation of Healthcare Organizations. 2005a. jcaho.org.

Joint Commission on Accreditation of Healthcare Organizations. 2005b (July 29). News release: Joint Commission hails enactment of patient safety and quality improvement act of 2005. Available online from jcaho.org/news+room/news+release+archives/nr_7_29_05.htm.

Joint Commission on Accreditation of Healthcare Organizations. 2000. *2001 Comprehensive Accreditation Manual for Hospitals.* Oakbrook Terrace, IL: JCAHO.

Joint Commission on Accreditation of Healthcare Organizations. 1999. *2000–2001 Comprehensive Accreditation Manual for Ambulatory Care.* Oakbrook Terrace, IL: JCAHO.

Joint Commission on Accreditation of Healthcare Organizations. 1998. *1998–2000 Comprehensive Accreditation Manual for Health Care Networks.* Oakbrook Terrace, IL: JCAHO.

Kohn, L. T., J. M. Corrigan, and M. S. Donaldson, eds. 1999. *To Err Is Human: Building a Safer Health System.* Washington, DC: National Academy Press.

Larsen-Denning, Lorie, et al. 1997. Clinical practice guidelines. In *Risk Management Handbook for Health Care Organizations,* 2nd ed., edited by Roberta Carroll. Chicago: American Hospital Publishing.

Licklighter, L. 1997. Safety and security. In *Risk Management Handbook for Health Care Organizations,* 2nd ed., edited by Roberta Carroll. Chicago: American Hospital Publishing.

Longo, D. 1990. Integrating quality assurance into a quality management plan. In *Quality Assurance in Hospitals: Strategies for Assessment and Implementation,* edited by N. Graham. Rockville, MD: Aspen Publishers.

McWay, D. 1997. *Legal Aspects of Health Information Management.* Albany, NY: Delmar.

Meisenheimer, C.G., ed. 1997. *Improving Quality: A Guide to Effective Programs,* 2nd ed. Gaithersburg, MD: Aspen Publishers.

Mon, D.T. 2005 (June). An Update on the NHIN and RHIOs. *Journal of American Health Information Management Association* 76(6):56-57,59.

Morrison, J. 1993. Total quality within the VA healthcare system: A case study. In *The Textbook of Total Quality in Healthcare,* edited by A. Al-Assaf and J. Schmele. Delray Beach, FL: St. Lucie Press.

National Committee for Quality Assurance. 2005. ncqa.com.

National Committee for Quality Assurance. 2000. *2001 Accreditation Manual.* Washington, DC: NCQA.

National Committee for Quality Assurance. 2000. *2001 HEDIS: Technical Specifications,* Vol. 2. Washington, DC: NCQA.

Office of Inspector General. 2005. Consecutive Medicare Inpatient Stays. Available online from oig.hhs.gov/oei/reports/oei-03-01-00430.pdf.

Pearson, S.D., Goulart-Fisher, D., and Lee, T.H. 1995 (Dec. 15). Critical pathways as a strategy for improving care: Problems and potential. *Annals of Internal Medicine* 123(12):941–948.

Scully, P. 1997. Statutes, standards, and regulations. In *Risk Management Handbook for Health Care Organizations,* 2nd ed., edited by Roberta Carroll. Chicago: American Hospital Publishing.

Sedwick, J. 1997. The risk manager role. In *Risk Management Handbook for Health Care Organizations,* 2nd ed., edited by Roberta Carroll. Chicago: American Hospital Publishing.

Shaw, P., et al. 2003. *Performance Improvement in Healthcare: A Programmed Learning Approach.* Chicago: AHIMA.

Smith, C., and M. Dougherty. 2001. Practice brief: Documentation requirements for acute inpatient records. *Journal of American Health Information Management Association* 72(3):327–28.

Spath, P. 2001. Reporting quality management results to the board. *The Quality Resource,* the Newsletter of the Quality Management Section of the American Health Information Management Association. Chicago: AHIMA.

Trombly, S.T. 1997. Technology management. In *Risk Management Handbook for Health Care Organizations,* 2nd ed., edited by Roberta Carroll. Chicago: American Hospital Publishing.

Watkins, S. 1999. Lecture Notes for HIT 240: Clinical Quality Assessment and Improvement. Santa Barbara, CA: Santa Barbara City College Health Information Technology Program.

West, J.C. 1997. Occupational and environmental risk exposures for health care facilities. In *Risk Management Handbook for Health Care Organizations,* 2nd ed., edited by Roberta Carroll. Chicago: American Hospital Publishing.

Chapter 12
Performance Improvement

Andrea Weatherby White, PhD

Learning Objectives

- To identify and explain performance improvement (PI) principles

- To understand the various philosophies and components of PI developed by quality management masters

- To understand how individuals or teams can use PI models to successfully plan, implement, and evaluate improvement initiatives

- To recognize how supervisors can use PI principles and concepts to motivate and manage their employees

- To discuss various PI tools and techniques that can be used to facilitate communication, identify root causes, and collect, analyze, and report data

- To understand how information management technologies enable and facilitate more effective PI activities

Key Terms

Affinity grouping

Brainstorming

Cause-and-effect diagram

Change agent

Checksheet

Common-cause variation

Customer

Dashboards

Fishbone diagram

Flowchart

Force-field analysis

Histogram

Inputs

Multivoting technique

Nominal group technique

Outcome indicators

Outputs

Pareto chart

Performance indicators

Process indicators

Processes

PDSA cycle

Root-cause analysis

Run chart

Scatter diagram

Scorecards

Special-cause variation

Statistical process control chart

Storyboard

Structure indicators

Introduction

Healthcare is an exciting and challenging field in which to work. Newspapers and magazines carry stories about new medical advances almost every week. Unfortunately, they also carry stories about medical errors almost as frequently. The public and those individuals working in healthcare have become increasingly aware of the problems healthcare faces and the urgent need to improve the way healthcare organizations and the people who work in them do business. Patients and their families, physicians, accreditation organizations, and communities are calling for improvements in the quality of healthcare services. As discussed in previous chapters, employers, government-sponsored health programs, and other third-party payers are demanding greater financial and patient safety accountability. The nation's changing demographic makeup and costly advances in healthcare technology have created perplexing social and ethical issues. In the face of these trends, healthcare organizations are working hard to provide high-quality healthcare services, and at the same time, control the cost of those services.

Healthcare organizations are using a number of strategies to meet the challenge of greater accountability. One effective strategy is to improve performance across a number of dimensions. The primary goal of performance improvement in healthcare is to improve customer service and patient care and simultaneously maintain the organization's financial stability. This chapter focuses on performance improvement and the strategies being used to facilitate it.

Theory into Practice

In the past, medical errors generally were kept quiet to avoid alarming the public or creating public relations problems for healthcare facilities and professionals. When mistakes were revealed, a great deal of finger-pointing followed, and the individuals involved were punished. Obviously, the incentive in this type of climate was to cover up mistakes. There was a climate of fear around errors.

Today, reports of medical mistakes are becoming more commonplace. Recent news stories have increased public concern about medical errors and their effect on patients. Efforts are under way to investigate the causes of errors and change systems to prevent similar errors in the future, rather than just covering them up. There is much greater emphasis on identifying the root causes of medical mistakes and less emphasis on punishing the individuals involved. We are working in healthcare to address mistakes openly as a way of preventing similar problems in the future.

The following fictional case was based on a number of actual events. It was developed by McClanahan, Goodwin, and Houser (1999). The events have been condensed for this chapter. It illustrates how errors occur as a result of system failures rather than the failure of any one individual.

The emergency department staff was busy tending a large number of patients. Mr. Murphy arrived at the hospital via ambulance a short time before a second ambulance arrived with another patient, Mr. Jenkins. Mr. Murphy was a heavyset, middle-aged man who had fallen on his right hip in the locker room at a golf course. He was in a great deal of pain. Mr. Jenkins was a frail, elderly patient who had fallen on his right hip in his room at a long-term care facility.

When the two patients arrived, the admissions registrar was behind in making patient identification bands. The equipment for making the bands was old, and the registrar had other duties that demanded her attention. As a result, neither Mr. Murphy nor Mr. Jenkins received an ID band until some time after they were evaluated. Tests were ordered for both men, including x-rays of their right hips. The nursing staff entered orders for the tests into the computer.

Mr. Murphy went to the radiology department first. By the time he arrived, a requisition for an x-ray of a right hip had printed out on the department's printer. Because Mr. Murphy did not have an ID band, the technician was unable to cross-check the name on the band with the name on the requisition as required by standard procedure. He also did not ask the patient for his name. The technician assumed that Mr. Murphy was the right patient because the patient transporter confirmed that the patient needed an x-ray of his right hip. However, the x-ray requisition that had come through was actually the requisition for Mr. Jenkins. That is how Mr. Jenkins's name came to be shown on Mr. Murphy's x-rays.

In the meantime, Mr. Jenkins, who was fairly incoherent, had been transported to the radiology department. A different technician had just returned from lunch. She retrieved the requisition order with Mr. Murphy's name on it from the printer. She then confirmed with the transporter that the patient lying on the gurney was there for an x-ray of the right hip. Unaware that another patient had had an x-ray done on his right hip while she was at lunch, the second technician performed the study and placed Mr. Murphy's name on Mr. Jenkins's x-ray. Thus, both x-rays were labeled with the wrong patient's name.

The radiologist called the emergency department and reported that the x-rays with Mr. Murphy's name on them indicated a fracture. The x-rays with Mr. Jenkins's name did not reveal a fracture; however, other studies performed on the real Mr. Jenkins revealed other medical problems. Mr. Jenkins was admitted to the hospital, but not for treatment of a fractured hip. Because the x-rays labeled Murphy revealed a fracture, the real Mr. Murphy also was admitted with a diagnosis of right hip fracture. The radiologist had seen neither Mr. Murphy nor Mr. Jenkins and had not been given clinical information about either patient. Had the radiologist been given clinical information, he might have noticed that Mr. Murphy's x-ray revealed very little soft tissue even though the patient was obese and that Mr. Jenkins's x-ray showed a great deal of soft tissue even though the patient was frail and thin.

Mr. Murphy was referred to the orthopedist. The orthopedist's physician's assistant (PA) conducted the preoperative history and physical examination. He noted a shortening of the right leg and an internal rotation in Mr. Murphy's medical record. Although the orthopedist had spoken to his PA about inadequately performed examinations in the past, he had not reported these performance problems to anyone else in the hospital. Even if he had, the hospital had no tracking system for performance data on allied health personnel. The orthopedist, who was very busy that day, did not conduct an examination of his own but, instead, relied on the PA's findings and scheduled Mr. Murphy for surgery the next day.

In the meantime, Mr. Jenkins continued to complain of pain in his right hip and could not put weight on his right leg. A second x-ray revealed a fracture. Despite the discrepancy in findings, however, no immediate investigation was done. The case was flagged for retrospective review to be conducted some time in the future.

The next day, Mr. Murphy went to the operating room. Although the x-rays were available in the surgical suite, they were not posted on the view box. Therefore, no discrepancy was noted between the lack of soft tissue on the x-ray and Mr. Murphy's rotund physique. Surgery was initiated. Upon discovering no fracture, the orthopedist quickly stopped the surgery and called risk management to determine what should be done next.

This case clearly demonstrates several system problems, as well as individual lapses in judgment. The following system elements contributed to the unnecessary surgery:

- Outdated equipment for making identification bands
- Inadequate mechanisms for managing heavy patient volume
- Inadequate procedures for verifying patient identification
- Lapses in communication between departments and technicians
- Inadequate performance-tracking mechanisms for nonphysician providers

Definition of Performance Improvement

The word *performance* has been defined as "the execution of an activity or pattern of behavior; the application of inherent or learned capabilities to complete a process according to prescribed specifications or standards" (Meisenheimer 1997, 700). Performance is not easy to measure because a data element may measure one component of performance, but not all the components inherent in performance. Performance is measured using one or more **performance indicators.** These indicators measure certain aspects of performance. For example, performance can be measured against financial indicators, such as the average cost per laboratory test, or productivity indicators, such as the number of patients seen per physician per day. There are numerous ways to measure various aspects of performance, but they all require time and effort. Therefore, when performance is measured, it is important to measure the most important aspects of performance, such as patient safety, patient outcome, and cost.

The term *performance improvement* (PI) can be defined as a "process for involving personnel in planning and executing a continuous flow of improvements to provide quality health care that meets or exceeds expectations" (McLauglin and Kaluzny 2006, 3). Although a number of terms and acronyms are frequently used to represent this concept (for example, continuous quality improvement [CQI] and total quality management [TQM]), this chapter uses performance improvement. Numerous improvement models and quality philosophies have been developed over the years. The key feature of the PI process performed in today's healthcare organizations is that it is a continuous cycle of planning and designing, measurement, analysis, and monitoring and evaluating.

Performance Improvement in Today's Healthcare Organizations

Performance improvement is intended to improve the quality and delivery of healthcare services. The traditional approach to ensuring quality was to view it as the absence of defects. In other words, quality was defined as performance that had attained a predetermined level of acceptability. Specific indicators helped organizations to determine whether they had reached that level.

For example, one indicator of quality might be that a physician sees patients within thirty minutes after their arrival at the facility. The organization could measure the minutes that it took from the time the patient stated his or her name to the time the physician first saw the patient. As long as patients were seen within that thirty-minute time frame, the organization could assume that it was providing high-quality care. No attempts would be made to analyze the process or take corrective action unless the number of minutes increased beyond the thirty-minute threshold. In this traditional approach, organizations actively addressed quality and performance issues only when they failed to meet the level of quality they had defined for themselves.

Donabedian (1988) contributed significantly to our understanding of measuring quality. He recognized that quality had multiple dimensions that needed to be measured using various types of indicators. He proposed three types of quality indicators:

- **Structure indicators,** which measure the attributes of the setting, such as number and qualifications of the staff, adequacy of equipment and facilities, and adequacy of organizational policies and procedures

- **Process indicators,** which measure the actual provision of care, from conducting appropriate tests, to making the diagnosis, to actually carrying out the treatment

- **Outcome indicators,** which measure the actual results of care for patients and populations, including patient and family satisfaction

In addition to identifying types of quality indicators, Donabedian introduced the idea that quality has both a technical and interpersonal dimension. The *technical* dimension recognizes that caregivers must have the knowledge and judgment to arrive at an appropriate strategy for providing service and the technical skills to carry it out. The *interpersonal* aspect recognizes that caregivers must have the communication skills and social attributes necessary to serve patients appropriately. The interpersonal aspect of quality recognizes the importance of empathy, honesty, respectfulness, tactfulness, and sensitivity to others. Donabedian acknowledged that it was far easier to measure quality's technical dimension than its interpersonal dimension.

The contemporary approach to PI is much more proactive than the traditional quality management approach. Although PI uses several traditional quality management techniques such as quality indicators, its primary focus is on continually making small, targeted changes for improvement, which over time, lead to significant improvement. Performance improvement is not a philosophy that is satisfied with the status quo; it is not based on the "if it ain't broke, don't fix it" assumption. Nor does PI operate on the theory of identifying "bad apples," where one conducts inspections to identify defects (that is, those bad apples that destroy the lot). PI does not attempt to find an individual to blame and punish for lapses in quality.

PI is based on the assumption that organizations should continuously and systematically identify and test small, planned changes in processes and systems. Over time, the theory proposes, these changes will improve the quality of care provided to patients (Berwick 1989). Opportunities for improvement are identified by gathering and analyzing data on an ongoing basis.

Performance improvement relies on effective teamwork and group processes. Teams accomplish change by striving to understand the elements of a system and identifying the root causes of potential problems. They then brainstorm, select, and test changes that might improve the process.

Check Your Understanding 12.1

Instructions: Indicate whether the following statements are true or false (T or F).

1. ____ Continuous performance improvement identifies the person responsible for a problem so that he or she can be held accountable and, if necessary, punished.

2. ____ TQM, CQI, and PI are acronyms for concepts based on the same general principles.

3. ____ An example of a structural indicator is the timely dictation of an operative report.

4. ____ Patient satisfaction is a useful outcome indicator.

5. ____ An example of a process indicator is whether or not health professionals have the appropriate credentials.

6. ____ According to Donabedian, healthcare professionals must have both technical skills and interpersonal skills in order to provide high-quality care.

7. ____ The traditional method of ensuring quality involves inspecting to make sure that indicator values are within an acceptable range and, when they are not, taking action to bring them in line.

8. ____ Continuous performance improvement promotes looking for ways to improve existing processes, even those processes that meet current performance standards.

9. ____ Opportunities for improvement are identified by gathering and analyzing data on an ongoing basis.

10. ____ Improvements in performance are best carried out by individual employees working alone in their areas of responsibility.

11. ____ The goal of performance improvement is to primarily improve customer service and patient care regardless of the cost to the organization.

12. ____ PI advocates that medical errors should be openly investigated so systems can change and problems can be corrected.

Principles and Concepts of Performance Improvement

Performance improvement is based on several fundamental principles, including:

- The structure of a system determines its performance. Therefore, problems are more often within systems than within individual people.

- All systems demonstrate variation. Some variation occurs because of common causes and some because of special causes.

- Improvements rely on the collection and analysis of data that increase knowledge.

- The focus is on customers, both internal and external.

- PI requires the commitment and support of top administration.

- PI works best when leaders and employees know and share the organization's mission, vision, and values.

- PI efforts take time and require a big investment in people.

- Excellent teamwork is essential.

- Communication must be open, honest, and multidirectional.

- Success must be celebrated to encourage more success.

The Problem Is Usually the System

As the case study at the beginning of this chapter showed, problems in patient care and other areas of the healthcare organization are usually symptoms of shortcomings inherent in a system or a process. Kelly defines a system as "a collection of parts that interact with each other to form an interdependent whole" (2003, 60). Practically everything one can think of (both entities and processes) can be viewed as systems. Human beings are systems (very complicated systems made up of a lot of subsystems). Families are systems. Shopping for the family's weekly groceries can be viewed as a system. Healthcare organizations are very large systems. Each department in a healthcare facility is a system with numerous subsystems.

Every system has **inputs.** The system **processes** the inputs and eventually produces **outputs.** One system's outputs may then become inputs for another system.

The hospital's admitting department is an example of a system. When a patient enters the hospital, he or she presents to the admitting clerk. The clerk uses a computer to collect data for the admitting system. The patient with knowledge of his or her condition, the admitting clerk with knowledge of the admitting process, and the computer with its admitting template can all be considered inputs for the admitting system. When the clerk begins asking for the patient's address, insurance coverage, and reason for admission and the patient begins responding, the admitting process is under way. The output of the process is the patient's admission to the hospital and a completed face sheet for his or her medical record. These outputs can then be viewed as inputs into the next system in the hospital, the patient care system.

Systems thinking is a vital part of performance improvement. Systems thinking requires individuals to think about patterns and interrelationships rather than simple units. Performance problems often occur because sources of problems were actually built into the system (Batalden and Stoltz 1993). Improvements must address the system's shortcomings. For example, if the admitting clerk had to follow a series of cumbersome procedures to obtain data about referring physicians in order to enter them into the admitting template, this could seriously affect the clerk's performance and produce a less-than-desirable output. Examples of poor-quality output might be inaccurate information or long delays in admissions. The problems in admitting then might create problems for other systems in the hospital.

Variation Is Constant

A second important principle to understand is that every system has some degree of variation built into it. No system produces the exact same output every time. It would be desirable to reduce variation within systems as much as possible so that system output could be more predictable or better controlled. However, there will always be some variation, albeit sometimes minor (Omachonu 1999). Variation that is inherent within the system is known as **common-cause variation.** For example, when a nurse takes a patient's blood pressure, she may believe that she is performing the procedure in exactly the same way every time, but she will get slightly different readings each time. Although the blood pressure cuff, the patient, and the nurse are all the same inputs into the system, variations can occur. For example, the cuff may be applied to a different place on the patient's arm. The patient may have a slightly different emotional or physiological status at the time of the measurement. The nurse may have a different level of focus or concentration. Any one of these factors, plus countless others, can affect the values obtained.

It is important to recognize that not every variation is a defect. The variation may just be an example of common-cause variation found inherently in the process.

Some variations are caused by factors outside the system. This type of variation is known as **special-cause variation.** If the special cause produces a negative effect, we will want to identify the special cause and eliminate it. If the special cause produces a positive effect, we will want to reinforce it so the good effect will continue. An example of this type of variation occurs when a patient is taking blood pressure medication and there is a substantial drop in the patient's values. The medication has caused the decrease in blood pressure values and can clearly be considered a special cause. In this situation, the variation is intentional and desired. In other situations, the variation may produce an undesirable and unintentional effect. For example, if a patient is upset about a phone call he received just before the nurse came in to take his vitals, his blood pressure could be exceptionally high. The change in values occurred due to a special cause (the phone call) and resulted in a blood pressure reading much higher than normally expected.

Similar examples of special-cause variation can be identified in our hospital systems. In the health information management (HIM) department, for example, there is always some common cause variation in the number of records that can be coded each day. On a day when one of the regular coders is out sick, however, the number of records coded might drop significantly. This would be an example of special-cause variation. As much as is possible, the goal should be to remove special causes if they are creating an undesirable effect.

Data Are Important

Data drive performance improvement. Omachonu states that "the ability to collect, analyze, and use data is a vital component of a successful performance improvement process. Healthcare organizations that do not devote sufficient attention to data collection may be able to speak of only marginal success in their process improvement journey" (1999, 71).

In the past, healthcare organizations relied on unsupported assumptions about which processes were functioning well and which ones were not. Without real data, however, no objective and accurate assessment can take place. Collecting data provides information about the current level of customer satisfaction, potential areas for improvement efforts, and the effectiveness of changes already implemented.

A number of methods can be used in data collection. PI activities must plan the best method for obtaining timely, accurate, and relevant data. Examples of data collection methods and instruments include retrospective record review with specific quality criteria, written surveys, direct observation, and individual or focus group interviews.

After adequate data have been collected, they must be carefully analyzed. Improvement efforts must be built on knowledge, and knowledge is gained through data analysis.

The Focus Is on the Customer

Many organizations and quality experts define *quality* as meeting or exceeding customer expectations. The term **customer** is used frequently in performance management activities. *External customers* are the people outside the organization for whom it provides services. For example, the external customers of a hospital would include patients, physicians, and third-party payers. Organizations also have *internal customers.* Employees are internal customers. They receive services from other areas in the organization that make it possible for them to do their jobs. For example, a nurse on an intensive care unit would be an internal customer of the hospital pharmacy. The nurse depends on the pharmacy to provide the medications needed to fill the physicians' orders for his or her patients.

Employees in one system or subsystem use the outputs from other systems or subsystems of the organization as inputs to their own system or subsystem. The employees then produce new outputs, which in turn may become inputs for still another system or subsystem. In this way, the performance of one system can affect the performance of many others.

The primary focus of PI efforts must be on the customer. The expectations and needs of both external and internal customers must be kept in mind throughout the PI process. Those involved in PI projects must know and understand their customers and involve them in the process so they can express their needs.

Support Must Come from the Top Down

PI as a vital, continuous process must be built into the organization's culture. The executive leaders of the organization must believe in its value in order for it to permeate the entire organization. Moreover, they must ensure that their management teams are well versed in the principles and techniques of continual performance improvement.

Training for managers and supervisors can be provided by outside consultants or through in-service training. Managers and supervisors then can train their own employees and model the continuous improvement philosophy. Every employee must understand the importance of continually improving processes so as to provide better service to the organization's customers.

The Organization Must Have a Shared Vision

The organization's executive leaders and board of directors are responsible for developing and communicating a clear vision of the organization's future. The organization's vision, mission, and values set its direction and support the norms it considers important. They communicate a constancy of purpose. Vision, mission, and values statements help employees to understand the vision and embrace it as their own. The statements also guide employees as they make their own contributions to the organization by fulfilling their professional responsibilities.

Staff and Management Must Be Involved in the Process

As mentioned earlier, executive leaders must be committed to the philosophy of continuous improvement and work to ensure that every manager and every employee are committed to its value. This commitment demands an investment in people and requires substantial time and training. PI depends on everyone in the organization actively seeking to meet internal and external customers' spoken or anticipated needs.

This is particularly important for employees who have direct contact with external customers. These employees are perhaps in the best position to recognize which needs of the customer are not being met. They often offer helpful ideas for improvement. It works to the organization's benefit when staff feel empowered to make a difference for their fellow workers and the patients they serve.

Teamwork Is Vital

The work of PI is accomplished through teamwork. Katzenbach and Smith define a team as "a small number of people with complimentary skills who are committed to a common purpose, set of performance goals, and approach for which they hold themselves mutually accountable" (1993, 112). PI teams should involve people from all levels of the organization and from any area that plays a role in the process to be improved. Each team member can contribute his or her own knowledge and unique perspective on the process.

The person who interacts most frequently with the customers often is the one who knows whether their needs are being met. Involving individuals who have different roles in a particular process can result in a better understanding of the process and the elements of the process that need improvement. A good team is made up of people with different skills and areas of expertise. It also relies on effective communication among its members.

Effective teams are composed of members who play varying roles. Some members play roles that contribute to accomplishing the task at hand. Examples of these roles include initiating and contributing, seeking information, providing information, coordinating, and evaluating. A good team also needs members who nurture the team and play roles that build and sustain its efforts. Examples of these roles include encouraging members, gate-keeping for discussions, summarizing perspectives, and building consensus among team members.

Good teams do not just happen. Getting to know each other, learning each other's strengths and shortcomings, and learning how to effectively use the skills and knowledge each member brings to the team take time.

Teams generally go through predictable stages as they develop:

1. The *forming* phase occurs when team members are first introduced. This stage is usually cordial, but not very productive regarding team output.

2. The *storming* phase occurs as team members learn whom they feel comfortable with and whom they do not. This phase is often a time of conflict and little productivity.

3. The *norming* phase occurs as team members better know each other and have come to understand the values, expectations, and "rules" of behavior within the group. At this point, the team begins to function fairly well.

4. The *performing* phase occurs when team members trust each other's abilities and talents. The team is now able to be creative and productive, to energize its members, and to produce results that far exceed what individual team members working alone could do (Fried and Carpenter, 2006).

Training Is Essential

For individuals to work in teams and carry out the functions of a PI program, training is essential. Employees must be trained in the specific aspects of PI and be thoroughly introduced to the principles and practices of how to improve the way people work. This may include learning about issue identification, problem solving, and other techniques.

However, simply understanding PI is not sufficient. Employees also must know and appreciate the elements of teamwork. This means recognizing the interdependence, shared responsibility, and accountability for outcomes of all team members. Training also must encompass team management. For example, teams must develop a charter, identify team norms, use techniques to arrive at team consensus, and evaluate their productivity and cohesiveness.

Setting Goals Is Crucial

All PI programs must have a set of goals. Goals are essentially targets that the organization and/or team strives to achieve. They should be specific and define measurable end results. An example of an organizational goal might be: "To provide high-quality patient care that is cost-effective."

After goals are established, it is important to identify specific, measurable objectives that can be completed within a certain time frame. An objective associated with the above goal might be: "By the end of the year, a high-quality, cost-effective care program will be designed for the management of diabetes patients."

Effective Communication Is Important

Effective communication is absolutely essential for the PI process to work. It must exist at all levels of the organization and in all directions. Managers must hear from staff how the organization is functioning. Staff must feel comfortable in telling management when things are going well and when there are problems. This level of communication requires trust and respect for all individuals and the recognition that everyone wants to do the best job possible.

Obviously, openly identifying and discussing problems is not always comfortable or easy. However, an organization that is committed to serving its customers must view problems as opportunities for improvement. The Japanese call it *kaizen:* the continuous search for opportunities for all processes to get better (Imai 1986). Defects are looked on as treasures because a chance for improvement lies in the discovery of imperfection (Berwick 1989). None of this can happen without effective communication.

Effective communication is two-way communication. It requires clear, articulate, and tactful speaking. Even more important, it requires careful, attentive listening and understanding. Organizations must take the time to listen to their customers, both internal and external, so they can hear information about where services need improvement.

Success Should Be Celebrated

Although PI demands that organizations focus on identifying and addressing problems, it also must celebrate the organization's successes. A celebration of success communicates to everyone that the participants' efforts are applauded, that success can occur from such efforts, and that others should be encouraged to participate in PI initiatives. Those people involved in improving the process need to be recognized and appreciated. One of the reasons organizations collect and analyze data is to let them know when they have reasons to celebrate. Achieving service excellence is certainly a great reason to celebrate.

One method for celebrating success is to create and display a poster for everyone in the organization to see. The poster is called a **storyboard.** It explains the problem, the plan for determining and testing a change for improvement, and the results of the effort.

Quality Masters

A number of individuals have contributed to the current philosophy of continuous performance improvement. This section discusses the contributions of Walter Shewhart, W. Edwards Deming, Joseph Juran, Armand Feigenbaum, Philip Crosby, and Brian Joiner.

Walter A. Shewhart

Walter Shewhart was a statistician and research engineer for Bell Laboratory from 1925 until 1956. During that time, he pioneered the use of a quality control mechanism called statistical process control. Its purpose was to reduce variation in processes. Shewhart was the first person to suggest that two types of variation could be at work in a process: variation that was the result of chance, and variation that was the result of a definable cause. He used this method to improve the stability of processes.

He also was the first to develop what he called the "act of control." This concept evolved into the plan–do–check–act cycle (discussed later in this chapter). W. Edwards Deming built on Shewhart's work.

W. Edwards Deming

W. Edwards Deming was an American statistician. He is often credited with revitalizing the Japanese economy after the Second World War. He wrote the book *Out of Chaos* in 1983. In his book, he described his methods for improving quality. Like Shewhart, Deming discussed variation and identified two types: common-cause variation (variation caused by chance) and special-cause variation (variation assigned a cause).

Deming believed that quality must be built in to the product. He made a number of controversial statements about standard management techniques. For example, he declared that he did not believe in performance appraisals, management by objectives, or work standards.

Deming also developed a fourteen-point plan to help executives lead their organizations. Several of his points can be recognized in the principles of performance improvement. He believed that senior administrators need to communicate a constancy of purpose in which the vision and mission statements are made known. He proposed focusing on the process and not the results. Another of the fourteen points was that organizations must not rely on inspection for defects but, rather, continually work to improve production and service.

According to Deming, the organization's leadership also must provide training, education, and self-improvement opportunities for employees and work to help employees achieve excellence in their jobs. Fear must be driven out of the organization because it impedes self-actualization. Barriers among departments and staff must be broken because barriers prevent people from communicating effectively and processes from being improved.

Joseph M. Juran

Joseph Juran also consulted with the Japanese in the 1950s and wrote several books on quality control. In the 1980s, he claimed that management could control over 80 percent of quality defects by using the three central principles of quality: planning, control, and improvement. He believed that training and hands-on management are basic requirements for meeting the needs of customers.

Armand F. Feigenbaum

Armand Feigenbaum built on Deming's statistical approach. In the early 1980s, he emphasized the necessity of integrating the functions of total quality control. Feigenbaum stated that the planning, design, and setup of the product or service must be integrated with its production and distribution. In turn, the product's production and distribution must be integrated with training, data analysis, and user feedback. Thus, customers and suppliers are all incorporated into the total quality concept. The goal is to meet the expectations and requirements of the organizations' customers.

Philip B. Crosby

Philip Crosby was a quality consultant working in the 1980s. He did not agree with his predecessors' focus on statistics. Instead, he proposed the concepts of zero defects and conformance to requirements. Crosby also proposed four absolutes of quality:

- Do it right the first time.

- Defect prevention is the only acceptable approach.

- Zero defects is the only performance standard.

- The cost of quality is the only measure of quality. This means that it is less costly to produce a high-quality product the first time than to manage the losses that result from producing a low-quality product.

Brian Joiner

Brian Joiner, also consulting in the 1980s, maintained that quality begins at the top and funnels down through the organization. He developed the Joiner triangle. This concept has three basic elements:

- Quality to ensure customer satisfaction and loyalty

- A scientific approach to root out underlying causes of problems

- The all-one-team method that encourages and empowers employees to work together to break down departmental barriers and creates buy-in to improvement, ownership in the process, and commitment to quality

---

Check Your Understanding 12.2

Instructions: Indicate whether the following statements are true or false (T or F) and correct the statement if it is false.

1. _____ Systems are entities that include inputs, processes, outputs, and feedback.

2. _____ All systems include some inherent variation known as common-cause variation.

3. _____ The manager's job is to remove all inherent variation from processes.

4. _____ Special-cause variation can sometimes produce good results in a system.

5. _____ PI activities require the collection and analysis of data.

6. ____ An example of an internal customer of a healthcare organization is the patient.

7. ____ Employees also are important customers of healthcare organizations.

Instructions: Match the quality masters listed below with the quality concepts for which they are known. Some masters are known for more than one concept.

a. Philip Crosby
b. W. Edwards Deming
c. Armand Feigenbaum
d. Brian Joiner
e. Joseph Juran
f. Walter Shewhart

1. ____ Two types of variation exist in systems: one type is caused by chance, and one type can be assigned a cause.

2. ____ Fear must be driven out of organizations so that ideas and efforts can flourish.

3. ____ Do things right the first time.

4. ____ Training and hands-on management are absolutely essential.

5. ____ Customers and suppliers are all part of the total quality concept. The goal is to meet customer expectations.

6. ____ PI must begin with top leadership and funnel down through the organization.

Managing Quality

Quality within an organization does not just happen. Quality and the entire PI cycle need to be managed. This means that the usual management processes such as planning, directing, and controlling must be applied to PI programs. This section examines the principal elements of performance improvement.

Organizational Components of Performance Improvement

To be successful in implementing PI programs, healthcare organizations may have to restructure and create a new learning culture to accommodate the enormous change and competition that exists in today's environment. Changes in customer expectations and the way that healthcare is financed demand organizational restructuring. Traditional, hierarchical management methods do not necessarily meet the needs of today's customer, the organization's employees, or the organization's operation.

PI must be encompassed in an environment of cooperation. It is most successful in organizations that have an interdisciplinary organizational management approach. As discussed previously, shared vision is one of the cornerstones of a successful PI program. A shared vision puts everyone, including the board, upper management, and employees, in the same ballpark.

In addition to an enterprise-wide vision, a shared leadership framework is essential for implementing PI. Shared leadership essentially means that organizations ensure that all employees participate in an integrated, continuous PI program. Various organizational frameworks or structures can be developed that encourage shared leadership. One suggested framework includes the following components:

- *Governing Board of Directors (GBOD):* The GBOD has overall responsibility and accountability for the successful operation of the organization.

- *Quality Management Board (QMB)*: The QMB has responsibility for the PI program throughout the organization.

- *Service Improvement Council (SIC):* The SIC is appointed by the QMB and has responsibility for all clinical patient services within the organization.

- *Practice Improvement Council (PIC)*: The PIC has responsibility for the practice improvement of all employees.

- *Governance Improvement Council (GIC):* The GIC has responsibility for the organization's day-to-day governance.

- *Performance Measurement Council (PMC):* The PMC has responsibility for receiving, collecting, and packaging all of the organization's data.

Changes in organizational structure to a shared leadership environment create a new organizational culture of shared vision, responsibility, and accountability. Because every employee is a vital part of this shared leadership, this type of environment helps to increase employee motivation and empowerment.

Change Management

The term *change management* refers to the process of planning for, implementing, and sustaining change. Organizations, as well as individuals, often find that making changes in the work environment is difficult. Employees sometimes resist change in processes, procedures, and policy. This is because proposed changes in work methods sometimes run counter to the expectations and attitudes of the work group or because employees feel threatened by the introduction of new systems and automation. Thus, to reduce potential conflict, management must plan for change implementation.

Usually, the organization identifies a **change agent** or a team of change agents whose principal responsibility is to facilitate the process of change. Sometimes the change agent is from outside the organization (for example, a consultant) and is hired temporarily to manage the change process. Frequently, however, the change agent is someone from inside the organization and a change team, such as the Quality Management Council mentioned earlier, oversees the change effort.

To be successful, several conditions need to be present in the manner in which organizational change is handled. Dyer (1989) cites the following as elements that are essential to change management:

- Management must have high visible commitment to the change effort.

- Employees affected by the change must have advance information so that they know what is to happen and why the change is occurring.

- The change must be directed by line managers and assisted by a change agent, if necessary.

- The change must be based on good diagnosis and be consistent with the conditions that already exist in the organization.

- Management must remain committed to the change effort throughout all its steps, from problem diagnosis through implementation and evaluation.

- Evaluation of the change is essential.

- Employees must see clearly the relationship between the change and the organization's mission and goals.

Supervisory Components of Performance Improvement

Supervisors work directly with employees and are in an excellent position to model and communicate the value of embracing a continuous improvement philosophy on a daily basis. As mentioned above, PI relies on effective communication, respect for individuals and their contributions to the workplace, recognition of the importance of continual learning, and emphasis on teamwork.

One of the goals of an effective supervisor is to motivate his or her employees to do the best job they can. Employees should be encouraged to point out situations and processes that might be improved. To effectively motivate their employees, supervisors themselves must convey a sense of respect and trust. They must indicate that they believe their employees are genuinely interested in performing well and providing the service their customers want. An environment that promotes open communication and expression of ideas is essential. Supervisors must create a climate in which suggestions for improvement can flow freely. As Deming indicated in his fourteen points, supervisors must give employees the freedom to identify problems and offer suggestions.

Supervisors play an important role in communicating the value of teamwork. It is important to offer each employee a chance to serve on an improvement team. Each member of the improvement team brings a unique perspective on the process designated for improvement. As team members communicate with each other and learn the bottlenecks and potential areas of difficulty and as they work toward solving the problems, they assume more ownership of the process. They tend to buy in to helping to make the processes work more efficiently. As teammates, they get to know each other better, begin developing cordial relationships with each other, and begin thinking more about the entire organization rather than their own individual departments. Supervisors can play valuable roles in both serving on teams and encouraging and selecting others to participate on teams.

Maximization of Individual Performance

An outgrowth of PI should be the design of more productive and motivating jobs for the employees affected by the change. The PI program should produce better job redesign. Employees should not only understand what they are expected to do and what tasks they are responsible for, but their jobs should provide for a certain degree of autonomy and for the development of trust and collaboration.

Inherent in process improvement is matching the employee's skills and attributes to the job. PI should result in a positive job environment and a quality of work life that enhances the dignity of all workers and improves their physical and emotional well-being (Gibson et al. 2000). Managers should strive to create work environments that encourage employees to use their knowledge, skills, and abilities in creative and innovative ways. Employees should not be afraid to initiate ideas or suggestions for improvement. Rather, they should be encouraged to give their best effort in providing high-quality service and to take pride in their accomplishments.

An environment that supports PI in the work product also should encourage striving for personal and professional effectiveness. Employees should be supported in their efforts to improve or maintain their own physical, mental, social, and spiritual well-being. Healthy employees are effective employees, and thus encouragement produces a beneficial situation for both the organization and the individuals. For example, employees might be encouraged to examine their time management techniques and to learn how to become more efficient. The use of day-timers and the realistic setting of time periods for accomplishing tasks help everyone become more organized.

In addition, employees might be encouraged to use stress management techniques to help them reach their potential more effectively. Taking time to engage in physical exercise and activities with friends and family is highly effective in reducing stress. Maintaining personal balance can help avoid burnout, which severely impedes individual performance.

Organizational Commitment to Learning

Peter Senge discussed the importance of personal and organizational learning for performance improvement. He stated that "the roots of the quality movement lie in assumptions about people, organizations, and management that have one underlying theme: to make continual learning a way of organizational life, especially improving the performance of the organization as a total system. This can only be achieved by breaking with the traditional authoritarian, command and control hierarchy where the top thinks, and the local acts, to merge thinking and acting at all levels" (1995, 250).

Improvement is built on knowledge. The organization's executive leadership must build a culture that promotes the importance of continuous learning. Similarly, everyone within the organization must strive to gain knowledge and expand their understanding to improve their own performance. Senge believed that each individual must be committed to personal mastery and must always seek to learn. A collective commitment to learning is built on individual learning. It is this individual learning that will enable an organization to create its own success in the future. Learning occurs in teams, where people can be encouraged to communicate freely, break down barriers, and solve problems as a group.

Performance Improvement Models

PI models are structured frameworks for planning, designing, implementing, and evaluating changes for improvement. This chapter presents an overview of four well-known models for improvement: The Langley, Nolan, and Nolan Foundation for Improvement Model; the FOCUS-PDCA Model; the Baldridge National Quality Program; and Six Sigma. Many other models and adaptations are used in health systems today. All the models incorporate basic principles of continuous improvement such as relying on teams of people who are familiar with the process to be improved, planning and designing a change strategy, gathering and analyzing data, and continuously learning.

Langley, Nolan, and Nolan Model for Improvement

One PI model that is very effective, partly due to its simplicity, is the Langley, Nolan, and Nolan model for improvement (1994). This model can be used for any improvement effort. It consists of two parts. The first part requires considering and answering three fundamental questions. The second part requires planning and conducting a "trial and learning" cycle, called a plan–do–study–act (PDSA) cycle.

Part 1: The Three Fundamental Questions

Three fundamental questions must be considered and answered for every improvement effort undertaken. The three fundamental questions are:

1. *What is the aim or goal?* By carefully considering and answering the first question, one can clearly articulate the goal of the project, what one hopes to accomplish, and what the end result will look like.

2. *How does one know that the change will be an improvement?* By carefully answering this question, one identifies some measures or indicators that will make it known that the changes being attempted are either working to create improvement or are failing to do so.

3. *What changes can one make that may result in improvement?* By brainstorming possible changes, one can identify various changes that can be tested before full implementation.

Not all changes actually bring about improvements. This is why it is important to first test small changes for improvement to see whether they actually bring the desired results. When they do, the changes should be continued. When they do not, the changes should be redeveloped. However, before testing the changes, it is important to specify measures (also known as metrics or indicators). Many models for improvement fail because they measure only whether the planned changes have been implemented, not whether they are actually resulting in improvements toward the goal.

After the goal has been established and measures of success have been developed, **brainstorming** can be used to come up with several potential changes. There is no way to know whether the proposed changes will actually lead to improvements. The changes must first be tested with the **PDSA cycle.** The model suggests that improvement efforts should start out slowly. Just one or two of the proposed changes should be tested to determine whether they are working toward progress on the goal.

Part 2: The PDSA Cycle

The four steps of the PDSA cycle are:

1. *Plan.* Planning requires the most mental effort. After the PI team has selected the change to be tested, the change must be carefully planned along with the method that will be used to evaluate its impact. This process includes considering the following questions:

    • When will the change or intervention start?

- Who will be involved in the change, and do they need any special training?

- How long will the change be tested?

- What method will be used to collect data about the process and outcomes of the change? What will the data collection form look like? Who will collect the data and when will the data be collected?

- When will there be enough data to determine whether the change is resulting in improvement?

2. *Do.* Doing requires implementing the change and beginning data collection efforts. In the discussion of continuous improvement principles, it was mentioned that PI efforts were always data driven. It is during this phase that the change occurs and data are actually collected.

3. *Study.* Studying requires an analysis of the collected data to determine whether the improvement effort is in fact making progress toward the goal. This assessment yields the knowledge needed to determine whether the change should be continued, modified, or stopped.

4. *Act:* The last part of the PDSA cycle requires the PI team to act on the knowledge it has gained. When the team believes the change is achieving the goal, it will want to continue the change and perhaps expand it. If the change is not achieving the goal, the team may want to modify or eliminate it and try something else. This segment requires action based on knowledge gained from testing the change.

It is interesting to note that this improvement model calls the third segment *study* rather than *check,* as in the Shewhart and Deming models. Langley, Nolan, and Nolan developed their model for healthcare applications. They believe that when the model is applied to a complex human service industry such as healthcare, the term *study* is more appropriate. One is not simply checking production points as one might do in an automobile industry but, rather, analyzing measures that may have created unplanned consequences. Thus, the term *study* is viewed as more appropriate because the cycle is a learning cycle rather than a simple inspection.

This model with its PDSA cycle permits individuals to gain knowledge through analysis of data. The more knowledge that is gained, the more improvement can be made. (See figure 12.1 for an illustration of the PDSA Learning Cycle.)

The FOCUS-PDCA Model

A PI model frequently used in hospitals is the FOCUS-PDCA model. It was originally developed in the 1980s by the Quality Resource Group, an internal consulting division of Hospital Corporation of America (HCA). This model provides a structured framework for change where PI team members follow a prescribed course of action. FOCUS-PDCA is an acronym that stands for:

- Find an opportunity for improvement.

- Organize an effort and assign a team familiar with the process.

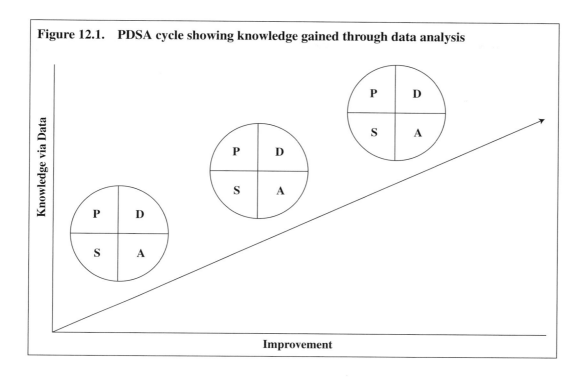

Figure 12.1.   PDSA cycle showing knowledge gained through data analysis

- Clarify current understanding of how the process works.

- Understand the process variation and capability.

- Select a strategy for improvement.

The PDCA cycle (Plan, Do, Check, and Act) tests the change to see if it results in improvement. As in the Langley, Nolan, and Nolan Model, the PDCA cycle is a trial and learning cycle.

The Baldridge National Quality Program

In 1987, the Malcolm Baldridge National Quality Program was established for businesses to encourage efforts leading to improved quality. In 1997, new healthcare-specific criteria were developed. Healthcare organizations also could use the criteria to help them "address challenges such as focusing on core competencies, introducing new technologies, reducing costs, communicating and sharing information electronically, establishing new alliances with health care providers, or just maintaining market advantage" (Baldridge National Quality Program 2003, ii). The Baldridge program also embraces many of the continuous improvement principles that were previously discussed, such as a commitment to organizational and personal learning, valuing the needs of customers and other partners, respecting the contributions of employees, managing by fact, and using a systems perspective to manage the organization.

The healthcare criteria provide a framework organized into seven interdependent categories. These include:

- Leadership
- Strategic planning
- Focus on patients, other customers, and markets
- Measurement, analysis, and knowledge management
- Staff focus
- Process measurement, and
- Organizational performance

Healthcare organizations that have undertaken the Baldridge program report they have made enormous strides in providing high-quality patient care and in achieving operational efficiency, regardless of whether they actually won the award. Just participating led to improvements. As of this writing, three healthcare facilities have actually been awarded the Malcolm Baldridge Award for Quality.

Six Sigma

Another system or model used in PI is Six Sigma. Originally developed by Motorola Corporation, this model has been used by Hewlett Packard and General Electric. In the past several years, it has been adopted by some healthcare organizations. The goal of Six Sigma is to significantly reduce variation in key processes so that management can better predict the outcome. It uses statistical tools to better understand key processes. The five steps used in Six Sigma are: define the process, measure the process and collect data, analyze the data, improve the process, and control the improved process.

Check Your Understanding 12.3

Instructions: Put the following steps of the Langley, Nolan, and Nolan Model for Improvement in the correct order (a–g).

1. _____ Plan the change thoroughly.

2. _____ Develop a goal.

3. _____ Brainstorm possible changes for improvement.

4. _____ Act on the knowledge gained.

5. _____ Study and analyze the results.

6. _____ Develop measures that will indicate whether progress is being made toward achieving the goal.

7. _____ Implement the change and collect the data.

Instructions: Indicate whether the following statements are true or false (T or F). If false, correct the statement to make it true.

1. _____ Performance improvement often requires changing structures or processes.

2. _____ Most people readily accept change because it invigorates them.

3. _____ An organization that promotes learning in all its employees is less likely to embrace the philosophy of continual performance improvement.

4. _____ Most organizations will gain in operational effectiveness and efficiency just by participating in the Malcolm Baldridge National Quality Program, regardless of whether they win an award.

5. _____ The goal of six sigma is to significantly reduce variation in key processes to prevent defects as much as possible.

Performance Improvement Tools and Techniques

A number of tools and techniques are used in PI initiatives (Brassard and Ritter 1993; Johnson and McLaughlin 1999; Cofer and Greeley 1993; Ransom, Joshi, and Nash 2005). Some of these are used to facilitate communication among employees. Others are used to help people determine the root causes of performance problems. Some tools indicate areas of agreement or consensus among team members. Others permit the display of data for easy analysis.

Brainstorming

Brainstorming is a technique used to generate a large number of creative ideas from a group. It encourages PI team members to think "out of the box" and offer original ideas. There are a number of approaches to brainstorming. Teams can use an unstructured method or a structured method.

The *unstructured method* results in a free flow of ideas. The team leader or facilitator writes the ideas on a flipchart as they are offered so that everyone can see the list as it forms. There should be no discussion or evaluation of the ideas at this point. The goal of brainstorming is to encourage creativity and to come up with a lot of ideas. Most brainstorming sessions are short (perhaps five minutes long). The ideas then are used as the basis for later discussions of the subject.

In *structured brainstorming,* the team leader or facilitator asks team members to generate their own list of ideas. Team members can work by themselves or in small groups. Again, the sessions are usually timed. Then, one by one, the team elicits a new idea from each member in turn. The process may take several rounds. As team members run out of new ideas, they pass. The next person then offers an idea until no team member can produce a fresh idea.

Brainstorming is highly effective for identifying a number of potential processes that may benefit from improvement efforts and for generating solutions to specific problems. It helps people to begin thinking in new ways and gets them involved in the process. It is an excellent method for facilitating open communication.

Affinity Grouping

A number of ideas are generated during the brainstorming process. Some of the ideas may be very similar to others. **Affinity grouping** allows the team to organize similar ideas into logical groupings. Ideas that are generated in a brainstorming session may be written on Post-it™ notes and arranged on a table or posted on a board. Without talking to each other, each team member is asked to walk around the table or board, look at the ideas, and place them in natural groupings that seem related or connected to each other. Each member is empowered to move the ideas in a way that makes the most sense.

As team members move the ideas back or place them in other groupings, the other team members consider the merits of the placements and decide whether further action is needed. The goal is to have the team become comfortable with the arrangement. Finally, the natural groupings that emerge are labeled with a category. The intent in using this tool is to bring focus to the new ideas. (See figure 12.2.)

Nominal Group Technique

Nominal group technique is a process used to develop agreement about an issue or an idea that the team considers most important. It helps the team visualize consensus. Each team member ranks each idea according to importance. For example, if there were six ideas, the idea that is most important would be given the number six. The second most important idea would be given the number five, and so on. After each individual team member has had a chance to rank the list of ideas, the numbers are totaled. The ideas ranked most important are clearly visible to all. Those ideas that people did not think were as important also become obvious owing to their low scores. The nominal group technique demonstrates where the team's priorities lie.

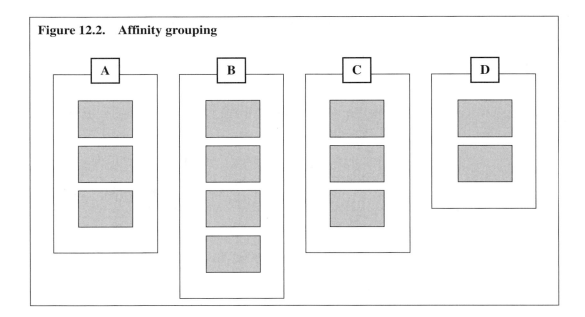

Figure 12.2.   Affinity grouping

Multivoting Technique

The **multivoting technique** is a variation of the nominal group technique and serves the same purpose. Instead of ranking each issue or idea, team members are asked to rate issues by marking them with a distribution of points. In weighted multivoting, a team member is asked to distribute his or her allotment of points among as few or as many issues as he or she wants. For example, the team member might give thirteen out of twenty-five points to one issue of particular importance, three points each to four other issues, and no points to the remaining issues. After the voting, the numbers are added. Thus, the team will be able to see which issue emerged as particularly important to the team as a whole.

This technique also can be done using colored dots. For example, if eight items are on a chart, the team members might be given four dots each to distribute among the four items that are most important to them. This method provides a visual demonstration of where the consensus lies and what issue has been ranked most important by the team as a whole.

Flowcharts

Whenever a team examines a process with the intention of making improvements, it must first understand the process thoroughly. Each team member has a unique perspective and significant insight about how a portion of the process works. **Flowcharts** help all the team members understand the process in the same way. (See figure 12.3 for an example of a flowchart.)

The work involved in developing the flowchart allows the team to thoroughly understand every step in the process as well as the sequence of steps. The flowchart provides a visual picture of each decision point and each event that must be completed. It readily points out places where there are redundancy and complex and problematic areas.

Cause-and-Effect Diagram

A **cause-and-effect diagram** facilitates **root-cause analysis.** The diagram is sometimes called a **fishbone diagram** because of its characteristic shape. (See figure 12.4.) The problem is placed in a box on the right side of the diagram. A horizontal line is drawn and diagonal lines resembling ribs are added to connect the boxes above and below the main horizontal line (or backbone). Each box contains a different category of information.

The categories may represent broad classifications of problem areas. For example, possible categories include people, methods, equipment, materials, policies, procedures, environment, measurement, and others. The team determines how many categories it needs to classify all the possible sources of the problem. Usually, there are four categories.

After constructing the diagram, the team brainstorms the possible root causes of the problem. These are then placed on horizontal lines extending from the diagonal category line. Brainstorming continues until all the team's ideas about causes are exhausted. The purpose of this tool is to permit the team to explore, identify, and graphically display all of the root causes of a problem.

After identifying a number of causes of a problem, the team may decide to begin working to remove one of them. PI efforts involve making efforts to improve processes by addressing one root cause at a time. However, the question may arise about which cause to remove first. The multivoting and nominal group techniques can help team members determine which root cause to work on first.

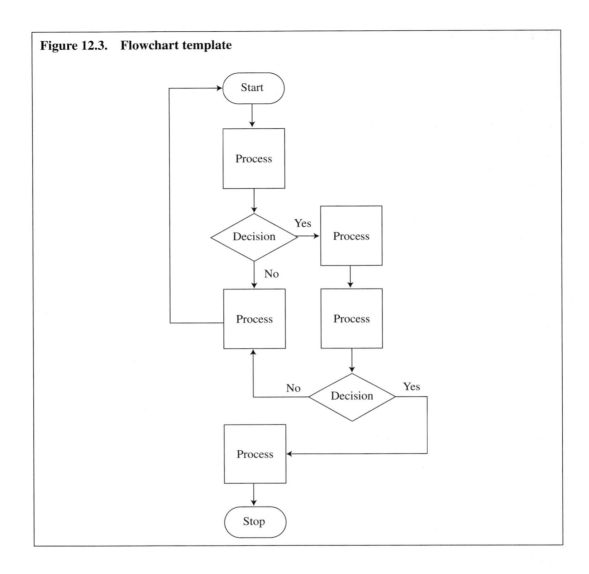

Figure 12.3.   Flowchart template

Pareto Charts

The PI team's ranking of potential changes for improvement can be displayed visually using a **Pareto chart.** (See figure 12.5.) A Pareto chart looks very much like a bar chart except that the highest-ranking item is listed first, followed by the second highest, down to the lowest-ranked item. Its purpose is to display how the team ranked the problems and to allow the team to focus on those problems that may have the biggest potential for improving the process. The chart is based on the Pareto principle. According to the Pareto principle, 20 percent of a problem's sources are responsible for 80 percent of its actual effects. By concentrating on the "vital few" sources, the team can eliminate a large number of undesirable results.

Force-Field Analysis

Force-field analysis is another tool used to visually display data generated through brainstorming. The team leader draws a large T shape on a board. (See figure 12.6.) The word *drivers* is written above the crossbar and on the left side of the T. The word *barriers* is written above the bar and on the right side of the T. Team members then brainstorm the reasons or factors that would encourage a change for improvement and those that might create barriers. The team leader places the factors in the appropriate column on the chart.

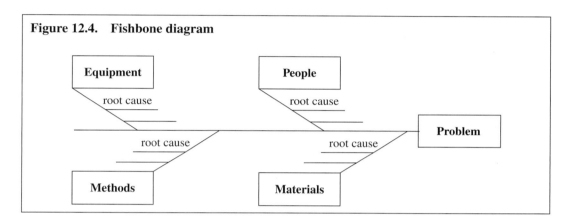

Figure 12.4. Fishbone diagram

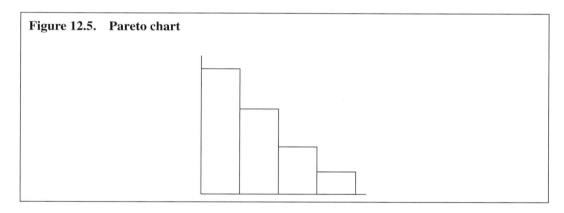

Figure 12.5. Pareto chart

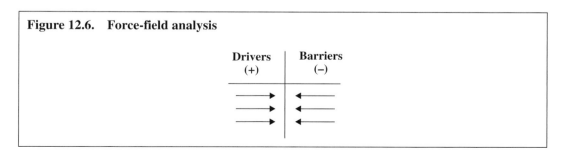

Figure 12.6. Force-field analysis

Force-field analysis enables team members to identify factors that support or work against a proposed solution. Often the next step after force-field analysis is to work on ways that would eliminate barriers or reinforce drivers.

Checksheets

A **checksheet** is a data collection tool that records and compiles observations or occurrences. It consists of a simple list of categories, issues, or observations on the left side of the chart and a place on the right for people to record checkmarks next to the item when it is observed or counted. (See figure 12.7.) After a period of time, the checkmarks are counted to reveal any patterns or trends.

A checksheet is a simple way to obtain a clear picture of the facts. After data have been collected, several tools can be used to display the data and help the team analyze them more easily.

Scatter Diagrams

Scatter diagrams are used to plot the points for two variables that may be related to each other in some way. For example, one might want to look at whether age and blood pressure are related. One variable, age, would be plotted on the vertical axis of the graph, and the other variable, blood pressure, would be plotted on the horizontal axis. (See figure 12.8.) After a number of blood pressures and patients' ages were plotted, a pattern might emerge. If the diagram indicated that blood pressure increased with age, it would reveal a positive relationship between these variables. In some cases, a negative relationship might exist, such as with the variables of age and flexibility or the number of hours of training and the number of mistakes made.

Whenever a scatter diagram indicates that the points are moving together in one direction or another, conclusions about the variables' relationship, either positive or negative, become evident. In other cases, however, the scatter diagram may indicate that there is no linear relationship between the variables because the points are scattered randomly and no pattern emerges. In this case, there would be no linear relationship between the two variables.

Figure 12.7.   Checksheet

	1	2	Total
A	~~////~~	/ / /	8
B	/ / / /	/ / / /	8
C	/ /	/	3

Histograms

A **histogram** can be used to display frequencies of responses. (See figure 12.9.) It is a much easier way to summarize and analyze data than using a table made up of numbers. A histogram displays data values that have been grouped into categories. The bars on the histogram reveal how the data were distributed. For example, a health information technician may wish to show the number of minutes it takes to respond to a patient's request for information. Minutes may be categorized into four groupings, such as one to thirty minutes, thirty-one to sixty minutes, sixty-one to ninety minutes, and over ninety minutes. Checkmarks may be recorded to indicate the category of minutes taken to respond to the request.

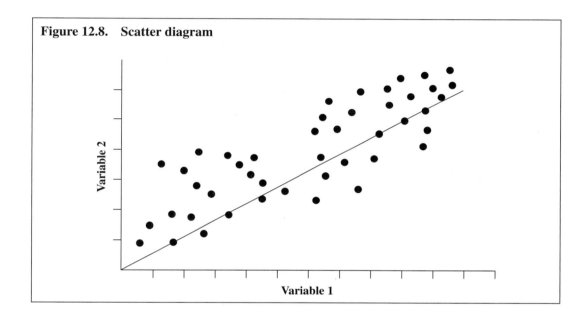

Figure 12.8.   Scatter diagram

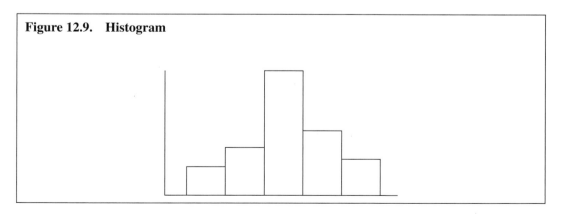

Figure 12.9.   Histogram

After a period of time, the checkmarks are added, and the histogram is plotted with the frequencies shown on the vertical (or y) axis and the minute intervals shown on the horizontal (or x) axis. The graph would indicate the different intervals that patients had to wait before having their requests filled. It can give PI teams an excellent idea of how well their process is performing. Thus, a histogram can show how frequently data values occur among the various intervals, how centered or skewed the distribution of data is, and what the likelihood of future occurrences will be.

Run Charts

A **run chart** displays data points over a period of time to provide information about performance. (See figure 12.10.) The measured points of a process are plotted on a graph at regular time intervals to help team members see whether there are substantial changes in the numbers over time. For example, suppose a health information technician wished to reduce the number of incomplete records in the HIM department. He might first plot the number of incomplete records each month for the past six months. He then might enact a change in the processing of records designed to improve the process. Following the improvement effort, he would continue to collect data on the number of incomplete records and plot the data on the graph. If the run chart showed that the number of incomplete charts had actually decreased, the health information technician could attribute the decrease to the improvement effort. A run chart is an excellent tool for providing visual verification of how a process is performing and whether an improvement effort has worked.

Statistical Process Control Chart

A **statistical process control chart** looks very much like a run chart except that it has lines drawn at the top and bottom. The upper line represents the upper control limit (UCL), and the lower line represents the lower control limit (LCL). (See figure 12.11.) These lines

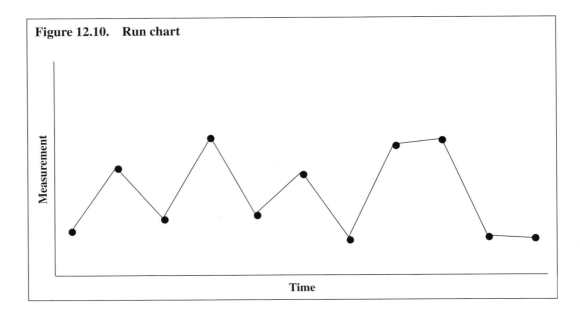

Figure 12.10.   Run chart

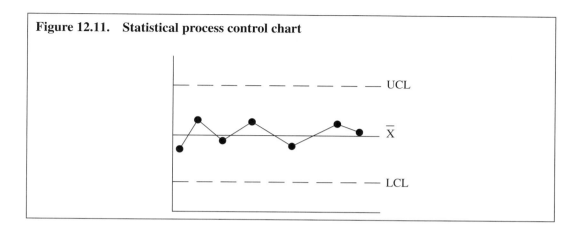

Figure 12.11. Statistical process control chart

represent values that have been statistically calculated from the data generated in the process. Like the run chart, the statistical process control chart plots points over time to show how a process is performing. However, the two control limit lines permit the evaluator to use rules for interpretation to determine whether the process is stable (in other words, predictable) or out of control.

As mentioned earlier, Deming and Shewhart talked about systems and how some variation always occurs within a system. The statistical process control chart makes it possible to see whether the variation within a process is the result of a common cause or a special cause. It lets the PI team know whether the team needs to try to reduce the ordinary variation occurring through common cause or to seek out a special cause of the variation and try to eliminate it.

Dashboards and Scorecards

As discussed earlier, quality has many dimensions. Healthcare leaders cannot just focus on one aspect of quality, such as the financial aspect, without also considering other aspects of quality such as patient satisfaction or clinical quality or they miss the whole picture. **Dashboards** and **scorecards** are tools that present metrics from a variety of quality aspects in one concise report. They may present measures of clinical quality (such as infection rates), financial quality, volume, and patient satisfaction. The indicators provide little snapshots of all areas of quality to give leaders a truer perspective of the service their facility is providing.

The terms *dashboard* and *scorecard* are often used interchangeably, but technically, dashboards (like dashboards on a car) are reports of process measures to help leaders know what is currently going on so that they can plan strategically where they want to go next, and scorecards (like baseball scorecards) are reports of outcomes measures to help leaders know what they have accomplished. These concise reports help leaders "align organizational effort to achieve higher levels of organizational performance" (Pugh 2005, 213).

JCAHO's Tracer Methodology

In 2004, the Joint Commission on Accreditation of Healthcare Organizations (JCAHO) developed a new and improved accreditation process. The intent now is to focus on continual operational improvement, helping to bridge the gap between the current state of health-care and the potential for safer, higher-quality care (Jackson 2005). The new technique for assessing the actual quality of care given to patients in healthcare facilities is called tracer methodology. In the Individual Tracer Activity, a patient is followed through the organization's systems and processes in the sequence in which he or she experienced the care. Patients and care providers also may be interviewed following the experience. This technique allows the organization to truly gain an appreciation of what the patient experiences as care is delivered.

JCAHO also has developed a Systems Tracer Activity that follows processes, systems, and functions that are influential to the patient care experience (Friedman 2004). The environment of care, the policies and procedures, personnel files, credentials and other documents can be reviewed as part of the process.

Information Technology and Performance Improvement

The U.S. healthcare system is notoriously behind other service industries in its development and use of information management technology. Perhaps the main reason for this lag is the system's fragmentation and complexity, but huge costs and resistance to change are likewise big inhibitors. Despite advances such as "word processors, handheld devices, Internet access, and increasingly broadband communication networks, the great majority of physician orders to hospitals, nursing homes, pharmacies, and other care settings still require paper, pen or pencil, and transmission through courier or FAX" (McLaughlin and Kaluzny 2006). The healthcare industry as a whole has invested a much smaller amount of its revenue in information technology than either the financial or insurance industry, and the inadequacy is apparent.

If we want to improve the quality of care that our healthcare system delivers and the efficiency of our healthcare processes, information systems must be developed that permit communication across disparate health facilities and across administrative and clinical systems. PI requires the collection and analysis of data, the transformation of those data into information, the use of that information to facilitate knowledge, and the use of knowledge to inform decision making. Vendors are aware of the need for integration and management of data and have developed information systems to facilitate PI in healthcare. By 1998, as JCAHO launched its ORYX initiative, it had approved more than 125 vendors that had developed outcomes and PI systems to meet its accreditation requirements.

Despite the underinvestment in information technology in the healthcare system overall, there have been some notable improvements. Even small medical offices and outpatient clinics are now using some information management technologies. For example, most practices and clinics use a practice management system for billing and accounting functions. Many also use office productivity software for clinical documents and personal digital assistants that may include medical reference sources. Copying machines and fax equipment are commonplace. Many practices and clinics also have Internet connections to local hospitals or corporate data centers. Many hospitals and a number of large ambulatory care practices are acquiring electronic health records (EHRs), which have the capability of dramatically improving patient care (McLaughlin and Kaluzny 2006). Indeed, there is evidence that some nonprofit consumer advocate groups are interested in promoting patient safety by providing data to consumers to make more informed hospital choices. For example, the Leapfrog Group has promoted the use of computerized physician order-entry systems and has suggested that consumers consider choosing only hospitals with this safety initiative in place. Their influence is promoting change.

The report from the Institute of Medicine (IOM), claiming that between 44,000 and 98,000 deaths occur each year in hospitals, has brought increased urgency in developing information systems that can improve the quality and delivery of care (2000). The development and use of EHRs and other information systems can produce numerous benefits. The IOM reports that EHR systems can contribute to improved quality, outcomes, and safety (Wager, Lee, and Glaser 2005). For example, practice guidelines and computerized reminders and alerts help physicians provide appropriate preventive care more frequently. They also increase effective drug prescribing and administration practices, improve the accuracy of drug dosing, and reduce adverse drug reactions. Clinical information systems permit medical information to be readily available to practitioners, thereby increasing their effectiveness in decision making.

Moreover, information systems can help improve efficiency and productivity and reduce costs. For example, they can make test results readily available, eliminating the need to reorder a test due to a lost result. They can reduce pharmaceutical costs by prompting physicians to use generic and formulary drugs. They can reduce the time and costs related to the retrieval and storage of medical records. Finally, they can produce higher-quality documentation, better coding, and, therefore, higher reimbursement.

Additionally, EHRs and information systems have been shown to increase service and satisfaction (Wager, Lee, and Glaser 2005). Patients whose physicians use EHRs report satisfaction that their physicians are innovative and progressive. Physicians and support staff also report that the improved documentation and the availability of patient and medical information has increased their own satisfaction at being able to provide a superior level of patient care and service than before they acquired the systems.

Organizational performance improvement requires information technology, but it does not require expensive, sophisticated equipment and software. In fact, a personal computer and office productivity software (word-processing, spreadsheet, and database applications) can meet the needs of most PI managers and teams. The technology is but one component. Involving the appropriate people, communicating effectively and getting everyone on the team to understand the goal and the process, understanding customers' needs and wants, and having knowledge of improvement practices and a positive attitude about continual improvement are all vital components of PI.

Data Quality

As mentioned previously, PI requires data, but not just any data. Data quality is critically important for any improvement effort. Data must be relevant, accurate, consistent, and timely for them to provide meaningful information upon which decisions can be based. Unfortunately, healthcare data are often of poor quality. Data for PI efforts come from a variety of sources and then are stored in electronic databases. Data may be accessed from EHRs, clinical information systems, customer satisfaction surveys, cost accounting systems, executive information systems, and decision support systems and then used to provide information for PI efforts.

To ensure the quality of information produced within an organization, data quality standards should be established. Both the American Health Information Management Association and the Medical Records Institute have published guidelines that may be useful to organizations establishing their own standards (Wager, Lee, and Glaser 2005). Technology also can assist in ensuring data quality. Increasingly, information systems are assisting data quality efforts by checking for data-entry errors and performing range validation, making it difficult for an end user to enter or send bad data to a software application. Accurate and relevant data are essential in PI activities.

Check Your Understanding 12.4

Instructions: Identify the appropriate category (a–e) for each of the following tools and techniques according to how they are used. Some tools and techniques may fit more than one category.

  a. Communication facilitators and idea generators
  b. Consensus builders
  c. Data collection methods
  d. Data analysis methods
  e. Data reporting methods

  1. _____ Force-field analysis

  2. _____ Histogram

  3. _____ Scatter diagram

  4. _____ Brainstorming

  5. _____ Affinity grouping

  6. _____ Nominal group technique

  7. _____ Run chart

  8. _____ Multivoting

  9. _____ Statistical process control chart

  10. _____ Checksheet

  11. _____ Dashboard

  12. _____ Fishbone diagram

  13. _____ Flowchart

  14. _____ Pareto chart

  15. _____ Scorecard

Instructions: Indicate whether the following statements are true or false (T or F). If false, correct the statement to make it true.

  1. _____ Healthcare information systems are much more state-of-the-art than information systems in the financial and insurance industries.

  2. _____ The Institute of Medicine has been actively advocating for the development and use of the EHR to facilitate improved patient care.

  3. _____ The use of practice guidelines and computerized reminders and alerts can aid physicians to provide appropriate preventive care more frequently.

  4. _____ For healthcare data to provide meaningful information, the data must be accurate, timely, relevant, and consistent.

  5. _____ Data and information are the same.

Real-World Case

An article in the *New York Times* (Kolata 2001) described several successful PI efforts. This case presents one of them.

Dr. Mark Murray is a family practice physician working at the Kaiser Permanente Medical Center in Roseville, California. A few years ago, the practice was similar to other practices in that it had an abundance of sick and irritated patients waiting for unacceptably long periods of time in the waiting room. When patients were finally able to see their doctors, the doctors often had to spend considerable amounts of time apologizing for the delays and trying to fix blame on someone for the long waits and the rushed visits. The process clearly was begging for improvement, but what could be done? This was the way successful physician practices were always run, with crowded waiting rooms ensuring that physicians have thriving practices and sufficient income.

Dr. Murray had heard of the work being done at a Boston-based nonprofit organization known as the Institute for Healthcare Improvement. This organization is committed to improving healthcare through the application of the principles of continuous improvement. Its proponents are physicians themselves. Dr. Murray had grown weary of facing irritated patients and decided to find ways to reduce the backlog and wait time and improve services.

He discovered that his patients had to wait an average of fifty-five days to obtain a nonemergency appointment. He also found out that there were a great many more patients on Mondays than on other days of the week. The fall and winter seasons produced more calls for appointments than spring and summer. Moreover, he found that if a physician took care of 2,500 patients, that physician would receive calls from sixteen to twenty-five of them each day and would see about twenty-one of them each day.

This information allowed Dr. Murray to make some informed decisions about supply and demand. One change he suggested was that the physicians in the practice plan to work longer hours on Mondays, particularly during the winter, so that more patients could be seen. As it was, the physicians had to work longer on Mondays anyway just to meet the additional patients squeezed into the schedule for emergency reasons. To reduce the existing backlog, Dr. Murray proposed to the staff and other physicians that they temporarily work longer hours until the oldest standing patient appointments were cleared off the books. The goal was to create an appointment book where each patient could be seen by his or her physician on the very day the patient called.

The goal seemed daunting. It also disturbed some physician colleagues who saw several weeks of patient appointments on the books as evidence of their practice's long-term viability. Patients were likewise suspicious of the goal of seeing patients on the same day they called because they had been conditioned to expect long wait times.

As with most PI projects, the change did not happen over night. It took about a year, but today patients can call and be seen by their physicians on the same day. Rarely do physicians in the practice work later than planned, their incomes have not changed, and their patients are no longer irritated and looking for care elsewhere. In fact, on some days, physicians vote to determine who gets to go home early.

Summary

Performance improvement is a management philosophy that eliminates the idea that it makes sense to ignore problems until they become so big they cannot be ignored. It is based on the theory that organizations should be continuously seeking ways to improve their systems by testing small, incremental changes. PI relies on the gathering and analysis of data to build knowledge on which informed decisions can be made.

PI is more than the latest buzzword in healthcare. It is a way of thinking, a way of being, a way of managing, a way of conducting business. It can be applied to the work of organizations as well as to the work of individuals. Key to its effectiveness is commitment from the organization's top management and its willingness to train and involve employees in the PI process.

Many individuals in the United States have proposed methods for ensuring quality management in healthcare. Shewart, Deming, and Juran introduced a number of tools and techniques that could be used to facilitate communication and the exchange of ideas, data collection, and data analysis.

The Joint Commission on Accreditation of Healthcare Organizations has incorporated PI concepts into its accreditation process and requires organizations to demonstrate that its principles are being implemented. Every health information management professional must become well acquainted with the principles of continuous improvement so as to take an active role in leading or participating in improvement efforts.

References

Baldridge National Quality Program. 2004. *Health Care Criteria for Performance Excellence.* Gaithersburg, MD: National Institute of Standards and Technology.

Batalden, P.B., and P.K. Stoltz. 1993. A framework for the continual improvement of health care: Building and applying professional and improvement knowledge to test changes in daily work. *Journal on Quality Improvement* 19(10):424–47.

Berwick, D.M. 1989. Continuous improvement as an ideal in health care. *New England Journal of Medicine* 320(1):53–56.

Brassard, M., and D. Ritter. 1993. *The Memory Jogger™ II.* Methuen, MA: GOAL/QPC.

Cofer, J.I., and H.P. Greeley. 1993. *Quality Improvement Techniques for Medical Records.* Marblehead, MA: Opus Communications.

Donabedian, A. 1988. The quality of care: How can it be assessed? *Journal of the American Medical Association* 260(12):1743–48.

Dyer, W.G. 1989 (Winter). Team building: A microcosm of the past, present, and future of O.D. *Academy of Management OD Newsletter,* pp. 7–8.

Elliott, C., et al. 2000. *Performance Improvement in Healthcare: A Tool for Programmed Learning.* Chicago: American Health Information Management Association.

Fried, B., and W. Carpenter. 2006. Understanding and improving team effectiveness in quality improvement. In *Continuous Quality Improvement in Health Care: Theory, Implementation, and Applications,* 3rd ed., edited by C. P. McLaughlin and A. D. Kaluzny, pp. 154-88. Boston: Jones and Bartlett.

Friedman, M. 2004. Tracer methodology and the new Joint Commission Home Care and Hospice Survey Process: Part 1. *Home Healthcare Nurse* 22(10):710–14.

Genovich-Richards, J. 1997. Selecting quality initiatives and methodologies. In *Improving Quality: A Guide to Effective Programs,* 2nd ed., edited by C. G. Meisenheimer, pp. 85–97. Gaithersburg, MD: Aspen.

Gibson, J.L., J.M. Ivancevich, and J H. Donnelly. 2000. *Organizations' Behavior, Structure, Processes,* 10th ed. Boston: Irwin McGraw-Hill.

Imai, M. 1986. *Kaizen: The Key to Japanese Competitive Success.* New York: Random House.

Institute of Medicine. 2000. *To Err Is Human: Building a Safer Health System.* Washington, DC: National Academy of Sciences, National Academies Press.

Jackson, R. 2005. Gearing up for the new accreditation process: Revised joint commission standards for 2004. *Health Care Food and Nutrition Focus* 20(3):1,3.

Johnson, S.P., and C. . McLaughlin. 1999. Measurement and statistical approaches in CQI. In *Continuous Quality Improvement in Health Care,* edited by C. P. McLaughlin and A. D. Kaluzny, pp. 70–101. Gaithersburg, MD: Aspen.

Joint Commission on Accreditation of Healthcare Organizations. 2005. jcaho.org.

Katzenbach, J.R., and D.K. Smith. 1993. *The Wisdom of Teams: Creating the High-performance Organization.* Boston: Harvard Business School Press.

Kelly, D. L. 2003. *Applying Quality Management in Healthcare: A Process for Improvement.* Chicago: Health Administration Press.

Kolata, G. 2001 (Jan. 4). Harried doctors try to ease big delays and rushed visits. *The New York Times.*

Langley, G.J., K.M. Nolan, and T.W. Nolan. 1994 (June). The foundation of improvement. *Quality Progress,* pp. 81–86.

McClanahan, S., S.T. Goodwin, and F. Houser. 1999. A formula for errors: Good people + bad systems. In *Error Reduction in Health Care: A Systems Approach to Improving Patient Safety,* edited by P. L. Spath, pp. 1–3. San Francisco: Jossey-Bass.

McLaughlin, C.P., and A.D. Kaluzny. 2006. *Continuous Quality Improvement in Health Care: Theory, Implementation, and Applications,* 3rd ed. Gaithersburg, MD: Aspen.

Meisenheimer, C.G. 1997. *Improving Quality: A Guide to Effective Programs,* 2nd ed. Sudbury, MA: Jones and Barlett.

Omachonu, V.K. 1999. *Healthcare Performance Improvement.* Norcross, GA: Engineering and Management Press.

Pugh, M.D. 2005. Dashboards and scorecards: Tools for creating alignment. In *The Healthcare Quality Book: Vision, Strategy, and Tools,* edited by S.B. Ransom, M.S. Joshi, and D.B. Nash, pp. 213–40. Chicago: Health Administration Press.

Racine, J.A. 1995. Double take on the history of quality in health care. In *Quality in Health Care: Theory, Application, and Evolution,* edited by N. O. Graham, pp. 15-31. Gaithersburg, MD: Aspen.

Ransom, S.B., M.S. Joshi, and D.B. Nash. 2005. *The Healthcare Quality Book: Vision, Strategy, and Tools.* Chicago: Health Administration Press.

Senge, P. 1995. Building learning organizations. In *Quality in Health Care: Theory, Application, and Evolution,* edited by N. O. Graham, pp. 249–64. Gaithersburg, MD: Aspen.

Stocklein, M. 2005. Quality improvement systems, theories, and tools. In *The Healthcare Quality Book: Vision, Strategy, and Tools,* edited by S. B. Ransom, M. S. Joshi, and D. B. Nash, pp. 63–86. Chicago: Health Administration Press.

Wager, K. A., F. W. Lee, and J. P. Glaser. 2005. *Managing Health Care Information Systems: A Practical Approach for Health Care Executives.* San Francisco: Jossey Bass.

Ward, R. E. 2005. Information technology applications for improved quality. In *The Healthcare Quality Book: Vision, Strategy, and Tools,* edited by S. B. Ransom, M. S. Joshi, and D. B. Nash, pp. 267–308. Chicago: Health Administration Press.

Part III
Health Services Organization and Delivery

Chapter 13
Healthcare Delivery Systems

Bonnie S. Cassidy, MPA, RHIA, FAHIMA, FHIMSS

Learning Objectives

- To understand the history of the healthcare delivery system from ancient times until the present

- To understand the basic organization of the various types of hospitals and healthcare organizations

- To recognize the impact managed care has had on healthcare providers

- To recognize the impact that external forces have on the healthcare industry

- To identify the various functional components of an integrated delivery system

- To describe the systems used for reimbursement of healthcare services

- To recognize the role of government in healthcare services

Key Terms

Allied health professionals

American Association of Medical Colleges (AAMC)

American College of Healthcare Executives (ACHE)

American Hospital Association (AHA)

American Medical Association (AMA)

American Nurses Association (ANA)

Average length of stay (ALOS)

Case management

Chief executive officer (CEO)

Chief information officer (CIO)

Chief nursing officer (CNO)

Chief operating officer (COO)

Clinical privileges

Commission on Accreditation for Health Informatics and Information Management Education (CAHIIM)

Continuous quality improvement (CQI)

Continuum of care

Extended care facility

Health savings accounts

Health systems agency (HSA)

Hill-Burton Act

Home healthcare

Hospice care

Integrated delivery network (IDN)

Integrated delivery system (IDS)

Investor-owned hospital chain

Managed care organization (MCO)

Medical staff bylaws

Medical staff classifications

Mission (statement)

National Institutes of Health (NIH)

National Practitioner Data Bank (NPBD)

Peer review organization (PRO)

Public health services

Quality improvement organization (QIO)

Reengineering

Rehabilitation services

Skilled nursing facility (SNF)

Subacute care

Utilization Review Act

Introduction

A broad array of healthcare services is available in the United States today, from simple preventive measures such as vaccinations to complex lifesaving procedures such as heart transplants. An individual's contact with the healthcare delivery system often begins before she or he is born, with family planning and prenatal care, and continues through the end of life, with long-term and hospice care.

Physicians, nurses, and other clinical providers who work in ambulatory care, acute care, rehabilitative and psychiatric care, and long-term care facilities provide healthcare services. Healthcare services also are provided in the homes of hospice and home care patients. In addition, assisted living centers, industrial medical clinics, and public health department clinics provide services to many Americans.

Integrated delivery systems (IDSs) offer a full range of healthcare services along a **continuum of care** to ensure that patients get the right care at the right time from the right provider. The continuum extends from primary care providers to specialist and ancillary providers. The goal of IDSs is to deliver high-quality, cost-effective care in the most appropriate setting (Sloane et al. 1999, 9).

Most hospitals are integrated into their communities through ties with area physicians and other healthcare providers, clinics and outpatient facilities, and other practitioners. Almost half the nation's hospitals also are tied to larger organizational entities such as multihospital and integrated healthcare systems (IHCSs), **integrated delivery networks** (IDNs), and alliances. An IDN comprises a group of hospitals, physicians, other providers, insurers, and/or community agencies that work together to deliver health services (AHA 2004).

In 2002, 1,343 acute care hospitals (27 percent of the total) were in IDNs (AHA 2004). Multihospital systems include two or more hospitals owned, leased, sponsored, or contract managed by a central organization. In 1985, 27.5 percent of hospitals were system members, which rose to 46 percent by 2002 (AHA 2004). An alliance is defined as a formal organization, usually owned by shareholders/members, that works on behalf of its individual members in the provision of services and products and in the promotion of activities and ventures (AHA 1999). In 2000, 3,344 hospitals were in group-purchasing organizations (the dominant kind of alliance). The same hospitals can be registered in more than one category (AHA 2004).

In 2002, the United States had 321 multihospital or integrated healthcare systems. Most were not for profit, including religious (56) and secular (209) systems. Fifty-one systems were investor owned, and five were operated by the federal government (Jonas and Kovner 2005).

This chapter traces the history of Western medicine to the present time. It discusses modern healthcare delivery in the United States, and how political, societal, and other factors have influenced its development. Well-known legislation affecting healthcare and healthcare information systems in the U.S. is examined. Different types of healthcare delivery facilities and the services they provide are explained.

Theory into Practice

In the 1990s, U.S. hospitals faced growing pressure to contain costs, improve quality, and demonstrate their contributions to the health of the communities they serve. They adapted to these pressures in various ways. Some merged with or bought out other hospitals and healthcare organizations. Others created IDSs to provide a full range of healthcare services along the continuum of care, from ambulatory care to inpatient care to long-term care. Still others concentrated on improving the care they provided by focusing on patients as customers. Many hospitals responded to local competition by quickly entering into affiliations and other risk-sharing agreements with acute and non–acute care providers, physicians' groups, and **managed care organizations** (MCOs).

History of Western Medicine

Modern Western medicine is rooted in antiquity. The ancient Greeks developed surgical procedures, documented clinical cases, and created medical books. Before modern times, European, African, and Native American cultures all had traditions of folk medicine based on spiritual healing and herbal cures. The first hospitals were created by religious orders in medieval Europe to provide care and respite to religious pilgrims traveling back and forth from the Holy Land. However, it was not until the late 1800s that medicine became a scientific discipline. More progress and change occurred in the twentieth century than during the preceding 2,000 years. The past few decades have seen dramatic developments in the way diseases are diagnosed and treated and in the way healthcare is delivered.

Before the advent of modern Western medicine, epidemics and plagues were common. Smallpox, measles, yellow fever, influenza, scarlet fever, and diphtheria killed millions of people. Bubonic plague spread periodically through Europe and killed millions more. Disease was carried by rodents and insects as well as by the travelers who moved along intercontinental trade routes.

The medical knowledge that had been gained by ancient Greek scholars such as Hippocrates was lost during the Middle Ages. The European Renaissance, a historical period beginning in the fourteenth century, revived interest in the classical arts, literature, and philosophy as well as the scientific study of nature. This period also was characterized by economic growth and concern for the welfare of workers at all levels of society. With this concept came a growing awareness that a healthy population promoted economic growth.

North America's First Hospitals

Early settlers in the British colonies of North America appointed commissions to care for the sick, to provide for orphans, and to bury the dead. During the mid-1700s, the citizens of Philadelphia recognized the need for a place to provide relief to the sick and injured. They also recognized the need to isolate newly arrived immigrants who had caught communicable diseases on the long voyage from Europe.

Benjamin Franklin and other colonists persuaded the legislature to develop a hospital for the community. The Pennsylvania Hospital was established in Philadelphia in 1752, the first hospital in the British colonies. (Almost 200 years earlier, Cortez established the first hospital in Mexico and it still serves patients today.)

In its first 150 years, the Pennsylvania Hospital was a model for the organization of hospitals in other communities. The New York Hospital opened in 1771 and started its first register of patients in 1791. Boston's Massachusetts General Hospital opened in 1821.

Standardization of Medical Practice

Human anatomy and physiology and the causes of disease were not well understood before the twentieth century. At one time, it was believed that four basic fluids, called humors, determined a person's temperament and health, and that imbalances in the proportion of humors in the body caused disease. The therapeutic bleeding of patients was practiced until the early twentieth century. Early physicians also treated patients by administering a variety of substances with no scientific basis for their effectiveness.

An individual's early medical education consisted of serving as an apprentice to an established practitioner. Just about anyone could hang out a shingle and call himself a physician. The medical profession recognized that some of its members achieved better results than others, and leaders in the profession attempted to regulate the practice of medicine in the late 1700s. The first attempts at regulation took the form of licensure. The first licenses to practice medicine were issued in New York in 1760. By the mid-1800s, however, efforts to license physicians were denounced as being undemocratic and penalties for practicing medicine without a license were removed in most states.

As the U.S. population grew and settlers moved westward, the demand for medical practitioners far exceeded the supply. To staff new hospitals and serve a growing population, private medical schools began to appear almost overnight. By 1869, there were seventy-two medical schools in the United States. However, these schools did not follow an established course of study and some graduated students with as little as six months of training. The result was an oversupply of poorly trained physicians.

The **American Medical Association** (AMA) was established in 1847 to represent the interests of physicians across the country. However, the AMA was dominated by members who had strong ties to the medical schools and the status quo. Its ability to lead a reform of the profession was limited until it broke its ties with the medical schools in 1874. At that time, the association encouraged the creation of independent state licensing boards.

In 1876, the **American Association of Medical Colleges** (AAMC) was established. The AAMC was dedicated to standardizing the curriculum for U.S. medical schools and to developing the public's understanding of the need to license physicians.

Together, the AMA and the AAMC campaigned for medical licensing. By the 1890s, thirty-five states had established or reestablished a system of licensure for physicians. At that time, fourteen states decided to grant licenses only to graduates of reputable medical schools. The state licensing boards discouraged the worst medical schools, but the criteria for licensing continued to vary from state to state and were not fully enforced.

By the early twentieth century, it had become apparent that improving the quality of American medicine required regulation through curriculum reform as well as licensure. However, the members of the AMA were divided on this issue. Conservative members continued to believe that the association should stay out of the area of regulation whereas progressive members supported continued development of state licensure systems and creation of a standardized model for medical education.

The situation attracted the attention of the Carnegie Foundation for the Advancement of Teaching. The president of the foundation offered to sponsor and fund an independent review of the medical colleges then operating in the United States. Abraham Flexner, an educator from Louisville, Kentucky, undertook the review in 1906.

Over the following four years, Flexner visited every medical college in the country and carefully documented his findings. In his 1910 report to the Carnegie Foundation, the

AMA, and the AAMC, he described the poor quality of the training being provided in the colleges. He noted that medical school applicants often lacked knowledge of the basic sciences. Flexner also reported how the absence of hospital-based training limited the clinical skills of medical school graduates. Perhaps most important, he reported that huge numbers of graduates were being produced every year and that most of them had unacceptable levels of medical skill. He recommended closing most of the existing medical schools to address the problem of oversupply.

Several reform initiatives grew out of Flexner's report and from recommendations made by the AMA's Committee on Medical Education. One of the reforms required medical school applicants to hold a college degree. Another required that medical training be founded in the basic sciences. Reforms also required that medical students receive practical, hospital-based training in addition to classroom work. These reforms were carried out in the decade following Flexner's report, but only about half the medical schools actually closed. By 1920, most of the medical colleges in the United States had met rigorous academic standards and were approved by the AAMC.

Today, medical school graduates must pass a test before they can obtain a license to practice medicine. The licensure tests are administered by state medical boards. Many states now use a standardized licensure test developed in 1968 by the Federation of State Medical Boards of the United States. However, passing scores for the test vary by state. Most physicians also complete several years of residency training in addition to medical school.

Specialty physicians also complete extensive postgraduate medical education. Board certification for the various specialties requires the completion of postgraduate training as well as a passing score on a standardized examination. The most common medical specialties include the following:

- Internal medicine
- Pediatrics
- Family practice
- Cardiology
- Psychiatry
- Neurology
- Oncology
- Radiology

The most common surgical specialties include:

- Anesthesiology
- Cardiovascular surgery
- Obstetrics/gynecology
- Orthopedics
- Urology
- Ophthalmology

- Otorhinolaryngology
- Plastic and reconstructive surgery
- Neurosurgery

Some medical and surgical specialists undergo further graduate training to qualify to practice subspecialties. For example, the subspecialties of internal medicine include endocrinology, pulmonary medicine, rheumatology, geriatrics, and hematology. Physicians also may limit their practices to the treatment of specific illnesses. For example, an endocrinologist may limit his or her practice to the treatment of diabetes. Surgeons can work as general surgeons or as specialists or subspecialists. For example, an orthopedic surgeon may limit his practice to surgery of the hand, surgery of the knee, surgery of the ankle, or surgery of the spine.

Some physicians and healthcare organizations employ physician assistants (PAs) and/or surgeon assistants (SAs) to help them carry out their clinical responsibilities. Such assistants may perform routine clinical assessments, provide patient education and counseling, and perform simple therapeutic procedures. Most PAs work in primary care settings, and most SAs work in hospitals and ambulatory surgery clinics. PAs and SAs always work under the supervision of licensed physicians and surgeons.

Standardization of Nursing Practice

In the nineteenth century and the first part of the twentieth century, religious organizations sponsored more than half the hospitals in the United States. Members of religious orders often provided nursing care in these organizations. As the U.S. population grew and more towns and cities were established, new hospitals were built. Older cities also grew, and city hospitals became more and more crowded.

In the late 1800s, nurses received no formal education and little training. Nursing staff for the hospitals was often recruited from the surrounding community, and many poor women who had no other skills became nurses. The nature of nursing care at that time was unsophisticated. Indeed, the lack of basic hygiene often promoted disease. Many patients died from infections contracted while hospitalized for surgery, maternity care, and other illnesses.

In 1868, the AMA called the medical profession's attention to the need for trained nurses. During the years that followed, the public also began to call for better nursing care in hospitals.

The first general training school for nurses was opened at the New England Hospital for Women and Children in 1872. It became a model for other institutions throughout the country. As hospital after hospital struggled to find competent nursing staff, many institutions and their medical staffs developed their own nurse training programs.

The responsibilities of nurses in the late nineteenth and early twentieth centuries included housekeeping duties. Nurses also cooked meals for patients in kitchens attached to each ward. Direct patient care duties included giving baths, changing dressings, monitoring vital signs, administering medications, and assisting physicians. During this time, nurses were not required to hold a license to practice.

In 1897, a group of nurses attending the annual meeting of the American Society of Superintendents of Training Schools for Nursing founded the Nurses Associated Alumnae of the United States and Canada. In 1911, the organization was renamed the **American**

Nurses Association (ANA). During the early meetings of the association, members established a nursing code of ethics and discussed the need for nursing licensure and for publications devoted to the practice of nursing.

At the turn of the twentieth century, nurses also began to organize state nursing associations to advocate for the registration of nurses. Their goal was to increase the level of competence among nurses nationwide. Despite opposition from many physicians who believed that nurses did not need formal education or licensure, North Carolina passed legislation requiring the registration of nurses in 1903. Today, all fifty states have laws that spell out the requirements for the registration and licensure of nursing professionals.

Modern registered nurses must have either a two-year associate's degree or a four-year bachelor's degree from a state-approved nursing school. Nurse practitioners, researchers, educators, and administrators generally have a four-year degree in nursing and additional postgraduate education in nursing. The postgraduate degree may be a master's of science or a doctorate in nursing. Nurses who graduate from nonacademic training programs are called licensed practical nurses (LPNs) or licensed vocational nurses (LVNs). Nondegreed nursing personnel work under the direct supervision of registered nurses. Nurses in all fifty states must pass an exam to obtain a license to practice.

Today's registered nurses are highly trained clinical professionals. Many specialize in specific areas of practice such as surgery, psychiatry, and intensive care. Nurse-midwives complete advanced training and are certified by the American College of Nurse-Midwives. Similarly, nurse-anesthetists are certified by the Council on Certification/Council on Recertification of Nurse Anesthetists. Nurse practitioners also receive advanced training at the master's level that qualifies them to provide primary care services to patients. They are certified by several organizations (for example, the National Board of Pediatric Nurse Practitioners) to practice in the area of their specialty.

Standardization of Hospital Care

In 1910, Dr. Franklin H. Martin suggested that the surgical area of medical practice needed to become more concerned with patient outcomes. He had been introduced to this concept in discussions with Dr. Ernest Codman. Codman was a British physician who believed that hospital practitioners should track their patients for a significant amount of time after treatment to determine whether the end result had been positive or negative. Codman also supported the use of outcome information to identify the practices that led to the best results for patients.

At that time, Martin and other American physicians were concerned about the conditions in U.S. hospitals. Many observers felt that part of the problem was related to the lack of organization in medical staffs and to lax professional standards. In the early twentieth century, before the development of antibiotics and other pharmaceuticals, hospitals were used mainly by physicians who needed facilities in which to perform surgery. Most nonsurgical medical care was still provided in the home. It was natural, then, for the force behind improved hospital care to come from surgeons.

The push for hospital reforms eventually led to formation of the American College of Surgeons in 1913. The organization faced a difficult task. In 1917, the leaders of the college asked the Carnegie Foundation for funding to plan and develop a hospital standardization program. The college then formed a committee to develop a set of minimum standards for hospital care. It published the formal standards under the title of the Minimum Standards.

During 1918 and part of 1919, the college examined the hospitals in the U.S. and Canada just as Flexner had reviewed the medical colleges a decade earlier. The performance of 692 hospitals was compared to the college's Minimum Standards. Only eighty-nine of the hospitals fully met the college's standards, and some of the best-known hospitals in the country failed to meet them.

Adoption of the Minimum Standards was the basis of the Hospital Standardization Program and marked the beginning of the modern accreditation process for healthcare organizations. Basically, accreditation standards are developed to reflect reasonable quality standards. The performance of each participating organization is evaluated annually against the standards. The accreditation process is voluntary; healthcare organizations choose to participate in order to improve the care they provide to their patients.

The American College of Surgeons continued to sponsor the hospital accreditation program until the early 1950s. At that time, four professional associations from the U.S. and Canada joined forces with the college to create a new accreditation organization called the Joint Commission on Accreditation of Hospitals. The associations were the American College of Physicians, the AMA, the **American Hospital Association** (AHA), and the Canadian Medical Association. The new organization was formally incorporated in 1952 and began to perform accreditation surveys in 1953.

The Joint Commission, under the name Joint Commission on Accreditation of Healthcare Organizations (JCAHO), continues to survey several different types of healthcare organizations today, including:

- Acute care hospitals

- Long-term care facilities

- Ambulatory care facilities

- Psychiatric facilities

- Home health agencies

Several other organizations also perform accreditation of healthcare organizations. These include the American Osteopathic Association (AOA), the Commission on Accreditation of Rehabilitation Facilities (CARF), and the Accreditation Association for Ambulatory Healthcare (AAAHC).

Professionalization of the Allied Health Professions

After the First World War, many roles previously played by nurses and nonclinical personnel began to change. With the advent of modern diagnostic and therapeutic technology in the mid-twentieth century, the complex skills needed by ancillary medical personnel fostered the growth of specialized training programs and professional accreditation and licensure.

According to the AMA, allied health incorporates the healthcare-related professions that function to assist, facilitate, and/or complement the work of physicians and other clinical specialists. The Health Professions Education Amendment of 1991 describes **allied health professionals** as health professionals (other than registered nurses, physicians, and physician assistants) who have received either a certificate, an associate's degree, a bachelor's degree, a master's degree, a doctorate, or postdoctoral training in a healthcare-related science. Such individuals share responsibility for the delivery of healthcare services with clinicians (physicians, nurses, and physician assistants).

Allied health occupations are among the fastest growing in healthcare. The number of allied health professionals is difficult to estimate and depends on the definition of allied health. Unlike the case in medicine, women dominate most of the allied health professions, representing between 75 and 95 percent in most of the occupations. All fifty states require licensure for some allied health professions (physical therapy, for example). Practitioners in other allied health professions (occupational therapy, for example) may be licensed in some states, but not in others.

The following list briefly describes some of the major occupations usually considered to be allied health professions (Jonas and Kovner 2005, 446–48):

- *Clinical laboratory science:* Originally referred to as medical laboratory technology, this field is now more appropriately referred to as clinical laboratory science. Clinical laboratory technicians perform a wide array of tests on body fluids, tissues, and cells to assist in the detection, diagnosis, and treatment of diseases and illnesses.

- *Diagnostic imaging technology:* Originally referred to as x-ray technology and then radiologic technology, this field is now more appropriately referred to as diagnostic imaging. The field continues to expand to include nuclear medicine technologists, radiation therapists, sonographers (ultrasound technologists), and magnetic resonance technologists.

- *Dietetics:* Dietitians (also clinical nutritionists) are trained in nutrition. They are responsible for providing nutritional care to individuals and for overseeing nutrition and food services in a variety of settings, ranging from hospitals to schools.

- *Emergency medical technology:* Emergency medical technicians (EMTs) provide a wide range of services on an emergency basis for cases of traumatic injury and other emergency situations and in the transport of emergency patients.

- *Health information management:* Health information management (HIM) professionals (formerly called medical record managers) oversee health record systems and manage health-related information to ensure that it meets relevant medical, administrative, and legal requirements. Health records are the responsibility of registered health information administrators (RHIAs) and registered health information technicians (RHITs).

- *Occupational therapy:* Occupational therapists (OTs) evaluate and treat patients whose illnesses or injuries have resulted in significant psychological, physical, or work-related impairment.

- *Physical therapy:* Physical therapists (PTs) evaluate and treat patients to improve functional mobility, reduce pain, maintain cardiopulmonary function, and limit disability. PTs treat movement dysfunction resulting from accidents, trauma, stroke, fractures, multiple sclerosis, cerebral palsy, arthritis, and heart and respiratory illness. Physical therapy assistants work under the direction of PTs and help carry out the treatment plans developed by PTs.

- *Respiratory therapy:* Respiratory therapists (RTs) evaluate, treat, and care for patients with breathing disorders. They work under the direction of qualified physicians and provide services such as emergency care for stroke, heart failure, and shock, and treat patients with emphysema and asthma.

- *Speech-language pathology and audiology:* Speech-language pathologists and audiologists identify, assess, and provide treatment for individuals with speech, language, or hearing problems.

Check Your Understanding 13.1

Instructions: Choose the word or term that correctly completes each of the sentences below.

1. ____ The ancient ____ developed surgical procedures, documented clinical cases, and created medical books.
    a. Egyptians
    b. Greeks
    c. Phoenicians
    d. Chinese

2. ____ The ____ was established in 1847 to represent the interests of physicians across the United States.
    a. American Association of Medical Colleges
    b. American College of Surgeons
    c. Committee on Medical Education
    d. American Medical Association

3. ____ Today, medical school students must pass a test before they can obtain a ____ to practice medicine.
    a. Degree
    b. Residency
    c. Specialty
    d. License

4. ____ The first general training school for ____ was opened at the New England Hospital for Women and Children in 1872.
    a. Nurses
    b. Physician assistants
    c. Surgical specialists
    d. Surgeons

5. ____ Modern ____ must have either a two-year associate's degree or a four-year bachelor's degree from a state-approved nursing school.
    a. Nurse practitioners
    b. Licensed vocational nurses
    c. Registered nurses
    d. Licensed practical nurses

6. ____ In 1910, Dr. Franklin H. Martin suggested that the surgical area of medical practice needed to become more concerned with ____
   a. Patient care
   b. Professional standards
   c. Patient outcomes
   d. Nonsurgical medical care

7. ____ The adoption of the Minimum Standards marked the beginning of the modern ____ process for healthcare organizations.
   a. Accreditation
   b. Licensing
   c. Reform
   d. Educational

8. ____ According to the AMA's definition, ____ incorporates the healthcare-related professions that function to assist, facilitate, and/or complement the work of physicians and other clinical specialists.
   a. Home health
   b. Nursing care
   c. Ambulatory care
   d. Allied health

Modern Healthcare Delivery in the United States

Until the Second World War, most healthcare was provided in the home. Quality in healthcare services was considered a product of appropriate medical practice and oversight by physicians and surgeons. Even the Minimum Standards used to evaluate the performance of hospitals were based on factors directly related to the composition and skills of the hospital medical staff.

The twentieth century was a period of tremendous change in American society. Advances in medical science promised better outcomes and increased the demand for healthcare services. But medical care has never been free. Even in the best economic times, many Americans have been unable to take full advantage of what medicine has to offer because they cannot afford it.

Concern over access to healthcare was especially evident during the Great Depression of the 1930s. During the Depression, America's leaders were forced to consider how the poor and disadvantaged could receive the care they needed. Before the Depression, medical care for the poor and elderly had been handled as a function of social welfare agencies. During the 1930s, however, few people were able to pay for medical care. The problem of how to pay for the healthcare needs of millions of Americans became a public and governmental concern. Working Americans turned to prepaid health plans to help them pay for healthcare, but the unemployed and the unemployable needed help from a different source.

Effects of the Great Depression

The concept of prepaid healthcare, or health insurance, began with the financial problems of one hospital, Baylor University Hospital in Dallas, Texas (AHA 1999, 14). In 1929, the administrator of the hospital arranged to provide hospital services to Dallas's schoolteachers for fifty cents per person per month. Before that time, a few large employers had set up company clinics and hired company physicians to care for their workers, but the idea of a prepaid health plan that could be purchased by individuals had never been tried before.

The idea caught on quickly, and new prepaid plans appeared across the country. Eventually, these plans became known as Blue Cross plans when the blue cross symbol used by some of the new plans was adopted officially as the trademark for all the plans in 1939.

Another type of prepaid plan, called the Blue Shield plan, was subsequently developed to cover the cost of physicians' services. The idea for the Blue Shield plans grew out of the medical service bureaus created by large lumber and mining companies in the Northwest. In 1939, the first formal Blue Shield plan was founded in California.

Growth in the number of Blue Cross/Blue Shield (BC/BS) plans continued through the Depression and boomed during the Second World War. During the war-related labor shortages, employers began to pay for their employees' memberships in the Blues as a way to attract and keep scarce workers.

The idea of public funding for healthcare services also goes back to the Great Depression. The decline in family income during the 1930s curtailed the use of medical services by the poor. In ten working-class communities studied between 1929 and 1933, the proportion of families with incomes under $150 per capita had increased from 10 to 43 percent. A 1938 Gallup poll asked people whether they had put off seeing a physician because of the cost. The results showed that 68 percent of lower-income respondents had put off medical care, compared with 24 percent of respondents in upper-income brackets (Starr 1982, 271).

The decreased use of medical services and the inability of many patients to pay meant lower incomes for physicians. Hospitals were in similar trouble. Beds were empty, bills went unpaid, and contributions to hospital fund-raising efforts tumbled. As a result, private physicians and charities could no longer meet the demand for free services. For the first time, physicians and hospitals asked state welfare departments to pay for the treatment of people on relief.

The Depression posed a severe test for the AMA. It was no easy matter to maintain a common front against government intervention when physicians themselves were facing economic difficulties. Because of the economic hardships, many physicians were willing to accept government-sponsored health insurance. In 1935, the California Medical Association endorsed the concept of compulsory health insurance because health insurance promised to stimulate the use of physicians' services and help patients pay their bills.

The AMA's response to the economic crisis emphasized restricting the supply of physicians, rather than increasing the demand for their services, by instituting mandatory health insurance. The AMA reacted by pushing for the closure of medical schools and reductions in the number of new medical students.

By the mid-1930s, however, the AMA began to adjust its position on health insurance. Instead of opposing all insurance, voluntary or compulsory, it began to define the terms on which voluntary programs might be acceptable. Although accepting health insurance plans in principle, the AMA did nothing to support or encourage their development.

The push for government-sponsored health insurance continued in the late 1930s during the administration of President Franklin D. Roosevelt. However, compulsory health insurance stood on the margins of national politics throughout the New Deal era. It was not made part of the new Social Security program, and it was never fully supported by President Roosevelt.

Postwar Efforts toward Improving Healthcare Access

After the Second World War, the issue of healthcare access finally moved to the center of national politics. In the late 1940s, President Harry S. Truman expressed unreserved support for a national health insurance program. However, the issue of compulsory health insurance became entangled with America's fear of communism. Opponents of Truman's healthcare program labeled it "socialized medicine," and the program failed to win legislative support.

The idea of national health insurance did not resurface until the administration of Lyndon Johnson and the Great Society legislation of the 1960s. The Medicare and Medicaid programs were legislated in 1965 to pay the cost of providing healthcare services to the elderly and the poor. The issues of healthcare reform and national health insurance were again given priority during the first four years of President Bill Clinton's administration in the 1990s. However, the complexity of American healthcare issues at the end of the twentieth century doomed reform efforts.

Influence of Federal Legislation

During the twentieth century, Congress passed many pieces of legislation that had a significant impact on the delivery of healthcare services in the United States.

Biologics Control Act of 1902

Direct federal sponsorship of medical research began with early research on methods for controlling epidemics of infectious disease. The Marine Hospital Service performed the first research. In 1887, a young physician, Joseph Kinyoun, set up a bacteriological laboratory in the Marine Hospital at Staten Island, New York. Four years later, the Hygienic Laboratory was moved to Washington, D.C. It was given authority to test and improve biological products in 1902 when Congress passed the Biologics Control Act. This act regulated the vaccines and sera sold via interstate commerce. That same year, the Hygienic Laboratory added divisions in chemistry, pharmacology, and zoology.

In 1912, the service, by then called the U.S. Public Health Service, was authorized to study chronic as well as infectious diseases. In 1930, reorganized under the Randsdell Act, the Hygienic Laboratory became the **National Institutes of Health** (NIH). In 1938, the NIH moved to a large, privately donated estate in Bethesda, Maryland (Starr 1982, 340).

Today, the mission of the NIH is to uncover new medical knowledge that can lead to health improvements for everyone. The NIH accomplishes its mission by conducting and supporting medical research, fostering communication of up-to-date medical information, and training research investigators. The organization has played a vital role in recent clinical research on the treatment of the following diseases:

- Heart disease and stroke
- Cancer
- Depression and schizophrenia
- Spinal cord injuries

Social Security Act of 1935

The Great Depression revived the dormant social reform movement in the United States as well as more radical currents in American politics. Unionization increased, and the American Federation of Labor (AF of L) abandoned its long-standing opposition to social insurance programs. The Depression also brought to power a Democratic administration. The administration of Franklin D. Roosevelt was more willing than any previous administration to involve the federal government in the management of economic and social welfare.

Even before Roosevelt took office in 1933, a steady movement toward some sort of social insurance program had been growing. By 1931, nine states had passed legislation creating old-age pension programs. As governor of New York State, Roosevelt endorsed unemployment insurance in 1930. Wisconsin became the first state to adopt such a measure early in 1932.

Although old-age pension and unemployment insurance bills were introduced into Congress soon after his election, Roosevelt refused to give them his strong support. Instead, he created a program of his own. On June 8, 1934, he announced that he would appoint a committee on economic security to study the issue comprehensively and report to Congress in January 1935. The committee consisted of four members of the cabinet and the federal relief administrator. It was headed by the secretary of labor, Frances Perkins.

Although Roosevelt indicated in his June message that he was especially interested in old-age and unemployment programs, the committee included medical care and health insurance in its research. From the outset, the prevailing sentiment on the committee was that health insurance would have to wait. Abraham Epstein was the founder of the American Association for Social Security and a leading figure in the social insurance movement. In an article published in October 1934, he warned the administration that opposition to health insurance was strong. He advised the administration to be politically realistic and go slow on health insurance.

Sentiment in favor of health insurance was strong among members of the Committee on Economic Security. However, many members of the committee were convinced that adding a health insurance amendment would spell defeat for the entire Social Security legislation. Ultimately, the Social Security bill included only one reference to health insurance as a subject that the new Social Security Board might study. The Social Security Act was passed in 1935.

The omission of health insurance from the legislation was by no means the act's only conservative feature. It relied on a regressive tax and gave no coverage to some of the nation's poorest people, such as farmers and domestic workers. However, the act did extend the federal government's role in public health through several provisions unrelated to social insurance. It gave the states funds on a matching basis for maternal and infant care, rehabilitation of crippled children, general public health work, and aid for dependent children under the age of sixteen.

Hospital Survey and Construction Act of 1946

Passage of the **Hill-Burton Act** was another important development in American healthcare delivery. Enacted in 1946 as the Hospital Survey and Construction Act, this legislation authorized grants for states to construct new hospitals and, later, to modernize old ones. The fund expansion of the hospital system was to achieve a goal for 4.5 beds per 1,000 persons. The availability of federal financing created a boom in hospital construction during the 1950s.

The hospital system grew from 6,000 hospitals in 1946 to a high of approximately 7,200 acute care hospitals.

Growth in Number of Hospitals
The number of hospitals in the United States increased from 178 in 1873 to 4,300 in 1909. In 1946, at the close of the Second World War, there were 6,000 American hospitals, with 3.2 beds available for every 1,000 persons.

In 2002, there were 4,927 hospitals in the U.S., with a total of 821,000 beds. Of the $1.4 trillion spent on healthcare in 2001, hospital costs totaled $415 billion, or 32 percent. Most U.S. hospitals are nonprofit or owned by local, state, or federal governments (Jonas and Kovner 2005, 224).

Decline in Number of Hospitals
During the 1980s, medical advances and cost-containment measures caused many procedures that once required inpatient hospitalization to be performed on an outpatient basis. Outpatient hospital visits increased by 40 percent with a resultant decrease in hospital admissions. Fewer patient admissions and shortened lengths of stay (LOS) resulted in a significant reduction in the number of hospitals and hospital beds. Healthcare reform efforts and the acceptance of managed care as the major medical practice style of U.S. healthcare resulted in enough hospital closings and mergers to reduce the number of government and community-based hospitals in the U.S. to approximately 5,000 (Sultz and Young 2004, 68).

The advent of diagnosis-related groups (DRGs) in the mid-1980s resulted in the closure of many rural healthcare facilities. DRGs are discussed later in this chapter.

Public Law 89-97 of 1965
In 1965, passage of a number of amendments to the Social Security Act brought Medicare and Medicaid into existence. The two programs have greatly changed how healthcare organizations are reimbursed. Recent attempts to curtail Medicare/Medicaid spending continue to affect healthcare organizations.

Medicare (Title XVIII of the Social Security Act) is a federal program that provides healthcare benefits for people 65 years old and older who are covered by Social Security. The program was inaugurated on July 1, 1966. Over the years, amendments have extended coverage to individuals who are not covered by Social Security but are willing to pay a premium for coverage, to the disabled, and to those suffering from chronic kidney disease.

The companion program, Medicaid, Title XIX of the Social Security Act, was established at the same time to support medical and hospital care for persons classified as medically indigent. Originally targeted recipients of public assistance (primarily single-parent families and the aged, blind, and disabled), Medicaid has expanded to additional groups so that it now targets poor children, the disabled, pregnant women, and very poor adults (including 65 and over). The only exception to these expansions was passage of the Personal Responsibility and Work Opportunity Reconciliation Act of 1996 (PRWORA, P.L. 104-193, 1996), which changed eligibility for legal/illegal immigrants (Jonas and Kovner 2005, 56).

Today, Medicaid is a federally mandated program that provides healthcare benefits to low-income people and their children. Medicaid programs are administered and partially paid for by individual states. Medicaid is an umbrella for fifty different state programs designed specifically to serve the poor. Beginning in January 1967, Medicaid provided federal funds to states on a cost-sharing basis to ensure that welfare recipients would be guaranteed medical services. Coverage of four types of care was required: inpatient and outpatient services, other laboratory and x-ray services, physician services, and nursing facility care for persons over 21 years of age.

Many enhancements have been made in the years since Medicaid was enacted. Services now include family planning and thirty-one other optional services such as prescription drugs and dental services. With few exceptions, recipients of cash assistance are automatically eligible for Medicaid. Medicaid also pays the Medicare premium, deductible, and coinsurance costs for some low-income Medicare beneficiaries.

Four million individuals were enrolled in Medicaid in 1966, its first year of implementation. By December 2002, 39.7 million people were enrolled in Medicaid programs. In 2002, the states and the federal government expended $250.4 billion on Medicaid, most of which was directed toward elderly, blind, or disabled participants. Elderly and disabled participants comprised about one quarter of the Medicaid rolls, yet the program expends almost three-quarters of all funds on this group (Jonas and Kovner 2005, 56–57).

Public Law 92-603 of 1972
Utilization review (UR) was a mandatory component of the original Medicare legislation. Medicare required hospitals and **extended care facilities** to establish a plan for UR as well as a permanent utilization review committee. The goal of the UR process was to ensure that the services provided to Medicare beneficiaries were medically necessary.

In an effort to curtail Medicare and Medicaid spending, additional amendments to the Social Security Act were instituted in 1972. Public Law 92-603 required concurrent review for Medicare and Medicaid patients. It also established the professional standards review organization (PSRO) program to implement concurrent review. PSROs performed professional review and evaluated patient care services for necessity, quality, and cost-effectiveness.

Three major eras occurred in healthcare policy from 1975 to 2000. Like an archeological site, these eras have accumulated mostly on top of one another, rather than fully replacing what has come before. The three health policy eras can be identified as the following:

- Age of Traditional Insurance (1965–1982), which began with the enactment of Medicare and Medicaid and which was based on open-ended, fee-for-service health insurance;

- Age of Regulated Prices for Government Programs (1983–1992), which was launched with the enactment of the Medicare DRG system; and

- Age of Markets, Purchasing and Managed Care (1993–2000), the era that has seen the population move to managed care plans in both the private and public coverage programs (Etheredge 2001).

Health Systems Agency
The Health Planning and Resources Development Act of 1974 called for a new type of organization, the **health systems agency** (HSA), to have broad representation of healthcare providers and consumers on governing boards and committees. Although the governance structure required participation by consumers, interested parties from the provider groups dominated the discussions. HSAs were fundamentally unsuccessful in materially influencing decisions about service or technology expansion. Their decisions became undeniably political and attempts to achieve consensus based on real service needs were counterbalanced by community interests in economic and employment expansions.

Concurrent with attempts to slow cost increases through a planning approach, a number of other legislative initiatives took shape that were directly related to concerns over Medicare costs and service quality (Sultz and Young 2004, 39,242). The legislation that created the HSAs or nationwide system of local health planning agencies was repealed in 1986.

Utilization Review Act of 1977
In 1977, the **Utilization Review Act** made it a requirement that hospitals conduct continued-stay reviews for Medicare and Medicaid patients. Continued-stay reviews determine whether it is medically necessary for a patient to remain hospitalized. This legislation also included fraud and abuse regulations.

Peer Review Improvement Act of 1982
In 1982, the Peer Review Improvement Act redesigned the PSRO program and renamed the agencies **peer review organizations** (PROs). At this time, hospitals began to review the medical necessity and appropriateness of certain admissions even before patients were admitted. PROs were given a new name in 2002 and now are called **quality improvement organizations** (QIOs). They currently emphasize quality improvement processes. Each state and territory, as well as the District of Columbia, now has its own QIO. The mission of the QIOs is to ensure the quality, efficiency, and cost-effectiveness of the healthcare services provided to Medicare beneficiaries in its locale.

Tax Equity and Fiscal Responsibility Act of 1982
In 1982, Congress passed the Tax Equity and Fiscal Responsibility Act (TEFRA). TEFRA required extensive changes in the Medicare program. Its purpose was to control the rising cost of providing healthcare services to Medicare beneficiaries. Before this legislation was passed, healthcare services provided to Medicare beneficiaries were reimbursed on a retrospective, or fee-based, payment system. TEFRA required the gradual implementation of a prospective payment system (PPS) for Medicare reimbursement.

In a retrospective payment system, a service is provided, a claim for payment for the service is made, and the healthcare provider is reimbursed for the cost of delivering the service. In a PPS, a predetermined level of reimbursement is established before the service is provided.

Prospective Payment Act (1982)/Public Law 98-21 of 1983
The PPS for acute hospital care (inpatient) services was implemented on October 1, 1983, according to Public Law 98-21. Under the inpatient PPS, reimbursement for hospital care provided to Medicare patients is based on diagnosis-related groups (DRGs). Each case is assigned to a DRG based on the patient's diagnosis at the time of discharge. For example, under inpatient PPS, all cases of viral pneumonia would be reimbursed at the same predetermined level of reimbursement no matter how long the patients stayed in the hospital or how many services they received.

PPSs for other healthcare services provided to Medicare beneficiaries have been gradually implemented in the years since 1983. Implementation of the ambulatory payment classification system for hospital outpatient services, for example, began in the year 2000.

Consolidated Omnibus Budget Reconciliation Act of 1985
The Consolidated Omnibus Budget Reconciliation Act made it possible for the Centers for Medicare and Medicaid Services (CMS) to deny reimbursement for substandard healthcare services provided to Medicare and Medicaid beneficiaries.

Omnibus Budget Reconciliation Act of 1986

The Omnibus Budget Reconciliation Act of 1986 requires PROs to report instances of substandard care to relevant licensing and certification agencies.

Healthcare Quality Improvement Act of 1986

The Healthcare Quality Improvement Act established the **National Practitioner Data Bank** (NPDB). The purpose of the NPDB is to provide a clearinghouse for information about medical practitioners who have a history of malpractice suits and other quality problems. Hospitals are required to consult the NPDB before granting medical staff privileges to healthcare practitioners. The legislation also established immunity from legal actions for practitioners involved in some peer review activities.

Omnibus Budget Reconciliation Act of 1989

The Omnibus Budget Reconciliation Act of 1989 instituted the Agency for Healthcare Policy and Research. The **mission** of this agency is to develop outcome measures to evaluate the quality of healthcare services.

Omnibus Budget Reconciliation Act of 1990

The Omnibus Budget Reconciliation Act of 1990 requires PROs to report actions taken against physicians to state medical boards and licensing agencies.

Health Insurance Portability and Accountability Act of 1996

The Health Insurance Portability and Accountability Act of 1996 (HIPAA) addresses issues related to the portability of health insurance after leaving employment, as well as administrative simplification. One of the provisions of HIPAA was creation of the Healthcare Integrity and Protection Data Bank (HIPDB). The mission of this data bank is to inform federal and state agencies about potential quality problems with clinicians and with suppliers and providers of healthcare services.

Biomedical and Technological Advances in Medicine

Rapid progress in medical science and technology during the late nineteenth and twentieth centuries revolutionized the way healthcare was provided. The most important scientific advancement was the discovery of bacteria as the cause of infectious disease. The most important technological development was the use of anesthesia for surgical procedures. These nineteenth-century advances laid the basis for the development of antibiotics and other pharmaceuticals and the application of sophisticated surgical procedures in the twentieth century.

To further medical advances in the twenty-first century, NIH sought the input of more than 300 recognized leaders in academia, industry, government, and the public to create a "Roadmap" program to accelerate biomedical advances, create effective prevention strategies and new treatments, and bridge knowledge gaps. The program, which involves a plethora of NIH institutes and centers, has three main strategic initiatives:

1. New Pathways to Discovery, which includes a comprehensive understanding of building blocks of the body's cells and tissues and how complex biological systems operate; structural biology; molecular libraries and imaging; nanotechnology; bioinformatics and computational biology;

2. Research Teams of the Future, including interdisciplinary research, high-risk research, and public-private partnerships; and

3. Re-engineering the Clinical Research Enterprise.

Through these efforts, NIH will boost the resources and technologies needed for 21st century biomedical science (NIH 2005). Figure 13.1 offers a time line of key biological and technological advances at a glance.

Surgical procedures were performed before the development of anesthesia, so surgeons had to work quickly on conscious patients to minimize risk and pain. The availability of anesthesia made it possible for surgeons to develop more advanced surgical techniques. The use of ether as an anesthetic was first recorded in 1842. At about the same time, nitrous oxide was introduced for use during dental procedures, and chloroform was used to reduce the pain of labor. By the 1860s, the physicians who treated the casualties of the American Civil War on both sides had access to anesthetic and pain-killing drugs.

In the 1860s, Louis Pasteur began studying a condition in wine that made it sour and unpalatable. He discovered that the wine was being spoiled by bacterial growths. His

Figure 13.1.   Key biological and technological advances in medicine

Time	Event
1842	First recorded use of ether as an anesthetic
1860s	Louis Pasteur laid the foundation for modern bacteriology
1865	Joseph Lister was the first to apply Pasteur's research to the treatment of infected wounds
1880s–1890s	Steam first used in physical sterilization
1898	Introduction of rubber surgical gloves, sterilization, and antisepsis
1895	Wilhelm Roentgen made observations that led to the development of x-ray technology
1940	Studies of prothrombin time first made available
1941–1946	Studies of electrolytes; development of major pharmaceuticals
1957	Studies of blood gas
1961	Studies of creatine phosphokinase
1970s	Surgical advances in cardiac bypass surgery, surgery for joint replacements, and organ transplantation
1971	Computed tomography first used in England
1974	Introduction of whole-body scanners
1980s	Introduction of magnetic resonance imaging
1990s	Further technological advances in pharmaceuticals and genetics; Human Genome Project
2000s	NIH creates roadmap to accelerate biomedical advances, create effective prevention strategies and new treatments, and bridge knowledge gaps in the 21st century

research proved that tiny, living organisms (called bacteria) increase through reproduction and cause infectious disease. Pasteur also demonstrated that heat and certain chemicals such as alcohol could destroy bacteria. In doing so, he laid the foundation for modern bacteriology. After twenty years of research into the biology of microorganisms, Pasteur began studying human diseases. In 1885, he developed a vaccine that prevented rabies.

Although the importance of cleanliness had been known since early times, the role that microorganisms played in disease was not understood until Pasteur conducted his research. In 1865, Joseph Lister was the first to apply Pasteur's research to the treatment of infected wounds. Lister began by protecting open fractures from infection by treating the wounds with carbolic acid (a disinfectant). His discovery was called the antiseptic principle. Antisepsis reduced the mortality rate in Lister's hospital after 1865 from 45 to 12 percent. He published his results in 1868, and soon carbolic acid was being used to prevent bacterial contamination during surgery.

During the 1880s and 1890s, physical sterilization using steam was developed. This technological advance had a major impact on surgery and in other areas throughout the hospital. The sterile operative technique was further advanced through the introduction of rubber surgical gloves in 1898. Other advances included the use of sterile gowns, masks, and antibiotics and other drugs.

In 1895, the well-known physicist Wilhelm Roentgen made observations that led to the development of x-ray technology. He found that he could create images of the bones in his hand by passing x-rays through his hand and onto a photographic plate. Radiographic technology is used extensively to diagnose illnesses and injuries today.

Many advances in laboratory testing occurred during the twentieth century. Equipment that allows the rapid laboratory processing of diagnostic and prognostic examinations was developed, and the number of diagnostic laboratory procedures increased dramatically. For example, studies of prothrombin time were first made available in 1940, electrolytes in 1941 through 1946, blood gas in 1957, creatine phosphokinase in 1961, serum hepatitis in 1970, and carcinoembryonic antigen (the first cancer-screening test) in 1974.

Diagnostic radiology and radiation therapy have undergone huge advances in the past fifty years. An enormous advance first used in 1971 in England is an imaging modality called computed tomography (CT). The first CT scanners were used to create images of the skull. Whole-body scanners were introduced in 1974. In the 1980s, another powerful diagnostic tool was added, magnetic resonance imaging (MRI). MRI is a noninvasive technique that uses magnetic and radio-frequency fields to record images of soft tissues.

Surgical advances have been remarkable as well. Cardiac bypass surgery was developed in the 1970s, as were the techniques for joint replacement. Organs are now successfully transplanted, and artificial organs are being tested. New surgical techniques have included the use of lasers in ophthalmology, gynecology, and urology. Microsurgery is now a common tool in the reconstruction of damaged nerves and blood vessels. The use of robotics in surgery holds great promise for the future (Sloane et al. 1999, 6–7).

Today, it is human genetics and progress toward sequencing the human genome that promise to change the healthcare paradigm. New research on cellular and molecular changes underlying disease processes will necessitate new approaches to diagnosis and treatment.

The current paradigm for treating disease is to meet with the patient, diagnose the patient's symptoms, and prescribe therapy to treat them. The hope is that genetic medicine will enable the provider to identify gene patterns that underlie the process of cellular dysfunction that leads to injury before even meeting with the patient. Thus, diseases will be diagnosed much earlier, enabling physicians to provide treatment to stop or slow down the disease process.

The study of cell-based technologies is particularly controversial. Cell-based technologies include:

- Tissue engineering, which involves the use of biomaterials to develop new tissue and even whole organs with or without transplanting cells

- Human embryonic stem cells and/or adult stem cells used for transplantation and in regenerative medicine

- Gene therapy/cell transplantation

Advances in cell-based technologies such as cell-signaling pathways, growth factors, and the human genome project are encouraging ongoing research in these areas (Elçin 2003).

The year 2003 saw completion of the Human Genome Project (HGP), a 13-year-long international effort with three principal goals: to determine the sequence of the three billion DNA subunits, to identify all human genes, and to enable genes to be used in further biological study. A process called parallel sequencing was used on selected model organisms to help develop the technology and interpret gene function. The U.S. Human Genome Project was a joint venture of the Department of Energy's HGP and the NIH's National Human Genome Research Institute. More information is available from ornl.gov/sci/techresources/Human_Genome/faq/faqs1.shtm.

Check Your Understanding 13.2

Instructions: Match the descriptions with the appropriate legislation.

1. _____ Hill-Burton Act
2. _____ Tax Equity and Fiscal Responsibility Act
3. _____ Public Law 89-79 of 1965
4. _____ Utilization Review Act
5. _____ Omnibus Budget Reconciliation Act of 1989
6. _____ Public Law 92-603 of 1972
7. _____ Healthcare Quality Improvement Act of 1986
8. _____ Omnibus Budget Reconciliation Act of 1990

a. Amendments to the Social Security Act that brought Medicare and Medicaid into existence
b. Authorized grants for states to construct new hospitals
c. Required concurrent review for Medicare and Medicaid patients
d. Required hospitals to conduct continued-stay reviews for Medicare and Medicaid patients
e. Established the National Practitioner Data Bank
f. Required PROs to report actions taken against physicians to state medical boards and licensing agencies
g. Required extensive changes in the Medicare program to control the rising cost of providing healthcare services to Medicare beneficiaries (PPS general implementation)
h. Instituted the Agency for Healthcare Policy

Professional and Trade Associations
Related to Healthcare

A number of trade and professional associations currently influence the practice of medicine and the delivery of healthcare services in the United States. Descriptions of a few of these associations are provided below.

American Medical Association

The AMA was founded in 1847 as a national voluntary service organization. Today, its membership totals approximately 300,000 physicians from every area of medicine. The organization is headquartered in Chicago. Its mission is to promote the science and art of medicine and to improve public health. Its key objectives are:

- To become the world leader in obtaining, synthesizing, integrating, and disseminating information on health and medical practice

- To remain the acknowledged leader in promoting professionalism in medicine and setting standards for medical ethics, practice, and education

- To continue to be an authoritative voice and influential advocate for patients and physicians

- To continue to be a sound organization that provides value to its members, related organizations, and employees

In addition, the AMA acts as an accreditation body for medical schools and residency programs. It also maintains and publishes the *Current Procedural Terminology* (CPT) coding system. CPT codes are the basis of reimbursement systems for physician's services and other types of healthcare services provided on an ambulatory basis.

American Hospital Association

The AHA was founded in 1899. At its first meeting, eight hospital superintendents gathered in Cleveland, Ohio, to exchange ideas, compare methods of hospital management, discuss economics, and explore common interests and new trends. Originally called the Association of Hospital Superintendents, its mission was "to facilitate the interchange of ideas, comparing and contrasting methods of management, the discussion of hospital economics, the inspection of hospitals, suggestions of better plans for operating them, and such other matters as may affect the general interest of the membership" (AHA 1999, 110).

The association adopted a new constitution in 1906 and a new name, the American Hospital Association. At that time, it had 234 members. Its major concerns were developing hospital standards and building the management skills of it members.

Today, the mission of the AHA is to advance the health of individuals and communities. The association's current membership includes approximately 5,000 hospitals and healthcare institutions, 600 associate member organizations, and 40,000 individual executives active in the healthcare field. Its headquarters are located in Chicago.

The AHA publishes *Coding Clinic,* which provides official ICD-9-CM coding advice.

Joint Commission on Accreditation of Healthcare Organizations

Since 1952, the Joint Commission has continually evolved to meet the changing needs of healthcare organizations. The organization changed its name from the Joint Commission on Accreditation of Hospitals (JCAH) to the Joint Commission on Accreditation of Healthcare Organizations (JCAHO) in the late 1980s in recognition of changes in the U.S. health delivery system. Today, it is the largest healthcare standards-setting body in the world. It conducts accreditation surveys in more than 19,500 facilities, including ambulatory care facilities, long-term care facilities, behavioral health facilities, healthcare networks, and MCOs in addition to acute care hospitals (JCAHO 2000).

In the late 1990s, the JCAHO moved away from traditional quality assessment processes and began emphasizing performance and quality improvement. The ORYX initiative reflected the new approach. The goal of the ORYX initiative was to incorporate the ongoing collection of quality and performance data into the accreditation process.

Today, JCAHO standards give organizations substantial leeway in selecting performance measures and improvement projects. Outcome measures document the results of care for individual patients as well as for specific types of patients grouped by diagnostic category. For example, an acute care hospital's overall rate of postsurgical infection would be considered an outcome measure. Outcome measures must be reported to the JCAHO via software from vendors that have been approved by the JCAHO for this purpose.

Blue Cross and Blue Shield Association

The forerunner of the Blue Cross and Blue Shield Association was a commission instituted by the AHA in 1929. In 1960, the commission was replaced by the Blue Cross Association and ties to the AHA were broken. In 1982, the Blue Cross Association merged with the National Association of Blue Shield Plans to become the Blue Cross and Blue Shield Association, often referred to as "the Blues."

"The purpose of Blue Cross and Blue Shield plans is to coordinate the activities of the local plans throughout the United States. More than 80 percent of hospitals and nearly 90 percent of physicians contract directly with Blue Cross and Blue Shield plans (3dquote.com/blue-cross-national-info.htm).

American College of Healthcare Executives

The **American College of Healthcare Executives** (ACHE) is an organization for healthcare administrators. Like most of the organizations already discussed, it is headquartered in Chicago. Its mission is to serve as "the professional membership society for healthcare executives; to meet members' professional, educational, and leadership needs; to promote high ethical standards and conduct; and to enhance healthcare leadership and management excellence."

ACHE has nearly 30,000 members internationally. It also publishes books and textbooks on healthcare services management.

American Nurses Association

The ANA was founded in 1897 and is headquartered in Washington, D.C. It is a professional association as well as the strongest labor union active in the nursing profession, representing the interests of the nation's 2.6 million registered nurses. The ANA's mission is to work for the improvement of health standards and the availability of healthcare services, to foster high professional standards for nurses, to stimulate and promote the professional development of nurses, and to advance the economic and general welfare of its members.

American Health Information Management Association

The American Health Information Management Association (AHIMA) is the professional membership organization for managers of health record services and healthcare information. It was founded in 1928 under the name of the Association of Record Librarians of North America. In 1929, the association adopted a constitution and bylaws. The name of the association was changed to the American Medical Record Association in 1970 and then to the American Health Information Management Association in 1991.

Headquartered in Chicago, the association currently has more than 50,000 members. Its mission is to be a "community of professionals engaged in health information management, providing support to members and strengthening the industry and profession." The association's vision is of "a world in which the public values the contribution of health information management professionals and the American Health Information Management Association, in the advancement of health through quality information."

AHIMA is the sponsoring organization for the **Commission on Accreditation for Health Informatics and Information Management Education** (CAHIIM), which accredits associate and baccalaureate programs in health information management. CAHIIM also oversees an approval program for master's degree programs in HIM. Certificate programs for coding specialists are approved through a special program offered by AHIMA, which also certifies health information professionals as registered health information technologists (RHITs) for graduates of associate degree programs and registered health information administrators (RHIAs) for graduates of baccalaureate degree programs. In addition, AHIMA offers credentialing examinations for coding professionals as certified coding associate (CCA), certified coding specialists (CCSs) and certified coding specialists for physicians' services (CCS-Ps). Certifications in healthcare information privacy (CHP), healthcare information security (CHS), and healthcare information privacy and security (CHPS) also are offered.

Other Healthcare-Related Associations

Many other healthcare-related associations serve their professional members by providing educational, certification, and accreditation services. The best known include:

- The American Osteopathic Association
- The American Dental Association
- The American College of Surgeons
- The American League for Nursing
- The American Society of Clinical Pathologists
- The American Dietetic Association
- The Commission on Accreditation of Rehabilitation Facilities
- The American Association of Nurse Anesthetists

Check Your Understanding 13.3

Instructions: Match each organization with the description that best describes it.

1. _____ American College of Healthcare Executives
2. _____ American Hospital Association
3. _____ American Medical Association
4. _____ American Nurses Association
5. _____ American Health Information Management Association
6. _____ Blue Cross and Blue Shield Association

a. Part of this organization's mission is to "enhance healthcare leadership and management excellence."
b. This organization was originally called the Association of Hospital Superintendents.
c. This organization was originally a commission instituted by the AHA in 1929.
d. This association was founded in 1928 under the name of the Association of Record Librarians of North America.
e. Part of this organization's mission is to work for the improvement of health standards and the availability of healthcare services.
f. This organization's mission is to promote the art and science of medicine and to improve public health.

Organization and Operation of Modern Hospitals

The term *hospital* can be applied to any healthcare facility that:

- Has an organized medical staff
- Provides permanent inpatient beds
- Offers around-the-clock nursing services
- Provides diagnostic and therapeutic services

Most hospitals provide acute care services to inpatients. Acute care is the short-term care provided to diagnose and/or treat an illness or injury. The individuals who receive acute care services in hospitals are considered inpatients. Inpatients receive room-and-board services in addition to continuous nursing services. Generally, patients who spend more than twenty-four hours in a hospital are considered inpatients.

The **average length of stay** (ALOS) in an acute care hospital is thirty days or less. (Hospitals that have ALOSs longer than thirty days are considered long-term care facilities. Long-term care is discussed in detail later in this chapter.) With recent advances in surgical technology, anesthesia, and pharmacology, the ALOS in an acute care hospital is much shorter today than it was only a few years ago. In addition, many diagnostic and therapeutic procedures that once required inpatient care now can be performed on an outpatient basis.

For example, before the development of laparoscopic surgical techniques, a patient might be hospitalized for ten days after a routine appendectomy (surgical removal of the appendix). Today, a patient undergoing a laparoscopic appendectomy might spend only a few hours in the hospital's outpatient surgery department and go home the same day. The influence of managed care and the emphasis on cost control in the Medicare/Medicaid programs also have resulted in shorter hospital stays.

In large acute care hospitals, hundreds of clinicians, administrators, managers, and support staff must work closely together to provide effective and efficient diagnostic and therapeutic services. Most hospitals provide services to both inpatients and outpatients. A hospital outpatient is a patient who receives hospital services without being admitted for inpatient (overnight) clinical care. Outpatient care is considered a kind of ambulatory care. (Ambulatory care is discussed later in this chapter.)

Modern hospitals are extremely complex organizations. Much of the clinical training for physicians, nurses, and allied health professionals is conducted in hospitals. Medical research is another activity carried out in hospitals.

Growth in Numbers of Hospitals

The number of hospitals in the U.S. increased from 178 in 1873 to 4,300 in 1909. In 1946, at the close of the Second World War, there were 6,000 hospitals, with 3.2 beds available for every 1,000 persons. By 2002, the number of hospitals in the U.S. had reached 4,927, with a total of 821,000 beds.

Of the $1.4 trillion spent on healthcare in 2001, hospital costs totaled $415 billion, or 32 percent. Most hospitals in the U.S. are nonprofit or owned by local, state, or federal governments (Jonas and Kovner 2005, 224).

Decline in Numbers of Hospitals

During the 1980s, medical advances and cost-containment measures enabled many procedures that once required inpatient hospitalization to be performed on an outpatient basis. Outpatient hospital visits increased by 40 percent, resulting in a decrease in hospital admissions. Fewer admissions and shortened lengths of stay for patients resulted in a significant reduction in the number of hospitals and hospital beds. Healthcare reform efforts and the rise of managed care resulted in enough hospital closings and mergers to reduce the number of governmental and community-based hospitals in the U.S. to approximately 5,000 (Sultz and Young 2004, 68).

Types of Hospitals

Hospitals can be classified in many different ways, including by:

- Number of beds
- Types of services provided
- Types of patients served
- For-profit or not-for-profit status
- Type of ownership

Number of Beds

A hospital's number of beds refers to the number of beds that are equipped and staffed for patient care. The term *bed capacity* sometimes is used to reflect the maximum number of inpatients the hospital can care for. Hospitals with fewer than a hundred beds are usually considered small. Most U.S. hospitals fall into this category. Some large, urban hospitals may have more than five hundred beds. The number of beds is usually broken down by adult beds and pediatric beds. The number of maternity beds and other special categories may be listed separately. Hospitals also can be categorized according to the number of outpatient visits per year.

Types of Services Provided

Some hospitals specialize in certain types of service and treat specific illnesses. For example:

- *Rehabilitation hospitals* generally provide long-term care services to patients recuperating from debilitating or chronic illnesses and injuries such as strokes, head and spine injuries, and gunshot wounds. Patients often stay in rehabilitation hospitals for several months.

- *Psychiatric hospitals* provide inpatient care for patients with mental and develop-mental disorders. In the past, the ALOS for psychiatric inpatients was longer than it is today. Rather than months or years, most patients now spend only a few days or weeks per stay. However, many patients require repeated hospitalization for chronic psychiatric illnesses. (Behavioral healthcare is discussed in more detail later in this chapter.)

- *General hospitals* provide a wide range of medical and surgical services to diag-nose and treat most illnesses and injuries.

- *Specialty hospitals* provide diagnostic and therapeutic services for a limited range of conditions such as burns, cancer, tuberculosis, or obstetrics/gynecology.

Types of Patients Served

Some hospitals specialize in serving specific types of patients. For example, children's hospitals provide specialized pediatric services in a number of medical specialties.

For-Profit or Not-for-Profit Status

Hospitals also can be classified based on their ownership and profitability status. Not-for-profit healthcare organizations use excess funds to improve their services and to finance educational programs and community services. For-profit healthcare organizations are privately owned. Excess funds are paid back to the managers, owners, and investors in the form of bonuses and dividends.

Type of Ownership

The most common ownership types for hospitals and other kinds of healthcare organiza-tions in the U.S. include:

- *Government-owned hospitals* are operated by a specific branch of federal, state, or local government as not-for-profit organizations. (Government-owned hospitals sometimes are called public hospitals.) They are supported, at least in part, by tax dollars. Examples of federally owned and operated hospitals include those oper-ated by the Department of Veterans Affairs to serve retired military personnel. The Department of Defense operates facilities for active military personnel and their dependents. Many states own and operate psychiatric hospitals. County and city governments often operate public hospitals to serve the healthcare needs of their communities, especially those residents who are unable to pay for their care.

- *Proprietary hospitals* may be owned by private foundations, partnerships, or investor-owned corporations. Large corporations may own a number of for-profit hospitals, and the stock of several large U.S. hospital chains is publicly traded.

- *Voluntary hospitals* are not-for-profit hospitals owned by universities, churches, charities, religious orders, unions, and other not-for-profit entities. They often provide free care to patients who otherwise would not have access to healthcare services.

Organization of Hospital Services

The organizational structure of every hospital is designed to meet its specific needs. For example, most acute care hospitals are made up of a board of directors, a professional medical staff, an executive administrative staff, medical and surgical services, patient care (nursing) services, diagnostic and laboratory services, and support services (for example, nutritional services, environmental safety, and HIM services).

Board of Directors

The board of directors has primary responsibility for setting the overall direction of the hospital. (In some hospitals, the board of directors is called the governing board or board of trustees.) The board works with the **chief executive officer** (CEO) and the leaders of the organization's medical staff to develop the hospital's strategic direction as well as its mission (statement of the organization's purpose and the customers it serves), vision (description of the organization's ideal future), and values (descriptive list of the organization's fundamental principles or beliefs).

Other specific responsibilities of the board of directors include:

- Establishing bylaws in accordance with the organization's legal and licensing requirements

- Selecting qualified administrators

- Approving the organization and makeup of the clinical staff

- Monitoring the quality of care

The board's members are elected for specific terms of service (for example, five years). Most boards also elect officers, commonly a chairman, vice-chairman, president, secretary, and treasurer. The size of the board varies considerably. Individual board members are called directors, board members, or trustees. Individuals serve on one or more standing committees such as the executive committee, joint conference committee, finance committee, strategic planning committee, and building committee.

The makeup of the board depends on the type of hospital and the form of ownership. For example, the board of a community hospital is likely to include local business leaders, representatives of community organizations, and other people interested in the welfare of the community. The board of a teaching hospital, on the other hand, is likely to include medical school alumni and university administrators, among others.

Increased competition among healthcare providers and limits on managed care and Medicare/Medicaid reimbursement have made the governing of hospitals especially difficult in the past two decades. In the future, boards of directors will continue to face strict accountability in terms of cost containment, performance management, and integration of services to maintain fiscal stability and to ensure the delivery of high-quality patient care.

Medical Staff

The medical staff consists of physicians who have received extensive training in various medical disciplines (internal medicine, pediatrics, cardiology, gynecology/obstetrics, orthopedics, surgery, and so on). The medical staff's primary objective is to provide high-quality patient care to the patients who come to the hospital. The physicians on the hospital's medical staff diagnose illnesses and develop patient-centered treatment regimens. Moreover, they may serve on the hospital's governing board, where they provide critical insight relevant to strategic and operational planning and policy making.

The medical staff is the aggregate of physicians who have been granted permission to provide clinical services in the hospital. This permission is called **clinical privileges.** An individual physician's privileges are limited to a specific scope of practice. For example, an internal medicine physician would be permitted to diagnose and treat a patient with pneumonia, but not to perform a surgical procedure. Most members of the medical staff are not actually employees of the hospital, although many hospitals do directly employ radiologists, anesthesiologists, and critical care specialists.

Medical staff classification refers to the organization of physicians according to clinical assignment. Depending on the size of the hospital and on the credentials and clinical privileges of its physicians, the medical staff may be separated into departments such as medicine, surgery, obstetrics, pediatrics, and other specialty services. Typical medical staff classifications include active, provisional, honorary, consulting, courtesy, and medical resident assignments.

Officers of the medical staff usually include a president or chief of staff, a vice-president or chief of staff-elect, and a secretary. These offices are authorized by a vote of the entire active medical staff. The president presides over all regular meetings of the medical staff and is an ex officio member of all medical staff committees. The secretary ensures that accurate and complete minutes of the meetings are kept and that correspondence is handled appropriately.

The medical staff operates according to a predetermined set of policies called the **medical staff bylaws.** The bylaws spell out the specific qualifications that physicians must demonstrate before they can practice medicine in the hospital. They are considered legally binding. Any changes to the bylaws must be approved by a vote of the medical staff and the hospital's governing body.

Administrative Staff

The leader of the administrative staff is the CEO or chief administrator. The CEO is responsible for implementing the policies and strategic direction set by the hospital's board of directors. He or she also is responsible for building an effective executive management team and coordinating the hospital's services. Today's healthcare organizations commonly designate a chief financial officer (CFO), a **chief operating officer** (COO), and a **chief information officer** (CIO) as members of the executive management team.

The executive management team is responsible for managing the hospital's finances and ensuring that the hospital complies with the federal, state, and local rules, standards, and laws that govern the delivery of healthcare services. Depending on the size of the hospital, the CEO's staff may include healthcare administrators with job titles such as vice-president, associate administrator, department director or manager, or administrative assistant. Department-level administrators manage and coordinate the activities of the highly specialized and multidisciplinary units that perform clinical, administrative, and support services in the hospital.

Healthcare administrators may hold advanced degrees in healthcare administration, nursing, public health, or business management. A growing number of hospitals are hiring physician executives to lead their executive management teams. Many healthcare administrators are fellows of ACHE.

Patient Care Services

Most direct patient care delivered in hospitals is provided by professional nurses. Modern nursing requires a diverse skill set, advanced clinical competencies, and postgraduate education. In almost every hospital, patient care services constitutes the largest clinical department in terms of staffing, budget, specialized services offered, and clinical expertise required.

Nurses are responsible for providing continuous, around-the-clock treatment and support for hospital inpatients. The quantity and quality of nursing care available to patients are influenced by a number of factors, including the nursing staff's educational preparation and specialization, experience, and skill level. The level of patient care staffing also is a critical component of quality.

Traditionally, physicians alone determined the type of treatment each patient would receive. However, today's nurses are playing a wider role in treatment planning and **case management.** They identify timely and effective interventions in response to a wide range of problems related to the patients' treatment, comfort, and safety. Their responsibilities include performing patient assessments, creating care plans, evaluating the appropriateness of treatment, and evaluating the effectiveness of care. At the same time that they provide technical care, effective nursing professionals also offer personal care that recognizes the concerns and emotional needs of patients and their families.

A registered nurse qualified by advanced education and clinical and management experience usually administers patient care services. Although the title may vary, this role is usually referred to as the **chief nursing officer** (CNO) or vice-president of nursing or patient care. The CNO is a member of the hospital's executive management team and usually reports directly to the CEO.

In any nursing organizational structure, several types of relationships can be identified, including:

- *Line relationships* identify the positions of superiors and subordinates and indicate the levels of authority and responsibility vested with each position. For example, a supervisor in a postop surgical unit would have authority to direct the work of several nurses.

- *Lateral relationships* define the connections among various positions in which a hierarchy of authority is not involved. For example, the supervisors of preop and postop surgical units would have parallel positions in the structure and would need to coordinate the work they perform.

- *Functional relationships* refer to duties that are divided according to function. In such arrangements, individuals exercise authority in one particular area by virtue of their special knowledge and expertise.

Diagnostic and Therapeutic Services

The services provided to patients in hospitals go beyond the clinical services provided directly by the medical and nursing staff. Many diagnostic and therapeutic services involve the work of allied health professionals. Allied health professionals receive specialized education and training, and their qualifications are registered or certified by a number of specialty organizations.

Diagnostic and therapeutic services are critical to the success of every patient care delivery system. Diagnostic services include clinical laboratory, radiology, and nuclear medicine. Therapeutic services include radiation therapy, occupational therapy, and physical therapy.

Clinical Laboratory Services

The clinical laboratory is divided into two sections: anatomic pathology and clinical pathology. Anatomic pathology deals with human tissues and provides surgical pathology, autopsy, and cytology services. Clinical pathology deals mainly with the analysis of body fluids, principally blood, but also urine, gastric contents, and cerebrospinal fluid.

Physicians who specialize in performing and interpreting the results of pathology tests are called pathologists. Laboratory technicians are allied health professionals trained to operate laboratory equipment and perform laboratory tests under the supervision of a pathologist.

Radiology

Radiology involves the use of radioactive isotopes, fluoroscopic and radiographic equipment, and CT and MRI equipment to diagnose disease. Physicians who specialize in radiology are called radiologists. They are experts in the medical use of radiant energy, radioactive isotopes, radium, cesium, and cobalt as well as x-rays, radium, and radioactive materials. They also are expert in interpreting x-ray, MRI, and CT diagnostic images.

Radiology technicians are allied health professionals trained to operate radiological equipment and perform radiological tests under the supervision of a radiologist.

Nuclear Medicine and Radiation Therapy

Radiologists also may specialize in nuclear medicine and radiation therapy. Nuclear medicine involves the use of ionizing radiation and small amounts of short-lived radioactive tracers to treat disease, specifically neoplastic disease (that is, nonmalignant tumors and malignant cancers). Based on the mathematics and physics of tracer methodology, nuclear medicine is widely applied in clinical medicine. However, most authorities agree that medical science has only scratched the surface in terms of nuclear medicine's potential capabilities.

Radiation therapy uses high-energy x-rays, cobalt, electrons, and other sources of radiation to treat human disease. In current practice, radiation therapy is used alone or in combination with surgery or chemotherapy (drugs) to treat many types of cancer. In addition to external beam therapy, radioactive implants, as well as therapy performed with heat (hyperthermia), are available.

Occupational Therapy

Occupational therapy is the medically directed use of work and play activities to improve patients' independent functioning, enhance their development, and prevent or decrease their level of disability. The individuals who perform occupational therapy are credentialed allied health professionals called occupational therapists. They work under the direction of physicians. Occupational therapy is made available in acute care hospitals, clinics, and rehabilitation centers.

Providing occupational therapy services begins with an evaluation of the patient and the selection of therapeutic goals. Occupational therapy activities may involve the adaptation of tasks or the environment to achieve maximum independence and to enhance the patient's quality of life. An occupational therapist may treat developmental deficits, birth defects, learning disabilities, traumatic injuries, burns, neurological conditions, orthopedic conditions, mental deficiencies, and psychiatric disorders. Within the healthcare system, occupational therapy plays various roles. These roles include promoting health, preventing disability, developing or restoring functional capacity, guiding adaptation within physical and mental parameters, and teaching creative problem solving to increase independent function.

Physical Therapy and Rehabilitation

Physical therapy and rehabilitation have expanded into many medical specialties. Physical therapy can be applied in most disciplines of medicine, especially in neurology, neurosurgery, orthopedics, geriatrics, rheumatology, internal medicine, cardiovascular medicine, cardiopulmonary medicine, psychiatry, sports medicine, burn and wound care, and chronic pain management. It also plays a role in community health education. Credentialed allied health professionals administer physical therapy under the direction of physicians.

Medical **rehabilitation services** involve the entire healthcare team: physicians, nurses, social workers, occupational therapists, physical therapists, and other healthcare personnel. The objective is to either eliminate the patients' disability or alleviate it as fully as possible. Physical therapy can be used to improve the cognitive, social, and physical abilities of patients impaired by chronic disease or injury.

The primary purpose of physical therapy in rehabilitation is to promote optimal health and function by applying scientific principles. Treatment modalities include therapeutic exercise, therapeutic massage, biofeedback, and applications of heat, low-energy lasers, cold, water, electricity, and ultrasound.

Respiratory Therapy

Respiratory therapy involves the diagnosis and treatment of patients who have acute and/or chronic lung disorders. Under the direction of qualified physicians and surgeons, respiratory therapists provide services such as emergency care for stroke, heart failure, and shock patients. They also treat patients with chronic respiratory diseases such as emphysema and asthma.

Respiratory treatments include the administration of oxygen and inhalants such as bronchodilators. The therapists set up and monitor ventilatory equipment and provide physiotherapy to improve breathing.

Ancillary Support Services

The ancillary units of the hospital provide vital clinical and administrative support services to patients, medical staff, visitors, and employees.

Clinical Support Services

The clinical support units provide the following services:

- Pharmaceutical services (provided by registered pharmacists and pharmacy technologists)

- Food and nutrition services (managed by registered dietitians who develop general and special-diet menus and nutritional plans for individual patients)

- HIM (health record) services (managed by RHIAs and RHITs)

- Social work and social services (provided by licensed social workers and licensed clinical social workers)

- Patient advocacy services (provided by several types of healthcare professionals, most commonly, registered nurses and licensed social workers)

- Environmental (housekeeping) services

- Purchasing, central supply, and materials management services

- Engineering and plant operations

Administrative Support Services

In addition to clinical support services, hospitals need administrative support services to operate effectively. Administrative support services provide business management and clerical services in several key areas, including:

- Admissions and central registration

- Claims and billing (business office)

- Accounting

- Information services

- Human resources

- Public relations

- Fund development

- Marketing

Check Your Understanding 13.4

Instructions: Indicate whether the statements below are true or false (T or F).

1. _____ Ambulatory care is the short-term care provided to diagnose and/or treat an illness or injury.

2. _____ The influence of managed care and the emphasis on cost control in the Medicare/Medicaid programs have resulted in shorter hospital stays.

3. _____ Hospitals can be classified based on type of ownership.

4. _____ Government hospitals are operated by a specific branch of federal, state, or local government as for-profit organizations.

5. ____ The board of directors has primary responsibility for setting the overall direction of the hospital.

6. ____ Medical staff classification refers to the organization of physicians according to clinical assignment.

7. ____ A registered nurse qualified by advanced education and clinical and management experience usually administers patient care services.

8. ____ Physicians who specialize in radiology are called radiology technicians.

9. ____ Occupational therapy is made available in acute care hospitals, clinics, and rehab centers.

10. ____ The ancillary units of the hospital provide vital clinical and administrative support services to patients, medical staff, visitors, and employees.

Forces Affecting Healthcare Delivery

A number of recent developments in healthcare delivery have had far-reaching effects on the operation of hospitals and other healthcare delivery facilities and services in the United States. Many of these developments are discussed below.

Growth of Subacute Care

Subacute care represents a new movement in healthcare. In the past, the term was used in reference to the services provided to hospitalized patients who did not meet the medical criteria for needing acute care. Today, it refers to the level of skilled care needed by patients with complex medical conditions, typically Medicare patients with multiple medical problems.

Traditionally, nursing homes, home care providers, and rehabilitation facilities have provided subacute care. Now some hospitals are developing subacute units in response to changing demographics that make it a cost-effective alternative to inpatient acute care.

Development of Peer Review and Quality Improvement Programs

The goal of high-quality patient care is to promote, preserve, and restore health. High-quality care is delivered in an appropriate setting in a manner that is satisfying to patients. It is achieved when the patient's health status is improved as much as possible. Quality has several components, including:

- Appropriateness (the right care is provided at the right time)
- Technical excellence (the right care is provided in the right manner)
- Accessibility (the right care can be obtained when it is needed)
- Acceptability (patients are satisfied)

Peer Review
In peer review, a member of a profession assesses the work of colleagues within that same profession. Peer review traditionally has been at the center of quality assessment and

assurance efforts. The medical profession's peer review efforts have emphasized the scientific aspects of quality. Appropriate use of pharmaceuticals, postoperative infection rates, and accuracy of diagnosis are among the measures of quality that have been used.

Peer review is a requirement of both CMS and the JCAHO.

Quality Improvement

Quality improvement (QI) programs have been in place in hospitals for years and have been required by the Medicare/Medicaid programs and accreditation standards. QI programs have covered medical staff as well as nursing and other departments or processes.

Efforts to encourage the delivery of high-quality care take place at the local and national levels. Such efforts are geared toward assessing the efforts of both individuals and institutions. Currently, professional associations, healthcare organizations, government agencies, private external quality review associations, consumer groups, MCOs, and group purchasers of care all play a role in trying to promote high-quality care.

Growth of Managed Care

Managed care is a generic term for a healthcare reimbursement system that manages cost, quality, and access to services. Most managed care plans do not provide healthcare directly. Instead, they enter into service contracts with the physicians, hospitals, and other healthcare providers who provide medical services to enrollees in the plans.

Managed care systems control costs primarily by presetting payment amounts and restricting patient access to healthcare services through precertification and utilization review processes. (Managed care is discussed in more detail in chapter 14.) Managed care delivery systems also attempt to manage cost and quality by:

- Implementing various forms of financial incentives for providers
- Promoting healthy lifestyles
- Identifying risk factors and illnesses early in the disease process
- Providing patient education

Although the most recent studies suggest that managed care results in lower costs with equal or better quality, most are limited because they have focused on short-term health outcomes (Weinerman et al. 1996). Very little is known about the long-term effects of specific reimbursement or organizational arrangements on quality of care. Further, recent evidence indicates that the quality of care provided under managed care systems may differ across population groups.

Efforts at Healthcare Reengineering

During the 1980s, healthcare organizations adopted **continuous quality improvement** (CQI) processes. Lessons learned from other areas of business were applied to healthcare settings. **Reengineering** came in many varieties, such as focused process improvement, major business process improvement and business process innovation, total quality management, and CQI. Regardless of approach, every healthcare organization attempted to look inside and to pratice "process" as opposed to traditional "department" thinking.

Healthcare organizations formed cross-functional teams that collaborated to solve organizational problems. At the same time, the JCAHO reengineered the accreditation process to increase its focus on process and systems analysis. Gone were the days of thinking in a "silo." All the silos were turned over, and healthcare teams learned from each other. The drivers of reengineering included cost reduction, staff shortages, and implementation of technology.

Emphasis on Patient-Focused Care

Patient-focused care is a concept developed to contain hospital inpatient costs and improve quality by restructuring services so that more of them take place in the nursing units (patient floors) and not in specialized units in dispersed hospital locations. The emphasis is on cross-training staff in the nursing units to perform a variety of functions for a small group of patients rather than one set of functions for a large number of patients. Some organizations have achieved patient-focused care by assigning multiskilled workers to serve food, clean patients' rooms, and assist in nursing care. However, some organizations have experienced low patient satisfaction with this type of worker because the patients are confused and do not know who to ask to do what.

Hospital staff spend most of their time performing activities in the following nine categories:

- Medical, technical, and clinical procedures
- Patient services
- Medical documentation
- Institutional documentation
- Scheduling and coordination
- Patient transportation
- Staff transportation
- Management and supervision
- Ready-for-action activities

A study at Lakeland Regional Medical Center, a 750-bed hospital in central Florida, found that medical, technical, and clinical activity consumed one-sixth of the center's personnel-related costs. The study also showed that almost twice that amount of time was spent writing things down. Scheduling and coordination took as much time as medical activity, and ready-for-action activities consumed even more.

The study suggested that restructuring services at Lakeland would reduce the number of staff required for patient care activities from 2,200 to 1,200 and improve care. The amount of physical space allotted to each unit would be sufficient to contain a minilab, diagnostic radiology rooms, linen and general supply, stockrooms, and so on. If such changes were carried out, medical documentation could be reduced by almost two-thirds, scheduling and coordination service by more than two-thirds, and ready-for-action time by two-thirds.

Hospitals have had difficulty in fully and rapidly implementing patient-focused care for the following reasons: the high cost of conversion; the extensive physical renovations required; resistance from functional departments; and other priorities for management, such as mergers and considering potential mergers.

Development of Integrated Healthcare Delivery Systems

An IDS is a healthcare provider made up of a number of associated medical facilities that furnish coordinated healthcare services. Most IDSs include a number of facilities that provide services along the continuum of care (ambulatory surgery centers, physician office practices, outpatient clinics, acute care hospitals, **skilled nursing facilities** [SNFs], MCOs, and so on).

The purpose of an IDS is to organize the continuum of care, maximize effectiveness, and reduce costs. The continuum of care includes services for patients at different levels of the healthcare system. In an IDS arrangement, the focus is on holistic care rather than on fragmented care among specialists. Examples of different levels of care across the continuum are:

- Health promotion and disease prevention
- Primary care
- Acute care
- Tertiary care
- Long-term care
- **Hospice care**

Integrated healthcare information systems are needed to manage the continuum of care. The electronic health record (EHR) is essential for meeting IDS goals of effectively managing and delivering high-quality care. Timely, accurate, and accessible information is needed to manage care across all the different continuum of care levels. (Chapters 4 and 5 discuss many communication and interoperability issues associated with EHRs.)

Licensure, Certification, and Accreditation of Healthcare Facilities

Licensure, certification, and accreditation have had an enormous impact on the standardization and quality of healthcare services in the U.S. Such programs require that high-performance standards be met in the provision of medical care and in the construction, maintenance, and management of the healthcare facility.

State Licensure

Licensure is a "process by which a governmental authority grants permission to an individual practitioner or healthcare organization to operate or to engage in an occupation or profession" (Quality Assurance Project 2005). State legislatures usually grant authority to a state agency to license healthcare facilities. For example, hospitals, nursing homes, home health agencies, ambulatory surgical facilities, and adult day-care/health facilities are usually licensed by state agencies.

Licensing agencies set standards that healthcare facilities must meet before being granted a license to operate. The standards are designed to promote the health, welfare, and safety of patients. Such standards may address staff levels, coordination of services, patient rights, quality assurance, safety of the environment, and adequacy of the physical plant. The licensing agency monitors compliance with the standards, usually through surveys and on-site inspections. The types of facilities licensed and the standards for licensure vary from state to state.

Although licensure requirements vary, healthcare facilities must meet certain basic criteria determined by state regulatory agencies. These standards address concerns such as adequacy of staffing, physical aspects of the facility (equipment, buildings), and services provided, including the maintenance of health records. Most licensing agencies perform reviews annually.

Certification for Medicare participation

Certification is the procedure conducted by an authorized body in evaluating and recognizing whether an individual or institution meets predetermined requirements. To receive Medicare and Medicaid reimbursement, providers must prove that they follow the rules and regulations for participating in the Medicare program. Called the Medicare Conditions of Participation, these rules are set forth by CMS. Facilities that must meet the standards in the Conditions of Participation include hospitals, home health agencies, ambulatory surgical centers, and hospices.

Certification for Medicare reimbursement is the responsibility of the states. However, the Medicare act specifies that those facilities accredited by the JCAHO and the AOA are "deemed" to be in compliance with the Conditions of Participation and do not have to undergo a separate certification process.

Voluntary accreditation

Accreditation is a voluntary system of institutional or organizational review performed by an independent body that has developed standards to measure and ensure the quality of healthcare services. Examples of accrediting organizations are the JCAHO and the AOA.

The JCAHO is a private, nonprofit organization that establishes guidelines and standards for the operation and management of healthcare facilities to ensure the quality and safety of care. It operates voluntary accreditation programs for hospitals, non-hospital-based psychiatric and substance abuse organizations, long-term care organizations, home care organizations, ambulatory care organizations, and organization-based pathology and clinical laboratory services.

Most state governments recognize JCAHO accreditation as a condition of licensure and receiving Medicaid reimbursement. Typically, organizations are inspected every three years with accreditation and survey findings made available to the public. When an organization is found to be in substantial compliance with the JCAHO standards, accreditation may be awarded for up to three years.

The AOA sponsors a voluntary accreditation program for osteopathic healthcare facilities and medical schools. Its purpose is to advance the philosophy and practice of osteopathy. The AOA has developed accreditation requirements for osteopathic hospitals, ambulatory care/surgery, mental health, substance abuse, and physical rehabilitation medicine facilities. Like JCAHO-accredited facilities, AOA-accredited facilities are considered to have "deemed" status and qualify to receive Medicare reimbursement.

Check Your Understanding 13.5

Instructions: Choose the best terms to complete the following sentences.

1. _____ Today, _____ refers to the level of skilled care needed by patients with complex medical conditions, typically Medicare patients who have multiple medical problems.
   a. Acute care
   b. Ambulatory care
   c. Subacute care
   d. High-quality care

2. _____ Quality has several components, including appropriateness, technical excellence, _____ and acceptability.
   a. Accuracy of diagnosis
   b. Continuous improvement
   c. Connectivity
   d. Accessibility

3. _____ _____ programs have been in place in hospitals for years and have been required by the Medicare/Medicaid programs and accreditation standards.
   a. Quality assurance
   b. Peer review
   c. Managed care
   d. Quality improvement

4. _____ _____ is a generic term for a healthcare reimbursement system that manages cost, quality, and access to services.
   a. Quality improvement
   b. Subacute care
   c. Managed care
   d. Patient-focused care

5. _____ Recent evidence indicates that the quality of care provided under managed care systems may differ across _____.
   a. Population groups
   b. Healthcare settings
   c. Medical facilities
   d. Integrated delivery systems

6. _____ _____ attempts to contain hospital inpatient costs and improve quality by restructuring services.
   a. Continuous quality improvement
   b. Patient-focused care
   c. Managed care
   d. Acute care

7. _____ Managed care and healthcare organization integration have placed enormous pressure on _____.
   a. Integrated delivery systems
   b. Acute care facilities
   c. Rehabilitation facilities
   d. Information systems

8. ____ The role of ____ has changed rapidly in healthcare organizations, just as it has in many service organizations.
   a. Reengineering
   b. Computers
   c. Quality improvement programs
   d. Peer review efforts

Other Types of Healthcare Services

Healthcare delivery is more than hospital-related care. It can be viewed as a continuum of services that cuts across care settings, including ambulatory, acute, subacute, long-term, and residential care, among others. This section describes several of the alternatives for healthcare delivery along this continuum.

Continuum of Care

In an IDN/IDS, providers strive to meet every healthcare consumer's needs. This can be described as a full-service model of meeting patient needs from the cradle to the grave. IDNs develop a full continuum of care model, including acute care inpatient and outpatient services, a home health agency, a long-term care facility, and hospital-based durable medical equipment (DME) services.

Ambulatory Care

Ambulatory care may be defined as:

> The preventive and/or corrective healthcare provided in a practitioner's office, a clinic, or a hospital on a nonresident (outpatient) basis. The term usually implies that patients go to locations outside their homes to obtain healthcare services and return the same day.

It encompasses all the health services provided to individual patients who are not residents in a healthcare facility. Such services include the educational services provided by community health clinics and public health departments. Primary care, emergency care, and ambulatory specialty care (which includes ambulatory surgery) all may be considered ambulatory care. Ambulatory care services are provided in a variety of settings, including urgent care centers, school-based clinics, public health clinics, and neighborhood and community health centers.

Current medical practice emphasizes performing healthcare services in the least costly setting possible. This change in thinking has led to decreased utilization of emergency services, increased utilization of nonemergency ambulatory facilities, decreased hospital admissions, and shorter hospital stays. The need to reduce the cost of healthcare also has led primary care physicians to treat conditions they once would have referred to specialists.

Physicians who provide ambulatory care services fall into two major categories: physicians working in private practice and physicians working for ambulatory care organizations. Physicians in private practice are self-employed. They work in solo, partnership, and group practices set up as for-profit organizations.

Alternatively, physicians who work for ambulatory care organizations are employees of those organizations. Ambulatory care organizations include health maintenance organizations (HMOs), hospital-based ambulatory clinics, walk-in and emergency clinics, hospital-owned group practices and health promotion centers, freestanding surgery centers, freestanding urgent care centers, freestanding emergency care centers, health department clinics, neighborhood clinics, home care agencies, community mental health centers, school and workplace health services, and prison health services.

Ambulatory care organizations also employ other healthcare providers, including nurses, laboratory technicians, podiatrists, chiropractors, physical therapists, radiology technicians, psychologists, and social workers.

Private Medical Practice

Private medical practices are physician-owned entities that provide primary care or medical/surgical specialty care services in a freestanding office setting. The physicians have medical privileges at local hospitals and surgical centers but are not employees of the other healthcare entities.

Hospital-Based Ambulatory Care Services

In addition to providing inpatient services, many acute care hospitals provide various ambulatory care services.

Emergency Services and Trauma Care

More than 90 percent of community hospitals in the U.S. provide emergency services. Hospital-based emergency departments provide specialized care for victims of traumatic accidents and life-threatening illnesses. In urban areas, many also provide walk-in services for patients with minor illnesses and injuries who do not have access to regular primary care physicians.

Many physicians on the hospital staff also use the emergency care department as a setting to assess patients with problems that may either lead to an inpatient admission or require equipment or diagnostic imaging facilities not available in a private office or nursing home. Emergency services function as a major source of unscheduled admissions to the hospital.

Outpatient Surgical Services

Generally, the term *ambulatory surgery* refers to any surgical procedure that does not require an overnight stay in a hospital. It can be performed in the outpatient surgery department of a hospital and in a freestanding ambulatory surgery center. During the 1980s and 1990s, the percentage of surgeries done on an outpatient basis rose dramatically and this trend continues today. The increased number of procedures performed in an ambulatory setting can be attributed to improvements in surgical technology and anesthesia and the utilization management demands of third-party payers.

Outpatient Diagnostic and Therapeutic Services

Outpatient diagnostic and therapeutic services are provided in a hospital or one of its satellite facilities. Diagnostic services are those services performed by a physician to identify the disease or condition from which the patient is suffering. Therapeutic services are those services performed by a physician to treat the disease or condition that has been identified.

Hospital outpatients fall into different classifications according to the type of service they receive and the location of the service. For example, emergency outpatients are treated in the hospital's emergency or trauma care department for conditions that require immediate care. Clinic outpatients are treated in one of the hospital's clinical departments on an ambulatory basis. Referral outpatients receive special diagnostic or therapeutic services in the hospital on an ambulatory basis, but responsibility for their care remains with the referring physician.

Community-Based Ambulatory Care Services

Community-based ambulatory care services are those services provided in freestanding facilities that are not owned by or affiliated with a hospital. Such facilities can range in size from a small medical practice with a single physician to a large clinic with an organized medical staff.

Among the organizations that provide ambulatory care services are specialized treatment facilities. Examples of these facilities include birthing centers, cancer treatment centers, renal dialysis centers, and rehabilitation centers.

Freestanding Ambulatory Care Centers

Freestanding ambulatory care centers provide emergency services and urgent care for walk-in patients. Urgent care centers (sometimes called emergicenters) provide diagnostic and therapeutic care for patients with minor illnesses and injuries. They do not serve seriously ill patients, and most do not accept ambulance cases.

Two groups of patients find these centers attractive. The first group consists of patients seeking the convenience and access of emergency services without the delays and other forms of negative feedback associated with using hospital services for nonurgent problems. The second group consists of patients whose insurance treats urgent care centers preferentially compared with physicians' offices.

As they have increased in number and become familiar to more patients, many freestanding ambulatory care centers now offer a combination of walk-in and appointment services.

Freestanding Ambulatory Surgery Centers

Freestanding ambulatory surgery centers generally provide surgical procedures that take anywhere from five to ninety minutes to perform and require less than a four-hour recovery period. Patients must schedule their surgeries in advance and be prepared to return home on the same day. Patients who experience surgical complications are sent to an inpatient facility for care.

Most ambulatory surgery centers are for-profit entities. Individual physicians, MCOs, or entrepreneurs may own them. Generally, ambulatory care centers can provide surgical services at lower cost than hospitals can because their overhead expenses are lower.

Public Health Services

The states have constitutional authority to implement public health, and many of them are assisted by a wide variety of federal programs and laws. The Department of Health and Human Services (HHS) is the principal federal agency that ensures health and provides essential human services. All HHS agencies have some responsibility for prevention. Through its ten regional offices, HHS coordinates closely with state and local government agencies and many HHS-funded services are provided by these agencies as well as by private-sector and nonprofit organizations.

Two units in the Office of the Secretary of HHS are important to public health: the Office of the Surgeon General of the U.S. and the Office of Disease Prevention and Health Promotion (ODPHP). ODPHP has an analysis and leadership role for health promotion and disease prevention.

The surgeon general is appointed by the president of the United States and provides leadership and authoritative, science-based recommendations about the public's health. He or she has responsibility for the Public Health Service (PHS) workforce (Jonas and Kovner 2005, 108–9).

Home Care Services

Home healthcare is the fastest-growing sector to offer services for Medicare recipients. The primary reason for this is increased economic pressure from third-party payers. In other words, third-party payers want patients released from the hospital more quickly than they were in the past. Moreover, patients generally prefer to be cared for in their own homes. In fact, most patients prefer home care, no matter how complex their medical problems. Research indicates that the medical outcomes of home care patients are similar to those of patients treated in SNFs for similar conditions.

In 1989, Medicare rules for home care services were clarified to make it easier for Medicare beneficiaries to receive them. Patients are eligible to receive home health services from a qualified Medicare provider when they are homebound, when they are under the care of a specified physician who will establish a home health plan, and when they need physical or occupational therapy, speech therapy, or intermittent skilled nursing care.

Skilled nursing care is defined as both technical procedures, such as tube feedings and catheter care, and skilled nursing observations. *Intermittent* is defined as up to twenty-eight hours per week for nursing care and thirty-five hours per week for home health aide care. Many hospitals have formed their own home healthcare agencies to increase revenues and at the same time to enable them to discharge patients from the hospital earlier.

Voluntary Agencies

Voluntary agencies provide healthcare and healthcare planning services, usually at the local level and to low-income patients. Their services range from giving free immunizations to offering family planning counseling. Funds to operate such agencies come from a variety of sources, including local or state health departments, private grants, and funds from different federal bureaus.

One common example of a voluntary agency is the community health center. Sometimes called neighborhood health centers, community health centers offer comprehensive, primary healthcare services to patients who otherwise would not have access to them. Often patients pay for these services on a sliding scale based on income or according to a flat rate, discounted fee schedule supplemented by public funding.

Some voluntary agencies offer specialized services such as counseling for battered and abused women. Typically, these are set up within local communities. An example of a voluntary agency that offers services on a much larger scale is the Red Cross.

Subacute Care

Patients needing ongoing rehabilitative care and/or treatments using advanced technology sometimes are eligible to receive subacute care. Subacute care offers patients access to constant nursing care while recovering at home. In the past, patients could receive comprehensive rehabilitative care only while in the hospital. Today, however, the availability of subacute care services allows patients to optimize their functional gain in a familiar and more comfortable environment. In essence, subacute care in most IDNs emphasizes patient independence. The patient is given an individualized care plan developed by a highly trained team of healthcare professionals. Patients considered appropriate for subacute care are those recovering from stroke, cardiac surgery, serious injury, amputation, joint replacement, or chronic wounds.

Long-Term Care

Generally speaking, long-term care is the healthcare rendered in a nonacute care facility to patients who require inpatient nursing and related services for more than thirty consecutive days. SNFs, nursing homes, and rehabilitation hospitals are the principal facilities that provide long-term care. Rehabilitation hospitals provide recuperative services for patients who have suffered strokes and traumatic injuries as well as other serious illnesses. Specialized long-term care facilities serve patients with chronic respiratory disease, permanent cognitive impairment, and other incapacitating conditions.

Long-term care encompasses a range of health, personal care, social, and housing services provided to people of all ages with health conditions that limit their ability to carry out normal daily activities without assistance. People who need long-term care have many different types of physical and mental disabilities. Moreover, their need for the mix and intensity of long-term care services can change over time.

Long-term care is mainly rehabilitative and supportive rather than curative. Moreover, healthcare workers other than physicians can provide long-term care in the home or in residential or institutional settings. For the most part, long-term care requires little or no technology.

Long-Term Care in the Continuum of Care

The availability of long-term care is one of the most important health issues in the U.S. today. There are two principal reasons for this. First, thanks to advances in medicine and healthcare practices, people are living longer today than they did in the past. The number of people who survive previously fatal conditions has been growing, and more and more people with chronic medical problems are able to live reasonably normal lives. Second, there was an explosion in birth rate after the Second World War. Children born during that period, the so-called baby-boomer generation, are today in or entering their fifties. These factors combined mean that the need for long-term care will only increase in the years to come.

As discussed earlier, healthcare is now viewed as a continuum of care. That is, patients are provided care by different caregivers at several different levels of the healthcare system. In the case of long-term care, the patient's continuum of care may have begun with a primary provider in a hospital and then continued with home care and eventually care in an SNF. The patient's care is coordinated from one care setting to the next.

Moreover, the roles of the different care providers along the patient's continuum of care are continuing to evolve. Health information managers play a key part in providing consultation services to long-term care facilities with regard to developing systems to manage information from a diverse number of healthcare providers.

Delivery of Long-Term Care Services

Long-term care services are delivered in a variety of settings, including skilled nursing facilities/nursing homes, residential care facilities, hospice programs, and adult day-care programs.

Skilled Nursing Facilities and Nursing Homes

The most important providers of formal, long-term care services are nursing homes. SNFs, or nursing homes, provide medical, nursing, and/or rehabilitative care, in some cases, around the clock. Most SNF residents are over age 65 and often are classified as the frail elderly.

Many nursing homes are owned by for-profit organizations. However, SNFs also may be owned by not-for-profit groups as well as local, state, and federal governments. In recent years, there has been a decline in the total number of nursing homes in the United States, but an increase in the number of nursing home beds.

Nursing homes are no longer the only option for patients needing long-term care. Various factors play a role in determining which type of long-term care facility is best for a particular patient, including cost, access to services, and individual needs.

Residential Care Facilities

New living environments that are more homelike and less institutional are the focus of much attention in the current long-term care market. Residential care facilities now play a growing role in the continuum of long-term care services. Having affordable and appropriate housing available for elderly and disabled people can reduce the level of need for institutional long-term care services in the community. Institutionalization can be postponed or prevented when the elderly and disabled live in safe, accessible settings where assistance with daily activities is available.

Hospice Programs

Hospice care is provided mainly in the home to the terminally ill and their families. Hospice is based on a philosophy of care imported from England and Canada that holds that during the course of terminal illness, the patient should be able to live life as fully and as comfortably as possible, but without artificial or mechanical efforts to prolong life.

In the hospice approach, the family is the unit of treatment. An interdisciplinary team provides medical, nursing, psychological, therapeutic, pharmacological, and spiritual support during the final stages of illness, at the time of death, and during bereavement. The main goals are to control pain, maintain independence, and minimize the stress and trauma of death.

Hospice services have gained acceptance as an alternative to hospital care for the terminally ill. The number of hospices is likely to continue to grow because this philosophy of care for people at the end of life has become a model for the nation.

Adult Day-Care Programs

Adult day-care programs offer a wide range of health and social services to elderly persons during the daytime hours. Adult day-care services are usually targeted to elderly members of families in which the regular caregivers work during the day. Many elderly people who live alone also benefit from leaving their homes every day to participate in programs designed to keep them active. The goals of adult day-care programs are to delay the need for institutionalization and to provide respite for caregivers.

Data on adult day-care programs are still limited, but there were about 3,000 programs in 2000. Most adult day-care programs offer social services, crafts, current events discussions, family counseling, reminiscence therapy, nursing assessment, physical exercise, activities of daily living, rehabilitation, psychiatric assessment, and medical care.

Behavioral Health Services

From the mid-nineteenth century to the mid-twentieth century, psychiatric services in the U.S. were based primarily in long-stay institutions supported by state governments and patterns of practice were relatively stable. During the past forty-five years, however, remarkable changes have occurred. These changes include a reversal of the balance between institutional and community care, inpatient and outpatient services, and individual and group practice.

Today, the number of long-stay residents in state mental hospitals is estimated to be well below 80,000. In 1955, it was more than 500,000. The shift to community-based settings began in the public sector and community settings remain dominant. The private sector's bed capacity increased in the 1970s and 1980s, including psychiatric units in non-federal general hospitals, private psychiatric hospitals, and residential treatment centers for children. Substance abuse centers and child and adolescent inpatient psychiatric units grew particularly quickly in the 1980s, as investors recognized their profitability. In the 1990s, the growth of inpatient private mental health facilities leveled off and the number of outpatient and partial treatment settings increased sharply.

Some patients with treatment-resistant schizophrenia, severe mood disorders, or chronic cognitive impairment may be dangerous to themselves or others. State and county hospitals may be returning to their traditional role by providing asylum to disabled patients who are unable function in their communities.

Residential treatment centers for emotionally or behaviorally disturbed children provide inpatient services to children under eighteen years of age. The programs and physical facilities of residential treatment centers are designed to meet patients' daily living, schooling, recreational, socialization, and routine medical care needs.

Day-hospital or day-treatment programs occupy one niche in the spectrum of behavioral healthcare settings. Although some provide services seven days a week, many programs provide services only during business hours, Monday through Friday. Day-treatment patients spend most of the day at the treatment facility in a program of structured therapeutic activities and then return to their homes until the next day. Day-treatment services include psychotherapy, pharmacology, occupational therapy, and other types of rehabilitation services. These programs provide alternatives to inpatient care or serve as transitions from inpatient to outpatient care or discharge. They also may provide respite for family caregivers and a place for rehabilitating or maintaining chronically ill patients. The number of day-treatment programs has increased in response to pressures to decrease the length of hospital stays.

Insurance coverage for behavioral healthcare has always lagged behind coverage for other medical care. Although treatments and treatment settings have changed, rising healthcare costs, the absence of strong consumer demand for behavioral health coverage, and insurers' continuing fear of the potential cost of this coverage have maintained the differences between medical and behavioral healthcare benefits.

Although most individuals covered by health insurance have some outpatient psychiatric coverage, the coverage is often quite restricted. Typical restrictions include limits on the number of outpatient visits, higher copayment charges, and higher deductibles.

Behavioral healthcare has grown and diversified, particularly During the past forty years, as psychopharmacologic treatment has made possible the shift away from long-term custodial treatment. Psychosocial treatments continue the process of care and rehabilitation in community settings. Large state hospitals have been supplemented—and in many cases replaced—by psychiatric units in general hospitals, new outpatient clinics, community mental health centers, day-treatment centers, and halfway houses. Treatment has become more effective and specific, based on our growing understanding of the brain and behavior. Recent advances in the biological and behavioral sciences continue to improve opportunities for diagnosing, treating, and preventing psychiatric disorders (Jonas and Kovner 1999, 243–73).

Check Your Understanding 13.6

Instructions: Match the descriptions provided with the terms to which they apply.

1. ____ Behavioral health service
2. ____ Public health service
3. ____ Home care service
4. ____ Hospice program
5. ____ Skilled nursing facility
6. ____ Voluntary agency
7. ____ Residential care facility
8. ____ Day-treatment program
9. ____ Continuum of care
10. ____ Freestanding ambulatory care center

a. Fastest-growing sector of Medicare
b. Provides emergency services and urgent care for walk-in patients
c. Represents a reversal in the balance between institutional and community care
d. Are designed to meet patients' daily living, schooling, recreational, socialization, and routine medical care needs
e. Has an analysis and leadership role for health promotion and disease prevention
f. Provides healthcare and healthcare planning services usually at the local level and to low-income patients
g. Provides alternatives to inpatient care or serves as a transition from inpatient to outpatient care or discharge
h. Care provided mainly in the home to the terminally ill and their families
i Care provided by different caregivers at several different levels of the healthcare system
j. Healthcare rendered in a nonacute care facility to patients who require inpatient nursing and related services for more than thirty consecutive days

---

Reimbursement of Healthcare Expenditures

Together, the Medicare and Medicaid programs and the managed care insurance industry have virtually eliminated fee-for-service reimbursement arrangements. (Reimbursement methodologies are thoroughly covered in chapter 7.)

Evolution of Third-Party Reimbursement

The evolution of third-party reimbursement systems for healthcare services began more than sixty years ago. It created a need for systematic and accurate communications between healthcare providers and third-party payers. Commercial health insurance companies (for example, Aetna) offer medical plans similar to BC/BS plans. Traditionally, Blue Cross organizations covered hospital services and Blue Shield covered inpatient physician services and a limited amount of office-based care. Today, Blue Cross plans and commercial insurance providers cover a full range of healthcare services, including ambulatory care services and drug benefits.

Most commercial health insurance is provided in the form of group policies offered by employers as part of their fringe benefit packages for employees. Unions also negotiate health insurance coverage during contract negotiations. In most cases, employees pay a share of the cost and employers pay a share.

Individual health insurance plans can be purchased but usually are expensive or have limited coverage and high deductibles. Individuals with preexisting medical conditions often find it almost impossible to get individual coverage.

Commercial insurers also sell major medical and cash payment policies. Major medical plans are directed primarily at catastrophic illness and cover all or part of treatment costs beyond those covered by basic plans. Major medical plans are sold as both group and individual policies. Cash payment plans provide monetary benefits and are not based on actual charges from healthcare providers. For example, a cash payment plan might pay the beneficiary $150 for every day he or she is hospitalized or $500 for every ambulatory surgical procedure. Cash payment plans are often offered as a benefit of membership in large associations such as the American Association of Retired Persons (AARP).

Like the Blues, commercial insurance companies are subject to supervision by state insurance commissioners. However, such supervision does not include rate regulation. One general requirement is that commercial plans establish premium rates high enough to cover all potential claims made under the insurance they provide.

Government-Sponsored Reimbursement Systems

Until 1965, most of the poor and many of the elderly in the United States could not afford private healthcare services. As a result of public pressure calling for attention to this growing problem, Congress passed Public Law 89-97 as an Amendment to the Social Security Act. The amendments created Medicare (Title XVIII) and Medicaid (Title XIX).

Medicare

Federal health insurance for the aged, called Medicare, was first offered to retired Americans in July 1966. Today, retired and disabled Americans who are eligible for Social Security benefits automatically qualify for Medicare coverage without regard to income. Coverage is offered under two coordinated programs: hospital insurance (Medicare Part A) and medical insurance (Medicare Part B).

Medicare Part A is financed through payroll taxes. Initially, coverage applied only to hospitalization and home healthcare. Subsequently, coverage for extended care in nursing homes was added. Coverage for individuals eligible for Social Security disability payments for over two years and those who need kidney transplantation or dialysis for end-stage renal disease also were added.

Medical insurance under Medicare Part B is optional. It is financed through monthly premiums paid by eligible beneficiaries to supplement federal funding. Part B helps pay for physician's services, outpatient hospital care, medical services and supplies, and certain other medical costs not covered by Part A. At the present time, Medicare Part B does not provide coverage of prescription drugs. (Medicare Parts A and B are discussed in greater detail in chapter 14.)

Medicaid

Medicaid is a medical assistance program for low-income Americans. The program is funded partially by the federal government and partially by state and local governments. The federal government requires that certain services be provided and sets specific eligibility requirements.

Medicaid covers the following benefits:

- Inpatient hospital care
- Outpatient hospital care
- Laboratory and x-ray services
- SNF and home health services for persons over twenty-one years old
- Physician services
- Family planning services
- Rural health clinic services
- Early and periodic screening, diagnosis, and treatment services

Individual states sometimes cover services in addition to those required by the federal government.

Services Provided by Government Agencies

Federal health insurance programs cover health services for several additional specified populations.

TRICARE, originally referred to as the Civilian Health and Medical Program for the Uniformed Services (CHAMPUS), pays for care delivered by civilian health providers to retired members of the military and the dependents of active and retired members of the seven uniformed services. The Department of Defense administers the TRICARE program. It also provides medical services to active members of the military.

The Department of Veterans Affairs (VA) provides healthcare services to eligible veterans of military service. The VA hospital system was established in 1930 to provide hospital, nursing home, residential, and outpatient medical and dental care to veterans of the First World War. Today, the VA operates more than 950 medical centers throughout the country. The medical centers are currently being organized into twenty-two Veterans Integrated Service Networks (VISNs) to increase the efficiency of their services.

Through the Indian Health Service, HHS also finances the healthcare services provided to native Americans living on reservations in the U.S.

State governments often operate healthcare facilities to serve citizens with special needs, such as the developmentally disabled and mentally ill. Some states also offer health insurance programs to those who cannot qualify for private healthcare insurance. Many county and local governments also operate public hospitals to fulfill the medical needs of their communities. Public hospitals provide services without regard to the patient's ability to pay.

Workers' Compensation

Workers' compensation is an insurance system operated by the individual states. Each state has its own law and program. In 1910, New York enacted the first workers' compensation law. Workers' compensation programs cover healthcare costs and lost income associated with work-related injuries and illnesses. Federal government employees are covered by the Federal Employees' Compensation Act (FECA). Individual states pass legislation that addresses workers' compensation coverage for nonfederal government employees. Some states exclude certain workers (for example, business owners, independent contractors, farm workers, and so on). Texas employers are not required to provide workers' compensation coverage. (FECA is discussed in more detail in chapter 7.)

Managed Care

Managed care is a broad term used to describe several types of prepaid healthcare plans. Common types of managed care plans include health maintenance organizations (HMOs), preferred provider organizations (PPOs), and point-of-service (POS) plans. MCOs work to control the cost of, and access to, healthcare services while striving to meet high-quality standards. They manage healthcare costs by negotiating discounted providers' fees and controlling patients' access to expensive healthcare services.

The development of managed care was an indirect result of the federal government's enactment of the Medicare and Medicaid laws in 1965. Medicare and Medicaid legislation prompted the development of **investor-owned hospital chains** and stimulated the growth of university medical centers. Both furthered the corporate practice of medicine by increasing the number of management personnel and physicians employed by hospitals and medical schools (Kongstevdt 1993, 3–5).

Reimbursement by MCOs varies depending on the type of organization and the contract negotiated. For example, members of HMOs pay a set premium and are entitled to receive a specific range of healthcare services. In most cases, employers and employees share the cost of the plan. HMOs control costs by requiring members of the plan to seek services only from a preapproved list of providers, who are reimbursed at discounted rates. The plans also control access to medical specialists, expensive diagnostic and treatment procedures, and high-cost pharmaceuticals. They generally require preapproval for specialty consultations, inpatient care, and surgical procedures. Many other examples of reimbursement in managed care arrangements are presented in detail in chapter 7.

Further federal support for the corporate practice of medicine resulted from passage of the HMO Act of 1973. Amendments to the act enabled managed care plans to increase in numbers and to expand enrollments through healthcare programs financed by grants, contracts, and loans.

After years of unchecked healthcare inflation, the government authorized corporate cost controls on hospitals, physicians, and patients for reimbursement of government-sponsored healthcare such as Medicare. DRGs, PPSs, and the resource-based relative value scale are examples of these controls.

The growth of managed care seemed to reduce inflation of healthcare costs during the early and mid-1990s. However, healthcare costs are again rapidly rising. Higher costs are making employers ask workers to pay a larger share for healthcare services. MCOs face major challenges in remaining fiscally strong in the coming years.

Consumer-Driven Healthcare

Consumer-driven healthcare is a new strategy in the private insurance market. This method allows employees more choice in their healthcare decision making. Consumer-driven plans vary, but basically employers provide employees with a personal care account. This account is a fixed amount and offered in the form of a voucher, refundable tax credit, higher wages, or some other transfer of funds (Jonas and Kovner 2005, 69).

Health Savings Accounts (HSA)

Health savings accounts, or HSAs (also called medical savings accounts, or MSAs), offer their members the opportunity to control how their healthcare dollars are spent with a tax-advantaged savings account and comprehensive medical insurance coverage.

HSAs are much like IRAs in that they combine high deductible health insurance with a tax-advantaged savings account. The money that a member saves in his or her account assists in paying the deductible. Most accounts limit the member to contributing the amount of the deductible into the tax- deferred account. This money is kept for medical expenses that qualify under the insurance plan.

The benefit of an HSA is that the member pays for this deductible with pretax dollars. This means that the member saves the money that ordinarily would have gone to pay taxes, which, in effect, decreases the cost of the deductible.

When the member has paid off the deductible, the insurance provider begins to pay. The money in the savings account earns interest and is owned by the member who holds the account. HSAs allow members to save approximately 70 percent or more on the cost of their health insurance (health-insurance-carriers.com/has.html).

Check Your Understanding 13.7

Instructions: Indicate whether the statements below are true or false (T or F).

1. ____ Blue Cross plans and commercial insurance providers cover a limited range of healthcare services.

2. ____ Most commercial health insurance is provided in the form of group policies offered by employers as part of their fringe benefit packages for employees.

3. ____ Today, retired and disabled Americans eligible for Social Security benefits automatically qualify for Medicare coverage.

4. ____ Medicaid is a medical assistance program for upper-income Americans.

5. ____ The Department of Defense administers the TRICARE program.

6. ____ Employers provide employees with a personal care account in consumer-driven healthcare.

7. ____ The development of managed care was a direct result of the federal government's enactment of the Medicare and Medicaid laws in 1965.

8. ____ The federal government became involved in the quality-of-care/malpractice issue through establishment of the National Practitioner Data Bank under the Healthcare Quality Improvement Act of 1986.

Real-World Case

This case study is extracted from a presentation at the 2004 IFHRO Congress and AHIMA Convention titled "e-HIM Framework and Case Study" (Cassidy 2004).

Evolution from e-Health Task Force to e-HIM Task Force

During the past decade, the Internet and its derived technologies have revolutionized the way business is conducted. In healthcare, the following examples illustrate this transformation:

- Increasing numbers of consumers access the Internet for information about health-care providers, treatment options, and their own personal health information.

- Health Web sites provide consumers with tools to develop and maintain their own online health records.

- Consumers and health providers correspond via e-mail.

- Businesses and consumers purchase supplies and equipment over the Internet.

- Health information management (HIM) business processes, such as transcription and coding, use the Internet for off-site transaction processing.

The Internet and its derived technologies create a plethora of opportunities for HIM professionals. HIM professionals who understand and embrace this technology will harness and direct it to improve health information and the efficacy of healthcare for consumers, providers, vendors, payers, and all those in the healthcare supply chain. Those who fail to understand and embrace this technology will be left behind, and their opportunities will be forfeited to faster-moving, better-focused professionals.

The work of the AHIMA e-Health Task Force (2001) resulted in the following vision statement.

Vision for e-Health Information Management

E-health presents a new frontier for managing health information. HIM professionals will reinvent traditional HIM functions for a health record model in which the patient is part of the documentation team. In this model, the health record will be designed and/or maintained by a trusted third-party organization or by the patient. Individually identifiable data will be transmitted and accessed via the Internet.

HIM professionals will clearly define the mission-critical role of a "cyber-health record practitioner." They will develop standards of practice that support the implementation of AHIMA's tenets that its e-Health Task Force developed in 2000 and address the security, privacy, and quality standards for personal health information on the Internet.

In early 2003, AHIMA appointed a task force of experts to develop a vision of the e-HIM future.

The task force developed the following vision of the future of health information: "The future state of health information is electronic, patient-centered, comprehensive, longitudinal, accessible, and credible."

The task force's vision is not only theoretical, but it also offers practical guidance for anyone traveling the road toward e-HIM. Advancing the recommendations of the e-HIM

Task Force, AHIMA created workgroups to develop practice standards that focus on areas that play an integral role in the transition from paper to electronic health records.

The following issues were selected for the initial standards development for the complete medical record in a hybrid electronic health record environment:

- Implementing Electronic Signatures
- E-mail as a Provider–Patient Electronic Communication Medium and Its Impact on the Electronic Health Record
- Electronic Document Management as a Component of the Electronic Health Record
- Core Data Sets for the Physician-Practice Electronic Health Record
- Speech Recognition in the Electronic Health Record

Note: The outcomes are presented in a series of documents that can be found on the AHIMA Web site. To view more information about the e-HIM initiatives, go to ahima.org and click on "HIM Resources."

From HIM to E-HIM

The knowledge and expertise for managing handwritten medical records containing source patient data have evolved through these steps:

- Independent management of paper medical records in settings across the continuum of care
- Scanning paper documents for multiple user access
- Entering data into automated systems that generate electronic patient data
- Integrated delivery systems that electronically manage the patient across the continuum of care
- Network integration and e-health information management

HIM professionals remain actively involved in developing effective processes to preserve patient privacy, confidentiality, and security. This is because the introduction of the Internet for accessing, transferring, and transmitting health information expanded the uses of source patient data (that is, the medical record as HIM professionals traditionally know it) as Internet-based business-to-business companies and business-to-consumer companies flourished.

Career Opportunities for e-HIM professionals

The application of HIM skills, expertise, and experience described in the previous section meet the job requirements of several roles in e-health businesses. This section discusses mission-critical functions and processes in e-health companies that HIM professionals can develop, manage, or perform. Some skills transfer easily into the e-health environment while some require translation due to the differences in the work setting or to accommodate differences in the capabilities of advanced technologies.

Many of these e-HIM processes are interrelated or complementary. Processes and/or functions may be decentralized in some e-health organizations and centralized in others in much the same way that HIM processes have always composed an HIM department in traditional healthcare provider organizations. In e-health companies as well as traditional settings, many HIM functions exist outside the HIM department. With e-health companies and providers varying in purpose and scope (from traditional healthcare provider organizations delivering services electronically, to clinical systems vendors, to application service providers, to consumer healthcare Internet Web sites), the concept of a professionally led HIM function or department will vary depending on the organization's structure, resources, and needs.

In the traditional and e-healthcare organizations, HIM professionals are responsible for managing two basic healthcare business objectives:

- Enabling the collection and storage of complete, accurate, and legal health information

- Facilitating the use of health information for patient care, quality evaluation, reimbursement, compliance, utilization management, education, research, funding, and in legal proceedings

The first objective is accomplished in the traditional setting through functions generally consolidated and managed under the auspices of the HIM director. It includes such functions as record assembly, analysis, coding and abstracting, correspondence, special registries, and medical transcription.

The second objective includes use of the information through functions such as creating and maintaining efficient filing and retrieval systems, master patient indices, chart and information retrieval and filing, release of information, and data retrieval for quality assurance, registries (for example, tumor, trauma), and other evaluative purposes.

These objectives are met within a highly regulated environment and managed with limited resources. This necessitates professional guidance by those with health information management skills, which includes knowledge in the administration of highly regulated activities.

Clearly, e-health companies having many of the same business objectives and challenges as traditional healthcare organizations need HIM knowledge and skills in developing processes that will meet their business objectives with a high level of quality and cost benefit.

Roles, Resources, and Competencies in e-HIM

"Revolution" is an overused word, but when applied to the effect of all that is digital, automated, or electronic in the healthcare industry, it is entirely accurate. Over the last decade, established relationships, value chains, and strategies have been radically altered or swept away.

As the revolution continues, the "front-line" challenge to HIM professionals is clear. They can allow the technologies to roll uncontrolled through and around their organizations, in effect, handing over their rich knowledge base and expert skills to faster-moving, better-focused professionals in professions that don't even exist yet. Or they can understand the potential of the Internet and control and direct its power to the benefit of their customers, health plan members, and patients.

Future of eHIM and Where You Might Work

Domain manager: Owns responsibility for a defined body of knowledge such as HIM, coding, laboratory, pharmacy, etc. Knowledge and authority may cross organizational lines as they maintain the integrity of the technical implementation of that body of knowledge. May work closely with product managers, operations staff, quality control, etc.

Project manager: Manages the implementation of systems necessary to support personal health records, Web site content, and other projects.

Medical language and classification expert: Employs skills in the design and use of medical vocabularies and classification; defines data and retrieves information from e-health systems.

Compliance officer: Designs, implements, and maintains a compliance program that assures conformity to all types of regulatory and voluntary accreditation requirements governing the provision of healthcare products or services via the Internet.

Information security expert: Designs, implements, or maintains an information security program that balances requirements of privacy, integrity, and availability of data. Understands the legal and social issues related to information security.

Patient information coordinator: Provides services to patients wanting to understand how to optimize their experience on the e-health Web site and create and maintain accuracy of their personal health records. Educates patients on protecting the privacy of their personal health information.

Reimbursement manager: Designs systems and procedures that assure generation of accurate clinical documentation needed to substantiate billing. Also involved in designing systems to efficiently classify information for billing. Develops and implements systems to assure the secure transfer of required data to billing centers, clearinghouses, or third-party payers.

Data quality manager: Ensures the quality of health information by performing quality reliability and validity checks. Develops reports and advises clinicians on identifying critical indicators.

Privacy officer: Oversees all ongoing activities related to the development, implementation, maintenance of, and adherence to the organization's policies and procedures covering the privacy of, and access to, patient health information in compliance with federal and state laws and the healthcare organization's information privacy practices.

Product manager: Responsible for overall implementation of a specific product or product line. This may include coordinating and managing the use, case design, development, quality control, version control, modifications and updates, etc.

The e-HIM Task Force (AHIMA) report outlines new roles and competency areas to help you envision ways to expand your scope of knowledge.

Business process engineer, information system designer, and consumer advocate are just a few new paths open to HIM professionals. Decision support is another important area where HIM professionals will be building, querying, and analyzing databases to give clinicians the information they need to decide how to treat current patients or analyze patterns in past patient care.

Coders will have several migration paths once code assignment becomes automated. Coders will play key roles as data quality and integrity monitors and data analysts. Others will become clinical vocabulary managers, helping to make the national information infrastructure a reality by ensuring consistency and linkages between different codes. Check out the AHIMA Web site to explore more information on these exciting emerging roles for HIM professionals.

Summary

Throughout history, humans have attempted to diagnose and treat illness and disease. As populations settled into towns and cities, early folk medicine traditions eventually led to the establishment of formalized entities specifically designed to care for the sick.

In the American colonies, enlightened thinkers such as Benjamin Franklin soon saw the need to establish hospitals and to regulate the practice of medicine. The nineteenth century saw the growth of organizations dedicated to standardizing medical practice and ensuring consistency in the quality of healthcare delivery. Organizations such as the American Medical Association and the American Nurses Association were created to represent the interests of their members and to further ensure the quality of their services.

The twentieth century ushered in a completely new concept in the provision of healthcare: prepaid health plans. For the first time, Americans could buy health insurance. However, during the Great Depression of the 1930s and the Second World War, it became obvious that millions of Americans could not afford to pay for healthcare. After the war, the federal government began to study the problem of healthcare access for all Americans. Finally, during the Johnson administration in the 1960s, Congress passed amendments to the Social Security Act of 1935 that created the Medicare and Medicaid programs. These programs were designed to pay for the cost of healthcare services for the elderly and the poor.

As the healthcare industry has grown, so have efforts to regulate it. Some regulation has come from professional and trade associations associated with the industry. However, much regulation has come from the federal government, particularly with regard to the Medicaid and Medicare programs. Moreover, the types and variety of healthcare services available today have increased dramatically. Every new type of service, and every new way to provide it, brings complex issues that must be addressed in order to ensure that Americans receive the highest-quality healthcare possible at the most affordable price.

Passage of the Medicare and Medicaid programs and establishment of the managed care industry have had a tremendous impact on the way that healthcare in the United States is delivered and paid for. The ramifications of these changes on the American healthcare industry have yet to be fully appreciated. The only thing that is certain is that the American healthcare system continues to be a work in progress.

References

American Hospital Association. 2004 (Oct. 25). Fast Facts on U.S. Hospitals from AHA Hospital Statistics. Available online from aha.org/aha/resource_center/fastfacts/fast_facts_US_hospitals.html.

American Hospital Association. 1999. *100 Faces of Healthcare.* Chicago: Health Forum.

Cassidy, Bonnie S. 2004 (October 15). E-HIM Framework and Case Study, AHIMA Convention. Available online from library.ahima.org/intradoc-cgi/idc_cgi_isapi.dll (proprietary content).

Centers for Disease Control. 2004. Health care in America: Trends in utilization. Available online from cdc.gov/nchs/datawh/nchsdefs/postacutecare.htm.

Centers for Medicare and Medicaid Services. 2002. U.S. Department of Health and Human Services. Available online from cms.hhs.gov/medicare/.

Cofer, Jennifer, ed. 1994. *Health Information Management,* 10th ed. Berwyn, IL: Physicians' Record Company.

Elçin, Y. Murat, ed. 2003. *Tissue Engineering, Stem Cells and Gene Therapies: Advances in Experimental Medicine and Biology.* New York: Springer.

Elliott, Chris, et al. 2000. *Performance Improvement in Healthcare: A Tool for Programmed Learning.* Chicago: AHIMA.

Etheredge, L. 2001. On the Archeology of Health Care Policy: Periods and Paradigms, 1975–2000. Washington, D.C.: The National Academies Press. Available online from nap.edu/books/NI000569/html/1.html.

HBS Consulting. 2003 (March 1). Telehealth: A keystone for future healthcare delivery. Available online from marketresearch.com/product/display.asp?ProductID=893831&xs=r#pagetop.

Human Genome Project. 2005 (Nov. 18). Frequently Asked Questions. Available online from ornl.gov/sci/techresources/Human_Genome/faq/faqs1.shtml.

Joint Commission on Accreditation of Healthcare Organizations. 2000. *2001 Comprehensive Accreditation Manual for Hospitals.* Oakbrook Terrace, IL: JCAHO.

Jonas, Steven, and Anthony R. Kovner. 2005. *Healthcare Delivery in the United States,* 8th ed. New York: Springer.

Jonas, Steven, and Anthony R. Kovner. 1999. *Healthcare Delivery in the United States,* 6th ed. New York: Springer.

Kongstevdt, Peter. 1993. *The Managed Care Handbook.* Gaithersburg, MD: Aspen.

Leavitt, Judith Walzer, and Ronald L. Numbers, eds. 1997. *Sickness and Health in America: Readings in the History of Medicine and Public Health,* 3rd ed. Madison, WI: University of Wisconsin Press.

National Institutes of Health. 2005. nih.gov

Plunkett Research. 2003 (December). *Plunkett's Healthcare Industry Almanac,* 2004 ed. Available online from plunkettresearch.com/health/health_almanac.htm.

President's Advisory Commission on Protection and Quality in the Health Care Industry; Final Report, Chapter 2. 1998 (July). Available online from nitrd.gov/pitac/.

Quality Assurance Project. 2005 (October 12). *Methods and Tools: A Glossary of Useful Terms.* Quality Research Project, University Research Company, LLC. Available online from qaproject.org/methods/resglossary.html.

Quality of healthcare, part 3: Improving the quality of care. 1996. *New England Journal of Medicine* 335:1062.

Shryock, R. H. 1947. The beginnings: From colonial days to the foundation of the American Psychiatric Association. In *One Hundred Years of American Psychiatry,* edited by J. K. Hall, G. Zilboorg, and H. A. Bunker. New York: Columbia University Press.

Sloane, Robert M., Beverly LeBov Sloane, and Richard Harder. 1999. *Introduction to Healthcare Delivery Organization: Functions and Management,* 4th ed. Chicago: Health Administration Press.

Starr, Paul. 1982. *The Social Transformation of American Medicine.* New York: Basic Books.

Stevens, Rosemary. 1999. *In Sickness and in Wealth.* Baltimore, MD: Johns Hopkins University Press.

Sultz, Harry A., and Kristina M. Young. 2004. *Healthcare USA—Understanding its Organization and Delivery,* 4th ed. Sudbury, MA: Jones and Bartlett.

Weinerman, E. R., R. S. Ratner, A. Robbins, and M. A. Lavenbar. 1996. Yale studies in ambulatory medical care: Five determinants of use of hospital emergency services. *American Journal of Public Health* 56:1037.

Chapter 14
Ethical Issues in Health Information Technology

Laurinda B. Harman, PhD, RHIA

Learning Objectives

- To identify the major ethical principles that guide health information management decision making

- To identify professional values and obligations inherent in the AHIMA Code of Ethics, including those important to patients, the healthcare team, employers, the public, peers and colleagues, and professional associations

- To understand how the steps in an ethical decision-making process are used to resolve ethical issues

- To recognize some of the core ethical problems, including those related to the release of health information and coding

Key Terms

Autonomy

Beneficence

Bioethics

Confidentiality

Ethicist

Ethics

Justice

Morality

Nonmaleficence

Privacy

Security

Introduction

The responsibilities of the health information technician (HIT) include a wide range of functions and activities. The HIT's core ethical obligation is to protect patient **privacy** and confidential communication. This obligation is at the center of his or her decision making, regardless of employment site or employment responsibilities.

Although most people probably have never undertaken a formal study of **ethics,** everyone is exposed to ethical principles, moral perspectives, and personal values throughout his or her lifetime. People learn about basic moral values from families, religious leaders, teachers, government and community organizations, and other groups that influence their experiences and perspectives. Ethical decision making requires everyone to consider the perspectives of others, even when they have different values.

The terms introduced in this chapter are specific to the study of ethics. They describe principles most people already know, such as doing good, not harming others, and treating people fairly. Using the terminology of ethics, **autonomy** means self-determination, **beneficence** means promoting good, **nonmaleficence** means not harming others, and **justice** means treating others fairly (Beauchamp and Childress 2001).

With regard to one of the HIT's primary functions, how might ethical principles apply in the case of deciding whether to release patient information?

- Autonomy would require the HIT to make certain that the patient, and not a spouse or third party, is making the decisions regarding access to the patient's health information.

- Beneficence would require the HIT to ensure that the information is released to individuals who need it to do something that will benefit the patient (for example, to the insurance company for payment of a claim).

- Nonmaleficence would require the HIT to ensure that the information is not released to someone who does not have authorization to access it and who might harm the patient if access were permitted (for example, a newspaper seeking information about a patient or an employer that uses health information for discriminatory purposes).

- Justice would require the HIT to apply the rules fairly and consistently for all, rather than responding more quickly to requests that have major financial implications.

This chapter discusses the role of ethical principles and professional values in health information management (HIM) decision making. It also offers a step-by-step process that HITs can use to make appropriate ethical choices, as well as an analysis of what is or is not justified from an ethical perspective.

Key Responsibilities of Health Information Technology Professionals

Some of the health information ethical responsibilities include (Harman 2006; LaTour and Eichenwald 2006):

- Protecting patient privacy and confidential information (Rinehart-Thompson and Harman 2006)

- Making appropriate decisions regarding the selection and use of clinical diagnostic and procedural codes (Schraffenberger and Scichilone 2006)

- Developing policies and procedures that ensure coding accuracy that supports clinical care and research and meets the requirements for reimbursement, while avoiding fraud and abuse violations (Rinehart-Thompson 2006)

- Reporting quality review outcomes honestly and accurately, even when the results might create conflict for an individual or an institution (Spath 2006)

- Ensuring that research and decision support systems are reliable (Johns and Hardin 2006)

- Releasing accurate information for public health purposes for patients with communicable diseases, such as AIDS or venereal disease, and assisting with the complexities of information management in the context of bioterrorism and the threat or reality of global diseases, such as smallpox or avian flu (Neuberger 2006)

- Supporting managed care systems by providing accurate, reliable information about patients/consumers, clinicians, healthcare organizations, and patterns of care, with special care devoted to the issues related to access to information (Schick 2006)

- Facilitating the exchange of information for patients, families, and providers of care (especially for those affected by chronic and terminal illness) that ensure patient autonomy and beneficence (Tischler 2006)

- Ensuring that the electronic health record meets the standards of privacy and security, according to the Health Insurance Portability and Accountability Act (HIPAA) and other federal and state laws (Hanken and Murphy 2006); meets the standards of information security (Czirr, Rosendale, and West 2006) and software development (Fenton 2006)

- Ensuring that clinical data repositories, data marts, data warehouses, and electronic health records meet the standards of the best practices of health information and database management (Lee, White, and Wager 2006)

- Participating in the development of integrated delivery systems so that patients can move across the continuum of care and the right information can be provided to the right people at the right time (Olson and Grant 2006)

- Working in the context of e-health technologies that allow consumers, patients, and caregivers to search for health information and advice, create and maintain personal health records, and conduct virtual consultations with their care providers (Baur and Deering 2006)

- Ensuring that health information technology systems, including electronic health records, electronic prescribing, bedside bar coding, computerized physician order entry (CPOE), and clinical decision support systems reduce errors and improve quality (Bloomrosen 2006)

- Managing the protection of sensitive information, including genetic (Fuller and Hudson 2006); drug, alcohol, sexual, and behavioral information (Randolph and Rinehart-Thompson 2006) and adoption information (Jones 2006)

- Developing moral awareness and nurturing an ethical environment in the context of managing a health information system (Flite and Laquer 2006)

- Serving as entrepreneur and advocate for patients, the healthcare team, and others who have interests in the information system (Gardenier 2006; Helbig 2006)

- Working with vendors in the development of business relationships that ensure ethical processes when selecting and communicating with the vendor, managing vendor relationships, and dealing with the contract negotiation process (Olenik 2006)

Because the HIT works with individuals and departments throughout the healthcare organization, his or her obligations extend into a variety of areas, as noted above. In fulfilling the responsibilities of the position, the HIT must apply ethical values when making decisions wherever he or she happens to be positioned within the organization.

Documentation and Access

Just a few years ago, only a few people created documentation in patients' health records and fewer still wanted access to patient information after the episode of care was complete. However, those days are over. In today's healthcare system, many providers document their decision-making process and patient outcomes in the health information system and many more people want access to that information. The HIT plays a critical role in ensuring that access to patient information is appropriate and authorized.

The HIT can serve many functions in this capacity, for example, as a member of the health information management (HIM) team. The HIM team designs and delivers educational sessions to the healthcare team to make them aware of the documentation and access rules and regulations. Sometimes educational sessions address the issue of participation in fraudulent or retrospective documentation practices. Retrospective documentation practices are those where healthcare providers add documentation, after care has been given, for the purpose of increasing reimbursement or avoiding suspension from the medical staff.

Unacceptable documentation practices include backdating progress notes or other documentation in the patient's record and changing the documentation to reflect the known outcomes of care (versus what was done at the time of the actual care). It is the HIT's responsibility to work with others to ensure that patient documentation is honest, accurate, and timely. The professional Code of Ethics requires the HIT's expertise to include the assurance of accurate documentation.

Protection of Privacy, Maintenance of Confidentiality, and Protection of Data Security

The terms *privacy, confidentiality*, and *security* are often used interchangeably. However, there are some important distinctions, including the following:

- **Privacy** is "the right of an individual to be let alone. It includes freedom from observation or intrusion into one's private affairs and the right to maintain control over certain personal and health information" (Harman 2006, 634).

- **Confidentiality** carries "the responsibility for limiting disclosure of private matters. It includes the responsibility to use, disclose, or release such information only with the knowledge and consent of the individual" (Harman 2006, 628). Confidential information can be written or verbal.

- **Security** includes "physical and electronic protection of the integrity, availability, and confidentiality of computer-based information and the resources used to enter, store, process, and communicate it. The means to control access and protect information from accidental or intentional disclosure" are elements of data security (Harman 2006, 628).

The Health Insurance Portability and Accountability Act of 1996 (HIPAA) is a statute that establishes national standards for privacy and security of health information. This law deals with privacy, information standards, data integrity, confidentiality, and data security (Rinehart-Thompson and Harman 2006; Harman 2005). HIPAA was passed in 1996. It took five years before the Privacy Rule became effective on April 14, 2001, with an April 14, 2003 compliance date. Congress passed the statute and the Department of Health and Human Services (HHS) developed the regulations contained within the HIPAA Privacy Rule (Standards for Privacy of Individually Identifiable Health Information 2003). The final HIPAA Security Rule regulations were published in the *Federal Register* on February 20, 2003, and became effective on April 21, 2005.

This legislation, which includes administrative simplification standards and security and privacy standards, has had a major impact on the collection and dissemination of information and will continue to do so in the coming years. It protects individuals from losing their health insurance when leaving and/or changing jobs by providing insurance continuity (portability) and increases the federal government's authority over fraud and abuse in the healthcare arena (accountability) (Harman 2005).

HIPAA was designed to guarantee that information transferred from one facility to the next would be protected. The National Committee on Vital and Health Statistics (NCVHS) supports a National Health Information Infrastructure (NHII) so that patient care information can be transferred and protected in our integrated healthcare systems. Patients can benefit from the continuity of the care, in addition to being able to control personal health information (NCVHS 2001; Gellman 2004; LaTour and Eichenwald 2006).

In an electronic environment, protecting privacy has become extremely difficult and patients are becoming increasingly concerned about the loss of privacy and the inability to control the dissemination of information about them. As patients become more aware of the misuses of information, they may become reluctant to share information with their healthcare team. This may, in turn, result in problems with the healthcare provided and information given to researchers, insurers, the government, and the many other stakeholders who legitimately need to gain access to patient information.

Release of Information

Three primary ethical problems are pertinent to the release of information (ROI):

- Violations of the need-to-know principle
- Misuse of blanket authorizations
- Violations of privacy that occur as a result of secondary release procedures

In the past, the standard for ROI was the need to know. If an insurance company had a patient request to pay for surgery, the request was sent to the healthcare facility and the HIM professional carefully examined it for legitimacy. He or she would:

- Compare the patient's signature to the one collected upon admission to the facility
- Check the date to ensure that the request was dated after the occurrence so that the patient was aware of what was being authorized for release
- Verify the insurance company as the one belonging to the patient
- Review the request for what was wanted and whether the requestor was entitled to the information

The HIT then reviewed the documentation and provided the information requested. For example, the admission and discharge dates, the diagnoses of cholecystitis and cholelithiasis, and the surgical procedure of cholecystectomy were provided to the insurance company so that the bill could be paid. The bottom line was: "Yes, insurance company, you can trust me as the health information professional. I reviewed the medical record, and you can pay for this surgery."

Today, the process of abstracting needed information is virtually nonexistent and documentation is copied above and beyond the criterion of need to know. For example, in response to the request to verify the admission for a cholecystectomy, a history and physical could be copied. That documentation could reveal social habits, genetic risks, and family history of disease that have nothing to do with the surgery. Further, patient privacy could be violated as a result of ROI through subsequent insurance discrimination.

Another common ethical problem is the misuse of blanket authorizations. Patients often sign a blanket authorization without understanding its implications. The requestor of the information then could use the authorization to receive health information for many years. The problem with the use of blanket authorizations is that there is no way for the patient to anticipate what future uses the information might be released for.

Responsibilities for technicians include ensuring that patient privacy and confidential information are protected and that data security measures are used to prevent unauthorized access to information. This responsibility includes ensuring that the release policies and procedures are accurate and up-to-date, that they are followed, and that all violations are reported to the proper authorities.

A third problem is that of secondary release to others. This problem has increased in frequency since the computerization of health information. A legitimate request might be processed to pay for an insurance claim, but there may not be adequate safety and protections for the information after it has been released. The initial requestor then could forward the information to others without patient authorization.

Patients are increasingly expressing concerns about the use of blanket authorizations and the secondary ROI by the initial requestor or receiving party. They fear that more information is being given out than is necessary or that it is being given to people whom they are not aware of. This situation has created an opportunity for HITs to participate with other HIM professionals in efforts to change these problems.

Coding

Before prospective payment systems were used to pay for healthcare services, clinical coding was performed for medical record identification for future clinical studies and quality assurance review processes. Although diagnosis and procedure codes were provided for health insurance claims, the healthcare facility was reimbursed for submitted costs rather than code assignments such as DRG codes. Over time, healthcare facilities continued to use the coding systems to retrieve information in health records for clinical and administrative studies and increasingly used codes for health insurance claims submission. After clinical codes became the basis for reimbursement, there were inherent incentives to assign selected codes so that maximum reimbursement could be claimed. This placed the importance of accurate and complete coding at the forefront of ethical issues facing HITs who have code assignment or code review responsibilities.

In selected circumstances, the health record documentation misrepresented the care that was actually rendered in order to optimize the reimbursement for an individual provider or a healthcare facility. Sometimes HIM professionals were tempted to assign certain codes in order to avoid conflicts. The increased complexity of the rules and regulations guiding the code assignment and reimbursement process made it difficult for coders to keep up-to-date. Additionally, there were instances where coders were pressured by their employers to engage in inappropriate or noncompliant coding practices. Pressure sometimes was in the form of an implied or even an actual threat of unemployment for failure to comply with the request to assign codes specifically for greater reimbursement or in violation of coding guidelines. Some common ethical coding problems include:

- Coding an inappropriate level of service for professional services
- Discovering misrepresentation in physician documentation
- Deliberately assigning inappropriate codes to avoid conflicts
- Discovering coding errors made by other staff members without taking action
- Lacking sufficient tools to do one's job
- Being required by the employer to engage in inappropriate coding
- Supporting and using application software that facilitates questionable results (Rinehart-Thompson 2006; Schraffenberger and Scichilone 2006)

These issues led to adoption of the Standards of Ethical Coding by the American Health Information Management Association (AHIMA). (See figure 14.1.)

Management of Sensitive Health Information

All health information must be protected, but ethical issues have emerged, particularly around the release of sensitive information such as genetic, drug and alcohol, communicable disease, and adoption information. At least two levels of genetic information can be reported in an information system: presence of a disease, such as cystic fibrosis; and presence of a risk of disease, such as a genetic risk for breast cancer. Various state laws govern the use of genetic information, and the HIT must be aware of them. Increasingly, there are concerns about discrimination in employment and insurance based on the misuse of genetic information (Fuller and Hudson 2006).

Federal and state laws also govern the use of behavioral health information and special concerns with its use. The HIT must respond to the government, the police, and other agencies that seek drug, alcohol, sexual, or other behavioral information (Randolph and Rinehart-Thompson 2006).

Figure 14.1.   1957 Code of Ethics for the Practice of Medical Record Science

[Note: Gender-neutral language was not used in the 1950s, so the male pronoun should be read as "he or she."]

As a member of one of the paramedical professions he shall:

1. Place service before material gain, the honor of the profession before personal advantage, the health and welfare of patients above all personal and financial interests, and conduct himself in the practice of this profession so as to bring honor to himself, his associates, and to the medical record profession.

2. Preserve and protect the medical records in his custody and hold inviolate the privileged contents of the records and any other information of a confidential nature obtained in his official capacity, taking due account of the applicable statutes and of regulations and policies of his employer.

3. Serve his employer loyally, honorably discharging the duties and responsibilities entrusted to him, and give due consideration to the nature of these responsibilities in giving his employer notice of intent to resign his position.

4. Refuse to participate in or conceal unethical practices or procedures.

5. Report to the proper authorities, but disclose to no one else, any evidence of conduct or practice revealed in the medical records in his custody that indicates possible violation of established rules and regulations of the employer or of professional practice.

6. Preserve the confidential nature of professional determinations made by the staff committee which he serves.

7. Accept only those fees that are customary and lawful in the area for services rendered in his official capacity.

8. Avoid encroachment on the professional responsibilities of the medical and other paramedical professions, and under no circumstances assume or give the appearance of assuming the right to make determinations in professional areas outside the scope of his assigned responsibilities.

9. Strive to advance the knowledge and practice of medical record science, including continued self-improvement, in order to contribute to the best possible medical care.

10. Participate appropriately in developing and strengthening professional manpower and in representing the profession to the public.

11. Discharge honorably the responsibilities of any Association post to which appointed or elected, and preserve the confidentiality of any privileged information made known to him in his official capacity.

12. State truthfully and accurately his credentials, professional education, and experiences in any official transaction with the American Association of Medical Record Librarians and with any employer or prospective employer.

The release of adoption information is another example of an issue that cannot be solved merely by following the legal rules. More and more, access to adoption information is being requested by adopted children seeking their biological parents, and vice versa. Biological parents often look for children who could be donors or sources of other medical assistance. Access to adoption information raises the larger issue of familial access to information, regardless of adoptive status (Jones 2006). HITs must be alert to these special needs and not process requests for adoption information without carefully considering the risks for violations of patient privacy, discrimination, or inappropriate access.

Check Your Understanding 14.1

Instructions: Match the following ethical principles with their definitions.

1. _____ Autonomy
2. _____ Beneficence
3. _____ Nonmaleficence
4. _____ Justice
5. _____ Moral values
6. _____ Ethics
7. _____ Privacy
8. _____ Confidentiality
9. _____ Data security
10. _____ HIPAA

a. Right or wrong
b. Reasoned discourse
c. Right to be let alone
d. Promote good
e. Self-determination
f. Healthcare communication
g. Do no harm
h. Fairness in applying rules
i. Establishes privacy and security standards
j. Electronic protection of information

Moral Values and Ethical Competencies

Morality is often described as actions that are either right or wrong. For example, some might consider it right to be nice to a neighbor and wrong to destroy the neighbor's property. However, these are not universal values. Others might consider it acceptable to be rude or mean to a neighbor and to destroy his or her property. Applying this language to health information management, it is right—and a moral obligation—to protect the neighbor's privacy if you learn about diseases and conditions while doing your job. It is wrong to share the neighbor's secrets with other neighbors, family, and friends.

Ethics is a process of reasoned discourse (discussion) among decision makers. They must carefully consider the shared and competing values and ethical principles that are important to the decision to be made. Ethical discussion provides a framework for resolving conflicts when competing values are at stake for the choices being considered. Ethical decision making requires people to explore options beyond the perspective of simple right or wrong (moral) options. According to Glover, "ethics refers to the formal process of intentionally and critically analyzing the basis for one's moral judgments, for clarity and consistency" (2006, 34). When making health information decisions, HIM professionals must go beyond the right or wrong moral perspective and evaluate the many values and perspectives of others engaged in the decision to be made.

Ethical discussions in nonhealthcare contexts can be theoretical in nature, and the analysis of a problem does not necessarily result in action. For example, **ethicists** could discuss whether to require all citizens living in a certain community to donate ten hours a week as part of their civic duty. One ethicist might argue for a decision based on the ethical principle of beneficence, which would guide action to do good things for others. Another ethicist might argue for the same decision, but based on the principle of justice in which every citizen should contribute his or her fair share for the good of the whole. Neither argument is right or wrong, just different. These discussions and decisions would not require action but would help frame the ethical justification for a certain action.

In contrast, **bioethics** involves problems or issues regarding clinical care or the health information system that are *never* strictly theoretical in nature and must *always* result in a decision. HITs cannot merely deliberate whether to release patient information. Instead, they must apply ethical principles and then perform an action—release the information requested or deny the request. In short, ethics applied in the work environment can never stay theoretical and always results in an action.

Moreover, HITs should not make ethical decisions based solely on personal moral values or perspectives. Not everyone shares the same moral perspectives or values. If one individual sees only one solution to a problem and others have different solutions, ethics can help with making a decision.

Ethical Foundations in Health Information Management

Ethical principles and values have been important to the health information management (HIM) profession since its beginning in 1928. The first ethical pledge was presented in 1934 by Grace Whiting Myers, the first president of the Association of Record Librarians of North America. The HIM profession was launched with a recognition of the importance of privacy and the requirement of authorization for the release of health information:

> I pledge myself to give out no information from any clinical record placed in my charge, or from any other source to any person whatsoever, except upon order from the chief executive officer of the institution which I may be serving (Huffman 1972, 135).

The most important value embedded in this pledge is the moral agency of the HIM professional to protect patient information.

The HIT has a clear ethical and professional obligation not to give any information to anyone unless its release has been authorized. Today, it is the patient who authorizes the release of information and not the chief executive officer (CEO), as stated in the original pledge.

Health Information Management's Codes of Ethics

HIM professionals used the pledge until 1957, at which time the American Association of Medical Record Librarians' (AAMRL) House of Delegates passed the first Code of Ethics for the Practice of Medical Record Science. (See figure 14.2.) The first Code of Ethics combined ethical principles with a set of professional values to help support the decisions that HIM professionals had to make at work. The original Code of Ethics has been revised many times. (See figures 14.3, 14.4, and 14.5, respectively, on the following pages.)

The fundamental values and professional obligations of all HIM professionals can be taken from AHIMA's ethical standards (Harman 2006):

- Providing service to others
- Protecting the privacy and confidentiality of both patient information and any committee deliberations
- Serving one's employer loyally and competently
- Refusing to participate in unethical behaviors or to take money for patient information
- Staying within the scope of responsibility as a health information practitioner
- Continuing to learn and study throughout one's career
- Representing the profession to the public
- Serving the professional association
- Being honest about educational degrees and credentials

Upon being awarded the credential of RHIT (registered health information technician) by AHIMA, the HIM professional agrees to follow the principles and values discussed in this chapter and to base all professional actions and decisions on those principles and values. Even if federal or state laws did not require the protection of patient privacy, the HIM professional would be responsible for protecting it according to AHIMA's Code of Ethics.

Professional Values and Obligations

Health information ethical and professional values are based on obligations to the patient, the healthcare team, the employer, the interests of the public, and oneself, one's peers, and one's professional associations.

Obligations to the Patient and the Healthcare Team

With regard to the patient and the healthcare team, the HIT is obligated to:

- *Provide service to those who seek access to patient information:* Individuals who may request access to patient information include healthcare providers, insurance or pharmaceutical companies, government agencies, and employers. The HIT must ensure the honor of the profession before personal advantage and the health and welfare of patients before all personal and financial interests. He or she also must balance the many competing interests of all the stakeholders who want patient information.

Figure 14.2.   1977 AMRA Bylaws and Code of Ethics

The medical record practitioner is concerned with the development, use, and maintenance of medical and health records for medical care, preventive medicine, quality assurance, professional education, administrative practices and study purposes with due consideration of patients' right to privacy. The American Medical Record Association believes that it is in the best interests of the medical record profession and the public which it serves that the principles of personal and professional accountability be reexamined and redefined to provide members of the Association, as well as medical record practitioners who are credentialed by the Association, with definitive and binding guidelines of conduct. To achieve this goal, the American Medical Record Association has adopted the following restated Code of Ethics:

1. Conduct yourself in the practice of this profession so as to bring honor and dignity to yourself, the medical record profession and the Association.

2. Place service before material gain and strive at all times to provide services consistent with the need for quality health care and treatment of all who are ill and injured.

3. Preserve and secure the medical and health records, the information contained therein, and the appropriate secondary records in your custody in accordance with professional management practices, employer's policies and existing legal provisions.

4. Uphold the doctrine of confidentiality and the individual's right to privacy in the disclosure of personally identifiable medical and social information.

5. Recognize the source of the authority and powers delegated to you and conscientiously discharge the duties and responsibilities thus entrusted.

6. Refuse to participate in or conceal unethical practices or procedures in your relationship with other individuals or organizations.

7. Disclose to no one but proper authorities any evidence of conduct or practice revealed in medical reports or observed that indicates possible violation of established rules and regulations of the employer or professional practice.

8. Safeguard the public and the profession by reporting to the Ethics Committee any breach of this Code of Ethics by fellow members of the profession.

9. Preserve the confidential nature of professional determinations made by official committees of health and health-service organizations.

10. Accept compensation only in accordance with services actually performed or negotiated with the health institution.

11. Cooperate with other health professions and organizations to promote the quality of health programs and advancement of medical care, ensuring respect and consideration for the responsibility and the dignity of medical and other health professions.

12. Strive to increase the profession's body of systematic knowledge and individual competency through continued self-improvement and application of current advancements in the conduct of medical record practices.

13. Participate in developing and strengthening professional manpower and appropriately represent the profession in public.

14. Discharge honorably the responsibilities of any Association position to which appointed or elected.

15. Represent truthfully and accurately professional credentials, education, and experience in any official transaction or notice, including other positions and duality of interests.

- *Protect both medical and social information:* Clinical information (diagnoses, procedures, pharmaceutical dosages, or genetic risk factors) must be protected as well as behavioral information (use of drugs or alcohol, high-risk hobbies, sexual habits). These days, it is increasingly important to protect social information to avoid risks of discrimination.

- *Protect confidential information:* This involves ensuring that the information collected and documented in the patient information system is protected by all members of the healthcare team and by anyone with access to the information while performing his or her job.

- *Preserve and secure health information:* This includes obligations to maintain and protect the medium that stores the information (hard copy, electronic, digital, imaged) and to secure the information for both manual and computerized information systems. All databases and detailed secondary records and registries also must be protected.

- *Promote the quality and advancement of healthcare:* As an important member of the healthcare team, the HIT provides valuable expertise in the collection of health information that will help providers improve the quality of care they deliver.

Figure 14.3.   1988 AMRA Code of Ethics and Bylaws

The medical record professional abides by a set of ethical principles developed to safeguard the public and to contribute within the scope of the profession to quality and efficiency in health care. This code of ethics, adopted by the members of the American Medical Record Association, defines the standards of behavior which promote ethical conduct.

1. The Medical Record Professional demonstrates behavior that reflects integrity, supports objectivity, and fosters trust in professional activities.

2. The Medical Record Professional respects the dignity of each human being.

3. The Medical Record Professional strives to improve personal competence and quality of services.

4. The Medical Record Professional represents truthfully and accurately professional credentials, education, and experience.

5. The Medical Record Professional refuses to participate in illegal or unethical acts and also refuses to conceal the illegal, incompetent, or unethical acts of others.

6. The Medical Record Professional protects the confidentiality of primary and secondary health records as mandated by law, professional standards, and the employer's policies.

7. The Medical Record Professional promotes to others the tenets of confidentiality.

8. The Medical Record Professional adheres to pertinent laws and regulations while advocating changes which serve the best interest of the public.

9. The Medical Record Professional encourages appropriate use of health record information and advocates policies and systems that advance the management of health records and health information.

10. The Medical Record Professional recognizes and supports the association's mission.

Copyright ©1988 by the American Medical Record Association.

Figure 14.4. 1998 AHIMA Code of Ethics and Bylaws

AHIMA's Mission

The American Health Information Management Association is committed to the quality of health information for the benefit of patients, providers and other users of clinical data. Our professional organization:

- Provides leadership in HIM education and professional development
- Sets and promotes professional practice standards
- Advocates patient privacy rights and confidentiality of health information
- Influences public and private policies including educating the public regarding health information
- Advances health information technologies

Guiding Principles

We are committed to the:

- Creation and utilization of systems and standards to ensure quality health information
- Achievement of member excellence
- Development of a supportive environment and provision of the resources to advance the profession
- Provision of the highest-quality service to members and health care information users
- Investigation and application of new technology to advance the management of health information

We value:

- The balance of patients' privacy rights and confidentiality of health information with legitimate uses of data
- The quality of health information as evidenced by its integrity, accuracy, consistency, reliability, and validity
- The quality of health information as evidenced by its impact on the quality of health care delivery

This Code of Ethics sets forth ethical principles for the HIM profession. Members of this profession are responsible for maintaining and promoting ethical practices. This Code of Ethics, adopted by the American Health Information Management Association, shall be binding on health information management professionals who are members of the Association and all individuals who hold an AHIMA credential.

I. Health information management professionals respect the rights and dignity of all individuals.

II. Health information management professionals comply with all laws, regulations, and standards governing the practice of health information management.

III. Health information management professionals strive for professional excellence through self-assessment and continuing education.

IV. Health information management professionals truthfully and accurately represent their professional credentials, education, and experience.

V. Health information management professionals adhere to the vision, mission, and values of the Association.

VI. Health information management professionals promote and protect the confidentiality and security of health records and health information.

VII. Health information management professionals strive to provide accurate and timely information.

VIII. Health information management professionals promote high standards for health information management practice, education, and research.

IX. Health information management professionals act with integrity and avoid conflicts of interest in the performance of their professional and AHIMA responsibilities.

Copyright ©1998 by the American Health Information Management Association.

Figure 14.5. 2004 American Health Information Management Association Code of Ethics

Preamble

The ethical obligations of the health information management (HIM) professional include the protection of patient privacy and confidential information; disclosure of information; development, use, and maintenance of health information systems and health records; and the quality of information. Both handwritten and computerized medical records contain many sacred stories—stories that must be protected on behalf of the individual and the aggregate community of persons served in the healthcare system. Healthcare consumers are increasingly concerned about the loss of privacy and the inability to control the dissemination of their protected information. Core health information issues include what information should be collected; how the information should be handled, who should have access to the information, and under what conditions the information should be disclosed.

Ethical obligations are central to the professional's responsibility, regardless of the employment site or the method of collection, storage, and security of health information. Sensitive information (genetic, adoption, drug, alcohol, sexual, and behavioral information) requires special attention to prevent misuse. Entrepreneurial roles require expertise in the protection of the information in the world of business and interactions with consumers.

Ethical obligations are central to the professional's responsibility, regardless of the employment site or the method of collection, storage, and security of health information. Sensitive information (genetic, adoption, drug, alcohol, sexual, and behavioral information) requires special attention to prevent misuse. Entrepreneurial roles require expertise in the protection of the information in the world of business and interactions with consumers.

Professional Values

The mission of the HIM profession is based on core professional values developed since the inception of the Association in 1928. These values and the inherent ethical responsibilities for AHIMA members and credentialed HIM professionals include providing service; protecting medical, social, and financial information; promoting confidentiality; and preserving and securing health information. Values to the healthcare team include promoting the quality and advancement of healthcare, demonstrating HIM expertise and skills, and promoting interdisciplinary cooperation and collaboration. Professional values in relationship to the employer include protecting committee deliberations and complying with laws, regulations, and policies. Professional values related to the public include advocating change, refusing to participate or conceal unethical practices, and reporting violations of practice standards to the proper authorities. Professional values to individual and professional associations include obligations to be honest, bringing honor to self, peers and profession, committing to continuing education and lifelong learning, performing Association duties honorably, strengthening professional membership, representing the profession to the public, and promoting and participating in research.

These professional values will require a complex process of balancing the many conflicts that can result from competing interests and obligations of those who seek access to health information and require an understanding of ethical decision-making.

Purpose of the American Health Information Management Association Code of Ethics

The HIM professional has an obligation to demonstrate actions that reflect values, ethical principles, and ethical guidelines. The American Health Information Management Association (AHIMA) Code of Ethics sets forth these values and principles to guide conduct. The code is relevant to all AHIMA members and credentialed HIM professionals and students, regardless of their professional functions, the settings in which they work, or the populations they serve.

The AHIMA Code of Ethics serves six purposes:

- Identifies core values on which the HIM mission is based.

- Summarizes broad ethical principles that reflect the profession's core values and establishes a set of ethical principles to be used to guide decision-making and actions.

(Continued on next page)

Figure 14.5. *(Continued)*

- Helps HIM professionals identify relevant considerations when professional obligations conflict or ethical uncertainties arise.
- Provides ethical principles by which the general public can hold the HIM professional accountable.
- Socializes practitioners new to the field to HIM's mission, values, and ethical principles.
- Articulates a set of guidelines that the HIM professional can use to assess whether they have engaged in unethical conduct.

The code includes principles and guidelines that are both enforceable and aspirational. The extent to which each principle is enforceable is a matter of professional judgment to be exercised by those responsible for reviewing alleged violations of ethical principles.

The Use of the Code

Violation of principles in this code does not automatically imply legal liability or violation of the law. Such determination can only be made in the context of legal and judicial proceedings. Alleged violations of the code would be subject to a peer review process. Such processes are generally separate from legal or administrative procedures and insulated from legal review or proceedings to allow the profession to counsel and discipline its own members although in some situations, violations of the code would constitute unlawful conduct subject to legal process.

Guidelines for ethical and unethical behavior are provided in this code. The terms "shall and shall not" are used as a basis for setting high standards for behavior. This does not imply that everyone "shall or shall not" do everything that is listed. For example, not everyone participates in the recruitment or mentoring of students. A HIM professional is not being unethical if this is not part of his or her professional activities; however, if students are part of one's professional responsibilities, there is an ethical obligation to follow the guidelines stated in the code. This concept is true for the entire code. If someone does the stated activities, ethical behavior is the standard. The guidelines are not a comprehensive list. For example, the statement "protect all confidential information to include personal, health, financial, genetic and outcome information" can also be interpreted as "shall not fail to protect all confidential information to include personal, health, financial, genetic, and outcome information."

A code of ethics cannot guarantee ethical behavior. Moreover, a code of ethics cannot resolve all ethical issues or disputes or capture the richness and complexity involved in striving to make responsible choices within a moral community. Rather, a code of ethics sets forth values and ethical principles, and offers ethical guidelines to which professionals aspire and by which their actions can be judged. Ethical behaviors result from a personal commitment to engage in ethical practice.

Professional responsibilities often require an individual to move beyond personal values. For example, an individual might demonstrate behaviors that are based on the values of honesty, providing service to others, or demonstrating loyalty. In addition to these, professional values might require promoting confidentiality, facilitating interdisciplinary collaboration, and refusing to participate or conceal unethical practices. Professional values could require a more comprehensive set of values than what an individual needs to be an ethical agent in their personal lives.

The AHIMA Code of Ethics is to be used by AHIMA and individuals, agencies, organizations, and bodies (such as licensing and regulatory boards, insurance providers, courts of law, agency boards of directors, government agencies, and other professional groups) that choose to adopt it or use it as a frame of reference. The AHIMA Code of Ethics reflects the commitment of all to uphold the profession's values and to act ethically. Individuals of good character who discern moral questions and, in good faith, seek to make reliable ethical judgments, must apply ethical principles.

The code does not provide a set of rules that prescribe how to act in all situations. Specific applications of the code must take into account the context in which it is being considered and the possibility of conflicts among the code's values, principles, and guidelines. Ethical responsibilities flow from all human relationships, from the personal and familial to the social and professional. Further, the AHIMA Code of Ethics does not specify which values, principles, and guidelines are the most important and ought to outweigh others in instances when they conflict.

Figure 14.5. *(Continued)*

Code of Ethics 2004

Ethical Principles: The following ethical principles are based on the core values of the American Health Information Management Association and apply to all health information management professionals.

Health information management professionals:

I. *Advocate, uphold and defend the individual's right to privacy and the doctrine of confidentiality in the use and disclosure of information.*

II. *Put service and the health and welfare of persons before self-interest and conduct themselves in the practice of the profession so as to bring honor to themselves, their peers, and to the health information management profession.*

III. *Preserve, protect, and secure personal health information in any form or medium and hold in the highest regard the contents of the records and other information of a confidential nature, taking into account the applicable statutes and regulations.*

IV. *Refuse to participate in or conceal unethical practices or procedures.*

V. *Advance health information management knowledge and practice through continuing education, research, publications, and presentations.*

VI. *Recruit and mentor students, peers and colleagues to develop and strengthen professional workforce.*

VII. *Represent the profession accurately to the public.*

VIII. *Perform honorably health information management association responsibilities, either appointed or elected, and preserve the confidentiality of any privileged information made known in any official capacity.*

IX. *State truthfully and accurately their credentials, professional education, and experiences.*

X. *Facilitate interdisciplinary collaboration in situations supporting health information practice.*

XI. *Respect the inherent dignity and worth of every person.*

How to Interpret the Code of Ethics

The following ethical principles are based on the core values of the American Health Information Management Association and apply to all health information management professionals. Guidelines included for each ethical principle are a non-inclusive list of behaviors and situations that can help to clarify the principle. They are not to be meant as a comprehensive list of all situations that can occur.

I. *Advocate, uphold, and defend the individual's right to privacy and the doctrine of confidentiality in the use and disclosure of information.*

Health information management professionals **shall:**

1.1. Protect all confidential information to include personal, health, financial, genetic, and outcome information.

1.2. Engage in social and political action that supports the protection of privacy and confidentiality, and be aware of the impact of the political arena on the health information system. Advocate for changes in policy and legislation to ensure protection of privacy and confidentiality, coding compliance, and other issues that surface as advocacy issues as well as facilitating informed participation by the public on these issues.

1.3. Protect the confidentiality of all information obtained in the course of professional service. Disclose only information that is directly relevant or necessary to achieve the purpose of disclosure. Release information only with valid consent from a patient or a person legally authorized to consent on behalf of a patient or as authorized by federal or state regulations. The need-to-know criterion is essential when releasing health information for initial disclosure and all redisclosure activities.

(Continued on next page)

Figure 14.5.   *(Continued)*

1.4.   Promote the obligation to respect privacy by respecting confidential information shared among colleagues, while responding to requests from the legal profession, the media, or other non-healthcare related individuals, during presentations or teaching and in situations that could cause harm to persons.

II.   *Put service and the health and welfare of persons before self-interest and conduct themselves in the practice of the profession so as to bring honor to themselves, their peers, and to the health information management profession.*

Health information management professionals **shall:**

2.1.   Act with integrity, behave in a trustworthy manner, elevate service to others above self-interest, and promote high standards of practice in every setting.

2.2.   Be aware of the profession's mission, values, and ethical principles, and practice in a manner consistent with them by acting honestly and responsibly.

2.3.   Anticipate, clarify, and avoid any conflict of interest, to all parties concerned, when dealing with consumers, consulting with competitors, or in providing services requiring potentially conflicting roles (for example, finding out information about one facility that would help a competitor). The conflicting roles or responsibilities must be clarified and appropriate action must be taken to minimize any conflict of interest.

2.4.   Ensure that the working environment is consistent and encourages compliance with the AHIMA Code of Ethics, taking reasonable steps to eliminate any conditions in their organizations that violate, interfere with, or discourage compliance with the code.

2.5.   Take responsibility and credit, including authorship credit, only for work they actually perform or to which they contribute. Honestly acknowledge the work of and the contributions made by others verbally or written, such as in publication.

Health information management professionals **shall not:**

2.6.   Permit their private conduct to interfere with their ability to fulfill their professional responsibilities.

2.7.   Take unfair advantage of any professional relationship or exploit others to further their personal, religious, political, or business interests.

III.   *Preserve, protect, and secure personal health information in any form or medium and hold in the highest regards the contents of the records and other information of a confidential nature obtained in the official capacity, taking into account the applicable statutes and regulations.*

Health information management professionals **shall:**

3.1.   Protect the confidentiality of patients' written and electronic records and other sensitive information. Take reasonable steps to ensure that patients' records are stored in a secure location and that patients' records are not available to others who are not authorized to have access.

3.2.   Take precautions to ensure and maintain the confidentiality of information transmitted, transferred, or disposed of in the event of a termination, incapacitation, or death of a healthcare provider to other parties through the use of any media. Disclosure of identifying information should be avoided whenever possible.

3.3.   Inform recipients of the limitations and risks associated with providing services via electronic media (such as computer, telephone, fax, radio, and television).

Figure 14.5.   *(Continued)*

IV.   Refuse to participate in or conceal unethical practices or procedures.

Health information management professionals **shall:**

4.1.   Act in a professional and ethical manner at all times.

4.2.   Take adequate measures to discourage, prevent, expose, and correct the unethical conduct of colleagues.

4.3.   Be knowledgeable about established policies and procedures for handling concerns about colleagues' unethical behavior. These include policies and procedures created by AHIMA, licensing and regulatory bodies, employers, supervisors, agencies, and other professional organizations.

4.4.   Seek resolution if there is a belief that a colleague has acted unethically or if there is a belief of incompetence or impairment by discussing their concerns with the colleague when feasible and when such discussion is likely to be productive. Take action through appropriate formal channels, such as contacting an accreditation or regulatory body and/or the AHIMA Professional Ethics Committee.

4.5.   Consult with a colleague when feasible and assist the colleague in taking remedial action when there is direct knowledge of a health information management colleague's incompetence or impairment.

Health information management professionals **shall not:**

4.6.   Participate in, condone, or be associated with dishonesty, fraud and abuse, or deception. A non-inclusive list of examples includes:

- Allowing patterns of retrospective documentation to avoid suspension or increase reimbursement

- Assigning codes without physician documentation

- Coding when documentation does not justify the procedures that have been billed

- Coding an inappropriate level of service

- Miscoding to avoid conflict with others

- Engaging in negligent coding practices

- Hiding or ignoring review outcomes, such as performance data

- Failing to report licensure status for a physician through the appropriate channels

- Recording inaccurate data for accreditation purposes

- Hiding incomplete medical records

- Allowing inappropriate access to genetic, adoption, or behavioral health information

- Misusing sensitive information about a competitor

- Violating the privacy of individuals

V.   Advance health information management knowledge and practice through continuing education, research, publications, and presentations.

Health information management professionals **shall:**

5.1.   Develop and enhance continually their professional expertise, knowledge, and skills (including appropriate education, research, training, consultation, and supervision). Contribute to the knowledge base of health information management and share with colleagues their knowledge related to practice, research, and ethics.

(Continued on next page)

Figure 14.5. *(Continued)*

5.2. Base practice decisions on recognized knowledge, including empirically based knowledge relevant to health information management and health information management ethics.

5.3. Contribute time and professional expertise to activities that promote respect for the value, integrity, and competence of the health information management profession. These activities may include teaching, research, consultation, service, legislative testimony, presentations in the community, and participation in their professional organizations.

5.4. Engage in evaluation or research that ensures the anonymity or confidentiality of participants and of the data obtained from them by following guidelines developed for the participants in consultation with appropriate institutional review boards. Report evaluation and research findings accurately and take steps to correct any errors later found in published data using standard publication methods.

5.5. Take reasonable steps to provide or arrange for continuing education and staff development, addressing current knowledge and emerging developments related to health information management practice and ethics.

Health information management professionals **shall not:**

5.6. Design or conduct evaluation or research that is in conflict with applicable federal or state laws.

5.7. Participate in, condone, or be associated with fraud or abuse.

VI. *Recruit and mentor students, peers and colleagues to develop and strengthen professional workforce.*

Health information management professionals **shall:**

6.1. Evaluate students' performance in a manner that is fair and respectful when functioning as educators or clinical internship supervisors.

6.2. Be responsible for setting clear, appropriate, and culturally sensitive boundaries for students.

6.3. Be a mentor for students, peers and new health information management professionals to develop and strengthen skills.

6.4. Provide directed practice opportunities for students.

Health information management professionals **shall not:**

6.5. Engage in any relationship with students in which there is a risk of exploitation or potential harm to the student.

6.1. Evaluate students' performance in a manner that is fair and respectful when functioning as educators or clinical internship supervisors.

6.2. Be responsible for setting clear, appropriate, and culturally sensitive boundaries for students.

6.3. Be a mentor for students, peers and new health information management professionals to develop and strengthen skills.

6.4. Provide directed practice opportunities for students.

VII. *Accurately represent the profession to the public.*

Health information management professionals **shall:**

7.1 Be an advocate for the profession in all settings and participate in activities that promote and explain the mission, values, and principles of the profession to the public.

Figure 14.5. *(Continued)*

VIII. ***Perform honorably health information management association responsibilities, either appointed or elected, and preserve the confidentiality of any privileged information made known in any official capacity.***

Health information management professionals **shall:**

8.1.   Perform responsibly all duties as assigned by the professional association.

8.2.   Resign from an Association position if unable to perform the assigned responsibilities with competence.

8.3.   Speak on behalf of professional health information management organizations, accurately representing the official and authorized positions of the organizations.

IX. ***State truthfully and accurately their credentials, professional education, and experiences.***

Health information management professionals **shall:**

9.1.   Make clear distinctions between statements made and actions engaged in as a private individual and as a representative of the health information management profession, a professional health information organization, or the health information management professional's employer.

9.2.   Claim and ensure that their representations to patients, agencies, and the public of professional qualifications, credentials, education, competence, affiliations, services provided, training, certification, consultation received, supervised experience, other relevant professional experience are accurate.

9.3.   Claim only those relevant professional credentials actually possessed and correct any inaccuracies occurring regarding credentials.

X. ***Facilitate interdisciplinary collaboration in situations supporting health information practice.***

Health information management professionals **shall:**

10.1.   Participate in and contribute to decisions that affect the well-being of patients by drawing on the perspectives, values, and experiences of those involved in decisions related to patients. Professional and ethical obligations of the interdisciplinary team as a whole and of its individual members should be clearly established.

XI.   Respect the inherent dignity and worth of every person.

Health information management professionals **shall:**

11.1.   Treat each person in a respectful fashion, being mindful of individual differences and cultural and ethnic diversity.

11.2.   Promote the value of self-determination for each individual.

Acknowledgement

Adapted with permission from the Code of Ethics of the National Association of Social Workers.

Resources

National Association of Social Workers. "Code of Ethics." 1999. Available online from socialworkers. org/pubs/code/code.asp.

Harman, L.B., ed.. 2001. *Ethical Challenges in the Management of Health Information.* Gaithersburg, MD: Aspen.

AHIMA Code of Ethics, 1957, 1977, 1988, and 1998.

Revised & adopted by AHIMA House of Delegates—July 1, 2004

Copyright ©2004 by the American Health Information Management Association.

- *Stay within the scope of responsibility and restrain from passing clinical judgment:* Sometimes healthcare data may indicate a problem with a provider of care, the treatment of a diagnosis, or some other problem. The HIT's obligation is to provide the data, no matter how often they are needed, but not to pass judgment on them. That obligation rests with the healthcare team that reviews the data. The HIT should repeatedly and consistently report accurate results of studies.

- *Promote interdisciplinary cooperation and collaboration:* As an important member of the healthcare team, the HIT should work with others to analyze and address health information issues, facilitate conflict resolution, and recognize the expertise and dignity of his or her fellow team members.

Obligations to the Employer

With regard to the employer, the HIT is obligated to:

- *Demonstrate loyalty to the employer:* The HIT can do this by respecting and following the policies, rules, and regulations of employment unless they are illegal or unethical. This obligation includes giving the employer adequate notice when the HIT decides to change employment sites.

- *Protect committee deliberations:* Examples of such committees include medical staff and employer committees. The HIT should be as committed to protecting committee conversations and decisions as he or she is to protecting patient information.

- *Comply with all laws, regulations, and policies that govern the health information system:* The HIT should keep up-to-date with state and federal laws, accrediting and licensing standards, employer policies and procedures, and any other standards that affect the health information system.

- *Recognize both authority and power associated with the job responsibility:* This obligation rests with the obligations to protect information, code accurately, release information appropriately, and other, similar functions.

- *Accept compensation only in relationship to work responsibilities:* The HIT must avoid the temptation to accept money for patient information or proprietary vendor secrets (which would clearly be an unethical behavior).

Obligations to the Public

With regard to the public interest, the HIT is obligated to:

- *Advocate change when patterns or system problems are not in the best interests of the patients:* The HIT should be proactive about protecting patients, the healthcare team, the organization, the professional association, peers, and him- or herself.

- *Refuse to participate or conceal unethical practices:* The HIT should be accountable for noticing trends and potential problems with regard to providers of care, diagnoses, procedures, and so on. Further, he or she should refuse to conceal illegal, incompetent, or unethical behaviors of individuals or organizations.

- *Report violations of practice standards to the proper authorities:* The HIT should not share information learned at work with family or friends or discuss such information in public places. He or she should report the results of audits to the proper authorities only. Moreover, the HIT should bring potential or actual problems to the attention of those individuals responsible for the delivery and assessment of care and services.

Obligations to Self, Peers, and Professional Associations

With regard to self, peers, and professional associations, the HIT is obligated to:

- *Be honest about degrees, credentials, and work experiences:* The HIT should only report an acquired academic degree (such as an AAS) or successfully earned credentials (such as an RHIT or a CCS). Work experiences must be reported accurately and honestly.

- *Bring honor to oneself, one's peers, and one's profession:* This obligation refers to personal competency and professional behavior (for example, at professional meetings). The HIT should try to ensure that peers and colleagues are proud to have him or her on the health information team.

- *Commit to continuing education and lifelong learning:* The HIT's education should not stop when he or she has earned a degree or a credential. Rather, he or she should continue to attend educational sessions to keep abreast of changing laws, rules, and regulations that affect the health information system. The HIT should be a lifelong learner and contribute to improving the quality of healthcare service delivery. HITs can keep their credentials by meeting the ongoing certification requirements of AHIMA. Maintaining competency through self-improvement is an important directive that ensures the continuance of the profession.

- *Strengthen the health information professional membership:* This obligation includes belonging to professional associations, actively participating in committees, making presentations, writing for publications, and encouraging others to seek health information as a career.

- *Represent the health information profession to the public:* The HIT has a responsibility to inform the public of the full range and importance of his or her job responsibilities.

- *Promote and participate in health information research:* When problems are discovered with the health information system, the HIT should conduct studies to clarify their sources and potential solutions.

Check Your Understanding 14.2

Instructions: Match the HIM professional's obligations to the following groups with the professional values expressed in AHIMA's 1998 Code of Ethics.

a.   Patients and the healthcare team
b.   Employer
c.   Public interest
d.   Oneself and one's peers and professional associations

1.   _____ Accept compensation only in relationship to responsibilities

2.   _____ Advocate change

3.   _____ Preserve and secure health information

4.   _____ Be honest

5.   _____ Commit to continuing education and lifelong learning

6.   _____ Promote interdisciplinary cooperation and collaboration

7.   _____ Promote and participate in research

8.   _____ Demonstrate loyalty to employer

9.   _____ Discharge association duties honorably

10.   _____ Protect committee deliberations

11.   _____ Stay within the scope of responsibility and restrain from passing clinical judgment

12.   _____ Bring honor to self, peers, and profession

13.   _____ Protect medical and social information

14.   _____ Promote the quality and advancement of healthcare

15.   _____ Represent profession to the public

16.   _____ Comply with laws, regulations, and policies

17.   _____ Report violations of practice standards to the proper authorities

18.   _____ Refuse to participate in or conceal unethical practices

19.   _____ Provide service

20.   _____ Strengthen professional membership

21.   _____ Recognize authority and power

22.   _____ Promote confidentiality

Ethical Decision-Making Model

HITs must factor several criteria into their decision making. These include, but are not limited to:

- *Cost:* Can the facility and the health information system afford the improvement in the system?

- *Technological feasibility:* Will the technological application provide accurate and reliable information for the decision-making process?

- *Federal and state laws:* Are there federal or state laws that must be considered before a change is made in the system?

- *Medical staff bylaws:* Are there rules or regulations unique to the facility that require or prohibit an action?

- *Accreditation and licensing standards:* Which agencies have standards that are important to the decision being made? Do the standards allow or prohibit a certain action?

- *Employer policies, rules, or regulations:* Does the facility have policies, rules, or regulations that require or prohibit an action?

Although these criteria must be assessed in the decision-making process, they cannot be used alone. Virtually every decision the HIT makes also must be based on ethical principles and professional values.

Ethicists provide assistance in this process. Glover (2006) has proposed a seven-step process to guide ethical decision making. When faced with an ethical issue, the HIT should ask and answer all the following questions:

1. What is the ethical question?

2. What facts do you know, and what do you need to find out?

3. Who are the different stakeholders, what values are at stake, and what are the shared or different obligations and interests of each stakeholder?

4. What options for action do you have?

5. What decision should you make, and what core HIM values are at stake?

6. What justifies the choice, and what are the value-based reasons to support the decision? What choice or choices cannot be justified?

7. What prevention options can be put in place so that this issue will not come up again?

Ethical Decision-Making Matrix

The ethical decision-making matrix is a tool to help you organize complex, ethical problems; however, there is no simple fill-in-the-box approach to ethical decision making. The objective is to follow each step of the process and not move from the question directly to what should be done or how to prevent it next time. If you skip steps, you will not fully understand all the values and options for action. There is more than one way to examine the problem. You can make an equally compelling ethical argument for a different decision—just be sure to follow all the steps of the matrix (figure 14.6). The questions represent the steps in the decision-making process.

If a decision must be made about an issue and only one choice is identified, the decision will most likely be based on the narrow moral perspective of right or wrong. However, a decision based solely on right and wrong does not take into account the perspectives of competing stakeholders and their values. Decisions that are made without this model will not benefit from an ethical decision-making process that considers multiple options.

Figure 14.6. Ethical decision-making matrix		
ETHICAL PROBLEM		
Steps	**Information**	
1. What is the question?		
2. What are the facts?	**KNOWN**	**TO BE GATHERED**
3. What are the values? Examine the shared and competing values, obligations, and interests in order to fully understand the complexity of the ethical problem(s).	**Patient:** **HIM Professional:** **Healthcare professionals:** **Administrators:** **Society:** **Other, as appropriate:**	
4. What are my options?		
5. What should I do?		
6. What justifies my choice?	*JUSTIFIED*	*NOT JUSTIFIED*
7. What can I do to prevent this ethical problem?		
Source: Glover 2006, p. 50.		

Check Your Understanding 14.3

Instructions: Using a, b, c, and so on, rearrange the steps of the ethical decision-making process in the correct order.

1. _____ What decision should you make, and what core HIM values are at stake?

2. _____ What facts do you know, and what do you need to find out?

3. _____ What options for action do you have?

4. _____ What is the ethical question?

5. _____ What justifies the choice, and what are the reasons to support the decision, based on values? What choice or choices cannot be justified?

6. _____ What prevention options can be put in place so that this issue will not happen again?

7. _____ Who are the different stakeholders, what values are at stake, and what are the different obligations and interests of each stakeholder?

Real-World Case

Health information technicians are frequently faced with ethical dilemmas on the job. One of the many ethical challenges they might face is detailed below (Rinehart-Thompson and Harman 2006, 52):

Mary is a health information management (HIM) student completing a clinical practice rotation in an acute care hospital in her community. This week she is learning about the release-of-information process. At the breakfast table, Mary's mother asks her to find out what is wrong with Ruth, their next-door neighbor. Ruth has been admitted to the hospital twice in the last three months, and Mary's mother wants to know why. While processing the requests for release of information that afternoon, Mary comes across one from Ruth's insurance company. Mary learns that Ruth was hospitalized due to physical abuse by her husband. Mary has been in trouble with her mother recently. She knows that if she tells her mother this information, she will score "big points." She is very tempted to tell her mother the information she has learned.

Later that same day, while responding to another request for information, Mary realizes that the medical record she is reviewing belongs to Ron, her best friend's fiancé. Mary learns that Ron has a drug abuse problem and was recently diagnosed with HIV. Mary will be the maid of honor at the wedding of Ron and Patricia two months from now, and she knows that Patricia does not know about Ron's problems. Mary becomes worried and wonders whether she should tell her best friend what she has learned, because Ron's conditions could affect Patricia's health and the quality of her married life.

Summary

Ethical decision making is one of the health information technician's most challenging and rewarding job responsibilities. It requires courage because there will always be people who choose not tell the truth or do the right thing. HITs must discuss these issues with their peer technicians and other health information management professionals and seek the advice of the professional association when necessary.

The HIT's job responsibilities inherently require an understanding of ethical principles, professional values and obligations, and the importance of using an ethical decision-making matrix when confronting difficult challenges at work. With this knowledge, the informed HIT can move from understanding problems based on a moral perspective only to understanding the importance of applying an ethical decision-making process. Ethical decision making takes practice, and discussions with peers will help the HIT to build competency in this important area.

When making ethical decisions, the HIT must use the complete ethical decision-making matrix to consider all the stakeholders and their obligations and the important HIM professional values. More than one response can be given for any ethical issue as long as the complete matrix is applied. Just as there can be more than one "right" answer to a problem, there can be "wrong" answers, especially when an answer is based only on a moral value or the perspective of one individual or results in an unethical action.

Bioethical decisions involving the use of health information require action, and such actions always require courage. The healthcare team, the patients, and the others who are served need to know that the HIT has the expertise and the courage to make the appropriate ethical decisions.

References

Baur, C., and M.J. Deering. 2006. e-Health for consumers, patients, and caregivers. Chapter 16 in *Ethical Challenges in the Management of Health Information,* 2nd ed., edited by L.B. Harman. Sudbury, MA: Jones and Bartlett.

Beauchamp, T., and J. Childress. 2001. *Principles of Biomedical Ethics.* New York: Oxford University Press.

Bloomrosen, M. 2006. E-HIM: Information technology and information exchange. Chapter 17 in *Ethical Challenges in the Management of Health Information,* 2nd ed., edited by L.B. Harman. Sudbury, MA: Jones and Bartlett.

Czirr, K., K. Rosendale, and E. West. 2006. Information security. Chapter 12 in *Ethical Challenges in the Management of Health Information,* 2nd ed., edited by L.B. Harman. Sudbury, MA: Jones and Bartlett.

Fenton, S.H. 2006. Software development and implementation. Chapter 13 in *Ethical Challenges in the Management of Health Information,* 2nd ed., edited by L.B. Harman. Sudbury, MA: Jones and Bartlett.

Flite, C., and S. Laquer. 2006. Management. Chapter 21 in *Ethical Challenges in the Management of Health Information: Process and Strategies for Decision-Making,* edited by L.B. Harman. Sudbury, MA: Jones and Bartlett.

Fuller, B.P., and K.L. Hudson. 2006. Genetic information. Chapter 18 in *Ethical Challenges in the Management of Health Information,* 2nd ed., edited by L.B. Harman. Sudbury, MA: Jones and Bartlett.

Gardenier, M. 2006. Entrepreneurship. Chapter 22 in *Ethical Challenges in the Management of Health Information,* 2nd ed., edited by L.B. Harman. Sudbury, MA: Jones and Bartlett.

Gellman, R. 2004 (June 23). When HIPAA meets NHII: A new dimension for privacy. Presentation to U.S. Department of Health and Human Services Data Council Privacy Committee, Washington, D.C. Available online from hhs.gov.

Glover, J.J. 2006. Ethical decision-making guidelines and tools. Chapter 2 in *Ethical Challenges in the Management of Health Information,* 2nd ed., edited by L.B. Harman. Sudbury, MA: Jones and Bartlett.

Hanken, M.A., and G. Murphy. 2006. Electronic patient record. Chapter 11 in *Ethical Challenges in the Management of Health Information,* 2nd ed., edited by L.B. Harman. Sudbury, MA: Jones and Bartlett.

Harman, L.B., ed. 2006. *Ethical Challenges in the Management of Health Information,* 2nd ed. Sudbury, MA: Jones and Bartlett.

Harman, L.B. 2005 (May 31). HIPAA: A few years later. *Online Journal of Issues in Nursing* 10(2): manuscript 2. Available online from nursingworld.org/ojin/topic27/tpc27_2.htm.

Harman, L.B. 1999. HIM and ethics: Confronting ethical dilemmas on the job, an HIM professional's guide. *Journal of American Health Information Management Association* 71(5):45–49.

Harman, L.B., and V.L. Mullen. 2006. Professional values and the Code of Ethics. Chapter 1 in *Ethical Challenges in the Management of Health Information,* 2nd ed., edited by L.B. Harman. Sudbury, MA: Jones and Bartlett.

Helbig, S. 2006. Advocacy. Chapter 24 in *Ethical Challenges in the Management of Health Information,* 2nd ed., edited by L.B. Harman. Sudbury, MA: Jones and Bartlett.

Huffman, E.K. 1972. *Manual for Medical Record Librarians,* 6th ed. Chicago: Physician's Record Company.

Johns, M.L. 2002. *Information Management for Health Professions,* 2nd ed. Albany, NY: Delmar.

Johns, M.L., and J.M. Hardin. 2006. Research and decision support. Chapter 7 in *Ethical Challenges in the Management of Health Information,* 2nd ed., edited by L.B. Harman. Sudbury, MA: Jones and Bartlett.

Jones, M.L. 2006. Adoption information. Chapter 19 in *Ethical Challenges in the Management of Health Information,* 2nd ed., edited by L.B. Harman. Sudbury, MA: Jones and Bartlett.

LaTour, K.M., and S.M. Eichenwald, eds. 2006. *Health information Management: Concepts, Principles, and Practice,* 2nd ed. Chicago: AHIMA.

Lee, F.W., A.W. White, and K.A. Wager. 2006. Data resource management. Chapter 14 in *Ethical Challenges in the Management of Health Information,* 2nd ed., edited by L.B. Harman. Sudbury, MA: Jones and Bartlett.

National Committee on Vital and Health Statistics. 2001. Information for health: A strategy for building the national health information infrastructure. Available online from aspe.hhs.gov/sp/nhii/Documents/NHIIReport2001/report11.htm.

Neuberger, B.J. 2006. Public health. Chapter 8 in *Ethical Challenges in the Management of Health Information,* 2nd ed., edited by L.B. Harman. Sudbury, MA: Jones and Bartlett.

Olenik, K. 2006. Vendor relationships. Chapter 23 in *Ethical Challenges in the Management of Health Information: Process and Strategies for Decision-Making,* edited by L.B. Harman. Sudbury, MA: Jones and Bartlett.

Olson, B., and K.G. Grant. 2006. Integrated delivery systems. Chapter 15 in *Ethical Challenges in the Management of Health Information,* 2nd ed., edited by L.B. Harman. Sudbury, MA: Jones and Bartlett.

Randolph, S.J., and L.A. Rinehart-Thompson. 2006. Drug, alcohol, sexual, and behavioral health information. Chapter 20 in *Ethical Challenges in the Management of Health Information,* 2nd ed., edited by L.B. Harman. Sudbury, MA: Jones and Bartlett.

Rinehart-Thompson, L.A. 2006. Compliance, fraud, and abuse. Chapter 4 in *Ethical Challenges in the Management of Health Information,* 2nd ed., edited by L.B. Harman. Sudbury, MA: Jones and Bartlett.

Rinehart-Thompson, L.A., and L.B. Harman. 2006. Privacy and confidentiality. Chapter 3 in *Ethical Challenges in the Management of Health Information,* 2nd ed., edited by L.B. Harman. Sudbury, MA: Jones and Bartlett.

Schick, I.C. 2006. Managed care. Chapter 9 in *Ethical Challenges in the Management of Health Information,* 2nd ed., edited by L.B. Harman. Sudbury, MA: Jones and Bartlett.

Schraffenberger, L.A., and R.A. Scichilone. 2006. Clinical code selection and use. Chapter 5 in *Ethical Challenges in the Management of Health Information,* 2nd ed., edited by L.B. Harman. Sudbury, MA: Jones and Bartlett.

Spath, P. L. 2006. Quality review. Chapter 6 in *Ethical Challenges in the Management of Health Information,* 2nd ed., edited by L.B. Harman. Sudbury, MA: Jones and Bartlett.

Standards for Privacy of Individually Identifiable Health Information. 2003 (April 17). 45 CFR Parts 160 and 164.

Thompson, T.G., and D. Brailer. 2004. The Decade of Health Information Technology: Delivering Consumer-centric and Information-rich Health Care. Washington, DC: HHS. Available online from hhs.gov/healthit/documents/hitframework.pdf.

Tischler, J.F. 2006. Clinical care: End of life. Chapter 10 in *Ethical Challenges in the Management of Health Information: Process and Strategies for Decision-Making,* edited by L.B. Harman. Sudbury, MA: Jones and Bartlett.

Chapter 15
Legal Issues in Health Information Technology

Laurie A. Rinehart-Thompson, JD, RHIA, CHP

Learning Objectives

- To become familiar with the legal issues pertaining to the confidentiality aspect of health information management

- To understand the significance of the roles that statutes, administrative laws, and regulatory agencies, including public health reporting requirements, have with regard to the use and disclosure of health information

- To identify issues related to ownership and control of the health record

- To discuss HIPAA privacy standards and rules with regard to health information use and disclosure

- To understand policies and procedures with regard to health information use and disclosure

Key Terms

Administrative law

Administrative simplification

Age Discrimination in Employment Act

Americans with Disabilities Act of 1990

Appeal

Appellate court

Arbitration

Authenticate

Authorization

Bench trial

Breach

Business associate

Causation

Collective bargaining

Complaint

Consent

Constitutional law

Counterclaim

Court order

Courts of appeal

Covered entity

Credentialing

Cross-claim

Defendant

De-identified information

Deposition

Designated record set

Discovery

District court

Diversity jurisdiction

Duty

Equal Employment Opportunity Act

Equal Pay Act

Fair Labor Standards Act

False Claims Act

Individually identifiable health information

Injury (harm)

Intentional tort

Joinder

Judicial law

Jurisdiction

Litigation

Malfeasance

Mediation

Medical malpractice

Minimum necessary

Misfeasance

National Labor Relations Act

Negligence

Nonfeasance

Notice of privacy practices

Occupational Safety and Health Act

Plaintiff

Preemption

Privacy officer

Private law

Public law

Rehabilitation Act

Right-to-work laws

Rules and regulations

Statutory law

Subject matter jurisdiction

Subpoena ad testificandum

Subpoena duces tecum

Summons

Supreme Court

Tort

Treatment, payment, and operations (TPO)

Trial court

Use, disclosures, and requests

Voir dire

Introduction

Every health information technician (HIT) should be familiar with the legal requirements concerning the compilation and maintenance of patient health records. In addition, every HIT must be concerned with how health information is used and when it can be disclosed. It is important for the HIT to be familiar with the pertinent state and federal regulations and statutes, including the federal Privacy Rule resulting from passage of the Health Insurance Portability and Accountability Act (HIPAA), that address these concerns.

The principal purpose of collecting and storing health information is to provide direct, high-quality patient care and serve the interests of the patient. To that end, the healthcare organization must ensure that the information in patient health records is complete, accurate, and timely. Healthcare organizations that do not abide by state regulations and laws could have their licenses suspended or revoked.

In addition to state and federal laws, healthcare organizations may be subject to the standards of accrediting bodies such as the Joint Commission on Accreditation of Healthcare Organizations (JCAHO) and the American Osteopathic Association (AOA). Organizations that fail to comply with the standards of the JCAHO and other such groups could lose their accreditation. As the customary custodian of patient records and health information, the HIT must be familiar with state and federal, accrediting, and other requirements for the maintenance of health records.

However, the use of personal health information (PHI) is not confined exclusively to the delivery of direct patient care. A hospital or healthcare organization may use such information internally to assess quality of care and operations (for example, for risk management, quality assessment, compilation of disease registries, and infection control). Hospitals also use health information internally to process billing information, support institutional research, and compile reports for government agencies and accrediting organizations.

Moreover, the use of personally identifiable information is not limited to organizations that provide direct patient care. Insurance companies, medical claims processing bureaus, third-party payers, employers, and pharmaceutical companies all may have access to patient health information. Further, because health information provides critical evidence in the legal process, the HIT must be familiar with the use of the health record and health information in judicial or quasi-judicial proceedings.

This chapter discusses the legal aspects surrounding the maintenance, use, and disclosure of personally identifiable health information. It identifies the HIT's role in these functions and emphasizes the importance of the HIT's ability to develop and/or follow policies and procedures that ensure the appropriate handling of health information in order to prevent abuse and improper disclosure.

Theory into Practice

The federal regulations resulting from passage of the Health Insurance Portability and Accountability Act of 1996 (HIPAA) require healthcare organizations to designate an individual to be responsible for the development and implementation of all health information privacy policies and procedures. Generally, this individual would have the title of **privacy officer.** The standards proposed in the HIPAA Privacy Rule are very complex. How does the health information management (HIM) professional begin to translate them into actual practice?

Jill Callahan Dennis, JD, RHIA, offered a peek into the game plan (Dennis 2001). First, the privacy officer must have the skills and knowledge appropriate to the job. These skills would include expertise in the HIPAA rules, familiarity with other applicable state and federal statutes and regulations, and a thorough understanding of how health information is used within the organization and disclosed outside the organization. Second, he or she must have excellent oral and written communication skills, experience with dealing with the public, and a good understanding of information technology.

Armed with these skills and expertise, the privacy officer's game plan consists of five principal elements:

- Compiling and evaluating existing policies and procedures against regulatory/ legal mandates

- Changing them where necessary and training staff on the changes

- Understanding how information flows within (and outside) the organization

- Determining what other tasks logically fit with those mandated duties

- Finding resources to assist in fulfilling the requirements

Turning theory into practice requires implementation of such a game plan. To accomplish this, the HIM professional must take an extremely organized and detailed approach. Using tools, checklists, and other resources, the HIM professional first must audit the current situation. He or she then must develop remedies, including policies and procedures, for any area that does not measure up to the specified standards of the regulations. However, developing policies and procedures is only one part of the battle. The real challenge lies in implementing and monitoring compliance with them.

Overview of Legal Issues in Health Information Management

For the HIM professional, dealing with the legal aspects of health records and health information presents three primary concerns:

- Compilation and maintenance of health records

- Ownership and control of health records, including use and disclosure

- Use of health records and health information in judicial proceedings

Compilation and Maintenance of Health Records

Requirements for compiling and maintaining health records are usually found in state rules and regulations. These rules and regulations, which are typically developed by the state administrative agency responsible for licensing hospitals and other health record organizations, usually say only that health records must be complete and accurate. However, others specify categories of information to be kept or, more specifically, outline the detailed contents of the health record. For example, Florida's statute states that:

> Each hospital . . . shall require the use of a system of problem-oriented medical records for its patients, which system shall include the following elements: basic client data collection; a listing of the patient's problems; the initial plan with diagnostic and therapeutic orders as appropriate for each problem identified; and progress notes, including a discharge summary (Showalter 2004, 391–92).

Moreover, in some circumstances, the federal government has stipulated specific requirements for maintaining health records. For example, the Medicare Conditions of Participation contain specific requirements and conditions that must be satisfied by healthcare provider organizations that treat Medicare or Medicaid patients.

In addition to state and federal requirements, various accrediting bodies have established standards for maintaining health records. Probably the most notable of these is the JCAHO. Specifically, the JCAHO has developed information management standards. Acute, long-term, home, and behavioral healthcare provider organizations must follow these standards if they are to be accredited by the JCAHO. The standards require that processes be "designed to facilitate the definition, capture and interpretation of data with the ultimate goal of transforming it into usable information for decision making, research, performance improvement and patient education" (Clark 2000, 46).

In addition to regulatory and accrediting body requirements, professional organizations such as the American Health Information Management Association (AHIMA) publish best practice information.

Besides defining the content of health records, states usually have laws that address how long records must be kept. Some state laws designate how long health records must be retained in their original form and specify whether they can be stored on other media, such as in digital or microfilm form.

HITs are responsible for knowing, understanding, and applying the pertinent state and federal laws as well as the voluntary standards that apply to their specific practice settings. Each practice setting (acute, long-term, and home healthcare) has different requirements. Thus, HITs must update their knowledge continuously through education and reading.

Further, HITs must be aware of the state and local laws that require information reporting to public authorities, such as state public health and vital statistics agencies. For example, state public health statutes may require hospitals to maintain records of births, deaths, and autopsies. In addition, they may require healthcare organizations to maintain records and report to the appropriate public health authority when patients are suffering from a specified communicable disease or have been involved in a violent crime or child abuse.

The importance of a complete, accurate, and timely health record cannot be overemphasized. Health record documentation not only helps to provide high-quality patient care but also can protect a healthcare facility or provider in civil malpractice litigation. Because health records are frequently admitted into evidence in medical malpractice suits, the absence of appropriate, complete, timely, and accurate entries can have severe adverse effects resulting in a verdict against the healthcare organization or provider.

Ownership and Control of Health Records, Including Use and Disclosure

HITs also must understand the rules, regulations, and statutes affecting the use and disclosure of health information. Use and disclosure are usually associated with the concepts of ownership and control. *Use* is how health information is used internally; *disclosure* is how health information is disseminated externally. Medical records, x-rays, laboratory reports, consultation reports, and other physical documents relating to the delivery of patient care are owned by the hospital or by the physician who orders them in connection with a private practice. However, ownership and physical control do not mean that the patient and other legitimately interested third parties do not have an ownership interest in the content and, therefore, a legal right of access to these documents (Showalter 2004).

State Laws Involving Use and Disclosure

More than half the states have statutes that address the patient's right to access, view, and/or copy his or her health records, although many qualify that right to some extent

(Johns 1997). Most recently, the HIPAA Privacy Rule established an individual's right to access his or her health information for as long as it is maintained, with limited situations where access may be denied. It also established standards by which others may access an individual's health information. The Privacy Rule is critical because it is a federal regulation that covers all types of healthcare providers and because it is central to the health information profession. As such, HITs must understand it well. It is discussed in detail later in this chapter.

State laws also usually govern the confidentiality of private information. Most states have enacted laws known as the privileged communication statutes. These vary in detail but, in general, medical practitioners are prohibited from disclosing information arising from the parties' professional relationship that relates to the patient's care and treatment (Showalter 2004, 417). Patients can waive their privilege, and in that event the medical provider would not be prohibited from making such disclosures.

Disclosure of health information without patient authorization may be required under specific state statutes. Examples include reporting vital statistics (births and deaths) and other public health, safety, or welfare situations. For example, healthcare providers may be required to provide information to the appropriate state agency about patients who suffer from venereal and other communicable diseases, have been injured by knives or firearms, or have wounds that would suggest some type of violent criminal activity. The treatment of infants who may be victims of child abuse or neglect also must be reported. Again, requirements vary state by state, so the HIT must bear responsibility for knowing and understanding the reporting requirements for the state in which he or she practices.

Because health information has a variety of purposes ranging from providing direct patient care to use by outside entities such as insurance and pharmaceutical companies, it is important that the use of such personally identifiable information be appropriate. Among the HIT's major responsibilities is that of ensuring conformance to legal requirements for appropriate use and disclosure, and adherence to the profession's ethical principles of practice.

Use of Health Records and Health Information in Judicial Proceedings

The health records of an individual who is a party to a legal proceeding are usually admissible in **litigation** or judicial proceedings provided they are material or relevant to the issue (Showalter 2004, 418–19). Either a **court order** or **subpoena duces tecum** is used to obtain medical information for a court that has **jurisdiction** over the pending litigation. When receiving a request for medical information in conjunction with litigation, HITs must be aware that a court order and a subpoena are not the same and must be handled differently. A court order, which is issued by a judge, must be complied with or the HIT faces contempt-of-court sanctions, possibly including jail time. Conversely, a subpoena is generated on behalf of a party to litigation. In most instances, a subpoena for the disclosure of an individual's health information must be accompanied by an **authorization** from that individual. Although court orders and subpoenas are official documents issued by the court, the HIT must carefully review any document when it is received to determine which type it is.

The method of response to court orders and subpoenas depends on state regulations. In some instances, states allow copies of health records to be certified and mailed to the clerk of the court or other designated individuals. In other instances, however, original records must be produced in person and the custodian of records is required to **authenticate** those records through testimony.

Check Your Understanding 15.1

Instructions: Select the phrase that best completes the following statements.

1. _____ HIT professionals must understand _____.
   a. Privacy issues with regard to the management of health information
   b. Laws affecting the use and disclosure of health information
   c. AHIMA's professional ethical principles of practice regarding the use and disclosure of health information
   d. All of the above

2. _____ A court order _____.
   a. Has the same force and effect as a subpoena
   b. Has greater legal weight than a subpoena
   c. Has less legal weight than a subpoena
   d. Must always be accompanied by patient authorization

3. _____ The HIPAA privacy rule _____.
   a. Applies only to certain states
   b. Applies only to healthcare providers operated by the federal government
   c. Applies nationally to healthcare providers
   d. Does not establish a standard to limit the amount of information that is disclosed

4. _____ When a health record is subpoenaed, _____.
   a. The original must always be produced
   b. A copy of the original may be allowed to be substituted
   c. A health information professional must always testify as to its authenticity
   d. Federal regulations determine the method of response

5. _____ The principal purpose of collecting and storing health information is to _____.
   a. Provide direct patient care and serve the patient's interests
   b. Support statistical analysis and research
   c. Serve as evidence in litigation
   d. Provide a record for reimbursement purposes

Introduction to the U.S. Legal System

With direct responsibility for the maintenance and use of business records (namely, health records and health information), HITs are likely to be involved in various situations involving state and federal regulations and statutes. Therefore, they need to have a basic understanding of the U.S. legal system.

The Source and Making of Laws

In the United States, law can be classified as either public or private. **Public law** involves the government and its relations with individuals and business organizations. Its purpose is to define, regulate, and enforce rights where any part of a government agency is a party (Showalter 2004, 2). Probably the most familiar type of public law is criminal law, where the government is a party against an accused who has been charged with violating a criminal statute. In healthcare, the Medicare law involves the government and its relationship with individuals in providing health insurance for the elderly with kidney failure and certain other groups with disabilities. Thus, Medicare is considered a public law.

Private law, on the other hand, is concerned with the rules and principles that define rights and duties among people and among private businesses. For example, private law applies when a contract for the purchase of a house is written between two parties. Normally, private law encompasses issues related to contracts, property, and **torts** (injuries). In the medical area, it often applies when there is a **breach** of contract or when a tort occurs through malpractice. There are four sources of public and private law: constitutions, statutes, **administrative law,** and judicial decisions.

Constitutions

Constitutional law is the body of law that deals with the amount and types of power and authority that governments are given.

The U.S. Constitution defines and lays out the powers of the three branches of the federal government. The legislative branch (the House of Representatives and the Senate) creates **statutory laws** (statutes). Examples include Medicare and HIPAA. The executive branch (the president and staff, namely cabinet-level agencies) enforces the law. For example, the Centers for Medicare and Medicaid Services (formerly the Health Care Financing Administration) is contained within the Department of Health and Human Services (HHS), a cabinet-level agency that reports to the president. It enforces the Medicare laws. The judicial branch (composed of courts) interprets laws passed by the Congress and signed by the president (at the federal level) and those passed by state legislatures and signed by governors (at the state level).

In addition to defining the three branches of government, the Constitution includes twenty-six amendments. These include the Bill of Rights (the first ten amendments) and sixteen additional amendments.

Each state also has a constitution. The state constitution is the supreme law of each state but is subordinate to the U.S. Constitution, the supreme law of the nation.

Statutes

Statutes (statutory laws) are enacted by a legislative body. The Congress and state legislatures are legislative bodies. Thus, Medicare and HIPAA are statutes because they were enacted by the Congress. Local bodies, such as municipalities, also can enact statutes, sometimes referred to as ordinances.

Administrative Law

Administrative law falls under the umbrella of public law. As already noted, the executive branch of government is responsible for enforcing laws enacted by the legislative branch. Frequently, the legislative body, which is Congress at the federal level and state legislatures at the state level, gives various administrative bodies the right to develop **rules and regulations** that carry out the intent of statutes. For example, Congress directed the secretary of

HHS to promulgate rules and regulations to carry out the intent of HIPAA. These rules and regulations constitute administrative law. As a second example, the Federal Food and Drug Administration (FDA), another agency contained within HHS, has the power to develop rules that control the manufacture of drugs. Thus, the legislative branch of the federal government has given a number of administrative agencies the power to establish regulations.

Judicial Decisions

The fourth major source of law is **judicial law,** which is the body of law created as a result of court (judicial) decisions. A primary decision-making responsibility of the courts is to interpret statutes and the Constitution. Judicial decisions are the primary source of private law (Showalter 2004, 5).

The Handling of Legal Disputes

The traditional method of resolving legal disputes is through court systems. In the United States, one court system exists at the federal level. As described below, certain requirements must be met for a case to be filed in the federal court system. The fifty states, the U.S. territories, and the District of Columbia have their own court systems as well. It is important to be aware that although the court system is the method we are most familiar with for the resolution of legal disputes, there is growing reliance on alternative dispute resolution methods to lessen the burden on typically overwhelmed court systems and to provide less costly alternatives by which opposing parties can settle their differences. These alternative dispute resolution methods are described below.

Court System

The U.S. court system consists of state and federal courts. The federal court system has a three-tier structure:

- **District courts** constitute the lowest tier in the federal court system. They have jurisdiction to hear cases involving felonies and misdemeanors that fall under federal statutes **(subject matter jurisdiction)** or suits where a citizen of one state sues a citizen of another state and the amount in dispute exceeds $75,000 **(diversity jurisdiction).** District courts are established geographically throughout the United States.

- **Courts of appeal** have the power to hear **appeals** on final judgments of the district courts.

- The **Supreme Court** is the highest court in the system. It hears appeals from the U.S. courts of appeal and from the highest state courts in cases generally involving federal statutes, treaties, or the U.S. Constitution.

As one might imagine, thousands of cases are submitted to the Supreme Court annually by parties who have lost at the lower court level with requests for review. Such requests are called *petitions for writ of certiorari.* The Supreme Court may deny the petition and refuse to review the case (informally referred to as *cert denied*) or grant the petition and agree to review the case (informally referred to as *cert granted*). The Supreme Court has broad discretion in deciding which cases to review and which to deny.

State court systems usually use the same three-tier system as the U.S. court system:

- **Trial courts** are at the lowest tier of state courts. In many states, trial courts are divided into two courts. Courts of limited jurisdiction hear cases that pertain to a particular subject matter (for example, landlord/tenant or juvenile) or that involve crimes of lesser severity or civil matters of lower dollar amounts. Courts of general jurisdiction hear more serious criminal cases or civil cases that involve large amounts of money.

- Many states have appellate courts similar to the federal courts of appeal. **Appellate courts** hear appeals on final judgments of the state trial courts.

- The state **supreme court** is the highest tier. It hears appeals from the appellate courts or from trial courts when the state does not have appellate courts.

In both the federal and state court systems, it is important to realize that cases presented to appellate courts in both the federal and state court systems are not reenactments of the trial. Legal documents are prepared by each party's attorney(s), who then argue the merits of the case before a panel of appellate judges. Witnesses are called and, generally, the facts of the case are not revisited. Appeals are designed to address solely legal errors or problems that are alleged to have occurred at the lower court.

Dispute Resolution

In addition to the court system, where disputes are resolved either as the result of trial or through settlement, disputes can be resolved through the legal system in three other ways: through an administrative agency, **arbitration,** or **mediation.** *Administrative agencies,* or tribunals, are created by statute or the Constitution. They may hear disputes arising from administrative law. A common example would be a case dealing with workmen's compensation. Such cases are settled by a state workmen's compensation commission. The HIT is often involved in such cases to the extent that the workmen's compensation board or commission subpoenas health records.

In *arbitration,* a dispute is submitted to a third party or a panel of experts outside the judicial trial system. The process only works when the parties to the dispute agree to have their differences heard and settled by an arbitrator or arbitration panel and agree that the settlement will be binding.

In *mediation,* a dispute is also submitted to a third party. However, the outcome of mediation occurs by agreement of the parties, not by a decision of the mediator. The role of the mediator is to facilitate agreement between the disputing parties.

Arbitration and mediation offer several advantages over the court system, including time and cost savings. These proceedings usually allow for more privacy than court proceedings do. Smaller tort claims are often handled through the arbitration process. Criminal misdemeanors, as an example, may be handled through mediation.

Legal Proceedings

HIT functions often involve copying health records for judicial proceedings that may be either civil or criminal in nature. These proceedings may involve accidents, workmen's compensation, physical abuse or other criminal activity, or malpractice. Consequently,

HITs should be familiar with various legal procedures, particularly those of deposition and other methods of **discovery.**

The Lawsuit

The individual who brings a lawsuit is the **plaintiff.** The individual or company that is the object of the lawsuit is the **defendant.** The plaintiff begins the lawsuit by filing a **complaint** in court. After the complaint is filed, a copy is served on the defendant along with a **summons.** Through this process, the defendant is given notice of the lawsuit and what it pertains to, and is informed that the complaint must be answered or some other action taken. If the defendant fails to answer the complaint or take other action, the court grants the plaintiff a judgment by default.

Usually, though, the defendant answers the complaint in one of four ways: by denying, admitting, or pleading ignorance to the allegations or by bringing a countersuit (**counterclaim**) against the plaintiff by filing a complaint. A defendant may file a complaint against a third party (**joinder**) or against a codefendant (**cross-claim**). Moreover, the defendant can ask the court to dismiss the plaintiff's complaint, but not without substantial reason.

The Discovery Period

The next stage of the litigation process is discovery. In the discovery stage, both parties use various strategies to "discover" information about a case prior to trial. The primary focus is to determine the strength of the opposing party's case. It is during this period that health records are usually subpoenaed. There are several different types of discovery methods, but the most common to the HIT's functions are the **deposition** and the subpoena duces tecum.

In a *deposition,* a subpoena is issued for an individual to appear at an appointed time and place and testify under oath before a reporter who transcribes the testimony. Usually, the attorneys for both plaintiff and defendant are present. Sometimes HITs are subpoenaed to testify as to the authenticity of the health records by confirming that they were compiled in the normal course of business and have not been altered in any way. A subpoena that is issued to elicit testimony is a **subpoena ad testificandum.**

Most frequently, however, in their position as custodian of records, HITs are served a subpoena duces tecum. Essentially, *duces tecum* means to bring documents and other records with oneself. Such subpoenas may direct the HIT to bring originals or copies of health records, laboratory reports, x-rays, or other records to a deposition or to court. Each state has different rules governing the production of health records in litigation. Often, the component state HIM association of AHIMA has a legal handbook that outlines the various conditions and how HITs should respond to a subpoena for deposition or a subpoena duces tecum.

The Trial

The next stage is the trial. A jury is selected through a process called **voir dire** or, if a jury is waived, a judge hears the case (**bench trial).** Evidence is then presented. The plaintiff's attorney is the first to call witnesses and present evidence. In turn, the defendant's attorney calls witnesses and presents evidence. Typically, the HIT is called as a witness by one party or the other to testify as to the authenticity of the medical record that is being sought as evidence. Testifying as to a record's authenticity means that the HIT is verifying that the record contains information about the individual in question and was compiled in the usual course of business and thus is reliable and truthful as evidence. Because individuals who document in a medical record do not typically falsify their entries, the truthfulness of a medical record is generally not questioned. As a result, the parties to litigation may agree (stipulate) as to a record's authenticity and allow it to be entered into evidence without requiring the HIT to appear in court and provide testimony. The parties may further agree to allow a photocopy of the record to be introduced into evidence, rather than the original. This generally requires the HIT to certify in writing that the photocopy being provided is an exact copy of the original medical record.

Many times, a case is settled before it reaches trial. This saves time, money, and emotional hardship on the parties. A settlement may be reached between or among parties to a lawsuit with or without intervention from a third party.

The Appeal and Collection of the Judgment

After the court has rendered a verdict, the next stage in the litigation process is the appeal. A case may or may not be appealed to the next court in the tiered system for a review of alleged legal errors at the lower court. The final stage of litigation is the collection of the judgment.

Professional Liability and the Physician–Patient Relationship

Medical malpractice refers to the professional liability of healthcare providers—physicians, nurses, therapists, or others involved in the delivery of patient care. Breach of contract, **intentional tort,** and **negligence** are all concepts that are related to professional liability. To understand how these concepts apply, it is first necessary to understand the elements of the physician–patient relationship.

A physician–patient relationship is established by either an implied contract or an express contract. A contract is usually created by the mutual **consent** of the parties involved, in this case, the patient and the physician or healthcare provider.

An example of an *implied contract* would be a case where an individual with symptoms of a cold comes to the doctor's office for treatment. If the doctor examines the patient and provides treatment, an implied contract exists between the two parties. An example of an express contract would be a case where an individual comes to the doctor's office with specific symptoms and agrees beforehand what the payment will be and what the physician will do in terms of the payment.

When either type of contract is established, an expectation of the scope of duty arises from the relationship. "In the typical physician-patient relationship, the physician has agreed to diagnose and treat the patient in accordance with the standards of acceptable medical practice and to continue to do so until the natural termination of the relationship" (Showalter 2004, 21). Termination of the contract usually occurs when the patient either gets well or dies, the patient and the physician mutually agree to terminate, or the patient dismisses the physician or the physician withdraws from providing care for the patient.

No medical liability for breach of contract can exist without a physician–patient relationship. However, when such a relationship does exist, the physician's failure to diagnose and treat the patient with reasonable skill and care may give the patient cause to sue the physician for breach of contract.

Healthcare providers also can be held responsible for professional liability when they harm another person. This is called a tort. A tort is a wrongful act that results in injury to another. An intentional tort is a circumstance where a healthcare provider purposely commits a wrongful act that results in injury. Usually, however, professional liability actions are brought against a healthcare provider because of the tort of negligence.

Negligence occurs when a healthcare provider does not do what a prudent person would normally expect the provider to do in similar circumstances. Negligence is of three types: failure to act (**nonfeasance**), a wrong or improper act (**malfeasance**), or improper performance during an otherwise correct act (**misfeasance**). An example of nonfeasance would be failure to order a standard diagnostic test. An example of malfeasance would be removal of the wrong body part. An example of misfeasance would be nicking the bladder during a surgery in which the gallbladder was appropriately removed.

For a negligence lawsuit to be successful, the plaintiff must prove four elements:

1. The existence of a **duty** to meet a standard of care

2. Breach or deviation from that duty

3. **Causation,** which is a relationship between the defendant's conduct and the harm that was suffered

4. **Injury/harm,** which may be economic (hospital expenses and loss of wages) and noneconomic (pain and suffering)

The causes of actions mentioned above are not the only ones that can be brought against a healthcare provider. Others include assault and battery, defamation, invasion of privacy, wrongful disclosure of confidential information, abandonment, and so on. Invasion of privacy and wrongful disclosure of confidential information are specific issues of concern for HITs and are discussed in greater detail later in this chapter.

Check Your Understanding 15.2

Instructions: Select the phrase that best completes each of the following sentences.

1. _____ Law can be classified as _____.
   a. Public or private
   b. Public or criminal
   c. Criminal or medical malpractice
   d. Trial or appeal

2. _____ The purpose of private law is to _____.
   a. Define, regulate, and enforce rights where any government agency is a party
   b. Define rights and duties among private parties
   c. Create statutes
   d. Convict individuals charged with crimes

3. _____ The sources of law are _____.
   a. Constitutions
   b. Statutes and administrative law
   c. Judicial decisions
   d. All of the above

4. _____ Statutes are laws _____.
   a. Created by administrative bodies
   b. Between private parties
   c. Created by trial and appellate courts
   d. Enacted by a legislative body

5. _____ Administrative law falls under the umbrella of _____.
   a. Criminal law
   b. Private law
   c. Public law
   d. Statutory law

6. _____ Arbitration is the submission of a dispute to a _____.
   a. Mediator
   b. Third party or a panel of experts outside the judicial trial system
   c. Judge, without a jury
   d. Judge, with a jury

7. _____ Medical malpractice _____.
   a. Refers to the professional liability of healthcare providers
   b. Includes breach of contract
   c. Includes intentional torts and negligence
   d. All of the above

8. _____ In a deposition, _____.
   a. A subpoena is issued
   b. An individual appears at an appointed time and place to testify under oath
   c. A reporter transcribes the testimony
   d. All of the above

9. _____ A lawsuit is filed by a plaintiff through a _____.
   a. Counterclaim
   b. Voir dire
   c. Cross-claim
   d. Complaint

10. _____ A tort is _____.
    a. A wrongful act that results in injury to another
    b. A purposeful wrongful act against another
    c. Mutual consent between two parties
    d. The professional liability of healthcare providers

Form and Content of the Health Record

The form and content of the health record are determined in a number of ways. Accrediting bodies such as the JCAHO, statutory laws such as state and federal statutes, and regulatory laws such as Medicare regulations, HIPAA regulations, and public health reporting requirements all play a significant role in determining the content and form of the health record. Failure to comply with the requirements of any these groups will likely result in some type of penalty such as loss of licensure or accreditation, fines, or even criminal penalties resulting in a jail sentence. Thus, the compilation and maintenance of health information must be performed appropriately and in conformance with all legal and ethical standards.

As mentioned earlier, states have specific statutes and regulations regarding the form and content of the health record. Furthermore, federal regulations such as the Conditions of Participation for Medicare and Medicaid specify the form and content of health records in various practice settings.

In addition to federal, state, and accreditation requirements, healthcare facilities establish their own requirements for the form, content, and handling of health records via policies and procedures. Thus, HITs also must be familiar with facility-specific requirements.

AHIMA has published guidelines on health record documentation and content requirements for a variety of settings. The following discussion recaps the documentation requirements for the acute care inpatient record (Smith 2001).

The primary purpose of the acute care health record is to document the care provided to the patient during his or her hospital stay. It also is used as a tool for providing:

- A means of communicating among the physician and the other members of the clinical team caring for the patient

- A basis for evaluating the adequacy and appropriateness of care

- Supporting data to substantiate insurance claims

- Protection of the legal interests of the patient, the facility, and the physician

- Clinical data for research and education

Every hospital should have policies that ensure the uniformity of both the content and the format of the health record based on all applicable accreditation standards, federal and state regulations, payer requirements, and professional practice standards. Following are general guidelines for determining acute care health record form and content:

- The health record should be organized systematically to facilitate the retrieval and compilation of data.

- Only persons authorized by the hospital's policies to document in the health record should do so. Such authority should be recorded in the medical staff rules and regulations and/or the hospital's administrative policies.

- Hospital policy and/or medical staff rules and regulations should specify who may receive and transcribe a physician's verbal orders.

- Health record entries should be documented at the time the treatment they describe is rendered.

- The authors of all entries should be clearly identifiable.

- Abbreviations and symbols should be used in the health record only when approved according to hospital and medical staff bylaws, rules, and regulations. JCAHO's list of prohibited abbreviations must be taken into consideration when the facility's approved list is updated.

- All entries in the health record should be permanent.

- To correct errors or make changes in the paper health record, a single line should be drawn in ink through the incorrect entry. The word error should be printed at the top of the entry along with a legal signature or initials; the date, time, title, and reason for the change; and the discipline of the person making the change. The existing entry should be left intact and corrections should be entered in chronological order. Late entries should be labeled as such. Error correction in electronic health records (EHRs) is particularly important because courts have historically viewed their integrity as suspect. Thus, procedures must be developed to control, check, and track changes made to data housed in the electronic record.

- In the event the patient wishes to change information in his or her record, the change should not be made to the original entry but, rather, should be made as an addendum. The information should be clearly identified as an additional document appended to the original health record at the direction of the patient, who will thereafter bear responsibility for explaining the change.

- The HIM department should develop, implement, and evaluate policies and procedures related to the quantitative and qualitative analysis of health records.

- Any requirements outlined in state law, regulation, or healthcare facility licensure standard should be reviewed as they relate to documentation requirements. Where the state requires verbal orders to be authenticated within a specified time frame, accrediting and licensing agencies will survey for compliance with that requirement.

Retention of the Health Record

Retention policies for the health record and health information depend on a number of factors. First, organizational retention policies must be in accordance with local, state, and federal statutes and regulations. Retention regulations vary from state to state and possibly by type of institution. Statutes of limitations for malpractice and other claims must be taken into consideration when determining the length of time to retain records as evidence. It is imperative that HITs know the laws of the state in which they practice. Further, they must be familiar with the retention standards developed by groups such as the JCAHO and the AOA.

In addition to laws and regulations and accreditation standards, health record retention depends on its uses within the healthcare institution. For example, a facility that provides care exclusively to children may have different retention policies than a home health agency does. An acute care facility may have very different retention policies than a long-term care facility that provides geriatric nursing care. Thus, the governing boards and medical staff organizations of every healthcare facility must analyze the facility's medical and administrative needs to ensure that health records are available for peer review, quality assessment, and other activities. Thus, in many instances, healthcare institutions retain health records longer than the law requires.

Retention Guidelines of AHIMA

AHIMA has developed guidelines for the retention of health records (AHIMA 2002). HITs can use the guidelines to determine how well their organizations measure up to industry-wide best practices. The guidelines include the following:

- Each healthcare provider should ensure that patient health information is available to meet the needs of continued patient care, legal requirements, research, education, and other legitimate uses.

- Each healthcare provider should develop a retention schedule for patient health information that meets the needs of its patients, physicians, researchers, and other legitimate users and complies with legal, regulatory, and accreditation requirements.

- The retention schedule should include guidelines that specify what information should be kept, the time period for which it should be kept, and the storage medium (paper, microfilm, optical disk, magnetic tape, or other).

- Compliance documentation:

  —Compliance programs should establish written policies to address the retention of all types of documentation, including clinical and medical records, health records, claims documentation, and compliance documentation. Compliance documentation includes all records necessary to protect the integrity of the compliance process and to confirm its effectiveness. Such records include employee training documentation, reports from hot lines, results of internal investigations, results of auditing and monitoring, modifications to the compliance program, and self-disclosures.

  —Documentation should be retained according to applicable federal and state laws and regulations and must be maintained for a sufficient length of time to ensure its availability to prove compliance with laws and regulations.

  —The organization's legal counsel should be consulted regarding the retention of compliance documentation.

Most states have specific retention requirements that should be used to establish a facility's retention policy. In the absence of specific state requirements, providers should keep health information for at least the period specified by the state's statutes of limitations or for a sufficient length of time to prove compliance with laws and regulations. If the patient is a minor, the health information should be retained until the patient reaches the age of majority (as defined by state law) plus the period of the statute of limitations, unless otherwise provided by state law. A longer retention period is prudent because the statute may not begin until a potential plaintiff learns of the causal relationship between an injury and the care received. In addition, under the **False Claims Act** (31 USC 3729), claims may be brought for up to ten years after the incident.

Unless state or federal law requires longer periods of time, specific patient health information should be retained for established minimum time periods.

Retention Guidelines of Accreditation Organizations

Table 15.1 shows AHIMA's retention standards for various types of health information. Table 15.2 shows the retention standards of various accrediting bodies.

Check Your Understanding 15.3

Instructions: Select the one best answer to each of the following questions.

1. _____ Which of the following determines the content of the health record?
    a. State law
    b. Federal regulations
    c. Accrediting body regulations
    d. All of the above

2. _____ What is the primary purpose of the health record?
    a. To document the care and treatment of the patient
    b. To provide data for research studies
    c. To protect the interests of the healthcare provider
    d. To provide public health data

3. _____ Which of the following is *not* true about correcting errors in the health record?
    a. Errors should be obliterated.
    b. The existing entry should be left intact with corrections entered in chronological order.
    c. Late entries should be labeled as such.
    d. The legal signature or initials of the individual making the correction should be included with the correction itself.

4. _____ A retention schedule for health information should include which of the following?
    a. Type of information to be retained
    b. Length of time the information should be retained
    c. Type of medium that should be used to retain the information
    d. All of the above

5. _____ Which of the following is *not* true with regard to health information retention?
    a. Retention depends on state, federal, and accreditation requirements.
    b. Retention is the same for all types of healthcare facilities.
    c. Retention depends on the needs of the healthcare facility.
    d. Retention periods are frequently longer for health information on minors.

Table 15.1.	AHIMA retention standards
Health Information	**Recommended Retention Period**
Diagnostic images (such as x-ray film)	5 years
Disease index	10 years
Fetal heart monitor records	10 years after the infant reaches the age of majority
Master patient/person index	Permanently
Operative index	10 years
Patient health/medical records (adults)	10 years after the most recent encounter
Patient health/medical records (minors)	Age of majority plus statute of limitations
Physician index	10 years
Register of births	Permanently
Register of deaths	Permanently
Register of surgical procedures	Permanently

Table 15.2.   Retention standards of accrediting bodies

Accreditation Agency	Retention Standard	Reference
Accreditation Association for Ambulatory Health Care (AAAHC)	Requires organizations to have policies that address retention of active clinical records, retirement of inactive clinical records, and retention of diagnostic images	*2001 Accreditation Handbook for Ambulatory Care*
American Accreditation Healthcare Commission/URAC	Member Protection Standard #7 states "the network shall have storage and security of confidential health information; access to hard copy and computerized confidential health information; records retention; and release of confidential health information."	*Health Network Accreditation Manual*
CARF . . . the Rehabilitation Accreditation Commission	Requires organizations to have policies that address record retention	*2002 Adult Day Services Standards Manual*
	Retention periods not specified for behavioral health, but policy must comply with applicable state, federal, or provincial laws	*2002 Behavioral Health Standards Manual*
	Retention periods not specified for employment and community services	
	Requires organizations to have policies that address retention of records and electronic records	*2002 Assisted Living Standards Manual*
	Requires organizations to have policies that address retention of records and electronic records	*2002 Medical Rehabilitation Standards Manual*
Community Health Accreditation Program (CHAP)	C25C—Elements 1 & 2: Records of adult patients must be retained for at least five years from the date of service and patient records for minors must be retained for seven years beyond the age of majority. C27C—Element 5: The records of occupationally exposed patients must be kept for 30 years.	*CHAP Core Standards of Excellence*
Joint Commission on Accreditation of Healthcare Organizations	IM.7.1.2—The retention time of medical record information is determined by the organization based on law and regulation and on its use for patient care, legal, research, and educational activities.	*2001–2002 Comprehensive Accreditation Manual for Ambulatory Care*
	IM.7.1.2—The retention time of clinical/ case record information is determined by the organization based on law and regulation and on its use for care, legal, research, and educational activities.	*2001–2002 Comprehensive Accreditation Manual for Behavioral Care*

Table 15.2. *(Continued)*

Accreditation Agency	Retention Standard	Reference
Joint Commission on Accreditation of Healthcare Organizations *(continued)*	IM.2.6—Data and information are retained for sufficient periods to comply with law and regulations and support member care, network management, legal documentation, research, and education.	*2001–2002 Comprehensive Accreditation Manual for Health Care Networks*
	IM.7—The organization initiates and maintains a record for every patient. Does the organization retain patient record information for the time period specified in policy and procedure and according to applicable law and regulations?	*2001–2002 Comprehensive Accreditation Manual For Home Care*
	IM.7.1.2—The hospital determines how long medical record information is retained, based on law and regulation and on its use for patient care, legal, research, and educational purposes.	*2001–2002 Comprehensive Accreditation Manual For Hospitals*
	IM.7.1.1—The retention time of medical record information is determined by law and regulation and by its use for resident care, legal, research, or educational purposes.	*2002–2003 Comprehensive Accreditation Manual for Long-Term Care*
	Intent of IM.7.1.1 Medical records are retained for the period of time required by state law, or five years from the discharge date when there is no requirement in state law. For a minor, the medical record is retained for the time period defined by state law or at least three years after a resident reaches legal age as defined by state law.	
National Commission on Correctional Health Care (NCCHC)	Inactive health records are retained according to legal requirements for the jurisdiction and are reactivated if a juvenile or inmate returns to the system or facility.	*Standards For Health Services in Juvenile Detention and Confinement Facilities (1999)* *Standards for Health Services in Jails (1996)* *Standards for Health Services in Prisons (1997)*
National Committee for Quality Assurance (NCQA)	Retention periods are not specified.	

The HIPAA Privacy Rule

The HIPAA Privacy Rule has become a key law governing the confidentiality of patient information. The following sections provide an overview of HIPAA legislation (namely, the Privacy Rule) that governs protected health information (PHI).

HIPAA Overview

HIM students and professionals often associate HIPAA with privacy, but the Privacy Rule is only part of the legislation passed by Congress in 1996. Much attention has rightfully been given to both the privacy and security aspects of HIPAA, but it is important for the HIT to understand the entire breadth of this legislation.

As shown in table 15.3, HIPAA contains five titles. As the figure demonstrates, HIPAA covers much more than patient information. As a result, several of these titles do not relate to the privacy of patient information. Title II is the most relevant title to the HIT. It contains provisions relating to the prevention of healthcare fraud and abuse and medical liability (medical malpractice) reform, as well as **administrative simplification.** The HIPAA Privacy Rule resides in the Administrative Simplification provision of Title II along with the HIPAA security standards and the transaction and code set standardization requirements. Because the complexity of HIPAA is well known, the term *administrative simplification* seems to be a misnomer. However, this term refers to HIPAA's attempt to streamline and standardize the healthcare industry's nonuniform and seemingly chaotic business practices, such as billing. A significant part of this simplification process is the electronic transmission of data.

Historical Context of the HIPAA Privacy Rule

The HIPAA Privacy Rule transformed the landscape of patient privacy. Before it was enacted, no federal statutes or regulations generally applied to protect the confidentiality of medical or personal information. Only specific legislation or regulations applied in particular circumstances, such as to providers of Medicare services or to those receiving federal funds, under federal legislation, to provide substance abuse treatment.

Table 15.3.   HIPAA components

Title I	Title II	Title III	Title IV	Title V
Health Care Access, Portability and Renewability	Preventing Health Care Fraud & Abuse	Tax-Related Health Provision	Group Health Plan Requirements	Revenue Offsets
	Medical Liability Reform			
	Administrative Simplification: 1. Privacy 2. Security, Identifiers, Code Sets			

Patient privacy protection laws governing access, use, and disclosure had largely resided with the individual states and they varied considerably, creating a patchwork of laws across the United States. Although many states had passed laws to protect highly sensitive health records such as mental health and HIV/AIDS, no laws existed in many states that protected health information generally. With passage of the Privacy Rule, such protection was achieved uniformly across all the states through establishment of a consistent set of standards that affected providers, healthcare clearinghouses, and health plans.

The legal doctrine of **preemption** applies to the Privacy Rule. Preemption means that federal law may supersede or preclude state law. However, the Privacy Rule provides a federal floor, or minimum, on privacy requirements. This means that the federal Privacy Rule does not preempt, or supersede, stricter state statutes (or other federal statutes, for that matter) when they exist. "Stricter" refers to state or federal statutes that provide individuals with greater privacy protections or give individuals greater rights with respect to their PHI. Thus, HITs must still review their state legal requirements and other federal requirements to determine which law prevails.

Basic Terms and Concepts

To understand the Privacy Rule, the HIT must understand its two key goals: first, to provide an individual with greater rights with respect to his or her health information; and second, to provide greater privacy protections for one's health information, which serves to limit access by others. While navigating the privacy rule's key terms, concepts, and many exceptions, keep in mind that the rule was written to accomplish these two goals.

Before discussing its specific requirements, it is necessary to understand some of the rule's basic terminology. One of the most fundamental terms used in the Privacy Rule is *protected health information.* The Privacy Rule defines PHI as **individually identifiable health information** that is transmitted by electronic media, maintained in any electronic medium, or maintained in any other form or medium (Section 164.501). To be individually identifiable, the information must either identify the person or provide a reasonable basis to believe the person could be identified from the information given. To meet the definition of PHI, the information also must relate to one's past, present, or future physical or mental health condition; the provision of healthcare; or payment for the provision of healthcare. The privacy extends to any information that a **covered entity** possesses in any form or medium, including paper and oral forms, that meets the PHI definition (Amatayakul 2001).

Another important term used in the privacy standards is *designated record set.* A **designated record set** includes the health records, billing records, and various claims records that are used to make decisions about an individual (Section 164.501).

The Privacy Rule affects three types of situations in which PHI is handled: **use, disclosures, and requests.** *Use* is internal to a covered entity or its **business associate.** *Disclosure* is the dissemination of PHI from a covered entity or its business associate. *Requests* for PHI refer to those made by a covered entity or its business associate. The reader of the Privacy Rule will notice an emphasis on use and disclosure.

The Privacy Rule introduced the standard of **minimum necessary** to limit the amount of PHI used, disclosed, and requested. Essentially, this means that healthcare providers and other covered entities must limit uses, disclosures, and requests to only the amount needed to accomplish the intended purpose. For example, for payment purposes, only the minimum amount of information necessary to substantiate a claim for payment should be disclosed.

The same standard of minimum necessary applies to use of information, even for individuals who work for the facility. For example, policies and procedures should be in place that identify those persons or classes of persons who work for the covered entity who need to access PHI to perform their duties. In addition, the categories of PHI that each person or class of persons can access and use should be identified. For example, employees working in the housekeeping department would not have the same level of access to PHI as a nurse working in critical care.

In the performance of their job responsibilities, HITs must understand what is meant by **treatment, payment, and operations,** commonly referred to as **TPO.** This term is important because the Privacy Rule provides a number of exceptions for PHI that is being used or disclosed for TPO purposes. First, *treatment* usually means providing, coordinating, or managing healthcare or healthcare-related services by one or more healthcare providers. For example, treatment would include the usual provision of care to patients admitted to the hospital or during an office appointment with a physician. Treatment in the Privacy Rule definition also covers healthcare provider consultations relating to a patient or the referral of a patient for healthcare from one provider to another.

Payment is defined in the Privacy Rule to mean a broad set of activities. For example, it can refer to activities by a health plan to obtain premiums or to activities by a healthcare provider or health plan to obtain reimbursement for care or services provided. Activities such as billing, claims management, claims collection, review of the medical necessity of care, and utilization review are all included under the term *payment.*

The Privacy Rule provides a broad list of activities that fall under the umbrella of healthcare operations. These activities include quality assessment and improvement, case management, review of healthcare professionals' qualifications, insurance contracting, legal and auditing functions, and general business management functions such as providing customer service and conducting due diligence. Because the list of activities that qualify as operations is so broad, one may question what does not fall under the TPO definition. Although health providers have argued otherwise, mandatory public reporting is not considered to be "operations" under the Privacy Rule. States universally require the reporting of certain events such as births (birth certificates); communicable diseases; and incidents of abuse or suspected abuse of children, mentally disabled individuals, and the elderly. As explained later in this chapter, one consequence of these activities not being classified as operations is that they must be included if an individual requests an accounting of disclosures. It is important that the HIT be able to distinguish activities that are operations versus those that are not.

Applicability of the Privacy Rule

Although it is broad, the scope of the HIPAA Privacy Rule is limited. This section discusses the individuals and organizations that are subject to the Privacy Rule, as well as the types of information that it protects.

Covered Entities

The privacy rule is applicable to all covered entities involved, either directly or indirectly, with transmitting or performing any electronic transactions specified in the act. Among these transactions are those relating to:

- Health claims and encounter information
- Health plan enrollment and disenrollment

- Eligibility for a health plan

- Healthcare payment and remittance advice

- Health plan premium payments

- Health claim status

- Referral certification

- Coordination of benefits

Covered entities include healthcare providers (hospitals, long-term care facilities, physicians, pharmacies, insurance carriers, and so on); health plans; and healthcare clearinghouses. Thus, HITs will likely be working for organizations that are covered by the privacy rule.

Business Associates

The privacy rule also applies to entities that have been identified by HIPAA-covered entities as business associates. A business associate is a person or organization, other than a member of a covered entity's workforce, that performs functions or activities on behalf of or to a covered entity that involve the use or disclosure of individually identifiable health information.

Can a covered entity such as a healthcare provider disclose PHI to business associates such as consultants, billing companies, accounting firms, or others that may perform services for the provider? The Privacy Rule allows PHI use and disclosure under these circumstances only when provider and business associate have signed a written contract, called a business associate agreement, in which the business associate agrees to abide by the provider's requirements to protect the information's security and confidentiality. In other words, the business associate must agree not to use or disclose the PHI in ways the provider would not permit.

At a minimum, the agreement between provider and business associate should (Cassidy 2000):

- Prohibit the business associate from using or disclosing the PHI for any purpose other than that stated in the contract

- Prohibit the business associate from using or disclosing the PHI in a manner that would violate the requirements of the HIPAA Privacy Rule

- Require the business associate to maintain safeguards, as necessary, to ensure that the PHI is not used or disclosed except as provided by the contract

- Require the business associate to report to the covered entity any use or disclosure of the PHI that is not provided for in the contract

- Require the business associate to ensure that any of its subcontractors that use PHI received from the covered entity agree to the same restrictions and conditions

- Establish how the covered entity would provide access to PHI to the individual whom the information is about when the business associate has made any material alterations to the information

- Require the business associate to make available its internal practices, books, and records relating to the use and disclosure of PHI received from the covered entity to the Department of Health and Human Services or its agents

- Establish how the entity would provide access to PHI to the individual whom the information is about in circumstances where the business associate holds the information and the covered entity does not

- Require the business associate to incorporate any amendments or corrections to the PHI when notified by the covered entity that the information is inaccurate or incomplete

- At termination of the contract, require the business associate to return or destroy all PHI received from the covered entity that it still maintains and prohibit the associate from retaining it

- State that individuals who are the subject of disclosed PHI are intended third-party beneficiaries of the contract

- Authorize the covered entity to terminate the contract when it determines that the business associate has repeatedly violated a term required in the contract

Workforce Members

A covered entity is responsible under the Privacy Rule for its workforce members. Inclusion in a covered entity's workforce is broad and consists not only of employees, but also volunteers, student interns, trainees, and even employees of outsourced vendors who routinely work on-site in the covered entity's facility.

Scenario: Ted is employed as a custodial worker by Tidy Team, a company that contracts with Mercy Hospital to provide janitorial services. Ted has been assigned to Mercy Hospital. As part of his duties, he routinely cleans the floors and empties the trash in the HIM department. What is Tidy Team's relationship with Mercy Hospital? What is Ted's relationship with Mercy Hospital? Does a business associate relationship exist here?

Some considerations: Tidy Team was contracted to clean the hospital, not to use or disclose individually identifiable health information. The fact that Ted is in close proximity to such information on a regular basis does not automatically place him (or Tidy Team) under the business associate definition. More appropriately, because he routinely works at Mercy Hospital, he would be treated as a workforce member and should be trained as such.

Because they handle confidential information daily, HITs must know the state and federal laws governing PHI use and disclosure. Certainly, the Privacy Rule has had a tremendous impact across the continuum of care. (The AHIMA Web site at ahima.org/ provides an analysis of the Privacy Rule by the AHIMA Policy and Government Relations Team.)

De-identified Information

In addition to applying to covered entities, their workforce members, and their business associates, the Privacy Rule limits applicability to PHI. A key part of the definition of PHI is that it either *identifies an individual or provides a reasonable basis to believe the person could be identified from the information given.* This definition does not include **de-identified information,** which therefore falls outside the scope of the Privacy Rule.

De-identified information is information that does not identify an individual. Essentially, it is information from which personal characteristics have been stripped. An important element associated with the de-identification of information is that it cannot be later constituted or combined to re-identify an individual. De-identified information is commonly used in research, in decision support, or for similar purposes.

Because of the power of current information technologies in assisting with the collection and analysis of data, it is possible to identify individuals by combining specific data. Therefore, the HIPAA Privacy Rule requires the covered entity to do one of following things to ensure the de-identification of information:

- The covered entity can strip off certain elements to ensure that the patient's information is truly de-identified. These elements are listed in figure 15.1 (HHS 2000, 82818).

- The covered entity can have an expert apply generally accepted statistical and scientific principles and methods to minimize the risk that the information might be used to identify an individual.

Figure 15.1.   Data elements to be removed for de-identification of information

- Names of individuals, relatives, employers, or household members

- Geographic identifiers including subdivisions smaller than a state, street addresses, city, county, and precinct

- The last six digits of the zip code, provided that the initial three digits of the zip code cover a geographic area of more than 20,000 people. If the geographic area covers 20,000 people or fewer, the zip code must be reported as 000.

- All elements of dates, except the year, or dates directly related to an individual, including birth, admission, discharge, and death dates. In addition, all ages over 89 and all elements of dates (including the year) that would identify such age cannot be used. However, individuals over 89 can be aggregated into a single category of 90 and over.

- Telephone numbers

- Fax numbers

- E-mail addresses

- Social Security numbers

- Medical record numbers

- Health plan beneficiary numbers

- Account numbers

- Certificate/license numbers

- Vehicle identifiers and serial numbers, including license plates

- Device identifiers and serial numbers

- Web universal resource locators (URLs)

- Internet protocol (IP) address numbers

- Biometric identifiers, including fingerprints and voiceprints

- Full-face photographic images and any comparable images

- Any other unique identifying number, characteristic, or code

---

What if the covered entity needs to re-identify information that has been stripped of individual identifiers? In other words, how might the entity match information back to the person it identifies? HIPAA allows an entity to assign a code to de-identified information to allow for re-identification. However, in doing so, the entity must ensure that the code assigned is not derived from or related to the information about the patient and cannot be translated to his or her identity. It also has to ensure that the code is not used for any other purpose and does not disclose in any way the mechanism for re-identification.

Individual Rights

The HIPAA Privacy Rule provides patients with significant rights that allow them to have some measure of control over their health information. Those rights include right of access, right to request amendment of PHI, right to accounting of disclosures, right to request restrictions of PHI, right to request confidential communications, and right to complain of Privacy Rule violations. These rights are described below. Further, table 15.4 details all individual rights except the right to complain of privacy rule violations.

Right of Access

Section 164.524 of the Privacy Rule states that an individual has a right of access to inspect and obtain a copy of his or her own PHI that is contained in a designated record set, such as a health record. The individual's right extends for as long as the PHI is maintained. However, there are exceptions to what PHI may be accessed. For example, psychotherapy notes; information compiled in reasonable anticipation of a civil, criminal, or administrative action or proceeding; or PHI subject to the Clinical Laboratory Improvements Act (CLIA) are all exceptions.

Grounds for Denial of Access
According to the Privacy Rule, there are times when a covered entity can deny an individual access to PHI without providing him or her an opportunity to review or appeal the denial. The HIT should be aware of such circumstances, particularly in the release of information area.

In what situations can denials to PHI occur that are not subject to an appeals process? One example of this type of situation was mentioned earlier: access to PHI contained in psychotherapy notes. Another situation would be covered entities that are correctional institutions or providers who have acted under the direction of a correctional institution. In these situations, an inmate's request to obtain a copy of his or her own PHI may be denied under certain circumstances without an appeal.

In some situations, PHI is created or obtained by a covered healthcare provider in the course of research that includes treatment. Sometimes an individual receiving treatment as part of a research study agrees to suspend his or her right to access PHI temporarily. This is usually for protection of the integrity of the research study. In such cases, the covered entity may deny access to PHI as long as the research is in progress.

There are two other circumstances where a covered entity may deny an individual access to his or her PHI without the benefit of an appeals process. One situation is when the PHI was obtained from someone other than a healthcare provider under a promise of confidentiality. If the covered entity decides that the access requested would be reasonably likely to reveal the source of the information, access might be denied without benefit of appeal. The other situation is when the PHI is contained in records that are subject to the federal Privacy Act (5 U.S.C. 552a) if the denial of access under the Privacy Act would meet the requirements of that law.

Table 15.4. Individual rights under the HIPAA Privacy Rule

		Patient Rights at a Glance				
Right	**Request**	**Acceptance**	**Termination**	**Timeliness**	**Fee**	**Denial**	**Review**
Right to request restriction of uses and disclosures	Provider must permit request, but does not have to be in writing	Provider not required to agree, but if accepted, must not violate restriction except for emergency care	Provider may terminate if individual agrees or requests in writing, oral agreement is documented, or written notice for information created after it has informed the individual.	There is no provision for addressing timeliness.	There is no provision for a fee.	There are no requirements associated with denying restriction.	Not applicable
Right to receive confidential communications	Provider may require written request for receiving communications by alternative means or locations.	Provider must accommodate reasonable requests and may condition how payment will be handled but may not require explanation.	There is no provision for termination.	There is no provision for addressing timeliness.	There is no provision for a fee.	Not applicable	Not applicable
Right of access to information	Provider must permit request for copying and inspection and may, upon notice, require requests in writing. Provider may supply a summary or explanation of information, instead, if individual agrees in advance.	Provider may deny access without opportunity for review if information is: psychotherapy notes, compiled for legal proceeding, subject to CLIA, about inmate and could cause harm, subject of research to which denial of access has been agreed, subject to Privacy Act, or obtained from someone else in confidence. Provider may deny access with opportunity to review if licensed professional determines access may endanger life or safety, there is reference to another person and access could cause harm, or request made by personal representative who may cause harm.	Individuals have right of access for as long as information is maintained in designated record set.	Provider must act upon a request within 30 days. If information is not maintained on site, provider may extend by no more than 30 days if individual is notified of reasons for delay and given date for access.	Provider may impose reasonable, cost-based fee for copying, postage, and preparing an explanation or summary.	If access is denied, provider must provide timely written explanation in plain language, containing basis for denial, review rights if applicable, description of how to file a complaint, and source of information not maintained by provider if known. Provider must also give individual access to any part of information not covered under grounds for denial.	An individual may request a review of a denial by a different healthcare professional.

(Continued on next page)

707

Table 15.4. *(Continued)*

Patient Rights at a Glance

Right	Request	Acceptance	Termination	Timeliness	Fee	Denial	Review
Right to amend information	Provider must permit requests to amend a designated record set and may, upon notice, require request in writing and a reason.	If amendment is accepted, provider must append or link to record set and obtain and document identification and agreement to have provider notify relevant persons with which amendment needs to be shared. Provider may deny amendment if information was not created by the provider unless individual provides reasonable basis that originator is no longer available to act on request, is not part of designated record set, would not be available for access, or is accurate and complete.	Amendment applies for as long as information is maintained in designated record set.	Provider must act upon a request within 60 days of receipt. If unable to act on request within 60 days, provider may extend time by no more than 30 days provided individual is notified of reasons for delay and given date to amend.	There is no provision for a fee.	If amendment is denied, provider must provide timely written explanation in plain language, containing basis for denial, right to submit written statement of disagreement, right to request provider include request and denial with any future disclosures of information that is subject of amendment, and description of how to file a complaint.	Provider must accept written statement of disagreement (of limited length). Provider may prepare written rebuttal and must copy individual. Provider must append or link request, denial, disagreement, and rebuttal to record and include such or accurate summary with any subsequent disclosure. If no written disagreement, provider must include request and denial, or summary, in subsequent disclosures only if individual has requested such action.

Table 15.4. *(Continued)*

Patient Rights at a Glance

Right	Request	Acceptance	Termination	Timeliness	Fee	Denial	Review
Right to accounting of disclosures	Provider must provide individual with written accounting including date of disclosure, name and address of recipient, description of information disclosed, purpose of disclosure or copy of individual's written authorization or other request for disclosure.	Provider must provide individual and retain documentation of written accounting of disclosures of PHI made in six years prior to date of request, except for disclosures (1) to carry out treatment, payment, and healthcare operations; (2) to the individuals themselves; (3) incident to a use or disclosure otherwise permitted or required; (4) pursuant to an authorization; (5) for the facility's director or to persons involved in the individual's care or other notification purposes; (6) for national security or intelligence purposes; (7) to correctional institutions or law enforcement as permitted; (8) as part of a limited data set; or (9) that occurred prior to the compliance date for the covered entity.	Not applicable	Provider must act upon request within 60 days of receipt. If unable to provide accounting, provider may extend time by no more than 30 days provided individual is notified of reasons for delay.	First accounting in any 12-month period must be provided without charge. A reasonable, cost-based fee may be charged for subsequent accountings in 12-month period if individual is notified in advance.	Provider must temporarily suspend right to receive an accounting of disclosures to health oversight agency or law enforcement official if agency or official provides written statement that accounting would impede their activities.	There is no provision for review of temporary suspension.

Source: Amatayakul 2001.

In two instances, the Privacy Rule requires a covered entity to give an individual the right to review a denial of access. These are situations where a licensed healthcare professional determines that access to PHI as requested by the individual or his or her personal representative (1) would likely endanger the life or physical safety of the individual or another person or (2) would reasonably endanger the life or physical safety of another person mentioned in the PHI.

According to the Privacy Rule, when a denial is made in the such circumstances, the covered entity has certain responsibilities. First, the denial must be written in plain language and include a reason for it. Second, it must explain that the individual has the right to request a review of the denial. Third, it must describe how the individual can complain to the covered entity and must include the name or title and phone number of the person or office to contact. Finally, it must explain how the individual can lodge a complaint with the secretary of HHS.

Moreover, when access to PHI is denied on the grounds mentioned above, the individual has the right to have the denial reviewed by a licensed healthcare professional. This must be someone who did not participate in the original denial and who is designated by the covered entity to act as the reviewing official. The covered entity then must grant or deny access in accordance with the reviewing official's decision.

Requesting Access to One's Own PHI

How does an individual go about requesting access to his or her own PHI? HITs will encounter such situations frequently.

The Privacy Rule specifies that the covered entity may require individuals to make their requests in writing, provided it has informed them of such a requirement. Timely response is an important part of the Privacy Rule. The rule specifies that a covered entity must act on an individual's request for review of PHI no later than thirty days after the request is made. The covered entity may extend the time period for response by no more than thirty days. It must have given the individual a written statement within the thirty-day time period explaining the reasons for the delay and the date by which the covered entity will complete its action on the request. The covered entity may extend the time for action on a request for access only once. If the PHI is not maintained or located on-site, the covered entity must respond to the request within sixty days of receiving it.

In responding to a patient or individual request for access to his or her PHI, the covered entity must arrange a convenient time and place of inspection with the individual or mail a copy of the PHI at the individual's request. One question that frequently arises is whether the covered entity can charge the individual for retrieving or copying the information. HIPAA allows the covered entity to impose a reasonable cost-based fee when the individual requests a copy of the PHI or agrees to accept summary or explanatory information. The fee may include the cost of:

- Copying, including supplies and labor
- Postage, when the individual has requested that the copy or summary or explanation be mailed
- Preparing an explanation or summary, if agreed to by the individual

It is important to note that charging retrieval fees to the patient is not allowed under HIPAA. However, charging them is possible in nonpatient requests.

Certain specifications must be met when requests for access to PHI are granted. Specifically, the covered entity must provide access to the PHI in the form or format requested when it is readily producible in such form or format. When it is not readily producible in the form or format requested, it must be produced in a readable hard-copy form or such other form or format agreed to by the covered entity and the individual.

Right to Request Amendment of PHI

Many states have laws or regulations that permit individuals to amend their health records. Section 164.526 of the Privacy Rule provides for the right of an individual to request that a covered entity amend PHI or a record about the individual in a designated record set (HHS 2000, 82824–82825). However, the covered entity may deny the request when it determines that the PHI or the record:

- Was not created by the covered entity

- Is not part of the designated record set

- Is not available for inspection as noted in the regulation of access (for example, psychotherapy notes, inmate of a correctional institution, and so on)

- Is accurate or complete as it stands

The covered entity may require the individual to make an amendment request in writing and provide a rationale for it. Such a process must be communicated in advance to the individual. The usual notice of such a process would be included in the covered entity's notice of information practice discussed earlier in this chapter.

The Privacy Rule provides requirements for timely response to an individual's request for amendment of PHI. Essentially, the covered entity must act on the individual's request no later than sixty days after its receipt by allowing the requested amendment or denying it in writing. The entity may extend the time for action by thirty days, provided that it explains the reasons for the delay in a written statement and gives a date by which it will complete its action on the request. Under no circumstances can there be any more extensions to action.

What kinds of specifications must the covered entity comply with when an amendment is granted? The Privacy Rule requires that the covered entity:

- Identify the records in the designated record set that are affected by the amendment and append the information through a link to the amendment's location. For example, if the diagnosis were incorrect, the amendment would have to appear and/or be linked to each record/report in the designated record set.

- Inform the individual that the amendment was accepted and have him or her identify the persons with whom the amendment needs to be shared and then obtain his or her agreement to notify those persons. The covered entity must make reasonable efforts to provide the amendment within a reasonable amount of time to anyone who has received the PHI.

What specifications must the covered entity meet when it denies the requested amendment? The Privacy Rule requires that several things happen under such circumstances.

First, the covered entity must deny the amendment within sixty days or less of the request. The denial must be written in plain language and contain the following information (HHS 2000, 82824–82825):

- The basis for the denial
- The individual's right to submit a written statement disagreeing with the denial
- The process by which the individual can submit his or her disagreement
- A statement explaining how, when the individual does not submit a disagreement, he or she may request that both the original amendment request and the covered entity's denial accompany any future disclosures of the PHI that is the subject of the amendment
- A description of how the individual may complain to the covered entity, including the name or title and telephone number of the contact person or office

The covered entity can prepare a written rebuttal to the individual's disagreement statement but must provide the individual with a copy of it.

All requests for amendments, denials, the individual's statement of disagreement, and the covered entity's rebuttal (if one was created) must be appended or linked to the record or PHI that is the subject of the amendment request. When any future disclosures of the subject information are made, this material or a summary of it must accompany them. However, if a request for amendment was denied and the individual did not write a statement of disagreement, the request for amendment and denial must only accompany future disclosures if the individual requests such action. In cases where the disclosure is made using a HIPAA standard electronic transaction, the covered entity may transmit the material that pertains to the standard transaction separately.

Right to Accounting of Disclosures

Maintaining some type of accounting procedure for monitoring and tracking PHI disclosures has been a common practice in HIM departments. However, the Privacy Rule has a specific standard with respect to such record keeping. Section 164.528 states that an individual has the right to receive an accounting of certain disclosures made by a covered entity within the six years prior to the date on which the accounting is requested (HHS 2000, 82826). Essentially, this means that the covered entity must maintain an ongoing accounting or record keeping of disclosures.

However, the type of disclosure for purposes of this record keeping is limited. Disclosures for which an accounting is *not* required and which are, therefore, exemptions are disclosures:

- Needed to carry out treatment, payment, and healthcare operations
- To individuals to whom the information pertains
- Incidental to an otherwise permitted or required use or disclosure
- Pursuant to an authorization
- For use in the facility's directory, to persons involved in the individual's care, or for other notification purposes

- To meet national security or intelligence requirements

- To correctional institutions or law enforcement officials

- As part of a limited data set

- That occurred before the compliance date for the covered entity

This extensive list does not seem to include many disclosures that do have to be included in an accounting. So, what is left? Despite arguments to the contrary, mandatory public health reporting is not considered part of a covered entity's operations. As a result, these disclosures must be included in an accounting of disclosures. For example, if a physician's office reports a case of tuberculosis to a public health authority, that disclosure must be included if the patient requests an accounting. If a covered entity provides PHI to a third-party public health authority to review, but the third party does not actually review it, the mere right of access must be included in an accounting of disclosures. Disclosure pursuant to a court order, without a patient's written authorization, also would be subject to an accounting. However, disclosure pursuant to a subpoena that is accompanied by a patient's written authorization would not be subject to an accounting because the authorization exempts the disclosure from the accounting requirement.

The accounting requirement includes disclosures made in writing, by telephone, or orally. Each disclosure described above that is not within the list of exemptions is still permitted by the Privacy Rule; however, a patient must be made aware of it if he or she so requests (hhs.gov/ocr/hipaa).

In some situations, an individual's right to an accounting of PHI disclosure may be suspended at the written request of a health oversight agency or law enforcement official. In these situations, the written request from the appropriate agency or law enforcement official must indicate that such an accounting would impede its activities. The oversight agency or the law enforcement official also must indicate how long such a suspension is required.

What type of information must be included in the accounting? HIPAA specifies that the date of disclosure, the name and address (when known) of the entity or person who received the information, and a brief statement of the purpose of the disclosure or a copy of the individual's written authorization or request must be included in the accounting process.

As with the request for amendment to PHI, certain time limits must be met for responding to a request for accounting of PHI disclosures. The covered entity must act on the request no later than sixty days after its receipt. When the entity is unable to provide the accounting within the time period required, it can extend the time period by no more than thirty days. Again, just as with the request for amendment, the thirty-day extension is permitted as long as the covered entity notifies the individual in writing of the reasons for the delay and the date by which the accounting will be made available.

Can the covered entity charge a fee for providing an accounting of disclosures? The first accounting within any twelve-month period must be provided without charge. For any other request within a twelve-month period, the covered entity may charge a reasonable, cost-based fee. However, the entity must inform the individual of the fee in advance and give him or her the opportunity to withdraw or modify the request for a subsequent accounting in order to avoid or reduce the fee.

The Privacy Rule requires documentation to be maintained on all accounting requests. This includes the information included in the accounting, the written accounting that was provided to the individual, and the titles of persons or offices responsible for receiving and processing requests for an accounting. Policies and procedures must be developed to ensure that PHI disclosed from all areas of an organization, which very likely may include departments outside HIM, be able to be tracked and compiled when an accounting request is received.

Since the April 14, 2003 Privacy Rule compliance date, this individual right has been the most controversial. Compliance with it requires a great deal of resources, and patients have infrequently requested such accountings. Interested parties have debated whether the disparity between the cost and the level of use might cause this individual right to be discontinued.

Right to Request Restrictions of PHI

Under the Privacy Rule, can an individual patient request that a covered entity restrict the uses and disclosures of PHI to carry out treatment, payment, or healthcare operations? Section 164.522(a) states that a covered entity must permit an individual to request such a restriction. However, the covered entity is not required to agree to such a provision and, in some cases, is restricted from doing so. The latter case would involve disclosures such as those required under law.

When, however, the covered entity does agree to such a restriction, it must live up to the agreement. The restriction can be terminated by either the individual or the covered entity. When the covered entity initiates termination of the agreement, it must inform the individual that it is doing so. However, the termination is only effective with respect to the PHI created or received after the individual has been informed (HHS 2000, 82822–82823).

Scenario: A patient, Mr. Smith, agrees to allow a hospital to tell callers that he has been admitted to the hospital and therefore is in the patient directory. Such notification is a hospital operation. However, he requests that this information be restricted/withheld only from his Aunt Mary and Uncle Jack, if they should call. What would you do if you were responsible for making the decision about a restriction such as this?

Some considerations: The hospital is not required to agree to this request for a restriction. In fact, the hospital probably should not agree with this request because of the administrative difficulty of informing certain individuals, but not others, as well as the risk of accidentally violating the request. Imagine how difficult it would be for every receptionist to recall this small restriction, particularly if other patients had similar restrictions on their information. The risk of violation simply becomes too great.

Right to Request Confidential Communications

Healthcare providers and health plans must give individuals the opportunity to request that communications of PHI be routed to an alternative location or by an alternative method under section 164.522(b) of the Privacy Rule. Healthcare providers must honor such a request without requiring a reason for it if it is reasonable. Health plans must honor such a request if it is reasonable and if the requesting individual states that disclosure could pose a safety risk. However, providers and health plans may refuse to accommodate requests if the individual does not provide either information as to how payment will be handled or an alternative address or method by which he or she can be contacted.

An example of a request for confidential communications would be a woman who requests that billing information from her psychiatrist, from whom she is seeking treatment because of a domestic violence situation, be sent to her work address instead of to her home.

Right to Complain of Privacy Rule Violations

As previously stated, the covered entity must provide a process whereby an individual can lodge a complaint about the entity's policies and procedures, its noncompliance with them, or its noncompliance with the Privacy Rule. This requirement is located in section 164.530(d). The covered entity's **notice of privacy practices,** described later in this chapter, must contain contact information at the covered entity level and inform individuals of the ability to submit complaints to HHS. All complaints must be documented along with the disposition of each complaint.

HIPAA Privacy Rule Documents

The Privacy Rule contains parameters for three key documents that serve to inform patients and give them a measure of control over their PHI. Two of these documents, the notice of privacy practices and the authorization, are required. The consent document is optional.

Notice of Privacy Practices

The Privacy Rule introduced the standard that individuals should be informed how covered entities use or disclose PHI. In general, section 164.520 requires that, except for certain variations or exceptions for health plans and correctional facilities, an individual has the right to a notice explaining how his or her PHI will be used and disclosed. This required document is the notice of privacy practices. Further, this notice is to explain the patient's rights and the covered entity's legal duties with respect to PHI. This information must be provided to an individual at his or her first contact with the covered entity (for example, first visit to a physician's office, first admission to a hospital, or first encounter at a clinic).

AHIMA outlines the requirements for the content of the notice of privacy practices (Hughes 2001b). The notice is to include the following elements:

- A header that reads: "This notice describes how information about you may be used and disclosed and how you can get access to this information. Please review it carefully."

- A description (including at least one example) of the types of uses and disclosures the covered entity is permitted to make for treatment, payment, and healthcare operations

- A description of each of the other purposes for which the covered entity is permitted or required to use or disclose PHI without the individual's written consent or authorization

- A statement that other uses and disclosures will be made only with the individual's written authorization and that the individual may revoke such authorization

- When applicable, separate statements indicating that the covered entity may contact the individual to provide appointment reminders or information about treatment alternatives or other health-related benefits and services that may be of interest to the individual; that the covered entity may raise funds; and that the group health plan or health insurance issuer or HMO may disclose protected health information to the sponsor of the plan

- A statement of the individual's rights with respect to PHI and a brief description of how the individual may exercise these rights, including:

  —The right to request restrictions on certain uses and disclosures as provided by 45 CFR 164.522(a), including a statement that the covered entity is not required to agree to a requested restriction

  —The right to receive confidential communications of PHI as provided by 164.522(b), as applicable

  —The right to inspect and copy PHI as provided by 164.524

  —The right to amend PHI as provided in 164.526

  —The right to receive an accounting of disclosures as provided in 164.528

  —The right to obtain a paper copy of the notice upon request as provided in 164.520

- A statement that the covered entity is required by law to maintain the privacy of PHI and to provide individuals with a notice of its legal duties and privacy practices with respect to PHI

- A statement that the covered entity is required to abide by the terms of the notice currently in effect

- A statement that the covered entity reserves the right to change the terms of its notice and to make the new notice provisions effective for all PHI that it maintains

- A statement describing how it will provide individuals with a revised notice

- A statement that individuals may complain to the covered entity and the secretary of HHS when they believe their privacy rights have been violated, a brief description of how to file a complaint with the covered entity, and a statement that there will be no retaliation for filing one

- The name or title and telephone number of a person or office to contact for further information

- An effective date, which may not be earlier than the date on which the notice is published

A sample notice of privacy practices is available from AHIMA (Hughes 2001b). As mentioned earlier, healthcare providers with a direct treatment relationship with an individual must provide the notice of privacy practices no later than the date of the first service delivery, including service delivered electronically. Notices must be available at the site where the individual is treated and must be posted in a prominent place where patients can reasonably be expected to read it. If the facility has a Web site with information on the covered entity's services or benefits, the notice of privacy practices must be prominently posted to it.

Consent to Use or Disclose PHI

Under the Privacy Rule, healthcare providers are not required to obtain the patient's consent to use or disclose personally identifiable information for the purposes of treatment, payment, and healthcare operations (section 164.506[b]). However, some providers may decide to obtain consents as a matter of policy. In such cases, patient consent is usually obtained at the time care is provided and has no expiration date. (See figure 15.2.)

If a covered entity elects to use it, when should the consent for use and disclosure of information be obtained from an individual? Except for some special circumstances discussed later in this chapter (such as emergencies), consent would be obtained at the time that healthcare services are provided. Because the consent for use and disclosure has no expiration date, in most cases it is indefinite unless specifically revoked by the individual.

Certain specifications should be followed with regard to content and language in the consent for use and disclosure of information. The content must:

- Be expressed in plain language so that the individual can understand its content

- Inform the individual that the PHI may be used and disclosed to carry out treatment, payment, or healthcare operations

- Refer the individual to the covered entity's notice of privacy practices for a more complete description of the uses and disclosures and state that the individual has the right to review the notice before signing the consent

- State that the terms of the notice of privacy practices may change and describe how the individual may obtain a revised notice if the covered entity has reserved the right to change its privacy practices

- State that the individual has the right to request that the covered entity restrict how PHI is used or disclosed to carry out treatment, payment, or healthcare operations (Note: The covered entity is not required to agree to the requested restrictions.)

- State that the restrictions are binding on the covered entity when it agrees to the requested restrictions

- State that the individual has the right to revoke the consent in writing, except to the extent that the covered entity has already taken action based on the consent

- Be signed and dated by the individual

As discussed earlier, an individual may revoke consent at any time. However, the revocation must be in writing and the covered entity must document and retain any signed consent as well as any revocation.

There are several situations when obtaining consent may be difficult or impossible. One example would be an emergency treatment situation where there are substantial barriers to communicating with the individual. Another example would be when the healthcare provider is required by law to treat the individual but is unable to obtain consent. In such circumstances, the provider would want to document its attempt to obtain consent and the reason it was unable to do so. In emergency treatment situations, the provider would want to obtain consent as soon as reasonably possible after the delivery of treatment.

Figure 15.2. Sample consent for the use or disclosure of individually identifiable health information

Consent to the Use and Disclosure of Health Information for Treatment, Payment, or Healthcare Operations

I understand that as part of my healthcare, this organization originates and maintains health records describing my health history, symptoms, examination and test results, diagnoses, treatment, and any plans for future care or treatment. I understand that this information serves as:

- A basis for planning my care and treatment

- A means of communication among the many health professionals who contribute to my care

- A source of information for applying my diagnosis and surgical information to my bill

- A means by which a third-party payer can verify that services billed were actually provided

- A tool for routine healthcare operations such as assessing quality and reviewing the competence of healthcare professionals

I understand and have been provided with a Notice of Information Practices that provides a more complete description of information uses and disclosures. I understand that I have the right to review the notice prior to signing this consent. I understand that the organization reserves the right to change its notice and practices and prior to implementation will mail a copy of any revised notice to the address I've provided. I understand that I have the right to object to the use of my health information for directory purposes. I understand that I have the right to request restrictions as to how my health information may be used or disclosed to carry out treatment, payment, or healthcare operations and that the organization is not required to agree to the restrictions requested. I understand that I may revoke this consent in writing, except to the extent that the organization has already taken action in reliance thereon. Therefore, I consent to the use and disclosure of my healthcare information.

☐ I request the following restrictions to the use or disclosure of my health information.

Signature of Patient or Legal Representative

_____

Witness _____

Date Notice Effective _____

Date or Version _____

☐ Accepted   ☐ Denied

Signature_____

Title _____

Date _____

Source: HHS 2000, 82818.

Authorization

In addition to the two forms just discussed, the notice of privacy practices and the consent for use and disclosure of information for TPO, section 164.508 of the Privacy Rule requires that an authorization for other uses and disclosures be obtained from an individual.

Essentially, except for the purposes and circumstances specifically mentioned in the Privacy Rule that do not require an authorization for use or disclosure (which are outlined later in this chapter and in table 15.5), all other uses and disclosures require an individual's authorization.

Under the Privacy Rule, an authorization must be written in plain language. A valid authorization is one that contains at least the following elements (HHS 2000, 82811):

- A description of the information to be used or disclosed that identifies the information in a specific and meaningful fashion

- The name or other specific identification of the person(s), or class of persons, authorized to make the requested use or disclosure

- The name or other specific identification of the person(s), or class of persons, to whom the covered entity may make the requested use or disclosure

---

Table 15.5.   Authorization requirements for use and disclosure of PHI

I.   **Patient Authorization Required:**

All situations except those listed in Part II

II.   **Patient Authorization Not Required:**

A.   **When use or disclosure is *required*, even without patient authorization**
- When the individual/patient or individual's/patient's personal representative requests access or accounting of disclosures (with exceptions)
- Dept. of HHS investigation, review, or enforcement action

B.   **When use or disclosure is *permitted*, even without patient authorization**
- Patient has opportunity to informally agree or object
  —patient directory
  —notification of relatives and friends
- Patient does not have opportunity to agree or object
  —Public interest and benefit (12 types)
    1. As required by law
    2. For public health activities
    3. To disclose PHI regarding victims of abuse, neglect, domestic violence
    4. For health oversight activities
    5. For judicial and administrative proceedings
    6. For law enforcement purposes (six specific situations)
    7. Regarding decedents
    8. For cadaveric organ, eye or tissue donation
    9. For research, with limitations
    10. To prevent or lessen serious threat to health or safety
    11. For essential government functions
    12. For workmen's compensation
  —TPO
  —To the individual/patient
  —Incidental disclosures
  —Limited data set

- An expiration date or event that relates to the individual or the purpose of the use or disclosure

- A statement of the individual's right to revoke the authorization in writing and the exceptions to the right to revoke, together with a description of how the individual may revoke it

- A statement that information used or disclosed pursuant to the authorization may be subject to redisclosure by the recipient and no longer protected by this rule

- Signature of the individual and date

- When the authorization is signed by a personal representative of the individual, a description of the representative's authority to act for the individual

An authorization is considered invalid (defective) when any one of the elements listed is missing, that is, when it has one or more of the following defects (HHS 2000, 82811):

- The expiration date has passed or the expiration event is known by the covered entity to have occurred.

- The authorization has not been filled out completely.

- The authorization is known by the covered entity to have been revoked.

- The authorization lacks a required element.

- The authorization violates the "compound authorization" requirements, if applicable.

- Any material information in the authorization is known by the covered entity to be false.

Authorizations are always required for the use or disclosure of psychotherapy notes except to carry out treatment, payment, or healthcare operations or to fulfill one of the following purposes (HHS 2000, 82811):

- Use by the originator of the psychotherapy notes for treatment

- Use or disclosure by the covered entity in training programs for students, trainees, or practitioners in mental health

- Use or disclosure by the covered entity to defend a legal action or other proceeding brought by the individual

- Use or disclosure that is required or permitted with respect to the oversight of the originator of the psychotherapy notes

An individual may revoke an authorization at any time, provided that he or she does so in writing. However, revocation does not apply when the covered entity has already taken action on the authorization.

The Privacy Rule requires that authorizations be obtained for uses and disclosures of PHI created for research that includes treatment of the individual. Exceptions would be instances where the covered entity obtains documentation showing that an alteration to or waiver of the requirement has been approved by the Institutional Review Board (IRB) or the privacy board. Under such circumstances, the Privacy Rule requires that the authorizations contain the core elements listed on the preceding page as well as a number of other specifications.

The Privacy Rule also provides other specifications for authorization, including authorizations requested by a covered entity for its own uses and disclosures and those requested by a covered entity for disclosures by others. This section of the Privacy Rule also includes a prohibition on requiring an authorization as a condition of treatment and allows authorizations to be combined only in certain situations. (Section 164.508 provides more information.) Covered entities must document and retain any signed authorization.

Differences among Notice of Privacy Practices, Consent, and Authorization

It is important to understand the differences among the notice of privacy practices, a consent, and an authorization for use and disclosure of information. The notice of privacy practices and authorization, which are required by the Privacy Rule, address a variety of uses and disclosures. The notice of privacy practices must include an explanation of TPO; authorizations are not required for uses and disclosures for TPO. A consent, which is optional, is limited to TPO.

The notice of privacy practices and consent provide *prospective* and *general* information about how PHI may be used or disclosed in the future. They seek to notify or obtain permission to use or disclose PHI that may or may not have already been created and for which there may not yet be a need. Neither of these documents has a time limit for as long as the document content stays the same. On the other hand, an authorization provides *specific* information about the PHI that an individual authorizes for use or disclosure, including the recipient of the PHI. It covers all uses and disclosures except those exempted by the Privacy Rule. It includes a time limit for the specific use and disclosure. The situation for which the PHI is being sought has generally already been created. In other words, an authorization generally (although not always) seeks information after it has been created and for which a specific need has arisen.

A healthcare provider may refuse treatment if the individual declines to sign the consent form. However, a healthcare provider may *not* refuse to treat an individual for declining to sign an authorization or a notice of privacy practices.

Uses and Disclosures of Health Information

As stated earlier in this chapter, one of the goals of the Privacy Rule is to provide greater privacy protections for one's health information by limiting access by others. This includes both use and disclosure. As table 15.5 shows, PHI may not be used or disclosed by a covered entity unless the individual who is the subject of the information authorizes the use or disclosure in writing or the Privacy Rule *requires or permits* such use or disclosure without the individual's authorization. The Privacy Rule *requires* such use or disclosure in only two situations: when the individual or individual's personal representative requests access to or an accounting of disclosures of the PHI (with the exceptions detailed earlier in this chapter), and when HHS is conducting an investigation, review, or enforcement action.

Uses and Disclosures for Which Authorization Is Not Required

In addition to the two situations where use or disclosure is *required* without the individual's authorization (section A in table 15.5), there are many situations where the Privacy Rule *permits* a covered entity to use or disclose PHI without an individual's authorization (HHS 2003). These are summarized in section B of table 15.5. Essentially, these provide a significant number of exceptions to the patient authorization requirement. As a result, critics of the Privacy Rule have argued that it actually diminishes patient privacy rather than improve it.

Permitted Uses and Disclosures without Patient Authorization:

Patient opportunity to agree or object (informal agreement)
   i.   patient directory
   ii. notification of relatives and friends

Patient does not have opportunity to agree or object
   i.   public interest and benefit (12 situations)
   ii.   treatment, payment and operations
   iii. to the individual
   iv.   incidental disclosures
   v.   limited data set

Patient Opportunity to Agree or Object

Section 164.510 of the Privacy Rule lists two circumstances in which PHI can be used without the individual's authorization, but where the individual must be informed in advance and given an opportunity to agree to use or disclosure or prohibit or restrict it. In such circumstances, the covered entity may inform the individual in a verbal communication and obtain his or her verbal agreement or objection.

The first circumstance is when the healthcare facility wants to keep a directory of patients. The information may include the patient's name, location in the facility, condition described in general terms, and religious affiliation. The purpose of the directory is to disclose such information to members of the clergy or other persons who ask for the individual by name. Disclosure of an individual's religious affiliation is limited to members of the clergy.

The covered entity must inform the patient of the information to be included in the directory and the people to whom the information may be disclosed. The patient must be given the opportunity to restrict or prohibit some or all of the uses or disclosures.

When it is impractical or impossible to inform the patient and obtain agreement (for example, in an emergency situation), the facility can use and disclose PHI for the purposes stated above. However, the disclosure must be consistent with the prior expressed preference of the patient or the facility must have determined that it is in the patient's best interest. When it becomes possible or practical after the emergency situation, the healthcare facility must inform the patient and give him or her the opportunity to object to such use and disclosure.

The second circumstance is the covered entity's ability under the Privacy Rule to disclose to a family member or a close friend the PHI directly relevant to his or her involvement with the patient's care or payment. Likewise, a covered entity may disclose

PHI, including the patient's location, general condition, or death, to notify or assist in the notification of a family member, personal representative, or some other person responsible for the patient's care (HHS 2000, 82812).

However, if the patient is present and otherwise able to make healthcare decisions, the covered entity may only use or disclose the PHI in the above situations if it has done one of the following:

- Obtained the patient's agreement

- Provided the patient with the opportunity to object to the disclosure and the patient has not objected

- Reasonably inferred from the circumstances that the patient does not object to the disclosure

The covered entity also may use or disclose PHI to a public or private entity authorized by law or by its charter to assist in disaster relief efforts.

Patient Does Not Have Opportunity to Agree or Object

There are sixteen circumstances where PHI can be used or disclosed without the individual's authorization and the individual does *not* have the opportunity to agree or object. Section 164.512 of the Privacy Rule refers to the first twelve circumstances as "public interest and benefit" circumstances. In other words, they have been identified as circumstances that benefit society. Although the Privacy Rule permits the twelve "public interest and benefit" uses or disclosures without an individual's authorization, if such use or authorization would violate a state law that otherwise protects the patient's information, the information cannot be legally used or disclosed.

In many cases, a disclosure meets more than one of the twelve public interest and benefit situations. The public interest and benefit circumstances are detailed in the following paragraphs.

1. As required by law: Disclosures are permitted when required by laws that meet the public-interest requirements of disclosures relating to victims of abuse, neglect, or domestic violence; judicial and administrative proceedings; and law enforcement purposes. These three areas are detailed more fully below.

2. Public health activities: Use or disclosure of PHI for public health purposes includes preventing or controlling diseases, injuries and disabilities, and reporting disease, injury, and vital events such as births and deaths. Examples include the reporting of adverse events or product defects to comply with FDA regulations and, when authorized by law, reporting a person who may have been exposed to a communicable disease and may be at risk for contracting or spreading it.

3. Victims of abuse, neglect, or domestic violence: An example is the reporting to authorities authorized by law to receive information about child or other abuse or neglect. In non-child abuse situations, the Privacy Rule does require the covered entity to promptly inform the individual that such a report has been or will be made. However, the entity does not have to inform the individual if it believes

that doing so would place the individual at risk of serious harm or not be in his or her best interest. An example might be when the covered entity would be informing the personal representative it reasonably believes is responsible for the abuse, neglect, or other injury.

4. Healthcare oversight activities: An authorized health oversight agency may receive PHI for activities authorized by law such as audits, civil or criminal investigations, licensure, and other inspections.

5. Judicial and administrative proceedings: Disclosures for judicial and administrative proceedings are permitted in response to an order of a court or an administrative tribunal, provided that the covered entity discloses only the PHI expressly authorized by such an order or in response to a subpoena, discovery request, or other lawful process. With regard to subpoenas and discovery requests, the party seeking the PHI must assure the covered entity that it has made reasonable efforts to make the request known to the individual who is the subject of the PHI. In this situation, the entity also must be assured that the time for the individual to raise objections to the court or administrative tribunal has elapsed and that either no objections have been filed, all objections have been resolved, or a qualified protective order has been secured.

6. Law enforcement purposes: The Privacy Rule specifies six instances when disclosures to law enforcement do not require patient authorization or the patient has no opportunity to agree or object:

    • Pursuant to legal process or otherwise required by law: Examples of legal process include a court order, a court-ordered warrant, a subpoena or a summons issued by a judicial officer. Relative to "otherwise required by law," for example, a law may exist that requires the reporting of certain types of wounds or other physical injuries to law enforcement.

    • In response to a law enforcement official's request for the purpose of identifying or locating a suspect, fugitive, material witness, or missing person: In such cases, only the following information may be disclosed:

    —Name and address

    —Date and place of birth

    —Social Security number

    —ABO blood type and Rh factor

    —Type of injury

    —Date and time of treatment

    —Date and time of death, if applicable

    —Description of distinguishing physical characteristics, including height, weight, gender, race, hair and eye color, and presence or absence of facial scars or tattoos

- In response to a law enforcement official's request about an individual who is, or suspected to be, a victim of a crime (when the individual agrees to the disclosure or when the covered entity is unable to obtain the individual's agreement because of incapacity or other emergency circumstance). The law enforcement official must represent that such information is needed to determine whether a violation of law has occurred, that immediate law enforcement activity depends on the disclosure, and that disclosure is in the best interest of the individual as determined by the covered entity.

- About a deceased individual when the covered entity suspects that the death may have resulted from criminal conduct

- To a law enforcement official when the covered entity believes in good faith that the information constitutes evidence of criminal conduct that occurred on the covered entity's premises

- To a law enforcement official in response to a medical emergency when the covered entity believes that disclosure is necessary to alert law enforcement to the commission and nature of a crime, the location or victims of such crime, and the identity, description, and location of the perpetrator of such crime. Further, it is permitted when the covered entity believes the medical emergency was the result of abuse, neglect, or domestic violence.

7. Decedents: Disclosures to a coroner or medical examiner are permitted to identify a deceased person, determine a cause of death, or accomplish other purposes as required by law. In accordance with applicable law, disclosures to funeral directors are permitted, as necessary, to allow them to carry out their duties with respect to the decedent. This type of information also may be disclosed in reasonable anticipation of an individual's death.

8. Cadaveric organ, eye, or tissue donation: PHI may be disclosed to organ procurement agencies or other entities to facilitate the procurement, banking, or transplantation of cadaveric organs, eyes, or tissue.

9. Research: PHI created for research is only subject to the Privacy Rule when the research includes treatment of an individual. An organization's IRB or privacy board plays a key role in this scenario because authorizations for the use of PHI in research are required except in instances where the covered entity obtains documentation that an alteration to or waiver of (in whole or in part) the individual authorization has been approved by its IRB or privacy board (HHS 2000, 82816). Many provisions must be met with regard to the documentation required for either board to make a decision about the waiver of individual authorization. (See section 164.512.) Table 15.6 provides a detailed analysis of the responsibilities of both the IRB and the researcher under the Privacy Rule requirements.

Table 15.6.   Actions required for use of PHI in research

Type of Information	IRB	Researcher	Research Subject (patient or decedent)
PHI preparatory to research	None*	Representation that use is solely and necessary for research and will not be removed from covered entity	None
Deidentified health information	None*	Removal of safe-harbor data or statistical assurance of deidentification	None
Limited data set	None*	Removal of direct identifiers and data use agreement	None
Individually identifiable on health information on decedents	None*	Representation that use is solely and necessary for research on decedents and documentation of death upon request of covered entity	None
PHI of human subjects (whether research is interventional or record review)	Waive authorization requirement if determined that risk to privacy is minimal	Representation that: 1. Privacy risk is minimal based on: • plan to protect identifiers • plan to destroy identifiers unless there is a health or research reason to retain • written assurance that PHI will not be reused or redisclosed 2. Research requires use of specifically described PHI 3. Justify the waiver 4. Obtain IRB approval under normal or expedited review procedures	None
	Approve alteration of authorization (e.g., to restrict patient's access during study) if determined that risk to privacy is minimal	Same as above	Sign altered authorization form
	Approve research protocol ensuring that there is an authorization for use either combined with consent for and disclosure of PHI research or separate		Sign authorization combined with consent for research or sign standard authorization for use and disclosure of PHI for research as described in authorization

* There may be requirements imposed by the IRB, but there are none imposed by HIPAA.

Source: Amatayakul 2003.

10. Threat to health and safety: Use or disclosure is allowed under circumstances where the covered entity believes it is necessary to prevent or lessen a serious and imminent threat to the health or safety of an individual or the public. In such cases, disclosure must be made to a person who can reasonably prevent or lessen the threat. Disclosures also are permissible when law enforcement officials must apprehend an individual who may have caused harm to the victim under treatment or when the individual appears to have escaped from a correctional institution or lawful custody.

    With regard to correctional institutions or to a law enforcement official who has lawful custody of an inmate, the Privacy Rule allows disclosures, provided that the institution states that the information is necessary to provide continuing healthcare; to secure the health and safety of the individual or other inmates, officers, employees, transportation personnel, or law enforcement on the premises; or to ensure the administration and maintenance of the institution's safety, security, and good order (HHS 2000, 82818).

11. Specialized government functions: Specialized government functions where uses and disclosures are permitted without authorization or opportunity to agree or object include information regarding armed forces personnel for military and veterans activities, for purposes of national security and intelligence activities, for protective services for the president of the United States and others, and for public benefits and medical suitability determinations (HHS 2000, 82817).

    How is PHI use and disclosure handled with regard to correctional institutions or to a law enforcement official who has lawful custody of an inmate? Essentially, the Privacy Rule allows such disclosures, provided that the correctional institution states that the information is necessary to provide continuing healthcare; to secure the health and safety of the individual or other inmates, officers, employees, transportation personnel, or law enforcement on the premises; or to ensure the administration and maintenance of the institution's safety, security, and good order (DHHS 2000, p. 82818).

12. Workers' compensation: The Privacy Rule permits the disclosure of PHI relating to work-related illness or injury or a workplace-related medical surveillance to the extent that such disclosure complies with workers' compensation laws.

The remaining four types of uses and disclosures that do not require patient authorization or an opportunity for the patient to agree or object are TPO; disclosure to the subject individual; incidental disclosures; and limited data set. It is important to note that the Privacy Rule does not specifically identify the four aforementioned circumstances as "uses and disclosures for which authorization or an opportunity to agree or object is not required." The first two have been discussed at length in this chapter; the latter two are examined here.

- *Incidental uses or disclosures* occur as part of a permitted use or disclosure (164.502[a][1][iii]). For example, calling out patients' names in a physician office is an incidental disclosure because it occurs as part of office operations. As long as the information disclosed is the minimum necessary (for example, the patient's name with no diagnostic information), it is permissible under the Privacy Rule.

- A *limited data set* is PHI that excludes direct identifiers of the individual, the individual's relatives, employers, or household members (164.514[e][2]). However, the exclusion is not great enough to de-identify the information. Such PHI may be used or disclosed, provided it is used or disclosed only for research, public health, or healthcare operations.

Check Your Understanding 15.4

Instructions: Select the phrase that best completes the following sentences.

1. _____ Ownership of the physical health record rests with _____.
   a. The patient who is the subject of the record
   b. The state Department of Health in which the healthcare provider is located
   c. The hospital, facility, or physician who keeps the records of patients
   d. No one

2. _____ The Privacy Rule establishes that a patient has the right of access to inspect and obtain a copy of his or her PHI _____.
   a. For as long as it is maintained
   b. For six years
   c. Forever
   d. For twelve months

3. _____ HIPAA regulations _____.
   a. Never preempt state statutes
   b. Always preempt state statutes
   c. Preempt less strict state statutes where they exist
   d. Preempt stricter state statutes where they exist

4. _____ The Privacy Rule applies to _____.
   a. All covered entities involved, either directly or indirectly, with transmitting or performing any electronic transactions specified in the act
   b. Healthcare providers only
   c. Only healthcare providers that receive Medicare reimbursement
   d. Only entities funded by the federal government

5. _____ The Privacy Rule extends to protected health information _____.
   a. In any form or medium, except paper and oral forms
   b. In any form or medium, including paper and oral forms
   c. That pertains to mental health treatment only
   d. That exists in electronic form only

6. _____ Under HIPAA privacy regulations, a patient does not have the right to access his or her _____.
   a. History and physical report
   b. Operative report
   c. Discharge summary
   d. Psychotherapy notes

7. _____ A provider may deny a patient's request to review and copy his or her health information if _____.
   a. The patient agreed to temporarily suspend access during a research study
   b. The patient requests his psychotherapy notes
   c. A licensed healthcare professional determines that access to PHI would endanger the life or physical safety of the patient or another person
   d. All of the above

8. ____ When an individual requests a copy of the PHI or agrees to accept summary or explanatory information, the covered entity may ____.
   a. Impose a reasonable cost-based fee
   b. Not charge the individual
   c. Impose any fee authorized by state statute
   d. Charge only for the cost of the paper on which the information is printed

9. ____ The Privacy Rule specifies that a covered entity must act on an individual's request for review of a copy of PHI no later than ____ after the request is made.
   a. Ninety days
   b. Sixty days
   c. Thirty days
   d. Six weeks

10. ____ An accounting of disclosures must include disclosures ____.
    a. To carry out treatment, payment, and operations
    b. For use in the facility's patient directory
    c. To the individual about whom the information pertains
    d. None of the above

11. ____ The term *minimum necessary* means that healthcare providers and other covered entities must limit use, access, and disclosure to the minimum necessary to ____.
    a. Satisfy one's curiosity
    b. Accomplish the intended purpose
    c. Treat an individual
    d. Perform research

12. ____ Notices of privacy practices must be available at the site where the individual is treated and ____.
    a. Must be posted next to the entrance
    b. Must be posted in a prominent place where it is reasonable to expect that patients will read it
    c. May be posted anywhere at the site
    d. Do not have to be posted at the site

13. ____ Inmates in correctional institutions ____.
    a. Must be provided with a notice of privacy practices with regard to their health information
    b. Are not considered "individuals" who receive privacy protection under the HIPAA Privacy Rule
    c. Are afforded most privacy protections under HIPAA
    d. Are covered entities per the HIPAA Privacy Rule definition

14. ____ A notice of privacy practices ____.
    a. Is to be given to patients upon their first contact with the covered entity
    b. Does not have to be given to inmates who are patients
    c. Explains an individual's rights under the HIPAA Privacy Rule
    d. All of the above

15. _____ The Privacy Rule requires that individuals be able to _____.
   a. Request restrictions on certain uses and disclosures of PHI
   b. Request amendment of their PHI
   c. Receive a paper copy of the notice of privacy practices
   d. All of the above

16. _____ A valid authorization must contain _____.
   a. A description of the information to be used or disclosed
   b. An expiration date or event
   c A statement that the information being used or disclosed may be subject to redisclosure by the recipient
   d. All of the above

17. _____ Consents _____.
   a. Are the same as authorizations
   b. Expire 60 days after they are executed
   c. Are required under the HIPAA Privacy Rule
   d. Are for the purpose of permitting use and disclosure of PHI for treatment, payment, or operations

18. _____ When a covered entity has given a patient a notice of privacy practices, _____.
   a. A consent to use or disclose information for purposes of treatment, payment, or operations is not required
   b. A consent to use or disclose information for purposes of treatment, payment, or operations is also required
   c. An authorization to use or disclose information for the purpose of treatment, payment, or operations is also required
   d. No authorizations are required for any subsequent use or disclosure of PHI

19. _____ Disclosure in a facility's patient directory _____.
   a. Can occur only with the patient's written authorization
   b. Is automatic upon a patient's admission to a healthcare provider
   c. Is subject to the patient having had the opportunity to informally agree or object
   d. Can include all PHI in the patient's designated record set

20. _____ An individual may _____.
   a. Revoke an authorization in writing
   b. Never revoke a valid authorization
   c. Not specify an expiration date on an authorization
   d. None of the above

21. _____ When an individual requests that PHI be routed to an alternative location, _____.
   a. A health plan may decline such a request if no reason is given
   b. Both health plans and healthcare providers may deny a request if it is unreasonable
   c. Both health plans and healthcare providers may deny a request if no alternative contact information is provided
   d. All of the above

22. _____ The Privacy Rule "public interest and benefit" purposes include _____.
   a. Facilitating organ donations
   b. Information about decedents
   c. Information provided to law enforcement
   d. All of the above

23. ____ Under the Privacy Rule, the release of PHI to a patient's relatives is ____.
    a. Never allowed
    b. Allowed when the information is directly relevant to their involvement with the patient's care or treatment
    c. Allowed only if the patient is declared incompetent by a court of law
    d. None of the above

24. ____ A covered entity's workforce can include ____.
    a. Employees
    b. Volunteers
    c. Employees of contractors
    d. All of the above

25. ____ De-identified information ____.
    a. Does not identify an individual
    b. Is information from which personal characteristics have been stripped
    c. Cannot be later constituted or combined to re-identify an individual
    d. All of the above

26. ____ Under the Privacy Rule, a code to re-identify de-identified information ____.
    a. Is never allowed
    b. Is allowed if it cannot be translated to the individual's identity
    c. May disclose the mechanism for re-identification
    d. None of the above

27. ____ Business associate agreements are developed to cover the use of PHI by ____.
    a. The covered entity's employees
    b. Organizations outside the covered entity's workforce that use PHI to perform functions for the covered entity
    c. The covered entity's entire workforce
    d. The covered entity's janitorial staff

28. ____ Release of birth and death information to public health authorities ____.
    a. Is prohibited without patient consent
    b. Is prohibited without patient authorization
    c. Is a "public interest and benefit" disclosure that does not require patient authorization
    d. Requires both patient consent and authorization

29. ____ Patient authorization is required to release ____.
    a. An individual's name and address to a law enforcement official who needs it to identify or locate a suspect
    b. PHI to the patient's family physician for follow-up treatment
    c. PHI that is relevant to national security
    d. PHI to the patient's attorney

30. ____ The Privacy Rule permits use or disclosure without written patient authorization ____.
    a. For specific law enforcement purposes specified by the Privacy Rule
    b. For incidental disclosures
    c. To prevent or lessen serious threats to health or safety
    d. All of the above

31. ____ Protected health information (PHI) ____.
    a Relates to one's past, present, or future mental health condition
    b. Relates to one's past, present, or future physical condition
    c. Relates to payment for the provision of healthcare
    d. All of the above

HIPAA Requirements Related to Marketing and Fundraising

The Privacy Rule defines marketing as communication about a product or service that encourages the recipient to purchase or use that product or service (section 164.501). PHI use or disclosure for marketing requires an authorization from the individual except in certain cases. Marketing activities that do not require authorization are those that (HHS 2000, 82819):

- Occur face to face between the covered entity and the individual, or
- Concern a promotional gift of nominal value provided by the covered entity.

Some activities look like marketing but do not meet the Privacy Rule's definition of marketing. As a result, no authorization is required for:

- Communications to describe health-related products and services provided by, or included in the plan of benefits of, the covered entity itself or a third party
- Communication for treatment of the individual
- Case management or care coordination for the individual, or to direct or recommend alternative treatments, therapies, healthcare providers, or care settings

If the covered entity has received—or will receive—direct or indirect remuneration in exchange for making a communication to an outside entity, this fact must be prominently stated.

In addition to the preceding specifications, when the communication is directed toward a specific target audience (for example, not a broad spectrum or cross section of patients), it must contain instructions on how the individual can opt out of receiving future communications of this type.

Whenever a covered entity uses PHI to target an individual or group based on health status or condition, it must meet certain requirements. For example, before making the communication, the entity must determine that the product or service being marketed may be beneficial to the health of the type of individual being targeted. Then, the communication must explain why the individual has been targeted and how the product or service relates to his or her health.

For fundraising activities that benefit the covered entity, the covered entity may use or disclose to a business associate or an institutionally related foundation, without authorization, demographic information and dates of healthcare provided to an individual. However, the covered entity must inform individuals in its notice of privacy practices that PHI may be used for this purpose. Moreover, it must include in fundraising materials instructions to the individual on how he or she may opt out of receiving such materials in the future. If a fundraising activity targets individuals based on diagnosis (for example, patients with kidney disease for a new kidney dialysis center), prior authorization is required.

HIPAA Privacy Rule Administrative Requirements

HIPAA provides several standards regarding administrative requirements that are important to the HIT, including:

- Designation of a privacy officer and a contact person for receiving complaints
- Requirements for privacy training

- Requirements for establishing privacy safeguards for handling complaints
- Standards for policies and procedures and changes to policies and procedures

Like most of the requirements discussed, HIT professionals may find that the scope of their responsibilities encompasses functions that relate to meeting the Privacy Rule requirements.

Designation of Privacy Officer and Contact Person

The Privacy Rule requires covered entities to designate an individual to be responsible for developing and implementing privacy policies and procedures. As mentioned earlier, this position is ideally suited to the background, knowledge, and skills of the HIM professional. (See appendix A of this textbook for a position description.)

In addition to a privacy officer, the covered entity must designate a person or office as the responsible party for receiving complaints. This individual must be able to provide further information about matters covered by the entity's notice of privacy practices.

Privacy Training

Every member of the covered entity's workforce must be trained in PHI policies and procedures according to the Privacy Rule. Thereafter, each new employee must be trained within a reasonable period of time after joining the workforce. In addition, whenever material changes are made to policies or procedures regarding privacy, employees must receive additional training.

Further, the covered entity must maintain documentation showing that privacy training has occurred. Although not required, a signed statement of training by each workforce member would be helpful in documenting such compliance.

Privacy Safeguards

A covered entity must have in place safeguards and mechanisms to protect the privacy of PHI. This includes appropriate administrative, technical, and physical safeguards. These safeguards should work hand in hand with those specified in the HIPAA Privacy Rule. (Chapter 17 of this text contains additional information on HIPAA security regulations.)

Standards for Policies and Procedures

The covered entity must implement policies and procedures to ensure that it is in compliance with all the standards, implementation specifications, and other requirements of the Privacy Rule. This process includes conducting an ongoing review of privacy policies and procedures and ensuring that all policy changes are consistent with changes in the privacy and security regulations. Any regulatory changes that materially affect the covered entity's notice of privacy practices must be reflected in the notice. This means that the notice must be updated as required. All revisions must be indicated as such on the policies, procedures, or notice of privacy practices. HIM professionals are ideally qualified for developing and overseeing such policies and procedures because of their background in health information management and privacy and security issues.

Medical Staff Appointments and Privileges

Another area that has significant legal implications in which the HIT may become involved is medical staff appointments, also referred to as **credentialing.** In some organizations, an HIT serves as the coordinator for the medical staff credentialing process. A basic understanding of the legal issues and some of the functions in the credentialing process is important.

As a legal entity, the healthcare facility is ultimately responsible for the quality of care it provides. A large part of this responsibility involves the quality of the medical staff. As described in chapter 13, the medical staff is the aggregate of physicians who have been given permission to provide a healthcare facility's clinical services. A healthcare facility's governing board is accountable for establishing policies and procedures that ensure that reasonable care has been taken in the appointment of medical practitioners to the facility's medical staff and the granting of clinical privileges, which is the defined set of services a physician is permitted to perform in that facility. Credentialing is the process that includes both the initial appointment and reappointment of individuals to the medical staff and determination of the extent of their privileges. Although the board of directors relies on the advice and recommendations of the medical staff, ultimate responsibility for making appointments and reappointments and for ensuring that the medical staff members are qualified to perform the functions for which they have been granted privileges rests with the board (Pozgar 2004, 172).

As described in chapter 9, an important part of the credentialing process is the National Practitioner Data Bank (NPDB) established by the federal Health Care Quality Improvement Act of 1986. One goal of the NPDB is to limit the movement of physicians throughout the United States where their negative histories such as medical malpractice lawsuits and loss of privileges at other healthcare facilities may go undetected. NPDB regulations include requirements for reporting information to the NPDB and querying information from the NPDB prior to granting medical staff privileges (Pozgar 2004).

How does this involve the HIT? As mentioned earlier, he or she may serve as the medical staff coordinator. The functions of this role can involve the collection, organization, verification, and storage of all information concerned with the credentialing process. This includes information on the individual staff member's professional background, credentials, previous professional experience, and quality profiles. All this information, including that obtained from the NPDB, is considered strictly confidential. Therefore, policies and procedures must be in place to specify who may have access to what information and under what circumstances. Additionally, the HIT should be aware of the penalties and liabilities that can result from failure to use the NPDB.

The customary process by which an application for medical staff appointment and privileges is reviewed involves several levels. These include the appropriate clinical departments, the credentials committee, the medical staff executive committee, and the board of directors.

Labor Laws and Unionized Personnel

In addition to the appointment of individuals to a health organization's medical staff, the HIT may be responsible for supervising his or her own staff. Additional requirements are present when an organization's employees belong to unions or professional associations that serve to represent their members through the **collective bargaining** process.

The most pervasive federal labor law is the **National Labor Relations Act** (NLRA) and its amendments. The act provides procedures for union representation and prohibits unfair labor practices by unions, such as coercing nonstriking employees, and by employers, such as interference with the union selection process and discrimination against employees who support a union. However, employers may restrict union activity to prevent the disruption of the organization's operations. Further, the NLRA allows employers to prohibit supervisors, as stewards of the employer, to be involved in union activity. Supervisors are thus differentiated from the NLRA definition of "employee" (Pozgar 2004).

Other federal labor laws that are significant to the HIT who supervises employees who are union members include (Pozgar 2004):

- The **Fair Labor Standards Act** (1938) defines the minimum wage and maximum hours of employment.

- The **Equal Pay Act** (1963) prohibits discrimination in payment of wages based on gender.

- The **Equal Employment Opportunity Act** (1972) is the amendment to the Civil Rights Act of 1964 (Title VII) that prohibits discrimination on the basis of age, race, color, religion, sex, or national origin.

- **The Age Discrimination in Employment Act** (1967) prohibits employment discrimination against workers at least 40 years of age.

- The **Occupational Safety and Health Act** (1970) was passed to develop and enforce safe and healthy workplace environments.

- The **Rehabilitation Act** (1973) was passed to protect handicapped employees against discrimination.

Managers also need to be familiar with state labor laws for several reasons. Because the NLRA does not apply to public organizations at the state or local level, individual state labor relations laws may fill that void. Other labor laws that are handled by the individual states include workers' compensation, child labor laws, and minimum wage laws where states have established a rate higher than the federal rate. States also may act to prohibit labor contracts that make union membership a condition of employment. Such laws are called **right-to-work laws** (Pozgar 2004).

Americans With Disabilities Act

The **Americans With Disabilities Act of 1990,** commonly referred to as the ADA, applies to the employment setting by prohibiting discrimination against qualified individuals who have disabilities with respect to hiring, promotion, and other employment actions. This law applies to both private and public employers. When reviewing the job application of an individual with a disability, it is important that the employer focus on the individual's ability to perform the required job duties rather than on his or her disability. For example, it is a violation of the ADA to ask whether an individual has a disability. However, it is appropriate to determine whether that person is able to perform the functions required by a particular job (Pozgar 2004).

An employer must, if possible, make "reasonable accommodations" or alterations that allow an individual with a disability to perform the necessary job functions. An example of a reasonable accommodation may be a larger computer monitor for a visually impaired employee. Accommodations may not be "reasonable" if an employer is able to show that they are cost prohibitive or negatively affect the completion of one's job duties. If an accommodation is not possible or is not "reasonable," an employer has a valid defense against a claim that the ADA was violated. However, what is considered "reasonable" differs from one court to another.

Check Your Understanding 15.5

Instructions: Select the answer that best completes the following statements.

1. _____ Under the Privacy Rule, a healthcare provider who chooses to obtain a patient's consent does so in order to use or disclose PHI for _____.
   a. Fundraising activities
   b. Marketing activities
   c. Treatment, payment, or healthcare operations
   d. None of the above

2. _____ An individual's request that a covered entity attach an amendment to his or her health record _____.
   a. Must always be honored
   b. Can always be denied
   c. Can be denied if the PHI in question was not created by the covered entity
   d. Must be acted on no later than six months after the request was made

3. _____ The use or disclosure of PHI for marketing _____.
   a. Always requires written authorization from the patient
   b. Does not require written authorization for face-to-face communications with the individual
   c. Requires written authorization from the patient when products or services of nominal value are introduced
   d. None of the above

4. _____ With regard to training in PHI policies and procedures, _____.
   a. Every member of the covered entity's workforce must be trained
   b. Only individuals employed by the covered entity must be trained
   c. Training only needs to occur when there are material changes to the policies and procedures
   d. Documentation of training is not required

5. _____ The Privacy Rule states that an individual has the right to receive an accounting of certain disclosures made by a covered entity _____.
   a. Within the twelve months prior to the date on which the accounting is requested
   b. Since the covered entity came into existence
   c. Within the six years prior to the date on which the accounting is requested
   d. None of the above

6. _____ The privacy officer is responsible for _____.
   a. Handling complaints about the covered entity's violations of the Privacy Rule
   b. Developing and implementing privacy policies and procedures
   c. Providing information about the covered entity's privacy practices
   d. All of the above

7. _____ Credentialing applies to _____.
   a. Medical staff appointments
   b. Medical staff reappointments
   c. The granting of specific clinical privileges
   d. All of the above

Real-World Case

Eunice Little is not nervous about HIPAA because she and her colleagues at UCLA Medical Center in Los Angeles have made major strides in their preparations for implementation of the privacy rules (Hagland 2001).

How did Eunice and her team orchestrate moving forward toward HIPAA privacy compliance? First, they established a steering committee responsible for HIPAA privacy planning. The committee focused on three broad tracks of development: education, assessment activities, and development of policies and procedures.

The steering committee recognizes that the scope of the project is huge. As Eunice reports, "The scope involves not just hospital information systems, but the operations of departments and manual processes. The various things that can be included in the scope of the assessment are the biggest challenge." Developing HIPAA-compliant policies and procedures is certainly not a one-time activity. Development and update means this is an ongoing effort.

Part of UCLA's key to success has been pulling together the right combination of people. The result is a multidisciplinary team that includes the director of HIM services and the chief compliance officer.

Experts in the area of HIPAA privacy suggest that healthcare organizations consider the following steps to become HIPAA privacy compliant:

- Inventory the organization's data as the first step in policy implementation.

- Read the *Federal Register* information on HIPAA.

- Focus on HIPAA as a business process issue.

- Secure the support of top management and the active involvement and participation of staff in all affected areas.

- Thoroughly review outside vendor contracts to ensure compliance with business associate requirements.

- Appoint a dedicated staff to the HIPAA privacy initiative.

Moving into HIPAA compliance will require a thorough, attic-to-basement evaluation and realignment of business and operational processes.

Summary

The health information technician is on the front line as a champion for health information privacy. Requirements for the maintenance of medical records and health information are only one important matter with which HITs must be concerned. How health information is used and under what circumstances it can be disclosed are equally important. The development of privacy standards under HIPAA has generated national awareness of the importance of informational privacy and increased the responsibilities of HIM professionals in terms of ensuring that their organizations meet these standards.

Thus, HITs must thoroughly understand the legal issues involved in the compilation and maintenance of health information as well as those involved in its use and disclosure. Knowing the contents of this chapter is only the beginning. Because practices and regulations are constantly evolving, the HIT must engage in constant learning. Keeping up-to-date in practice in this essential and important area is among the HIT's key responsibilities.

References

Amatayakul, M. 2003. HIPAA on the Job: Another layer of regulations: Research under HIPAA. *Journal of American Health Information Management Association* 74(1):16A–D.

Amatayakul, M. 2001. HIPAA on the Job: Five steps to reading the HIPAA rules. *Journal of American Health Information Management Association* 72(8):16A–C.

Amtayakul, M. 2001. HIPAA on the Job: Managing individual rights requirements under HIPAA privacy. *Journal of American Health Information Management Association* 72(6):16A–D.

American Health Information Management Association. 2001. Sample (chief) privacy officer job description. *Journal of American Health Information Management Association* 72(6):39.

American Health Information Management Association. 2002. Practice brief: Retention of health information (Updated). *Journal of American Health Information Management Association* 73(6). Available online from ahima.org.

Black's Law Dictionary, abridged 5th ed. 1983. St. Paul, MN: West Publishing.

Cassidy, B. 2000. HIPAA on the job: Update on business partner/associate agreements. *Journal of American Health Information Management Association* 71(10):16A–D.

Clark, J.S. 2000. Mastering the information management standards. *Journal of American Health Information Management Association* 71(2):45–50.

Dennis, J.C. 2001. The new privacy officer's game plan. *Journal of American Health Information Management Association* 72(2):33–40.

Department of Health and Human Services. 2003. OCR privacy brief: Summary of the HIPAA Privacy Rule 2003. Available online from hhs.gov/ocr/privacysummary.pdf.

Department of Health and Human Services. 2000 (December 28). *Federal Register* 65(250):82811–82826.

Fletcher, D.M. 1999. Practice brief: Retention of health information. *Journal of American Health Information Management Association* 70(6). Updated June 2002, Web extra (Harry Rhodes).

Hagland, M. 2001. The journey of 1,000 miles: Are providers really ready for HIPAA privacy requirements? *Journal of American Health Information Management Association* 72(2):28–32.

Hughes, G. 2001a. Practice brief: Consent for the use or disclosure of individually identifiable health information. *Journal of American Health Information Management Association* 72(5):64E–G.

Hughes, G. 2001b. Practice brief: Notice of information practice. *Journal of American Health Information Management Association* 72(5):64I–M.

Johns, M.L. 1997 (June 5). Testimony to the Subcommittee on Government Management, Information, and Technology, Government Reform and Oversight Committee. Fair Health Information Practices Act 1997.

Office of Civil Rights, Department of Health and Human Services. hhs.gov/ocr/hipaa/.

Pozgar, G.D. 2004. *Legal Aspects of Health Care Administration,* 9th ed. Sudbury, MA: Jones and Bartlett Publishers.

Showalter, J.S. 2004. *The Law of Healthcare Administration,* 4th ed. Chicago: Health Administration Press.

Smith, C.M. 2001. Practice brief: Requirements for the acute care inpatient record. *Journal of American Health Information Management Association* 72(3):56A–G.

Standards for Privacy of Individually Identifiable Health Information. 2003 (April 17). *Code of Federal Regulations* 45 CFR 160 and 164.

Part IV
Information Technology and Systems

Chapter 16
Fundamentals of Information Systems

Merida Johns, PhD, RHIA

Learning Objectives

- To discuss the three major functions of an information system
- To identify the three components of information technology
- To describe the major types of information systems and give an example of each
- To describe the steps in the systems development life cycle
- To compare the functions of systems analysis with the functions of systems design
- To identify the three main types of system software and provide an example of each
- To discuss the major types of databases
- To understand the functions of a communications system's components
- To compare and contrast clients and servers
- To compare and contrast local-area networks, wide-area networks, intranets, extranets, and the Internet
- To become acquainted with the policies that must be incorporated into the use of an information system
- To identify four criteria used to evaluate an information system
- To understand how to use the Internet to conduct research on health-related topics

Key Terms

Actor

Artificial intelligence

Assembler

Assembly language

Bugs

Business process

Change management

Client

Column/field

Communications technology

Compiler

Data type

Data warehouse

Database

Encoder

Extranet

Foreign key

Graphical user interface (GUI)

Hardware

Information system (IS)

Information technology (IT)

Internet

Interpreter

Intranet

Key field

Language translator

Local-area network (LAN)

Machine language

Mainframe

Management support information systems

Minicomputer

Natural language

Network

Network protocol

Object

Object-oriented database

Object-relational database

Operating system

Operation support systems

Peripheral

Primary key

Productivity software

Programming language

Relational database

Row/record

Screen prototype

Secondary storage

Sequence diagram

Server

Software

Specialty software

Structured query language (SQL)

Supercomputer

Systems testing

Telecommunications

Transaction-processing system (TPS)

Unified modeling language (UML)

Use case diagram

Utility program

Web appliance

Wide-area network (WAN)

Workstation

Introduction

Computer use is essential in the healthcare industry. Computers comprise a major portion of an organization's **information system (IS).** The IS helps healthcare organizations meet the growing demands of patients, providers, and payers for information. Efficient management and distribution of information are indispensable to a healthcare organization's operation. Because of the principal role that computers play in an organization's healthcare information system, it is important that HIT professionals understand what makes up a well-constructed computer IS.

It is essential that health information technicians (HITs) understand their role and responsibilities in working in an electronic health record (EHR) environment. To be effective workers, HITs must know the basic structure of an electronic information system and how it is applied to the healthcare environment. This chapter introduces the primary components of an IS and discusses its essential elements, including data, people, processes, and computer systems. The chapter serves as a foundation for chapters 4, 17, 18, and 19 of this text.

Theory into Practice

This case study from the January 2004 edition of the Journal of American Health Information Management Association shows how one health information professional has participated in the change from a paper to an EHR environment (Duggan 2004, 40).

Change is constant in Kathleen Cleary's career and something she welcomes and embraces. Throughout her 15-year medical-records career, she has helped implement electronic records management systems for two large ambulatory clinics.

In addition to change, there's another constant in Cleary's career—her enthusiasm for the benefits of electronic medical records. "The more information that's available on the patient, and the more readily available that information, the better the quality of patient care."

Kathleen began her career in a traditional inpatient setting. After two years as supervisor of the HIM department at Milwaukee County Medical complex, Kathleen accepted a position as assistant director at the Palo Alto Medical Foundation (PAMF), a large ambulatory clinic with four satellite offices. After four years she advanced to director.

In her position as director, Kathleen managed 60 employees and was responsible for approximately 170,000 patient medical records. "Initially we worked with a paper-based system—multiple chart pulls, multiple competing appointments. One central record would travel wherever the patient was." Soon, Kathleen concentrated on quality improvement initiatives and the organization transitioned to an electronic bar-code chart-tracking system.

In 1999, PAMF decided to transition to an electronic medical records system. Selecting a vendor took six years. One satellite office served as the pilot for implementing the new electronic medical records system and eventually the other offices were added. "This new system was wonderful," says Kathleen. "I had reached a point with the old system where going to work wasn't fun anymore. We were always behind, we couldn't catch up, charts were in constant motion. Electronic medical records created efficiency and improved patient care."

After leaving PAMF, Kathleen took a position as the HIM director and privacy officer at the Austin Diagnostic Clinic (ADC), a large ambulatory care clinic. ADC has several satellite offices and approximately 200,000 active patient records. When she first began her job at ADC, the medical records were paper-based, and ADC was in the beginning phase of implementing electronic records.

One year into the implementation, they stopped filing progress notes, radiology reports, letters, prescription refills, and telephone encounters into the paper chart because the information was available in the electronic record. "Now all exam rooms have PCs, as do the nurses' stations and doctors' offices—the EMR is visible and useable to all," says Kathleen. "Using a paper-based system means that only one person could view the record at a time, but now the e-record is readily available."

How did Kathleen make the transition professionally from an expert in a paper-based medical records system to an electronic health record? Learning and listening have added to Kathleen's continued success. "I read a lot." She also attends AHIMA conventions and educational seminars. Networking with other HIM professionals is important to Kathleen, but looking beyond HIM is crucial, too. "I talk to people in the MIS department, business services, nursing services and risk management. . . . Being informed in other areas helps me do my job."

Basic Concepts of an Information System

An information system (IS) is the integration of several elements of a **business process** to effect a specific outcome. The system receives and processes input and provides output.

For instance, a physician ordering a lab test is a business process. The input is the order for the lab test. The outcome is a report from the laboratory. An IS is essential in integrating all the elements of the process so that the laboratory test is performed. For example, the physician must provide the laboratory with specific information about what test is to be performed, when it needs to be performed, and on whom it is to be performed. The laboratory must schedule the requested test, collect the sample, analyze the sample (usually with the aid of a computer system), and finally report the test results to the physician. As you can see, the IS integrates all of the steps of the test-ordering process.

An IS receives and processes input and provides output. A well-designed and well-managed IS is critical to the success of the healthcare industry. Accurate data can provide physicians, nurses, and administrators with information to make sound decisions. Bad data, on the other hand, can create bad decisions that can affect the health of patients.

In Computers, Communications & Information, Hutchinson and Sawyer (2000, 9.2) define an information system "as a collection of related components that interact to perform a task in order to accomplish a goal." All organizations generate information that must be managed and used in ways that allow them to accomplish their goals. "In addition to coordination among elements, systems must also be adaptive. That is, they must be able to respond to environmental changes by self-correcting the relationships among their internal elements" (Johns 1999, 368). Computers often are used to assist organizations with this challenging task.

Information System Components

An IS consists of data, people, and work processes and a combination of **hardware** (machines and media), **software** (computer programs), and **communications technology** (computer networks) known as **information technology (IT).**

Data, or raw facts, are provided to the IS by end users. These raw facts (also called input) have no meaning of their own. The IS refines them into meaningful information. For example, an end user may input the number 103 into the IS. The raw fact of 103 does not have any specific meaning of its own. However, when the IS system associates the fact as a patient's temperature and compares the fact to the normal temperature range, the raw fact is transformed into meaningful information, in this case, indicating that the patient's temperature is above normal.

In addition to data, an IS also consists of people. Users work with the IS to accomplish a variety of tasks. In healthcare, users include providers such as doctors and nurses, health data managers, technicians, therapists, oncology registrars, unit secretaries, case managers, chief information officers, and others who add data to the patient's health record. Because the IS must satisfy their needs and solve their problems, users should be a part of the team that designs the IS. Their tasks and goals should be included in the system's initial concept, and the users should be able to suggest changes as the system is being developed.

The last component of an IS is work processes. Processes are the policies and procedures that users must follow to do their work. An IS automates many processes that are performed by end users. For example, procedures that are followed to assign an ICD code to a diagnosis would be considered a process. A coding **encoder** automates many of the procedures used to assign an ICD code number.

Information System Activities

An IS performs five specific activities: input, processing, output, storage, and controlling. Typically, the first activity an IS performs is accepting input (for example, a patient's identification, temperature, blood pressure, and heart rate).

The second activity is processing the input. Processing can include performing calculations, making comparisons, or selecting alternative actions. For instance, the patient's temperature and blood pressure readings may be compared against the normal values to determine if his or her vital signs are within normal range.

The third activity is producing meaningful output (for example, providing a report of a patient's vital signs). The output of an IS is usually considered information to be used in making decisions.

In addition to accepting input and processing it into meaningful output, an IS performs storage and control activities. For example, in an EHR, the computer would store a patient's physical exam on specific storage media such as a hard disk so that many users can retrieve it or so that it can be accessed at a later time.

The final activity of an IS is to control its own performance. For example, a hospital administrator might discover that the daily census output does not add up to the correct monthly census. This may indicate that data-entry or data-processing procedures need to be corrected.

Check your understanding 16.1

Instructions: Choose the correct answer for the following questions.

1. ____ What is an information system?
   a. A collection of related components that interact to perform a task in order to accomplish a goal
   b. The integration of several elements in a business process to effect a specific outcome
   c. A process that refines raw facts into meaningful information
   d. All of the above

2. ____ What are the components of an information system?
   a. Computer servers, networks, and wiring along with personal computers
   b. A combination of hardware, software, and communications technology
   c. Data, people, and processes and a combination of hardware, software, and communications technology
   d. Collecting, maintaining, analyzing, and disseminating information

3. ____ What is the difference between data and information?
   a. Data are composed of numbers, and information is composed of words.
   b. Data represent raw facts and figures, and information represents the meaningful interpretation of data.
   c. There is no difference between data and information.
   d. All of the above

Types of Information Systems

In healthcare organizations, computer-based information systems are used to help managers at different levels to do their work. For example, physicians use specialized computer systems called decision support systems (DDSs) to help them make important decisions about the care of patients. The heads of the nursing, physical therapy, and health information management (HIM) departments often use computer systems called management information systems (MISs) to manage budgets, create work schedules, perform employee evaluations, and so on.

Coders, on the other hand, use transaction systems. Every record is coded and entered into the database as part of an ongoing, daily activity. Eventually, the billing department uses the codes to submit bills to insurance companies and patients. The computer system stores this vast amount of data and makes them available for reuse for a variety of purposes. The following sections examine the different types of information systems in detail.

Operation Support Systems

When ISs are used to process data created and used by business operations, they are referred to as **operation support systems.** The role of an operations support system is to efficiently process business transactions, support communication and collaboration among business units, and update business databases (O'Brien, 2002, 26). A registration, admission, discharge, and transfer (R-ADT) system is an example of an operation support systems. It is used to process data created and used for the registration, admission, discharge, and transfer of patients. Outputs of an R-ADT system would include the daily admission, census, and discharge reports.

Transaction–Processing System

A **transaction-processing system (TPS)** is an example of an operations support system. A TPS manages the different kinds of transactions that occur in a healthcare facility. Patient admissions, employee time cards, and supply purchases are examples of transactions that take place in a healthcare facility.

The characteristics of a TPS include the following:

- Inputs and outputs: Examples include patient admissions, discharges, and transfers.

- Users: The users of a TPS are mainly lower-level managers who make daily operational decisions.

- Products: These are detailed reports on transactions. A dictation-monitoring system reports the number of dictated events by type and by physician. A transcription supervisor can see how much work is left to do, what each transcriptionist has done, and other important data that can be used to determine how many transcriptionists are needed, how much overtime is required to handle the workload, and so on.

- Support MISs and DSSs (discussed below): For example, the database for the ADT transaction system in a hospital supports higher-level decision-making support systems. The ADT system does this by interfacing the daily number of transactions with software that can calculate average daily census, average length of stay, percentage of occupancy, and bed turnover rates.

Enterprise Collaboration Systems

Enterprise collaboration systems are another type of operations support system. These systems typically enhance teamwork and are sometimes called office automation systems. Examples include electronic mail and appointment scheduling, project management software to coordinate tasks and schedules, and videoconferencing systems to hold electronic meetings.

Enterprise-wide System

An enterprise-wide system is a large IS that manages data for an entire healthcare business. It helps automate information at the point of service, supports patient care, and analyzes clinical practices for outcome and cost improvements. An example of an enterprise-wide system is PeopleSoft. PeopleSoft is a product that allows an organization to perform activities such as:

- Human resource management
- Financial management
- Supply chain planning
- Sales and logistics

Management Support Information Systems

Information systems that provide information primarily to support manager decision making are called **management support information systems.** Three major information systems fall into this category: management information systems (MIS), decision support systems (DSS) and executive information systems (EIS).

Management Information System

An MIS is supported by TPS data to help middle managers make decisions about their departments' objectives. The features of an MIS include the following:

- Example inputs of an MIS include admission, discharge, and transfer data; dictated reports; coded records; filed records; and incomplete records. Examples of the outputs include structured reports, production schedules, and productivity analysis.

- The users of an MIS include middle managers, such as directors of HIM departments.

- The products of the system include summary, exception, periodic, and on-demand reports. An exception report, for example, might be a monthly report that lists the percentage of incomplete records by clinical department specialty.

Decision Support System

A DSS provides information to help users make accurate decisions. To the healthcare provider, this means using a product that goes beyond supplying facts about a patient's medical condition. For example, a clinical DSS is a special type of DSS that helps a provider make decisions about patient care. It may alert the physician when a lab result is outside the normal range, for instance.

Moreover, reminders help physicians comply with clinical practice guidelines in the management of certain disease processes, such as diabetes mellitus. In addition, DSSs are used to link physicians via the World Wide Web to clinical knowledge databases. One such database is the National Library of Medicine, which enables physicians to search the literature to learn about the latest research. Top management also uses DSSs in planning for the future.

The general characteristics of a DSS include the following:

- The inputs and outputs of a DSS include summarized reports, transaction data, and perhaps external data such as the ORYX performance measurement data developed by the Joint Commission on Accreditation of Healthcare Organizations (JCAHO).

- The users of a DSS include top and middle managers and clinicians. Information from the system can help users make decisions about unexpected, and sometimes isolated, problems.

- The products of a DSS include analytic models. Analytic models are mathematical interpretations of real systems such as pharmacy drug inventory systems. They help users manage inventory, predict customer needs, and make informed business decisions.

Executive Information System

An executive information system (EIS) is an easy-to-use DSS made especially for top managers. Several databases are attached to this type of system, including external operations, internal operations, and special management. These databases allow senior executives to project trends in the healthcare organization's services using what-if scenarios. An EIS provides summarized information on every aspect of the organization's work.

Other Information systems

Several other types of information systems may support a healthcare facility's operations or decision making. Examples of these include expert systems and knowledge management systems.

An expert system is a knowledge system built from a set of rules applied to specific problems. It can take the place of a human expert when it comes to problem solving. The system simulates the reasoning process of human experts in certain well-defined areas. "Knowledge engineers interview the expert or experts and determine the rules and knowledge that must go into the system. Programs incorporate not only surface knowledge ('textbook knowledge') but also deep knowledge ('tricks of the trade')" (Hutchinson and Sawyer 2000, 11.19).

Dr. Larry Weed's "knowledge coupler" system (Weed 1991) is an example of an expert system applied to the practice of internal medicine. Much of the knowledge built into the system comes from his experience as a practicing physician as well as from common medical theory. Expert systems are discussed in more detail in chapters 17 and 18.

A knowledge management system (KMS) is a more recent type of information system that has the potential to increase work effectiveness. This type of system supports the creation, organization, and dissemination of business or clinical knowledge and expertise to providers, employees, and managers throughout the healthcare enterprise.

A KMS is usually composed of an electronic library or central repository of best practices that offers enhanced search capabilities. Information is organized by specific business domain in the electronic library. Employees can access the electronic library through the **Internet** or an **extranet** to search for information. KMSs also use special software that enables employees to collaborate in teams to use or add to the knowledge in the electronic library.

An example of a KMS is one developed at Partners Healthcare in Boston. This system integrates the clinical database and patient electronic records and embeds drug information into the physician order-entry process. Using this type of system, the physician is alerted to potential drug interactions before an order is processed. This system has reportedly reduced medication errors by 55 percent (Davenport and Glaser 2002).

Check your understanding 16.2

Instructions: Match the type of information system with the scenario in which it would be used.

a.   Transaction-processing system
b.   Management information system
c.   Executive information system
d.   Expert system
e.   Decision support system

1.   _____ Dr. J is treating a patient with a rare disease. He enters the patient's signs and symptoms into a computer program that indicates the probability of the correct diagnosis with its treatment regime. The doctor then uses this information to determine the best treatment protocol for the patient.

2.   _____ Every week, an HIM department director receives statistical information on the number of incomplete medical records for discharged patients. Summary reports show totals and trends by the physician responsible for completing each patient record.

3.   _____ Dr. J orders a series of lab tests on his patient with a rare disease. The computer-generated results signal several abnormal values. This prompts the physician to add three new medications to the patient's treatment protocol. The computer then reminds Dr. J that serious drug interactions could occur when the new medications are combined with the original drug protocol. In response to this reminder, he stops the order for the new medications.

4.   _____ The HIM department director receives daily reports on the number of new admissions to, and discharges from, the hospital.

Development of Information Systems

Information systems must be created in a logical manner. The system development life cycle (SDLC) is the traditional way to plan and implement an IS in an organization. The four major phases of the cycle are planning and analysis, design, implementation, and maintenance. Figure 16.1 shows the twelve steps of the cycle.

Figure 16.1.   Steps in the system development life cycle

1. Request for development	7. Development of system documentation
2. Requirements and system analysis	8. User training
3. System design	9. System conversion
4. Specification of functions	10. Operation of the system
5. Coding of computer programs	11. System maintenance
6. Testing of system	12. System changes and upgrades

Planning and Analysis Phase

The planning and analysis phase of the SDLC process involves performing a systems analysis. It is very likely that the HIM professional will be involved in the planning and analysis phase of systems development. HITs may participate in this phase as end users who identify necessary functions of a new or existing IS. If the system is part of the HIM department, the HIT may be a member of the HIM team that determines the costs and benefits of the new system and prepares a report that justifies proceeding with analysis and design of the new system. Therefore, it is important that the HIT be familiar with the various steps in the systems development life cycle.

The systems analysis defines the whats of the project. The whats are based on asking some of the following questions:

- What are the current healthcare business practices?

- Which current organizational structure of the healthcare organization will be using this product?

- What are the project's schedule and budgetary constraints?

- What training methodologies are used currently in the healthcare organization?

- What are the users' needs for this project?

- What system interfaces are used in this project (for example, user interfaces, system-to-system interfaces, and so on)?

- What legal issues are involved with this project (for example, patient confidentiality, physicians' signatures, and so on)?

How do systems analysts collect information about the requirements for an IS project? Several methods are available to them. One very useful method for collecting data is to review existing documentation, forms, and databases. In the healthcare industry, paper forms are vital tools in understanding healthcare processes.

Another useful method is to do research and make site visits. Systems analysts must observe the work environment and learn how forms are used in the organization. The users of an IS can be invaluable to analysts. Users know their jobs well and can help analysts determine the system's requirements. Users sometimes even teach analysts how to do the jobs in question. This enables the analysts to understand the processes in question firsthand.

Conducting a joint application development (JAD) session is a valuable technique used to identify the goals, objectives, and required functions of a proposed IS. A JAD session is made up of a group of end users, system analysts, and technical development professionals who are brought together to analyze the strengths and weaknesses of the current IS and to propose functionalities for the new system. It is very likely that an HIT will participate as an end user in a JAD session.

A trained facilitator conducts the JAD session, which usually spans a period of several days. The session is held away from the organizational campus in a specially prepared meeting room so that participants will not be distracted or interrupted. At the conclusion of the

JAD session, the essential functions of a new IS have been identified. The strength of the JAD method is that end users, analysts, and developers are brought together to collaborate in analysis of the IS. This allows for the free exchange and input of information among all concerned groups. The premise underlying JAD is that a group of individuals working together at the same time can perform an analysis faster and better than individuals working independently.

Prototyping is another analysis technique. A prototype is a model or example of what a completed IS may look like. Prototyping a system allows for maximum end-user input while speeding up the analysis and development process. End users and analysts work together to develop the external features of the IS, such as input screens and reports. These external features provide the look and feel of the proposed system but do not include actual program application codes that would make the IS work. The strength of the prototyping method is that it allows the end user to critique the functionalities of the system before time and expense are put into programming efforts. When the basic functionality of the system is prototyped, developers and computer programmers can develop application program codes and databases to support the new system.

As the systems analyst collects data for the IS project, he or she needs a way to document the system's requirements in an easy-to-use graphical manner. Many graphical techniques are available to assist systems analysts. One technique is the **unified modeling language (UML).** The UML is an object-oriented modeling language that assists in the documentation of a software project. It is used by companies around the world and became a standard in 1997. An HIT will not likely develop the diagrams discussed below; however, a general knowledge of the process is helpful in helping the HIT understand how a systems analyst might document end-user requirements.

Using UML, a systems analyst can use two diagrams to document the functions of an information system:

- A **use case diagram** captures the functions of a system from a user's point of view.

- A **sequence diagram** captures the interaction among different pieces of an IS.

Use Case Diagram

In a use case situation, the systems analyst works with the user to document the IS requirements. Figure 16.2 shows an example of a use case diagram.

A use case diagram consists of two parts: an actor and the use case itself. The **actor** is the role the user plays in the system. For example, the actor may represent the role of a principal user of the system (for example, a physician) or the role of a secondary user (for example, an administrator who handles the system's maintenance functions). In addition, it

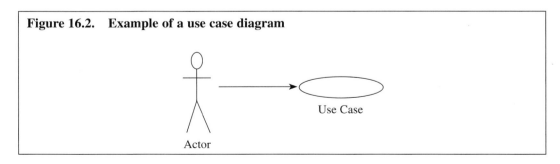

Figure 16.2.   Example of a use case diagram

may represent another system that interacts with the main system. An example of another system could be a COBOL program running on a **mainframe** or another program providing health data to the system.

The use case part of the diagram represents a function of the system. For example, the function may be to add a patient, search for a patient, or remove a patient. The use case diagram shows the interaction between the actor and functions of the system but does not show the interaction between the actor and the system itself.

Sequence Diagram

A sequence diagram or a sequence table is a tool the systems analyst can use to document the interaction between the actor and the system. Figure 16.3 shows examples of a use case diagram, a sequence diagram, and a sequence table.

The use case diagram shows the interaction between a physician and the function of searching patient data. The sequence diagram uses arrows to show the interaction between actor and system over time. The sequence table shows how the interaction between actor and system unfolds in a tabular format. The elements of a sequence table include the following:

- Use case name: Identifies the function by name (in this case, search patient data)

- Description: Defines the purpose of the use case

- Successful course: Describes the steps in a successful interaction between actor and use case

- Unsuccessful course: Describes an unsuccessful interaction between actor and use case

- Precondition: Describes any use case(s) the user must follow before going to the use case

- Postcondition: Describes any use case(s) the user must follow after going to the use case

- Assumptions: Describes any assumptions made during the use case

The systems analyst creates as many use cases as he or she thinks the system should have. Basically, the systems analyst decides when all functions are defined in the system. Each use case and sequence diagram or sequence table provides the basis for the requirements document. This document fully describes the system's requirements and, if required, also includes the project's schedule and budget.

Design Phase

When the analysis phase has been completed and IS functions identified, the system must be designed. The systems design describes the system's hows. The hows of the project are based on asking some of the following questions:

- How do the actors interact with the system? What do the user interfaces look like?

- How do the data collected in the use cases relate to each other? What are the logical and physical data models for this project?

Figure 16.3.   Example of a complete use case with sequence diagram and sequence table

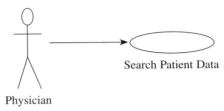

Search Patient Data

Physician

a. Use Case Diagram

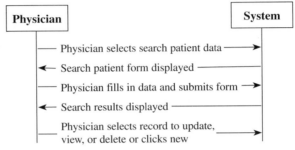

b. Sequence Diagram

Use Case Name	Search Patient Data
Description	Allows the user to search for a patient

Successful Course	1. User clicks on link for search patient data
	2. The system displays a form to input the data
	    Last name
	    First name
	    or
	    Social Security number
	3. The user fills in data and submits the form
	4. The system displays the search results
	5. The user selects a record to update, view, or delete or selects new

Unsuccessful Course	1. User clicks on link for search patient data 2. The system displays a form to input the data 3. The user submits the form 4. The system displays no data for search results; user can select to create a new record
Precondition	Authentication
Postcondition	Add a patient, modify a patient, delete a patient, or view a patient
Assumptions	N/A

c. Sequence Table

- How do the pieces of the system interact with each other? What does the solutions model look like?

- How do you code this project? What languages, databases, and tools will be used in this project?

The systems designer works with the system's requirements and the systems analysts to determine a model for the problem being analyzed. He or she may use several models, including an object design or logical design, a physical design, and **screen prototypes.** The choice of design depends on the use cases created earlier. The use cases provide a function-by-function analysis of the system. The system's design combines similar use cases into a model.

The IS design can be compared to a blueprint of a house. The blueprint tells the contractor how the house should be built; the IS design, including all the models developed by the systems analysts, tells the programmers and database administrators how to develop the information system.

Implementation Phase

After the system's design is done, it is given to the programmers to code. This is the implementation phase. The programmers must make a working application from the user requirements and design. The systems analysts and designers work with the programmers throughout the process.

Another part of the implementation phase is testing. At the basic level, there are unit testing and systems testing. Unit testing occurs when the programmers test their own code; **systems testing** is performed by an organization that is independent of the project team. The independent organization's job is to look for **bugs** (problems) in the software and to make the software stable for use. It is very likely that an HIT will participate in systems testing, particularly when the IS is part of the HIM department. For example, the HIT may be asked to put test data into the new IS, such as an electronic master patient index, and determine whether the system provides the expected output.

Systems testers test the use cases against the system's requirements. If a requirement fails, the tester reports the problem to the programmers. The programmers then fix the problem and complete their report. Based on this report, the testers retest the requirement until it passes.

After systems testing, training and system documentation begin. Users attend training sessions to learn how the IS works. Technical writers work on user documentation.

Maintenance Phase

The maintenance phase begins after the testing has validated all the system's requirements. This phase consists of operating the system and working with users on any problems that occur. Depending on severity, the maintenance team fixes the problems and runs the changes. The maintenance phase is really a help desk, where systems analysts, designers, and programmers answer users' questions and work on any problems the users find while operating the system.

Check your understanding 16.3

Instructions: Choose the best answer to complete the following statements.

1. _____ The systems development life cycle (SDLC) _____.
   a. Is the traditional way to plan and implement an IS
   b. Takes at least three years to complete
   c. Is primarily transaction oriented
   d. Is a never-ending process

2. _____ The first phase of the SDLC is the _____ phase.
   a. Design
   b. Planning and analysis
   c. Implementation
   d. Maintenance

3. _____ End-user requirements are identified in the _____ phase of the SDLC.
   a. Design
   b. Planning and analysis
   c. Implementation
   d. Maintenance

4. _____ The method(s) used to identify requirements for a proposed IS is(are) _____.
   a. Conducting site visits
   b. Conducting a JAD
   c. Developing a prototype
   d. All of the above

5. _____ Testing the new IS system is part of the _____ phase.
   a. Design
   b. Planning and analysis
   c. Implementation
   d. Maintenance

Information Technology

Information technology (IT) can encompass a wide range of topics. This section examines the basic functions of the hardware and software used in information systems.

Categories of Computers

Even though they perform basically the same functions, computers come in various size categories. The different-size computers are discussed in the following subsections.

Supercomputers
Supercomputers are the fastest and highest-capacity machines built today. They can cost millions of dollars and are used in large-scale activities such as weather forecasting and mathematical research. The fastest computer in the world is located at Los Alamos Laboratory in New Mexico.

Mainframe Systems
Mainframes were the only computers available until the late 1960s. They can perform millions of instructions per second, and hundreds of users can be connected at the same

time. Mainframe systems vary in size from middle to large capacity, depending on the number of concurrent stations they serve. They are generally used in healthcare to handle input/output-intensive transactions.

Most hospitals use mainframes dating back to the 1960s and 1970s to store payroll, personnel, billing, and accounting data. The challenge for today's systems engineers is to interface newer technologies for clinical information systems with the older legacy systems stored within the mainframes.

Midrange Systems

There are two types of midrange systems: minicomputers and workstations. **Minicomputers** were introduced in the 1960s and can support up to 4,000 connected users at the same time via terminals consisting of a keyboard and a video screen. They are cheaper than mainframes.

A more recent introduction in the 1980s was the workstation. A **workstation** is a very powerful desktop computer used mainly by power users such as graphics specialists for multimedia production. Workstations are comparable to midsize mainframes but sit on a desktop. They also may be used as servers to microcomputers connected through a network.

Microcomputers

Microcomputers, also called personal computers (PCs), were introduced in the early 1970s and are the fastest-growing type of computer today. They come in a variety of sizes, including desktop, laptop, palmtop, and pen-based. Microcomputers can be used in a stand-alone environment or connected to a network.

Web Appliances

Web appliances are used in conjunction with the Internet. One device sits on top of a television and allows the user to surf the Internet using a remote control device. Web appliances have no processing unit or storage device. Their main purpose is Web navigation.

Computer Peripherals

The different pieces of hardware that are connected to central processing units (CPUs) to make them more functional and user-friendly are called peripherals. **Peripherals** are usually described in terms of the five basic computer functions: input, processing and memory, output, storage, and communications.

Input Devices

Input devices include keyboards; microphones; scanners; pointing devices such as "mice," trackballs, light pens, and intelligent tablets; sensors; and biometrics such as fingerprints, handprints, and iris scans. Sensors are important in healthcare because they can read a patient's physiological data and transmit them to a computer database. A common example is the use of monitoring systems in critical care units.

The selection of the appropriate type of input device for an IS depends on the user's work flow. If the user moves around a lot (as a nurse does, for example), an input device that allows data entry while moving from place to place is ideal. Headsets with speech input are often used in a mobile work environment.

Output Devices

Output devices include printers, monitors, and speakers.

Storage Devices

Secondary storage devices include a floppy disk drive, a hard disk drive, magnetic tape, and an optical disk drive. The drives may be internal or external. Digital data can be stored permanently on any of these media, although the life span of each medium varies.

Optical storage allows for extremely large quantities of data to be stored on one CD. This medium is very useful for storing image and sound data and has the longest life span of secondary storage media.

Communications Devices

Communications devices are used to assist communications among different computers. Modems translate digital data into analog data so that the data can be transmitted over telephone lines and received by a remote computer. At the receiving end, the modems reverse the process by turning the analog signal back to digital.

Transmission speeds are very important to the transmission of data. They are expressed in terms of bits per second (bps) or kilobits per second (kbps). Many phone lines max out at 28.8 kbps. Thus, even though the user may have a 56K modem, the rate of transmission will still be 28.8K. Newer technologies in communications include integrated services digital network (ISDN) lines that allow digital data to be transmitted through copper wire telephone lines. This is a dedicated line that can be very costly compared to normal telephone service, but it is five times faster than the fastest modem.

Another recently developed technology is the asymmetric digital subscriber line (ADSL). This is thought to be the successor to the ISDN and also functions on standard telephone lines.

Cable modems are connected through TV cable lines. This technology is faster than ADSL. Cable modems can download data in a million bits per second (mbps).

Finally, satellite dishes offer the fastest transmission. Clients subscribe through a service provider, but it is a wireless connection. DirectPC is an example of such a service.

Trends in Technology

From the preceding discussion, it is obvious that the future will be faster and more adaptable to a variety of work environments. According to the February 2000 issue of Healthcare Informatics, some of the hot technology trends include increasing the use of wireless technology: "For example, many organizations are fielding in-house cellular phone systems to replace nurse call buttons" (DeJesus 2000, 67). Another example is the use of wireless graphic data transmission that permits clinicians to see both text and pictures. This is particularly useful in radiology.

According to the same article, another vision is the increased use of interactive technologies: "Continuous speech recognition, intelligent and optical character recognition, touch screen and multimedia technologies are poised for widespread adoption in the healthcare industry. . . . Voice-controlled robotic operating equipment from Santa Barbara, Calif.-based Computer Motion allows surgeons to dim the lights, move the camera closer or adjust the height of an operating table without relying on the scrub nurse" (DeJesus 2000, 70).

The October 16, 2000 Washington Post reported that software developers are working diligently to refine talking computers:

Boston-based SpeechWorks is one of a number of companies with its sights on a far broader landscape: The now text-centered global computer network. . . . SpeechWorks founded six years ago, is one of a group of companies producing the building blocks for the voice boom. Using a "voice recognition engine" that breaks words into digital bits and matches them with words in a database, it already has launched automated services for several major companies, including United Airlines and Federal Express. . . . But if voice on the Internet is suddenly fashionable, it has its share of skeptics.

"That promise has been out there for 20 years," scoffed Thomas J. Trimneer, vice president of data product development at AT&T Wireless, one of the nation's largest mobile telephone carriers. "If you have a high voice, a low voice, if you have an accent, if you have a lot of ambient noise, voice recognition doesn't work." Despite the criticism, most experts believe that the future of the net will contain both text and speech (Goodman 2000).

Computer Software

To make all these fantastic devices work, the equipment must use a set of instructions called software. The software programs (or directs) the hardware components to perform the tasks required of them. The earliest computers required rewiring to perform tasks. The next step involved punch cards to feed instructions to the computer. Today, there are two basic types of software: system and application.

System Software

In an orchestra, the different musical instruments are played in complete synchronization. How does this happen? A composer writes a set of instructions for each instrument using the language of music. In a sense, a computer programmer is a composer except that the programmer writes a set of instructions for computer hardware. Like the conductor guiding the orchestra through a musical composition, the system software acts as the conductor for all the hardware components and the application software. Without system software, nothing would happen.

System software has three basic pieces. These are discussed in the following subsections.

Operating System
The **operating system** "consists of the master programs, called the supervisor, that manage the basic operations of the computer. These programs reside in RAM [random access memory] while the computer is on and provide resource management services of many kinds; for example, they run and store other programs and store and process data. The operating system includes BIOS (the basic input/output system), which manages the essential peripherals such as the keyboard, screen disk drives, and parallel and serial ports" (Hutchinson and Sawyer 2000, 5.4–5.5).

Common microcomputer operating systems include DOS (disk operating system), Windows 2000, and earlier versions—OS/2, Unix, and Macintosh.

Utility Programs
Utility programs "are generally used to support, enhance, or expand existing programs in a computer system" (Hutchinson and Sawyer 2000, 5.8). Examples of utilities include:

- Backup processes that store data in more than one location

- Virus protection that prevents computer catastrophes

- Data recovery that prevents the loss of data in the event of physical or software accidents

Language Translator

The **language translator** "is software that translates a program written by a programmer in a language such as C++ into **machine language,** which the computer can understand. All system software and applications software must be turned into machine language for execution by the computer" (Hutchinson and Sawyer 2000, 5.12). According to Hutchinson and Sawyer (2000, 10.15–10.16):

> Language translators are of three types: assemblers, compilers, [and] interpreters. **Assemblers** translate assembly-language programs into machine language. **Compilers** look at an entire high-level language program before translating it into machine language.
>
> **Interpreters** convert high-level language statements into machine language statements one at a time in succession. Unlike compilers, which must look at an entire program before converting it into machine language, interpreters provide programmers with immediate feedback regarding the accuracy of their coded instructions.

User interfaces are an important software support for an operating system because they determine how the user communicates with the computer. The DOS system, for example, uses a command-driven interface that requires instructions to be typed in at a command prompt. A second type of interface is the menu-driven approach. This approach allows the user to select choices using a mouse or some other non-keyboard pointer.

Presently, the **graphical user interface (GUI)** is the standard microcomputer interface. It operates on the basis of icons that represent different computer tasks and programs. The GUI allows for keyboard as well as point, click, and drag functions.

Application Software

Application software can be categorized into four different types:

- **Productivity software** products are used in almost all businesses to assist with word processing, accounting, database management, graphics presentations, scheduling, e-mail, time management, and other functions performed in offices and homes.

- **Specialty software** includes programs designed for a specific industry. For example, in health information management, encoders are designed to accelerate the medical coding process. Other types of specialty software in other industries include multimedia authoring, desktop publishing, and CAD/CAM products.

- Education and reference software includes encyclopedias, anatomy atlases, and library searches. One very successful library search program is Medline, which is offered through the Internet site of the National Library of Medicine.

- Entertainment software includes games and audio/video entertainment.

Programming Languages

Software programmers who write instructions to the computer use highly specialized languages. The relative ease with which people can interact with and instruct computers has progressed dramatically—from very difficult hardwiring instructions to the use of natural languages.

Since they were introduced in 1945, **programming languages** have gone through five generations of development, including:

1. **Machine languages:** The first generation of programming languages, machine language, consisted of ones and zeros.

2. **Assembly languages:** The second generation, assembly language, used a standard set of abbreviations to replace some of the ones and zeros of machine language.

3. High-level languages: High-level languages used words and arithmetic phrases to construct programs. Examples of third-generation languages include COBOL and BASIC.

4. Very high-level languages: The fourth generation of programming languages included report generators, query languages, and application generators. These languages were easy to use and required fewer commands to execute programs. **SQL (structured query language)** is an example of a fourth-generation language.

5. **Natural languages:** Natural programming languages allow users to speak in a more conversational way with the computer and are part of the expanding field of **artificial intelligence** (AI). "One of the most successful natural language systems is LUNAR, developed to help users analyze the rocks brought back from the moon" (Hutchinson and Sawyer 2000, 13.14). AI is used widely to develop expert systems that help physicians manage patient care, telemedicine, teleradiography, and other e-health and telemedicine activities.

Check your understanding 16.4

Instructions: Indicate whether the following statements are true or false (T or F).

1. _____ Computer peripherals such as mouses, printers, and monitors control the computer's operating system.

2. _____ Common utility programs include virus checkers, backup, and recovery.

3. _____ An interpreter program must look at an entire program before beginning its translation into machine language.

4. _____ DOS stands for disk operating standard.

5. _____ The user communicates with the computer through an interface (Windows, for example).

6. _____ Machine languages use a standard set of abbreviations to replace some of the ones and zeros used in assembly language.

7. _____ The increasing use of wireless technology is one of the hottest technology trends today.

8. _____ Artificial intelligence is one type of natural programming language.

9. _____ Education and reference software is one category of application software.

10. _____ The three basic pieces of system software are the operating system, the language translator, and the utility program.

Database Management

The most critical resource in healthcare is patient data. The most important functions of any healthcare information system involve being able to create, modify, delete, and view patient data. And the most important storage mechanism used to perform these functions is a database. As discussed in chapter 4, databases are essential in the development of EHR systems.

A **database** is an organized collection of data saved as a binary-type file on a computer. Users cannot read a binary-type file because it contains only ones and zeros. A database management system provides the ability to perform the functions mentioned earlier. Many different kinds of database management system vendors are available in the marketplace, including Oracle, SQL Server, Sybase, and Access.

Database Approach

Today, three main types of databases are available: relational databases, object-oriented databases, and object-relational databases.

A **relational database** stores data in predefined tables that contain rows and columns similar to a spreadsheet. The kinds of data that can be stored in a relational database are currency, real numbers, integers, and strings (characters of data). This type of database is a popular model used in healthcare applications.

An **object-oriented database** stores objects of data. An **object** is a discrete or abstract thing such as a car or a line at the grocery store. Data objects can model relational data or advanced **data types** such as graphics, movies, and audio.

Finally, the **object-relational database** combines the best of the relational and object-oriented databases. It uses both traditional data types (such as currency, integers, and strings) and advanced data types (such as graphics, movies, audio, and so on).

Database Activities

The purpose of a database is to store and retrieve data. All database vendors use a common language called structured query language (SQL) to store and retrieve data. SQL gives the information system the ability to query and report on data and to insert, update, and delete data from the database.

Some database vendors include their own development tools to create a complete system with such development as report generators. Some database management system vendors include a report generator that allows a user or programmer to create reports from the data in the database.

Relational databases perform the following activities:

- Store data in tables consisting of rows and columns. Figure 16.4 shows the hierarchy of data in a relational database. A column consists of a name and a data type (the kind of data being stored in the column). A row in a table consists of data values in the various columns. A row would be the values of these columns, such as "John" for the first name and "Smith" for the last name.

- Reduce redundancy in tables. If a table were created in Excel, some data would be duplicated.

- Retrieve and store data in tables using SQL to insert, update, delete, and query data from tables.

- Provide a level of security, usually by user and by table and column that each user is allowed to access. In healthcare systems, access to health records must be limited to only certain users in order to protect patient privacy.

A table is a two-dimensional structure made up of rows and columns. Table 16.1 shows an example of a table that stores information about a patient.

A **column/field** is a basic fact such as LAST_NAME, FIRST_NAME, DOB, RACE. A **row/record** is a set of columns or a collection of related data items. An example of a row in the PATIENTS table is: Smith, Keith, 2/13/70, White.

A **key field** uniquely identifies each row in a table. There are two types of keys:

- **Primary keys** ensure that each row in a table is unique. A primary key must not change in value. Typically, a primary key is a number that is a one-up counter or a randomly generated number in large databases. A number is used because a number processes faster than an alphanumeric character. In large tables, this makes a difference. In the PATIENTS table, the PATIENT_ID is the primary key. It is good programming practice to create a primary key that is independent of the data in a table.

- A **foreign key** is a column of one table that corresponds to a primary key in another table. Together, they allow two tables to join together.

The cancer registry is an example of a health record database that can be computerized. A manual registry is already organized logically by site of the neoplasm. Imagine

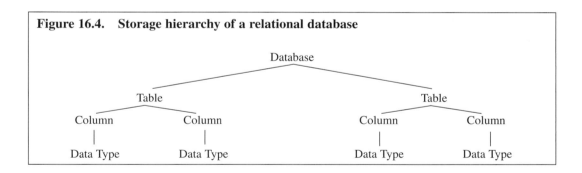

Figure 16.4. Storage hierarchy of a relational database

Table 16.1. Example of a PATIENTS table

PATIENT_ID	LAST_NAME	FIRST_NAME	DOB	RACE	DOCTOR_ID
1	Smith	Keith	2/13/70	White	1
2	Roberts	Debbie	7/30/70	Black	1
3	Morrison	Rebecca	2/4/99	White	1
4	James	Sally	7/29/50	Black	1

that a two-drawer file cabinet is being used for the cancer registry. The entire file cabinet is considered the database. The first drawer contains a set of abstracts by site of the neoplasm. Within each file folder are the abstracts or records kept on each patient. Each record contains a collection of data fields or facts about the patient.

The second file drawer is organized by month. Each month is one file folder. Within each month's folder are the cases that need to be followed for that month. Each case is considered a record. Within each record are the necessary pieces of information, or data fields, required to contact the patient and update the medical data.

In a computerized IS, each case is stored in one table and each patient is stored in another table. Case and patient have to be related to each other so that the user can look up the case and also locate the patient information. For example, if the cases were stored in a CASES table (with a primary key of CASE_ID) and the patients were stored in a PATIENTS table (with a primary key of PATIENT_ID), a foreign key would be needed to relate the case to the patient. If the patient were to have many cases, a foreign key of PATIENT_ID would have to be located in the CASES table in order to create the one-to-many relationship. Thus, when a user queries a case, he or she can easily use the foreign key PATIENT_ID to find the patient information.

To be able to use a database, the user first must create a database structure (the definitions of the tables, columns, and keys) and then insert, update, or delete data in the database. SQL is the language used to create the database structure as well as to store and manipulate the data.

One technique to describe the structure of a database is to use a data dictionary. (See table 16.2.) A data dictionary is the equivalent of a detailed road map of the database. Maintaining the data dictionary frequently is an HIM function. A data dictionary is essential in ensuring consistent definitions of what data names mean and making sure that data are accurate. A data dictionary is essential in the development of EHR systems. A good dictionary defines each data field or column according to the following information:

- Name of computer
- Type of data field
- Length of data field
- Edits placed on the data field
- Values allowed to be placed in the data field
- A clear definition of each value

The data fields themselves usually evolve from a predetermined data set, such as the Universal Hospital Discharge Data Set or the UB-92.

Data sets are typically developed by groups of people who have a legitimate use for collecting the data. The purpose of carefully defining a data set is to help ensure the accuracy of the data collected and the usefulness of the statistics obtained from the collection of the data. HITs can play a vital role in the development of data sets and data dictionaries. Their involvement will help healthcare organizations to create clear and nonredundant electronic patient records in the future.

Table 16.2. Sample data dictionary	
Data Element	**Variables (Attributes)**
Sex	Male, female
Race	American Indian Alaskan Native Asian or Pacific Islander African American White
Ethnicity	Hispanic origin (not Hispanic)
Type of provider practice	Solo practice Group practice Hospital Neighborhood health center Other
Place of encounter	Private office Clinic or health center Hospital outpatient department Hospital emergency department Other
Disposition	No follow-up planned Follow-up planned Return when necessary Return to the current provider Telephone follow-up Return to referring provider Referred to other provider Admit to acute care hospital Admit to residential healthcare facility Other
Principal source of payment	Workers' compensation Medicare Medicaid CHAMPUS CHAMPVA Blue Cross/Blue Shield Private or commercial insurance Prepaid group practice Medical foundation Self-pay No charge Other
Living arrangement (optional)	Alone With spouse or unrelated partner With children With parent or guardian With relative other than spouse, children, or parents With nonrelatives Unknown

Databases and Client Server Computing

Database management systems (DBMSs) fall into two categories: a personal DBMS, which runs on a client; and a server-based DBMS, which runs on a server.

Personal DBMS

A personal DBMS is used for small projects such as storing contact information (for example, in a personal address book). It should not be used for systems that require large amounts of storage and 24/7 access. Most healthcare systems would not use a personal DBMS. Personal DBMSs are tempting to use because (1) they are inexpensive and (2) most people already have access to one with an office software package such as Microsoft Office. Microsoft Access only supports a few gigabytes of storage. Today, databases span terabytes of storage. These types of databases require the use of a server-based DBMS.

Server-Based DBMS

A server-based database management system runs on a server computer. It also runs as a separate application from a personal system. This allows the DBMS to run faster and more efficiently than the personal DBMS. A question might take minutes to answer on a personal DBMS, but only seconds on a server-based DBMS. Examples of a server-based DBMS are Oracle, SQL Server, Sybase, and Informix. A server-based DBMS also allows data to be retrieved by multiple end users. Such a database system is essential in an EHR system.

Server-based database management systems provide support for 24/7 access with large amounts of storage in the terabyte range or higher. They are very expensive compared to personal database management systems.

Data Warehouses

Today, most organizations use multiple databases in their daily business operations. **Data warehouses** provide organizations with the ability to access data from multiple databases and to combine the results into a single question-and-reporting interface. Chapter 4 discussed how data warehouses (sometimes referred to as data repositories) are necessary for EHR systems. Figure 16.5 shows how a data warehouse is organized.

Typically, different databases are used in a healthcare organization to serve different functions. Some store patient data, and others store lab results. In some cases, these databases are separate from each other. A data warehouse is able to take data from the DBMS and store them in an intermediary format that any user can use. The user then can create specific reports and queries on data that might be useful in making a decision. For example, cost data are very important in determining the right costs to charge patients.

The November 1999 issue of Health Management Technology offers an example of how a data warehouse is used. The director of data warehousing practice at Sysix Technologies, located in Oakbrook, Illinois, created a data warehouse to document the effectiveness of a disease management program. He did this using questions such as: Do DASI scores improve more for patients on a program that lasts more than ninety days, or do the improvements level off after sixty days?

Organizations can use information from data warehouses to determine whether programs are working and to tailor them to better meet patient needs. This gives such organizations a competitive edge in the marketplace.

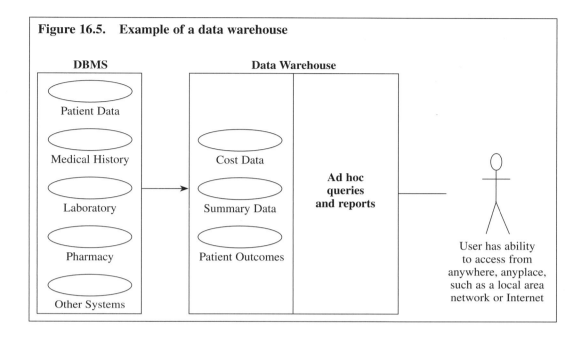

Figure 16.5. Example of a data warehouse

Telecommunications and the Internet

The 1990s experienced tremendous growth in the areas of telecommunications and the Internet. Advances in telecommunications systems allowed data to be transmitted over telephone lines. These advances made connecting to the Internet faster and more efficient.

Role of Telecommunications

Telecommunications is the term used to describe voice and data communications within an organization. It is fast becoming a central and critical aspect of any healthcare organization. Telecommunications provides the technology infrastructure that enables people in any type of organization to talk with each other using a telephone, access a database, and send e-mail to each other using a computer.

In a healthcare organization, the efficiency of the technology infrastructure sometimes means life or death for patients. Thus, a properly designed technology infrastructure is needed to provide instant and highly reliable access to data with 24/7 security.

Network Fundamentals

To understand the nature of a computer network, it is important to first understand the nature of communications systems. As shown in figure 16.6, every type of communications system is made up of four components:

- The transmitter is the device that sends information.

- The receiver is the device that receives information.

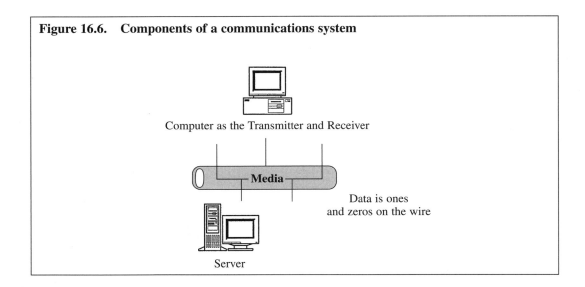

Figure 16.6.   Components of a communications system

- The medium is the mechanism that connects the transmitter to the receiver. It may be a cable (for example, the twisted-pair cable commonly used to connect workstations in an office building) or the air (in the case of cellular phone transmissions).

- Data create the message that is transferred from the transmitter to the receiver as electrical pulses.

One very common communications system is the telephone. The handset of a typical telephone acts as both transmitter and receiver. The cables and telephone wires that connect one telephone to another are the media. Voice signals, such as words and other sounds, are the data.

It is possible to create a specialized type of communication system by connecting one computer to another to form a network. The users of computers in the network then can share information and resources. In a computer network, a computer functions as both transmitter and receiver.

The specific type of communication that takes place on a computer network is often called data communication. Data communication involves transferring information in binary form, which is the electronic equivalent of ones and zeros. In addition to computers, a network can incorporate a variety of computer devices such as printers, fax modems, scanners, CD-ROM drives, tape backup units, and plotters. The collection of computers and devices that make up a network are sometimes called the network's resources.

The purpose of a **network** is to allow users to share its resources easily and efficiently. For example, any network user can access the network printer, not just the user sitting behind the computer to which the printer is attached.

Clients, Peers, and Servers

Network computers play one of two roles: client or server. **Clients** are computers that access shared resources. **Servers** are computers that share resources such as printers or hard-disk space across the network. For example, a user interacts with the client computer to request something from the network (for example, e-mail messages). The server responds by supplying the e-mail messages the user requested. People often refer to this interaction as the client–server relationship. (See figure 16.7.)

The term services refers to tasks that a network server performs, such as facilitating e-mail, Web, Internet, and printer connections; providing database access; performing backups; providing network communication; coordinating security; and managing files. The various services a server provides include:

- Application services that allow different pieces of application software to reside on a specialized type of server called an application server

- Communication services that allow different systems to communicate with each other

- E-mail services that permit the exchange of correspondence electronically

- Internet services that let users transfer files and other information via the Internet

- Web services that allow users to use a browser and a server to access the World Wide Web (a system of Internet servers that support specially formatted documents called Web pages, although some Internet servers are not part of the Web)

- Printer services that enable users to access a printer from anywhere on the network

- Database services that store and retrieve information such as accounting and financial data

- Backup services that routinely create backup copies of information

- Network management services that make it possible to manage network resources from a central location

- Security services that prevent unauthorized users from accessing the network

- File services that allow anyone with access to a server to store and retrieve files

Because network computers can act in only one of two roles, the peer-to-peer relationship is an extension of the client–server model. In a peer-to-peer relationship, a networked computer acts as both client and server.

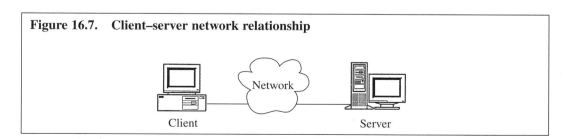

Figure 16.7.   Client–server network relationship

Network

Client   Server

Network Architectures

The way a computer network is set up is its basic design or architecture. There are two main types of network architectures: local-area networks and wide-area networks.

Local-Area Networks

The **local-area network (LAN)** connects computers in a relatively small area (for example, within one room or one building). It can take the form of a client–server network, a peer-to-peer network, or a hybrid network. A hybrid network is a mixture of client–server and peer-to-peer networks.

One special form of a LAN is an intranet. An **intranet** is a specialized client–server network that uses Internet technologies. Intranets let corporations supply Internet services over their LANs. Essentially, Intranets are private Internets with the security required to protect a corporation's assets. An extranet, on the other hand, provides network connectivity between suppliers to allow direct connection to each other's network.

Wide-Area Networks

The **wide-area network (WAN)** connects devices across a large geographical area (for example, across a state or even the world). WANs can take several forms but often simply consist of two or more LANs connected by telephone lines.

The world's largest public WAN is the Internet. The Internet consists of hundreds of thousands, if not millions, of interconnected LANs around the world. By connecting private LANs to the Internet, individuals and corporations can create a relatively inexpensive WAN. However, the Internet is a very insecure environment. Thus, LANs connected via the Internet may be subject to intrusion from unauthorized users.

Network Protocols

Network protocols enable computers on the network to communicate with each other. The computers have to use the same language, just as people have to speak the same language in order to understand each other. Network protocols provide computers with a common language.

The variety of network types, computers, operating systems, and browsers available today greatly complicates the exchange of information between computers. To facilitate this exchange, networks rely on some basic protocols, or rules, to govern the organization and transmission of data. Most protocols apply to three distinct phases of the data exchange process:

1. Connection setup phase: Just as a telephone uses ringing to request a connection to another telephone, a protocol must first initiate a connection between computers on the network.

2. Data transfer phase: After setting up the connection, the protocol allows the computers to transfer data. After the data are transmitted, the receiving computer decides whether to accept or reject them.

3. Connection release phase: After the data transfer is complete, the protocol allows the computers to terminate the connection.

Check your understanding 16.5

Instructions: Match the following terms with their definitions.

1. _____ Intranet

2. _____ World Wide Web

3. _____ Extranet

4. _____ LAN

5. _____ WAN

6. _____ Data warehouse

7. _____ Clients

8. _____ Telecommunications

9. _____ Relational database

10. _____ Data dictionary

a. Type of database that stores data in predefined tables made up of rows and columns
b. Storage device for multiple databases that can be accessed via a single question-and-report interface
c. Type of network that works as a private Internet
d. Computer network that connects devices in a small geographical area
e. System of Internet servers that supports specially formatted documents
f. Description of the structure of a specific database
g. Type of network that allows the networks of separate organizations to communicate with one another
h. Term used to describe a system of voice and data transmission
i. Computers that are used to access shared resources in a network
j. Computer network that connects devices across a large geographical area

Electronic Commerce Revolution in Healthcare

Electronic commerce (e-commerce) has revolutionized healthcare. Some e-commerce sites allow consumers to learn about the medicines they are taking, buy medicines over the Internet, learn about diseases and disease prevention, and so on. Some e-commerce sites enable phycians to learn about new procedures and practices and to keep up with the ever-changing nature of healthcare.

One site that is becoming prominent on the Internet is WebMD. WebMD describes its services this way:

> WebMD provides connectivity and a full suite of services to the healthcare industry that improve administrative efficiencies and clinical effectiveness enabling high-quality patient care. The company's products and services facilitate information exchange, communication, and transactions between the consumer, physician, and healthcare institutions. The company's technology head-quarters are located in Santa Clara, and its corporate headquarters are located in Atlanta. For more information, visit Webmed.com.

Another prominent site is CVS.com. This site allows people to refill prescriptions, learn about prescriptions, read about medical news, and so on.

Even insurance companies have an e-commerce presence on the Web. One healthcare organization that provides health information to its members is Kaiser Permanente at kaiser permanente.org. The Kaiser site provides information on prevention, diet, and health issues.

Electronic sites such as those mentioned above provide consumers with more information on their health and healthcare than they have had at any time in history. Consumers can learn about their diagnoses and find information on drugs and other issues that affect their healthcare.

Management of Information Technology

Information technology (IT) in the healthcare environment is essential for the delivery of patient care. The various types of IT discussed above are necessary for various departmental information systems and for EHR systems. Therefore, management of an organization's health information technology is extremely important.

How a healthcare organization manages its IT depends on a number of factors. Whether the IT considered is for a departmental system (pharmacy, HIM, laboratory, dietary, and so on), enterprise-wide system (R-ADT), or an EHR system, all the following factors are important to consider.

Structure of the Organization

As mentioned earlier, a good information system (IS) is critical to the overall healthy state of a healthcare organization. To achieve a healthy state, extensive planning must take place at every level of the organization. The HIT may be involved in helping to plan or administer an IS at the departmental level.

The type of IS an organization uses depends on its overall mission and strategic objectives. For example, a solo practitioner's office would have a very different mission than a community-based, large-scale healthcare enterprise trying to deliver a full array of healthcare products. Various organizational structures are covered in chapter 17.

Planning Phase

Planning is essential to an information system's success. The type of planning needed ensures that the organization's overall vision, IT priorities, dollars, and resources are in line. It would be a mistake for an organization to concentrate on using technology without first analyzing its business and clinical needs (Hoehn 1999, 25).

Evaluate Organizational Readiness

Evaluating organizational readiness is one of the first steps in managing change to an IS. It includes evaluating processes, user acceptance, and the technology infrastructure:

- Processes: It is important to identify the processes that will have the most impact on the organization. Focusing on those processes as priorities in the implementation phase is vital to the system's success.

- User acceptance: The users who were the early adopters of technology will play a significant role in ensuring the system's success. They should be selected as key players in the process-identification activity described above. In addition, they will be helpful in spreading information about the new system throughout the organization and ensuring its acceptance. Using **change management** techniques and providing training for new users are critical components in the planning phase.

- Technology infrastructure: Evaluating the technology infrastructure involves examining the existing software and hardware components at the enterprise, department, and desktop levels. Also included is evaluation of connectivity among applications, including both local- and wide-area network capability.

Identify Barriers to Change

According to Amatayakul, change management is "the formal process of introducing change, getting it adopted, and diffusing it through the organization" (1999, 241–42). Identifying the barriers to technology acceptance by future users is critical to the success of the project. Andrews and Stalick (2000) have identified four hurdles that affect acceptance of change:

1. Lack of cross-organizational commitment: Lack of user buy-in can ruin the best-laid plans.

2. Deliverable complexity: The more complex the change, the higher the probability of failure.

3. Environmental complexity: Transformation does not happen overnight. Usually, it is phased in over time and may require the temporary use of both old and new systems.

4. Unrealistic expectations: Users often believe that computers can accomplish miracles overnight. They must be taught to deal with frustration, ambiguity, and downtime while learning new ways to perform their tasks.

Some suggest that the secret to success is a team model (illustrated in figure 16.8) that includes the roles of executive sponsors, the project director, part-time project champions, project advisors (subject matter experts), and the core group.

In a healthcare organization, it is important to select highly respected professional specialists to be the project champions. These would be people who believe in the organization's vision and who can lead and persuade others within their specialty of the value and importance of the change.

Establish Policies and Procedures

Information systems must be controlled, and users must be controlled in their use of systems. Within healthcare, the confidentiality and security of the collected data are of utmost concern. (See chapter 14.) Experts agree that organizational policies and standards should be developed and maintained in the following areas:

- Identification, authentication, and certification: Standards in these areas should cover the use of hardware tokens, personal ID numbers, and other password systems that restrict access to a system.

- Authorization: Authorization standards should require that access be approved/granted by the information owner.

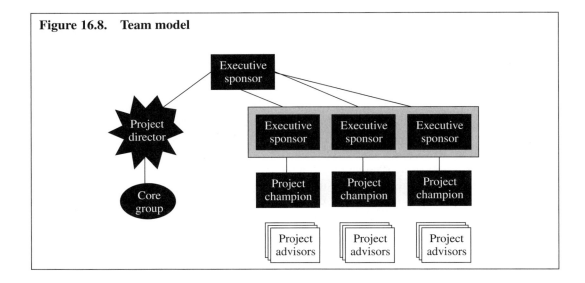

Figure 16.8. Team model

- Tracking, detection, and monitoring: Standards in these areas should establish logging processes for identifying failed log-on attempts.

- Management or measurement systems: Standards covering management or measurement systems should dictate when users should change their passwords.

- Disaster preparation and recovery: Standards should require that backup copies be easily generated and available within a prescribed window of time.

- Physical security: Standards should dictate how the organization's IT resources are protected from theft and damage.

The organization's employees must be instructed in such policies from the first day of employment and must be aware of the sanctions that can be imposed if security procedures are violated. Many facilities require employees to sign a confidentiality agreement that is kept in their personnel file. The organization's policy statement should be a part of every orientation program and the personnel policy manual.

Acquisition Phase

After the organization has established goals and specific requirements, it can search for vendors that match their requirements. Figure 16.9 illustrates the various steps an organization should take in purchasing or leasing a new information system.

Amatayakul (1999, 178) lists a number of questions to incorporate in the selection criteria, including:

- Does the vendor share the organization's vision?

- Does the vendor's product provide the key functionality necessary to achieve the organization's vision?

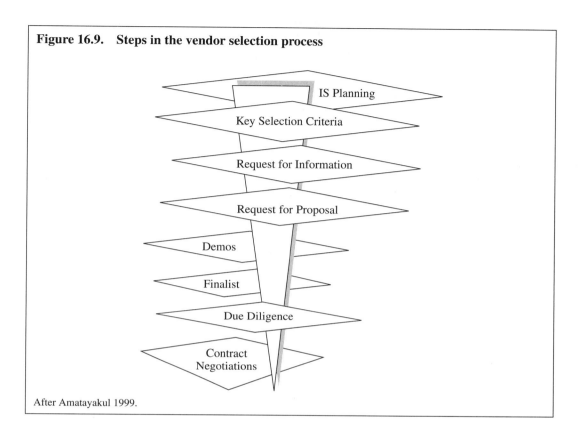

Figure 16.9. Steps in the vendor selection process

IS Planning

Key Selection Criteria

Request for Information

Request for Proposal

Demos

Finalist

Due Diligence

Contract Negotiations

After Amatayakul 1999.

- Does the vendor use the desired technology?

- Does the vendor qualify under the organization's acquisition policies?

- Can the vendor support the organization's desired implementation strategy?

- What is the vendor's track record with regard to operations and maintenance support?

The request for information might include data on the company's background, product information, market information, installed base, and clients.

Standard information in the request for proposal (RFP) would include organizational profile, vendor information, functional specifications, operational requirements, technical requirements, application support, licensing and contractual details, and evaluation criteria. (Chapter 17 discusses the RFP process for selecting a vendor.)

After a vendor has passed the RFP selection process, the organization should schedule a demonstration of the vendor's products and follow up with site visits to its clients to assess its product in action. Further, the organization should check out the vendor's references and ask the vendor to develop an implementation plan. This allows the organization to compare various approaches to implementation and select the one that best matches its vision.

Due diligence involves not only scrutiny of the product, but also the vendor's financial background. Careful inquiries into all aspects of the finalist's operations will help to ensure a successful implementation (Amatayakul 1999, 178–92).

Implementation of New Systems

According to the 1999 Comprehensive Guide to Electronic Health Records, successful implementation of an IS in a healthcare environment constitutes "the ability to demonstrate to the physician community that the computer-based patient record will deliver immediate and obvious value. Physicians are receptive to technology if it is practical, effective and user-friendly. Technology must provide the physician with tangible benefits, including enhanced patient care and reduced administrative burdens" (Hoehn 1999). In addition,

> Physicians must be continually educated in the benefits of electronic records and must be kept informed about implementation plans. They must also be involved in system procurement and implementation. The organization should choose a leader from the physician staff to head the steering committee or share leadership with the CIO (Hoehn 1999, 34–35).

Other critical success factors include:

- Manage the expectations of all end users as well as top executives. Organizers must make sure that senior management and end users agree on the final functionality provided to the clinicians from an information perspective. They also must be certain that all participants understand how the system will affect clinical practice and are willing and able to make the clinical process changes necessary to effectively use the computer-based patient record.

- Educate end users on how to integrate the use of the system into their clinical practices. The use of an electronic record will enable clinicians to work differently and document care decisions differently and provide them with the ability to make quicker, more timely decisions. Some changes in the clinician work flow will need to be made to effectively use an electronic record.

- Assess the business processes that will be affected by the computer-based patient record and plan to redesign those processes to make them more effective and efficient.

- Develop a strategic relationship with those vendors whose computer-based patient record vision is similar to the organization's vision and work with the vendor to define new and more robust functionality.

- Understand that an electronic record implementation may never be truly complete. Developing the computer-based patient record is an evolutionary process. As clinical knowledge, technology, and the provider organization itself change, so will the focus of the project. This means that the goals will need to be updated continually.

- Ensure collaborative participation of interdisciplinary clinical teams. Clinicians and physicians must be involved from the start of the project. The organization must determine how departments will be informed of the progress of the projects and upcoming tasks. Users must believe they are key decision makers in the process and that they have made valuable contributions to the success of the project.

Evaluation of Existing Systems

Whether evaluating an existing IS or selecting a new one to integrate with an existing system, the system's ability to meet the organization's vision must not be overlooked. The Computer-based Patient Record Institute (CPRI) recognized the need for standard criteria when it established the Nicholas E. Davies CPR Recognition program. The criteria can be applied universally to any IS project. Projects are categorized by management function, system functionality, technology, and the system's impact on the organization and its mission. According to the CPRI's Web information:

> The management section addresses strategic planning, implementation, operation, and evaluation processes guiding the CPR systems project. The functionality section focuses on the CPR systems' users and their information needs, the process for identifying and prioritizing functional requirements, and evidence that user needs are being met. The technology section is directed to the technical design of the CPR system, security and data integrity, use of standards and system performance. The impact section looks at quantitative results concerning the impact of the system on the care recipient, particularly access to needed information for direct care, research, and other purposes and on the processes and outcomes of care delivery (cpri.org/davies/criteria).

In examining an existing system, the following subjects should be included (Welch 1999):

- Security: List the levels of security and access mechanisms. Are they adequate?

- Compatibility: List the existing systems such as lab, pharmacy, and scheduling. Determine whether they are interfaced with each other and whether their interfaces match proposed systems on the horizon.

- User-friendliness: What do users currently think of the existing system? What changes would they make in data entry, results reporting, and comfort level with the technology?

- Portability: Does it exist? Should it exist?

- Storage: How many data can be stored now? What is needed for the future? What backup capability does the system have?

- Remote access: Are wide-area networks functioning or available?

- Ad hoc query and reporting capabilities: Does the system allow for customized reporting?

According to the CPRI:

> Creating a CPR system in a health care enterprise is a very complex, long-term undertaking. There are many challenges and barriers to be overcome and no absolute models of success, either in technology or in the many organizational aspects of implementation. Innovation and experimentation are needed to achieve breakthroughs and these are inherently risky. An important element of achieving incremental, forward progress is the ability to leverage successes, to learn from failures, and to continue to improve. Progress is almost never totally linear, and, in projects of this type, one strength of management is the ability to change strategy and direction (2000, p. 4).

The ongoing evaluation of existing systems will help make the end result more acceptable and usable to everyone affected by its impact.

Check your understanding 16.6

Instructions: Indicate whether the following statements are true or false (T or F).

1. _____ Change management should be part of the process of planning the implementation of new information technology.
2. _____ Most physicians are very receptive to changes in technology that affect the way they practice medicine.
3. _____ Three main factors affect the acceptance of change: deliverable complexity, environmental complexity, and cross-organizational commitment.
4. _____ It would be a mistake for an organization to focus on using technology without first analyzing its business and clinical needs.
5. _____ Nicholas E. Davies developed a set of criteria that can be applied universally to any IS project.

Real-World Case

The Health Technologies Division of Northern Virginia Community College (NVCC) provides free nurse-managed healthcare services at ten clinics located in the Northern Virginia area. Each clinic has its own staff of nurse practitioners and nursing students who see patients several times a week.

One of the clinics' challenges is to capture and maintain records on every patient they see. Currently, this is done manually with paper forms. The paper forms are sent to the college and stored in filing cabinets. The clinics are unable to access data on any patient and do not even know whether a patient has been seen before. The grants supporting the project require special statistical reports of patient activity to be generated on a quarterly basis.

In 2000, the Health Technologies Division began to work with the Information Systems Technology Program to provide a solution to this information problem. The solution would allow clinics access to patient data at any time and anywhere in a secure fashion.

The hope is to provide an inexpensive system that is able to capture patient data and also generate the needed reports from the source document. Every clinic in Northern Virginia is equipped with a low-end Gateway Pentium 133MHz computer with 32MB of RAM and a 2GB hard drive that was donated by the college. Each computer has a modem that allows the clinic to connect to the Internet.

At the Annandale campus, a server stores the patient data for all the clinics. The server is powerful enough to handle the ten clinics and also securely transmits data over the Internet. This requires the server to encrypt the data as they are transmitted. Figure 16.10 shows the layout of the network infrastructure of the project.

At each clinic, data entry currently takes place as the patient is treated and leaves the clinic. On the server, a Web application is being designed to provide the clinics with an electronic view of the forms that once were created manually. The Web application will require the clinics to enter patient data on the computer instead of on paper. This would reduce the amount of paper generated and also provide patient data to the clinics on an as-needed basis.

The Web application will use a technology by Microsoft called Active Server Pages (ASP). ASP is a scripting technology that allows coders to generate HTML automatically. The ASP pages will connect to an Access database for the prototype and a server-based database management system called SQL Server.

This project requires knowledge of the data set captured at each clinic as well as how to conduct a systems analysis of the information problem to achieve a solution.

The system development life cycle can be applied to arrive at an appropriate solution. As mentioned earlier, the SDLC consists of four phases: analysis, design, implementation, and maintenance.

The analysis phase requires an understanding of how the theNetwork works today. As mentioned earlier, each clinic has several nursing students and at least one nurse

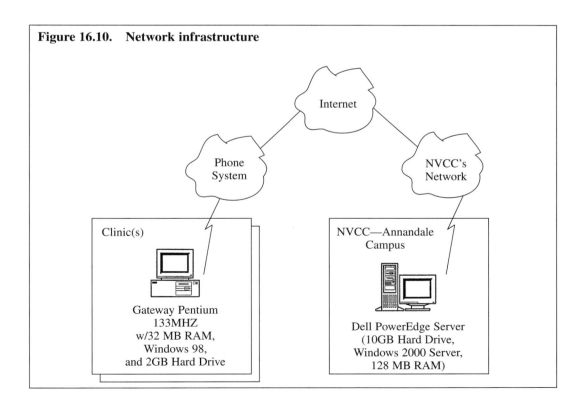

Figure 16.10.   Network infrastructure

practitioner. Patients line up and are treated on a first-come, first-serve basis. Because the number of patients who can be seen in a single day is limited, one nursing student surveys the line to determine the maximum number for a given day. With the help of the nurse practitioner, the nursing student estimates each patient visit and selects the number of patients on the basis of the estimate. Each nursing student is assigned to a patient and stays with him or her throughout the entire visit. The nursing students help the patients fill out the top of the paper form. (See figure 16.11.)

Each nursing student then brings his or her patient to see the nurse practitioner, and the nurse practitioner fills out the medical portion of figure 16.11. Before the patient leaves, the student helps him or her fill out a patient survey form. (See figure 16.12, p. 782.)

In a systems analysis, the paper forms are the first step in determining the users' needs. The analyst uses them to create use cases and sequence diagrams. But before getting to the details of the use cases, the analyst needs to review some other requirements for this system. To create a system to support the two paper forms, the data need to be secured during any transmission. Thus, the Web application will encrypt data during any transmission between client and server.

The actors of this system are the system administrator, the medical provider, and the nursing student. The system administrator is responsible for the overall operation of the system and for setting up the user accounts. The medical provider is the provider of the medical service.

The overall structure of the system is a search page that allows the user to search for a particular item. When the search takes place, the results are displayed in the search results page. This page allows the user to create, edit, delete, or just view an item. Whatever the user selects, an item's form page displays to allow the user to view, create, edit, or delete. When the action is submitted, a form response page appears detailing the results of the action.

The theNetwork system can be split into several subsystems, including the following:

- The medical subsystem contains the medical demographics, medical records, pap results, and patient survey subsystems.

- The patient subsystem is the top of the Screening Results/Health Education Form that tracks patient information.

- The medical demographics subsystem is the middle part of the form.

- The medical record is the bottom part of the same form. If the reason for the visit is to have a pap test done, the pap results subsystem is responsible for tracking its outcomes.

- The patient survey subsystem is the patient survey form. This subsystem tracks the patient outcomes from a clinic visit. Some of this information is already duplicated from the screening form and will not appear in the electronic form. This information can be looked up easily. Examples of duplicate information are the gender, race, and insurance questions.

Table 16.3 (p. 783) provides an example of a patient survey use case. The flow for each subsystem is search, search results, main form, and form response. This use case illustrates how user and system can interact to search for a particular patient record.

Table 16.4 (p. 783) shows how user and system interact when a search has been completed. Table 16.5 (pp. 784–85) shows the patient survey use case for create, edit, and delete.

Figure 16.11. theNetwork screening results/health education form

Screening Results/Health Education Form

Mobile Nurse-Managed Health Center: AL ☐   AN ☐   LO ☐   MA ☐   WO ☐   CCC ☐   GT South ☐   ECDC ☐

Administrative Data
(Please print, CAPITAL LETTERS ONLY)   GW Mammo ☐   FFRC ☐   LAMB ☐   Asthma ☐   LRC ☐   Other ☐ _____

Date of Service [| | | |]   Gender   M ☐ F ☐   Insurance   Y ☐ N ☐

[| | | | | | | |]   [ ]   [| | | | | | | | | | | | | | | | |]
       First   Middle Initial   Last

[| | | | | |]   [| | | | | | | | | | | |]
   Street Number   Street name

[| | | | | | | | |]   [| | | |]   [| | | | |]
            City   State   Zip

Date of Birth [| | | | |]   Phone [| | |] [| | |] [| | | |]

Reason for Visit   Pap ☐   Mammo ☐   CBE ☐   HTN ☐   HIV/AIDS ☐   PE ☐ Diabetes ☐

Cholesterol ☐   Preg Test ☐   F/U Pap ☐   Annual Mammo ☐   Minor Illness ☐   Other ☐

Referral Source   MD ☐   Health Dept. ☐   ACS ☐   GW Mammo ☐   ER ☐   Friend/Family ☐   School ☐   Clinic ☐

Last Visit   Never ☐   <1 year ☐   >2 years ☐   3–4 years ☐   5–6 years ☐   7–8 years ☐   >9 years ☐

Place of Last Visit   NVCC ☐   MD ☐   Other Clinic ☐   Health Dept. ☐   Hospital ER ☐   Other Country ☐

Referring NP   Cruz ☐   Dooley ☐   Missett ☐   Morales ☐   Riha ☐   Spinelli ☐   Raj ☐   Other ☐ _____

Referrals Made   ACS ☐   Arlington Free Clinic ☐   Prince William H.D. ☐   Fairfax Hospital ☐   County ☐   GW ☐   ER ☐

Type of Interpreter   Not Needed ☐   Clinic Staff ☐   Family/Friend ☐   NVCC ☐   AHEC ☐

Clinical Data

Normal Physical Exam   Yes ☐   No ☐   Comments _____

_____

_____

Test Results: [| |] / [| |]   [| |]   [| |]   Normal ☐ Abnormal ☐   [| |] • [ ]   [| |]
                  BP   Glucose   Cholesterol   UA   Hg   PPD

Vision Exam [| |] / [|]   [| |] / [|]   [| |] / [|]   W/Correction ☐
                  OD   Os   OU   W/O Correction ☐

CBE   Normal ☐   [| | |]   [| | |] • [|]
      Abnormal ☐   WT (LBS)   HT (IN.)

Referral (note reason) _____

Comments _____

Provider Signature _____

Page number 1

Figure 16.12.   theNetwork patient survey form

Patient Survey Form

OFFICE USE ONLY

Mobile Nurse-Managed Health Center: AL ☐   AN ☐   LO ☐   MA ☐   WO ☐   CCC ☐

GT South ☐   GW Mammo ☐   FFRC ☐   LRC ☐   LAMB ☐   Asthma ☐   ECDC ☐   Health Mobile ☐   Other ☐ _____

Today's Date [| | | |]
MM   DD   YY

Thank you for participating in our survey.

Please mark an "X" in the correct box for each question.

1. Gender: Male ☐   Female ☐

2. Race/Ethnicity:
   African ☐   Arabic ☐   Asian/ Pacific Islander ☐   European ☐
   Latino ☐   U.S. Black ☐   U.S. White ☐   Other ☐

3. Do you have health insurance?   Yes ☐   No ☐

4. Did your visit to this clinic and the treatment you received save you a trip to a hospital or emergency room?   Yes ☐   No ☐

5. Did the healthcare worker talk to you about your visit and explain all instructions to you clearly?   Yes ☐   No ☐

6. How did you find out about us?
   Friend/Family ☐   School ☐   Clinic ☐
   American Cancer Society ☐   Health Dept. ☐   Other ☐

7. How would you rate your overall visit to the clinic today?
   Excellent ☐   Good ☐   Fair ☐   Poor ☐

8. Is there anything else we could have done to improve your visit to the clinic?   Yes ☐   No ☐
   If yes, please explain here:

   _____
   _____
   _____

Table 16.3.   Search patient survey use case

Use Case Name	Search Patient Form
Description	Allows user to enter patient name and to search for patient record.

Successful Course	1. User clicks on link for patient survey form in the home page.
	2. System displays a search form.
	3. User enters patient information:
	    Last name
	    First name
	    Middle Initial
	4. User submits form.
	5. System searches database for the patient name entered by user.
	6. If patient exists, system displays patient search results form with last name, first name, and middle initial entered.
	7. If patient does not exist, system displays message that patient does not exist.

Unsuccessful Course	Do steps 1–4 above. 5. System searches the database for the patient entered by user. 6. If patient exists, system displays patient search results form with last name, first name, and middle initial entered. 7. If patient does not exist, system displays message that patient does not exist.
Precondition	Authentication
Postcondition	System displays patient search results form.
Assumptions	Patient and form objects exist.
Courtesy of Saroja Ullagaddi.	

Table 16.4.   Patient survey search results use case

Use Case Name	Patient Search Results Form		
Description	Allows user to click on links for create, edit, delete, or view patient survey form for the date of service selected. Form also can be used for medical records, medical demographics, and pap results.		
Date of Visit	*Search Results*	*Action*	
Today is: date	Medical Demographics	Create	
	Medical Records	Create	
	Patient Survey	Create	
	Pap Results	Create	
10/26/00:	Medical Demographics	Edit	Delete	View
	Medical Records	Edit	Delete	View
	Patient Survey	Edit	Delete	View
	Pap Results	Edit	Delete	View
09/23/00:	Medical Demographics	Edit	Delete	View
	Medical Records	Edit	Delete	View
	Patient Survey	Edit	Delete	View
	Pap Results	Edit	Delete	View
Successful Course	1. Displays patient name and links for various actions. 2. System displays appropriate (main) form for the link selected by user.		
Unsuccessful Course	Displays search patient form again.		
Precondition	Authentication		
Postcondition	System displays appropriate (main) form for the action select by user.		
Assumptions	Patient and form objects exist.		
Courtesy of Saroja Ullagaddi.			

Table 16.5.   Create, edit, and delete patient survey use cases

Create Patient Survey Use Case

Use Case Name	Create Patient Survey Form
Description	Allows user to enter patient survey information.
Successful Patient Survey Form	1. User requests to create (clicks the create button on the search results form). 2. System displays patient survey form. 3. User fills out form by choosing appropriate buttons (only one for each): 　　Save a trip to hospital (SAVE_ER_VISIT) 　　Clarity of instructions (INSTRUCTIONS) 　　Rating of clinic (CLINIC_RATING) 　　Improve visit (VISIT_IMPROVEMENT) 　　Additional comments (COMMENTS) 4. User submits form. 5. System validates data on form. 6. System saves the create information. 7. System displays successful save create message.
Unsuccessful Course	Do steps 1–4. 5. System displays error message.
Precondition	Authentication
Postcondition	System displays completed survey form.
Assumptions	Patient and form objects exist.

Edit Patient Survey Use Case

Use Case Name	Edit Patient Survey Form
Description	Allows user to edit patient survey information.
Successful Patient Survey Form	1. User requests to edit (clicks the edit button on the search results form). 2. System displays patient survey form completed earlier. 3. User chooses the form by selecting appropriate buttons (only one for each): 　　Save a trip to hospital (SAVE_ER_VISIT) 　　Clarity of instructions (INSTRUCTIONS) 　　Rating of clinic (CLINIC_RATING) 　　Improve visit (VISIT_IMPROVEMENT) 　　Additional comments (COMMENTS) 4. User submits form. 5. System validates data on form. 6. System saves edited information. 7. System displays successful Save Edit message.
Unsuccessful Course	Do steps 1–4. 5. System displays error message.
Precondition	Authentication
Postcondition	System displays completed survey form.
Assumptions	Patient and form objects exist.

Table 16.5. *(Continued)*	
Delete Patient Survey Use Case	
Use Case Name	Delete Patient Survey Form
Description	Allows user to delete patient survey information.
Successful Course	1. User requests to delete (clicks delete button on search results form). 2. System displays patient survey form completed earlier. 3. User submits form. 4. System deletes information. 5. System displays successful delete message.
Unsuccessful Course	Do steps 1–4. 5. System displays error message.
Precondition	Authentication
Postcondition	System displays delete message.
Assumptions	Patient and form objects exist.
Courtesy of Saroja Ullagaddi.	

After creating use cases for each of the subsystems, the analyst needs to create a requirements document containing the use cases, schedule, and budget for the system.

The next phase of the SDLC is the systems design. This includes the logical and physical designs and the screen prototypes.

The logical design consists of an UML class diagram for theNetwork. The systems analyst will need a UML diagram for patient demographics, medical record, and patient survey. Figure 16.13 (p. 786) illustrates the UML class diagram for patient surveys.

The next step is to determine the business rules for the patient survey class. These rules are shown in table 16.6 (p. 786). As part of determining the business rules, the analyst will need to determine, at a minimum, the mandatory fields and their respective maximum lengths. There may be additional rules depending on the object.

After completing the object model, it must be translated into the logical data model for the database structure. Figure 16.14 (p. 787) shows the logical data model, including the business rules for patient surveys.

The class diagram is changed to a table with columns. A table in a database contains a primary key and sometimes a foreign key, depending on the database. The primary key is PATIENT_SURVEY_ID. The foreign key is MED_DEM_ID, which provides a relationship to the MEDICAL_DEMOGRAPHICS table. Because only one patient survey form is filled out for every completed screening form, the relationship is one to one.

The physical design contains the physical data model, which is how the logical model is implemented in an Access database, and screen prototypes of the forms. Table 16.7, p. 787) shows the physical data model of patient surveys.

Figures 16.15 through 16.17 show the screen prototypes for search, search results, and patient survey forms.

After the logical and physical data models and screen prototypes are complete, the design must be formalized into a design document. In the implementation/maintenance phase, the coding begins, testing takes place, and deployment occurs. (A discussion of the writing of software is beyond the scope of this book.) After coding is complete, testing begins toward the use cases developed in the requirements. Any bugs are documented and fixed until the software becomes stable. The software then is deployed on the server described above.

Figure 16.18 (p. 790) shows the start page of the theNetwork Web application that solves the above problem.

Figure 16.13.   Patient survey UML class diagram

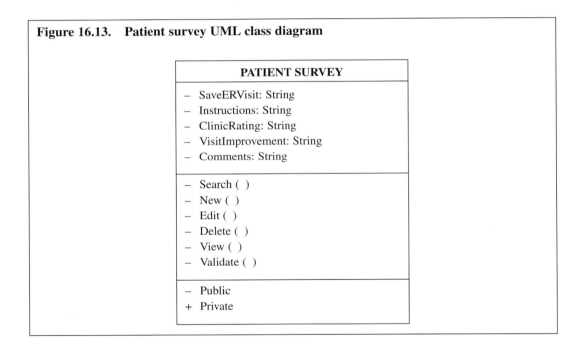

Table 16.6.   Business rules for patient survey class

Class	Attribute	Business Rule
Patient Survey	SaveErVisit	Choose only one answer
	Instructions	Choose only one answer
	ClinicRating	Choose only one answer
	VisitImprovement	Choose only one answer
	Comments	Maxlength 64,000 bytes

Figure 16.14.   Logical data model for patient surveys

Patient Surveys
PATIENT_SURVEY_ID: INTEGER
SAVE_ER_VISIT: STRING
INSTRUCTIONS: STRING
CLINIC_RATING: STRING
VISIT_RATING: STRING
COMMENTS: STRING
MED_DEMO_ID: LONG INTEGER

Business Rules

RELATION	COLUMN	BUSINESS RULE
Patient Survey Form	Patient_Survey_Id: Integer Save_Er_Visit: String Instructions: String Clinic_Rating: String Visit_Rating: String Comments: String Med_Demo_Id: Long Integer	For every patient survey, there must be one row Medical Demographics table. The Patient_Survey_Id, Must be number with one Counter up.

Table 16.7.   Physical data model of patient surveys

Field Name	Data Type	Field Size	Constraint
Patient_Survey_Id	Autonumber	Long Integer	Not Null & is Primary Key
Save_Er_Visit	String	1	Choose only one (yes or no)
Instructions	String	1	Choose only one (yes or no)
Clinic_Rating	String	1	Choose only one (yes or no)
Visit_Rating	String	1	Choose only one (yes or no)
Comments	Memo	65,535 characters	
Med_Demo_Id	Autonumber	Long Integer	Not Null & is Foreign Key

Figure 16.15.   Medical search form

Patient Data			
PATIENT_ID	LAST_NAME	FIRST_NAME	ACTION
2	Barker	Sherry	Select

Figure 16.16.   Patient search results form

Patient: Lindsay E. Jones

DOB: Dec 25th, 1976   Gender: F

Race: US White   Insurance?   No

Site Name	Form Number	Date of Visit	Search Result	Action			
AN	9999	1/2/00	*Medical Demographics*	Create	Edit	Delete	View
			Medical Records	Create	Edit	Delete	View
			Patient Surveys	Create	Edit	Delete	View
			Pap Results	Create	Edit	Delete	View
AL	9860	12/2/99	*Medical Demographics*	Create	Edit	Delete	View
			Medical Records	Create	Edit	Delete	View
			Patient Surveys	Create	Edit	Delete	View
			Pap Results	Create	Edit	Delete	View

Summary

A well-managed information system (IS) is critical to the success of today's healthcare organizations. Information systems are the integration of people, data, processes, and technology to effect specific outcomes in a business process. They can be categorized as operation support, enterprise-wide, and management systems. The traditional way to implement an IS is to use the systems development life cycle. The SDLC is a four-step process that takes the organization from system planning and design through maintenance.

Key to the successful operation of an IS is the type of technology used. A variety of computer hardware and software components are currently available to ensure the effective storage, management, and transmission of healthcare data both within the organization and outside. Moreover, advances in programming languages are enabling users to communicate with and through computers with greater ease and efficiency.

Patient data are organized and stored in databases. The three types of databases available today are relational databases, object-oriented databases, and object-relational databases. The relational database is the most common type of database system. Most healthcare organizations maintain several different databases to serve different functions

---

Figure 16.17.   Patient survey form

Patient: Lindsay E. Jones
DOB: Dec 25th, 1976   Gender: F
Race: US White   Insurance?   No

1. Did your visit to this clinic and the treatment you received save you a trip to a hospital or emergency room?

   ☐ Yes   ☐ No

2. Did the healthcare worker talk to you about your visit and clearly explain all the instructions to you?

   ☐ Yes   ☐ No

3. How would you rate your overall visit to clinic today?

   ☐ Excellent   ☐ Good   ☐ Fair   ☐ Poor

4. Could we have done anything else to improve your visit to the clinic?

   ☐ Yes   ☐ No

   If yes, please explain here:

---

in their day-to-day operations. Data warehouses enable organizations to access data from the different databases and to combine them into a single interface.

Moreover, healthcare organizations must have a technology infrastructure in place that provides the users of healthcare data with a communications system that enables them to share information and resources. One example of such a system is a computer network in which computers are either clients or servers. The two main types of computer network setups are local-area networks (LANs) and wide-area networks (WANs).

Implementing an IS or changing from an existing system to a new one is a complex undertaking. The healthcare organization must evaluate the processes that will have the greatest impact on the organization, assess its current technology infrastructure to determine what must be done to accommodate the new system, and ensure user acceptance of the change. Further, the organization will have to develop policies and procedures to ensure the confidentiality and security of the information entrusted to its care.

References

Amatayakul, M. 1999. *The Role of Health Information Managers in CPR Projects.* Chicago: AHIMA.

Andrews, D., and S. Stalick. 2000. BPR project management: A radical approach to project team organization. *American Programmer* 8(6). Available online from gslink.com/~brri/article.html.

Briggs, B. 1999. *1999 Comprehensive Guide to Electronic Health Records,* edited by Barbara Hoehn. New York: Faulkner and Gray.

Burke, L., and B. Weill. 2000. *Information Technology for the Health Professions.* New York: Prentice-Hall.

CPRI-HOST. 2000. Criteria for the Davies Award. Available online from cpri.org/davies/criteria.html.

Davenport, T.H., and J. Glaser. 2002 (July). Just-in-time delivery comes to knowledge management. *Harvard Business Review.*

Degoulet, P., and M. Fieschi. 1997. *Introduction to Clinical Informatics.* New York: Springer-Verlag.

DeJesus, E. 2000 (February). The wireless e-connection. *Healthcare Informatics* 2:67–70.

Duggan, C.M. 2004 (January) The Constancy of Change. *Journal of American Health Information Management Association* 75(1):40.

Goodman, P.S. 2000 (Oct. 16). Hello, Internet? Talking Web sites next challenge. *Washington Post.*

Hoehn, B, ed. 1999. *1999 Comprehensive Guide to Electronic Health Records.* New York: Faulkner and Gray.

Hutchinson, S.E., and S.C. Sawyer. 2000. *Computers, Communications & Information.* Boston: Irwin McGraw-Hill.

Johns, M. 1999. The electronic health record process for health services delivery. In *Electronic Health Records: Changing the Vision,* edited by G.F. Murphy, M.A. Hanken, and K.L. Waters. Philadelphia: W. B. Saunders.

Figure 16.18.   Screen view of nurse-managed health center network

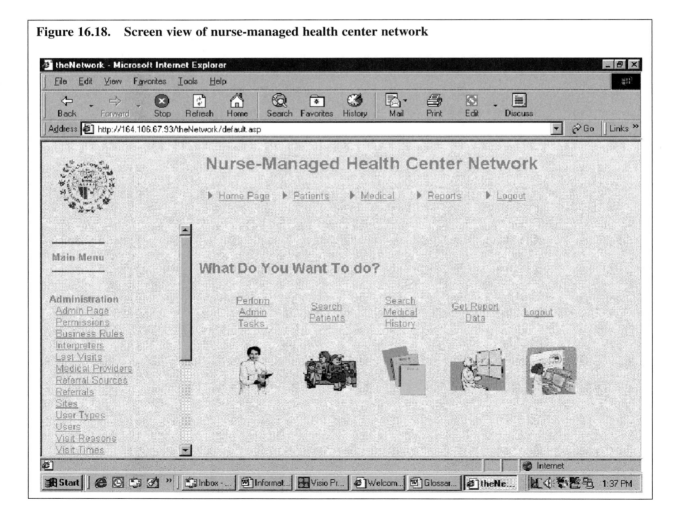

Morneau, K. 2000. *MCSD Guide to Solutions Architectures.* Boston: Thompson Course Technology.

Murphy, G.F., M.A. Hanken, and K.A. Waters. 1999. *Electronic Health Records: Changing the Vision.* Philadelphia: W.B. Saunders Company.

Nakamoto, G. 2000. Building a legacy system. *Health Management Technology* 21(10):56.

O'Brien, J.A. 2002. *Management Information Systems Managing Information Technology in the E-Business Enterprise.* New York: McGraw-Hill.

Weed, L. 1991. Knowledge Coupling. New York: Springer-Verlag.

Welch, J.J. 1999. CPR systems: Which one is right for your organization? *Journal of American Health Information Management Association* 70(8):24–26.

Wyderka, K.C. 1999 (Nov.) Data warehouse techniques for patient outcomes management. *Health Management Technology.* Available online from healthmgttech.com.

Chapter 17

Introduction to Healthcare Information Systems

Karen A. Wager, DBA
Frances Wickham Lee, DBA

Learning Objectives

- To describe the evolution of information systems in healthcare

- To identify the major types of information system applications used in healthcare organizations

- To recognize the importance of strategic information systems planning to a healthcare organization

- To understand the systems development process and its role in the planning, selection, implementation, and evaluation of healthcare information systems

- To identify the key elements needed to manage information resources effectively

- To recognize emerging trends affecting the development of healthcare information systems

- To understand the role of the health information technician in information systems planning and development

Key Terms

Administrative information systems

Application service provider (ASP)

Chief financial officer (CFO)

Chief information officer (CIO)

Chief information security officer (CISO)

Chief medical informatics officer (CMIO)

Chief privacy officer

Clinical information systems

Cost–benefit analysis

Health information services department

Information resource management

Information services department

Microcomputer

Regional health information organization (RHIO)

Request for information (RFI)

Request for proposal (RFP)

Shared systems

Strategic information systems planning

System design

System implementation

System maintenance and evaluation

System planning and analysis

Systems development life cycle (SDLC)

Turnkey system

Introduction

Healthcare information systems (ISs) run the gamut from patient-specific clinical ISs to administrative or financial systems to fully integrated systems that combine clinical and administrative/financial information. Such systems can exist within a single institution or across organizations. The development and use of healthcare information systems is not new. ISs were first introduced in healthcare in the 1960s. Since then, advances in computer technology coupled with the increasing demand for clinical and administrative information have grown exponentially. Despite these advances, however, many healthcare organizations today continue to maintain paper-based medical record systems.

The reasons for the predominance of paper-based medical records are many. Healthcare organizations are enormously complex, both overall and in terms of the information they manage. The complexity makes it difficult to implement healthcare information systems effectively. Healthcare ISs can be costly to implement and support, and many small community-based providers may not have the resources or technical expertise to maintain and support them. For those able to overcome these initial barriers, experts report that 50 percent of IS projects will fail despite best-made plans and efforts (Anderson and Aydin 2005).

Our intention is not to paint a bleak picture. In fact, we predict a steady rise in the extent to which healthcare ISs are adopted and used in the future. Unprecedented attention at the national level has been directed toward the expanded use of information technology (IT) in healthcare and, most recently, the adoption of electronic health records (EHRs). Two years ago, President Bush called for adoption of the EHR within the next decade. Soon afterward, he appointed a leader for the Office of the National Coordinator Health Information Technology (ONC) within the Office of the Secretary of Health and Human Services. Resources in terms of people, technology, and infrastructure are being allocated to lay the road map necessary for widespread adoption and use of EHR systems—tools that have the potential to reduce medical errors, improve patient safety, ensure quality, and facilitate efficiency. Numerous reports support the need for radical change in how we manage patient information (Bates 2005; IOM 2001, 2000). Local communities and regions are establishing **regional health information organizations** (RHIOs), or networks for sharing clinical and administrative information across organizational boundaries for the purposes of improving patient care and managing costs.

In addition to the national and regional efforts directed toward the president's call for widespread use and adoption of EHR systems, a great deal of work must be done at the institutional or organizational level. Healthcare organizations must learn from their successes and failures. They must adopt appropriate planning strategies and methods and put the necessary resources in place to support any healthcare IS, large or small. Selecting the most up-to-date and appropriate IS is not always adequate to ensure successful implementation of a new system. Healthcare organizations must continually evaluate the extent to which their ISs are meeting the needs of users. Sufficient financial, personnel, and other resources must be available to support the system and its users.

Health information management (HIM) professionals play an important role in the selection, development, implementation, and support of healthcare ISs. Their roles depend on individual work responsibilities and on the size, scope, and complexity of the organization in which they work. In one setting, a health information technician (HIT) whose main responsibility is coding may be asked to participate in evaluating an automated coding system as a component of an integrated health record system. In another setting, an HIT in a supervisory position may offer input on user needs and expectations of an EHR system. Regardless of the setting, HIM professionals should understand the major types of healthcare ISs available, the process of selecting and implementing such systems, and the resources needed to support them.

This chapter reviews the history of healthcare ISs and describes the major IS applications used by healthcare organizations today. It also describes the process that many organizations use in planning, selecting, developing, and implementing ISs. Because selecting the right system is not enough to ensure its success, the chapter also discusses the resources needed to ensure that systems are adequately maintained and supported. This discussion includes a description of the people, policies, and organizational structure needed to manage information resources in today's healthcare environment. Several examples that demonstrate the importance of appropriate planning and user buy-in also are offered.

Theory into Practice

This case comes from a comprehensive study of five primary care physician practices that implemented the same electronic medical record (EMR) product (Wager et al. 2000). In this chapter, EMR refers to computer-based patient record systems that are used within an organization and EHR refers to systems that share patient information across different organizations (not under the same governance and ownership).

Family Medicine Center (FMC) was the one practice out of the five studied that was dissatisfied with its choice of EMR. This brief synopsis provides a good illustration of the notion that factors beyond the functionality of the healthcare IS may cause a system failure (or success).

FMC implemented its EMR system in 1994. The practice purchased the system from a reputable vendor. It expected the system to reduce personnel costs and to enable it to realize numerous other efficiencies. FMC invested more than $400,000 in the system and spent several years trying to get it to work. Eventually, key personnel within the clinic became so frustrated that they started pushing the idea of starting again with a new system (Wager, Lee, and White 2001).

What went wrong? As with most system failures, many factors contributed to the frustrations and dissatisfactions with the EMR implemented at FMC. One factor may have been the disastrous implementation phase. The practice's lead physician selected the system based on advice from a colleague in the field. The other physicians in the practice knew very little about computers and trusted their partner's judgment. A planning group was not organized, and the choice of system was not based on a strategic decision-making process.

To complicate matters further, the lead physician agreed with the EMR distributor that it was best to implement the scheduling and billing components of the system concurrently with the EMR components. It was the distributor's first sale, and much of his time was spent handling conversion problems from the old billing system to the new one. Little time was invested in training the nurses, physicians, and support staff.

Years later, common complaints among the nurses and physicians include the following:

- The initial training was grossly inadequate.
- The system is too cumbersome to use.
- Our patients do not like us typing in the exam room.
- Half the record is electronic; half is on paper.
- It has not saved time but actually created more work.
- No one is available to help when we have problems with the system.

It would be easy to assume that FMC's EMR system failed because the choice of product was inappropriate. However, this conclusion seems too simplistic when examined within the context of the larger study. The majority of practices were pleased or very pleased with the same EMR product that was installed at FMC. What could FMC have done to improve its chances for a successful implementation? Subsequent sections of this chapter outline some of the ways healthcare organizations can improve their chances of successfully implementing healthcare information systems.

Evolution of Information Systems in Healthcare

Information systems (ISs) are not new to healthcare. Early automated systems were implemented almost forty years ago. Despite this long history, the majority of health record systems in place today are still predominately paper based (Hillestad et al. 2005). An overview of the evolution of healthcare IS may explain why full implementation is taking so long. (See figure 17.1.)

The first computer systems used in healthcare date to the early 1960s. A small number of hospitals began to develop in-house administrative and/or financial systems. The systems were used primarily to perform payroll and patient accounting functions (Austin and Boxerman 2003; Wager, Lee, and Glaser 2005). The reason these early systems focused on financial applications was primarily because financial applications were being used in other industries and it made sense to transfer this technology to healthcare.

The nature and scope of computer technology at the time also supported data-processing systems rather than more sophisticated information systems (Johns 1997). Hospitals with sufficient resources maintained data-processing departments with in-house computer programmers. The data-processing unit typically reported to the finance department or the **chief financial officer** (CFO) because healthcare institutions relied on revenue generation and volume-of-service statistics. This reporting structure may have contributed to the slow growth of **clinical information systems** (Johns 1997). Little clinical information was collected and maintained, and few clinical information systems were available during this time.

The administrative and financial systems used in hospitals during this era ran on large, centralized mainframe computers. The cost of the computers made it prohibitively expensive to develop multiple departmental systems (Kennedy, Davis, and Heda 1992).

The expense barrier in the 1960s and 1970s led to the emergence of so-called **shared systems.** Shared systems were developed by data-processing companies to provide computing power simultaneously to several healthcare organizations within a local or regional area. Healthcare organizations were charged for using the shared-system company's data-processing centers and, usually, their applications. Like the mainframe systems used by hospitals that could afford them, most shared-system products began as administrative and financial systems. During the 1970s, the systems gradually migrated toward department-level clinical systems such as laboratory, radiology, and pharmacy systems.

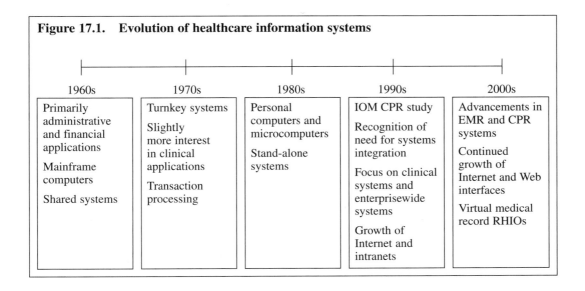

Figure 17.1. Evolution of healthcare information systems

1960s	1970s	1980s	1990s	2000s
Primarily administrative and financial applications	Turnkey systems	Personal computers and microcomputers	IOM CPR study	Advancements in EMR and CPR systems
Mainframe computers	Slightly more interest in clinical applications	Stand-alone systems	Recognition of need for systems integration	Continued growth of Internet and Web interfaces
Shared systems	Transaction processing		Focus on clinical systems and enterprisewide systems	Virtual medical record RHIOs
			Growth of Internet and intranets	

Turnkey systems also began to emerge in the 1970s. All a healthcare institution needed to do was to turn on the system, and it was fully operational. Turnkey systems were actually developed by IS vendors and installed on the hospitals' computers. Typically, the hospital's data-processing staff maintained the systems (Johns 1997; Wager, Lee, and Glaser 2005). However, most turnkey systems could not be modified.

By the 1980s, healthcare institutions were beginning to change their focus from maximizing revenues to minimizing expenses. There was still a financial focus, but more progress was being made in the development of clinical systems. Hospitals were under pressure to decrease their average lengths of stay and to shift patient care from inpatient to outpatient settings. Clinical departments also were under pressure to increase productivity.

At the same time, advances were being made in computer technology. The development of **microcomputers,** also called personal computers, enabled healthcare institutions to purchase relatively inexpensive desktop computers. The new computers had computing power and storage capacity equivalent to that of the early mainframe computers.

Stand-alone systems supported functional tasks for specific departments and units. Departments controlled their own information because they collected and maintained it. However, the use of stand-alone systems led to duplication of effort and redundant files. There was little, if any, effort to integrate the data among systems. Even today, hospitals and other healthcare organizations struggle with integrating data from separate ISs within the same organization.

The early 1990s brought further changes in the healthcare industry with the advent of market-driven healthcare reform, the growth of managed care, and the development of integrated delivery systems. As a result, much more attention was given to the development of clinical systems and the integration of clinical and financial data for decision-making purposes.

In 1991, the Institute of Medicine (IOM) published its landmark report outlining the need for computer-based patient record (CPR) systems (Dick and Steen 1991). The IOM report brought national attention to the problems with paper-based systems. It also challenged private and public sectors to work together to develop an electronic, longitudinal health record. The goal of developing longitudinal records was to capture information about the health of individuals throughout their lifetime.

By the late 1990s, the widespread use of home computers and the Internet began to change how healthcare institutions delivered services and managed health-related information. The growth of the World Wide Web (WWW) and other Internet technologies led to the development of easy-to-access healthcare ISs in many organizations. These systems range from Web pages that provide consumers with information on health issues and the services provided by the sponsoring healthcare organization to sophisticated, interactive, Web-based clinical ISs.

Clinicians and others no longer need to be physically present in the healthcare organization to view and, in some cases, record patient data. Web interfaces have led to the development of virtual health records. In these systems, the Web-based interface brings together information from different databases and data repositories, links the data by patient, and displays them on a single workstation.

Today, less than 25 percent of healthcare providers and organizations have EMR systems in place (Hillestad et al. 2005). However, the number of new EMR systems and similar ISs will continue to grow as managing clinical and administrative information on paper becomes increasingly difficult. Additionally, various initiatives such as changes in reimbursement systems (for example, pay for performance), increased availability of EMR products and vendors, financial incentives, advances in portable technology (for example, wireless, bar coding, and so on) are paving the way for further adoption and use.

Check Your Understanding 17.1

Instructions: Indicate the time period during which each of the following systems, technologies, or events was first implemented in healthcare organizations.

a.   1960–1970s
b.   1980s
c.   1990s and beyond

1.   _____ Turnkey systems

2.   _____ Mainframe computers

3.   _____ Administrative and financial systems

4.   _____ IOM study on CPR

5.   _____ Microcomputers

6.   _____ Shared systems

7.   _____ Enterprise-wide information systems

8.   _____ Clinical information systems

9.   _____ Internet technology

10. _____ Wireless technology

Overview of Healthcare Information Applications

Many IS applications are used in healthcare today and can be classified in many ways. For simplicity's sake, this chapter groups them into three broad categories:

- Clinical information systems
- **Administrative information systems**
- Management support systems

Many of the functions identified for the following categories apply regardless of whether the system supports healthcare delivery in an inpatient or outpatient setting. Clinical ISs include systems that support the following functions:

- EMRs, EHRs, and CPRs
- Patient care management
- Computer-based provider order entry (CPOE)
- Results reporting
- Nursing services

- Departmental clinical management
- Laboratory services
- Medication administration (using bar-coding technology)
- Pharmacy services
- Radiology services
- Clinical decision support

Administrative ISs support the following functions:

- Patient registration
- Financial management
- Human resource management
- Materials management
- Facilities management

Management support systems are applied in the following areas:

- Executive decision making
- Financial modeling
- Planning and marketing
- Resource allocation (labor, supplies, and facilities planning)
- Expert systems

To realize the full potential of each system, the system must be fully integrated. In other words, it must be possible to combine information from any system with information from any other system. For example, when healthcare practitioners are expected to control costs and provide high-quality care at the same time, they must have access to both clinical *and* financial information. Similarly, when administrators are making difficult decisions about the future direction of their enterprises, they need access to decision support systems that provide timely, relevant, and meaningful clinical and administrative information.

The course of hospital care for a typical patient illustrates how several different systems or applications might be used to collect information during an encounter.

Carlson Medical Center is a large, academic medical center. Mrs. Emily Mason, a 65-year-old woman, was admitted to Carlson for coronary bypass surgery. Prior to admission, she had experienced severe chest pain and was brought to the emergency department by her husband. Upon their arrival, Mr. Mason gave information about his wife's health history, current medications, and insurance coverage. This clinical information, along with demographic information about Mrs. Mason (her address, age, marital status, and so on), was entered into the patient registration system by the registration staff. Mrs. Mason's insurance carrier was notified immediately of her need for medical services and possible bypass surgery.

A nurse then entered Mrs. Mason's vital signs and clinical notes into the nursing IS. The attending physician on duty obtained additional information on Mrs. Mason's health history and ordered a comprehensive battery of laboratory tests. The physician's orders were submitted electronically through the order-entry system to the laboratory. The results of the tests were made available through the laboratory IS within a few hours. As the various tests were run, the charges for the tests were added automatically to the patient accounting system and eventually appeared on Mrs. Mason's hospital bill.

The attending physician recommended that Mrs. Mason be admitted immediately. He also ordered a cardiac catheterization and several medications. The cardiac catheterization laboratory was notified of the admission, and the procedure was scheduled through the hospital's scheduling system. The pharmacy component of the hospital's IS alerted the physician to a possible drug interaction. In response to the pharmacy alert, the physician altered his medication order for Mrs. Mason.

During her stay, Mrs. Mason had two chest x-rays. Radiology staff performed the procedures and made the results available to the physician through the radiology IS.

Upon discharge from the hospital, Mrs. Mason was scheduled to have a follow-up visit at the hospital's ambulatory care clinic. The clinic was located in a building adjacent to the medical center.

This case illustrates the use of several different information systems. What is not obvious from this case is the extent to which these systems operate independently or as parts of the whole. The following section discusses the various types of ISs as well as some other IS applications that are commonly used in healthcare facilities. It should be kept in mind that the goal in today's healthcare environment is to create fully integrated ISs. Although these systems can be described as separate entities with specific functions, they should be viewed as part of the enterprise-wide IS.

Inpatient Clinical Information Systems

The first major category of information systems used in healthcare is the clinical information system. Clinical ISs are designed primarily to support patient care by providing healthcare practitioners with access to timely, complete, and relevant clinical information. Healthcare practitioners use clinical information to diagnose, treat, and manage patient care.

In addition to patient care, clinical ISs also may be used for quality improvement, peer review, research, and other purposes. Clinical ISs include a broad range of applications such as patient records, patient care management, departmental clinical management (also known as ancillary systems), computerized provider order entry, medication administration, and clinical decision support.

Electronic Medical Records

The terms *EMR, EHR (electronic health record),* and *CPR (computer-based patient record)* are often used interchangeably to describe many different levels of computer systems used to maintain patient care information. (See chapter 4 for additional information on EMRs, EHRs, and CPRs.) One of the first definitions and uses of the term *CPR* appeared in the IOM's landmark study on the state of health records in 1991. According to the IOM, a CPR was "an electronic patient record that resides in a system specifically designed to support users by providing accessibility to complete and accurate data, alerts, reminders, clinical decision support systems, links to medical knowledge, and other aids" (Dick and Steen 1991). (By the mid-1990s, the term *CPR* began to wane and the terms *EMR* and *EHR* become more widely used.)

As noted in chapter 4, the EMR is more than scanned documents or replication of paper forms made available electronically. Its structure allows for electronic information storage, exchange, and retrieval. EMR systems generally include clinical decision support capabilities, reminders, and access to knowledge databases.

The major advantages to EMR systems can be categorized into three major groups: (1) improved quality, outcomes and safety (Bates and Gawande 2003), (2) improved services and satisfaction (Wager et al. 2000), and (3) improved efficiency, productivity, and cost reduction. In fact, a recent report indicated that adoption of interoperable EMR systems could produce efficiency and safety savings of $142 to $371 billion (Hillestad et al. 2005). Despite the many advantages of adopting EMR systems, however, less than 15 percent of healthcare organizations have fully implemented them. The major barriers to implementation include user acceptance, insufficient standards, security and privacy concerns, high cost, and lack of organizational support and leadership.

Patient Care and Departmental Clinical Systems

Even though electronic record keeping systems are still evolving and not yet the standard in healthcare, other patient care and departmental clinical systems are widely available. They collect and maintain a significant portion of the clinical data captured during a patient visit or encounter in an electronic form. Common patient care systems include order entry, results reporting, and department-based clinical systems in specific areas of the hospital such as laboratory, pharmacy, nursing, and radiology. To have an accurate and complete picture of the patient's health history and care, the provider must have access to all relevant clinical information from each of these ancillary systems.

Laboratory Information Systems

Laboratory ISs are used for collecting, verifying, and reporting test results. Systems today use computer technology to process specimens and analyze data, monitor test quality, control inventory, monitor work flow, and assess laboratory productivity (Hunter 1999).

Pharmacy Information Systems

Most pharmacy ISs simplify and streamline the dispensing of medications, control inventory, automatically compare drug orders with dosages appropriate for the patient, and provide information about contraindications. Common functions in a pharmacy IS include online order entry, automatic refill dispensing reports, and drug compatibility checks.

Radiology Information Systems

Major advances in diagnostic imaging technologies have led to radiology ISs that can generate, analyze, and manage images. Picture archiving and communication systems (PACSs) are being used widely in managing digital images. Moreover, they are making it unnecessary to store radiological images on film.

Nursing Information Systems

Nursing ISs are used to automate the nursing process from assessment to evaluation, including patient care documentation. Common features of a nursing IS include patient care decision support, management applications, and nursing education and research.

Clinical Decision Support Systems

The more advanced clinical information systems generally include decision support capabilities. Clinical decision support (CDS) systems assist healthcare providers in the actual diagnosis and treatment of patients. CDS systems analyze data from clinical ISs, search for unusual patterns or possible adverse effects, and recommend alternative actions to remedy the situation (Teich and Wrinn 2000). These alerts or reminders can perform a wide range of functions from indicating potential drug–drug interactions to recommending a complete plan of care based on the patient's health history and clinical assessment.

Studies have shown that CDS systems can save lives, reduce healthcare costs, improve communication, increase clinician and patient satisfaction, and enhance the overall process of care (Bates and Gawande 2003).

Computerized Provider Order Entry Systems

A computerized provider order entry (CPOE) system is a computer application that accepts physician orders electronically, replacing handwritten or verbal orders and prescriptions. Most CPOE systems provide physicians with decision-support capabilities during the ordering process (Wager, Lee, and Glaser 2005) and are used to facilitate patient care and decrease medical errors.

Medication Administration Systems

Like CPOE systems, medication administration (bar code–enabled point-of-care) systems are designed to improve patient safety. Using bar code–enabled devices at the point of care, these systems are designed to ensure that the right patient gets the right dose at the right time and through the right route. Medication administration systems that use bar code–enabled point-of-care technology can be highly effective in reducing all types of medication errors (Barlas 2002).

Administrative Information Systems

Administrative information systems comprise the second major category of IS used in healthcare. Often called management information systems (MISs), these systems are used to manage the financial, personnel, materials, facilities, and other resources used in the delivery of healthcare services. In other words, administrative information systems support the daily management-related operations of the healthcare enterprise.

Patient Registration Systems

According to the Office of the National Coordinator,

> Going to the doctor or hospital often requires filling out multiple forms. These forms collect information such as name, address, insurance, medications, allergies, etc. Then, when an individual requires lab work or other testing, the same information has to be collected again. A single electronic health registration will make it easier for individuals to give their information and for clinicians to use it. Additionally, the consumer could update the information once and share it with all providers immediately as needed (ONC 2005).

Today, most hospitals and other healthcare facilities use computer systems for registering patients and tracking their encounters that require multiple points for data input. Within hospitals, these systems are commonly known as admission–discharge–transfer (ADT) systems. Diagnostic and length of stay (LOS) information also can be stored in

ADT systems. In ambulatory care and outpatient settings, similar registration systems are used to collect relevant demographic and insurance information.

Patient registration systems must be linked with other ancillary departments in order to coordinate the patient's care. Similarly, they are often used to generate a set of documents that require the patient's signature when the patient is unable to consent to treatment. Examples of such documents are a consent to treatment, an authorization to release medical information for insurance purposes, and advance directives for care.

Financial Information Systems

As discussed earlier, administrative systems and financial information systems were the first computer systems used by healthcare organizations. Financial ISs typically include functions such as payroll preparation and accounting; accounts payable; patient accounting, including billing and accounts receivable processing; cost accounting; general ledger accounting; budgeting; and financial statement preparation (Malec 1998). All these functions provide essential information to the healthcare managers who plan, monitor, and control the financial resources of the enterprise.

Human Resource Management Systems

Today, personnel expenses make up 60 to 70 percent of the operating budgets of healthcare institutions. Consequently, healthcare managers rely increasingly on ISs not only to maintain personnel records, but also to enable them to create management reports.

A wide range of human resource management applications is available. Reports can be created to track staff productivity, analyze labor expenses by cost center, monitor turnover and absenteeism, assess training and continuing education needs, and forecast staffing needs. Some healthcare organizations use human resource management programs to review applicants' qualifications and experience and match them with current job openings.

Materials Management Systems

Healthcare organizations also use computer systems to manage materials and supplies. Materials management systems may include electronic purchasing and inventory control software and bar coding and wireless devices for tracking supplies and materials. The benefits of using materials management systems include cost savings, reductions in inventory, greater efficiency, fewer lost charges, and lower labor costs (Bockle et al. 1996).

Facilities Management Systems

In today's competitive environment, well-maintained physical facilities are critical to providing high-quality patient care and a safe, comfortable environment for patients and their families. In fact, in recent years, many healthcare organizations have invested considerable resources in upgrading their physical facilities in an effort to make patients feel more at home. Automated facilities management systems can help organizations plan, manage, and maintain physical facilities. Common functions include preventative maintenance, energy management, and project management and scheduling (Malec 1998).

Management Support Systems

Management support systems comprise the third major category of information systems used by healthcare organizations. Management support systems produce reports for the organization's day-to-day operation and allow data to be manipulated to provide information for strategic decision making. There are several subcategories of management support systems, including management information systems (MISs), executive information systems (EISs), and strategic decision support (SDS) systems.

Management Information Systems

MISs focus on providing reports and information to managers for day-to-day operations of the organization. The types of common reports produced by an MIS include:

- *Periodic, scheduled reports:* Periodic, scheduled reports are the most traditional type of reporting system. The content and the time schedule for production of the reports are prespecified. Examples of periodic, scheduled reports are the daily hospital census and the financial monthly reports of the organization. The content and the format of these reports are specified in advance, as is the time period in which they will be produced.

- *Exception reports:* An MIS also may include reports that are produced only when exceptional or out-of-the-ordinary conditions are met or occur. An example of an exception report is an accounting report of past-due bills. In this case, the report is only generated for accounts that are past due. The out-of-the-ordinary occurrence and content and format of the report are predefined, and only cases or records meeting the predefined criteria are reported.

- *Demand reports:* As opposed to periodic and exception reports, demand reports are produced, as needed, whenever a manager "demands" or asks for it. Usually, demand reports are produced through report generators or database query languages and are customized by the manager.

Strategic Decision Support System

Another category of management reports is the SDS system. There are several differences between an MIS and a DSS. A DSS is geared toward supporting strategic decisions whereas the MIS produces reports for operational and tactical decision making. MIS reports are less dynamic than DSS reports. However, DSS reports allow managers to manipulate data and conduct what-if, sensitivity, and optimization analyses.

Some common features of SDS systems include the ability to:

- Monitor and evaluate key performance indicators and trends

- Perform simulations of revenue and expense patterns based on various assumptions

- Estimate potential demand for services within different market areas

Moreover, SDS systems may be used to allocate resources or improve overall operations and efficiency within the healthcare enterprise. Although these systems are not currently used as widely as clinical and administrative ISs, they are emerging as a vital resource that helps healthcare executives make sound strategic decisions. (The application of such systems is described more fully in chapter 18.)

Executive Information Systems

EISs are a type of decision support system used by high-level managers. Like other decision support systems, an EIS draws data from the organization's other databases. The EIS is programmed to reorganize and distill large quantities of data into a form that meets the executive's information needs. Executive information systems are essential tools for financial management in modern organizations. The EIS yields financial information at the summary level, but it also allows a user to "drill down" to more detailed information when necessary. In an acute care hospital, for example, the EIS typically provides yearly LOS and average daily census statistics in addition to financial data. These types of ISs are often referred to as "dashboard reports" or "balanced scorecard" reports.

Outpatient Information Systems

As mentioned previously, outpatient information systems have many functions associated with inpatient systems. For example, outpatient systems often feature EHR components. However, outpatient systems must be tailored to the needs of the ambulatory care environment. Depending on the type of outpatient service (physician office, clinic, dental office, and so on), the type of functionality in the ISs will vary. In general, however, outpatient IS will include the following functionalities:

- Appointment scheduling
- Patient billing
- Electronic claims submission for health plans
- Automatic charge and payment posting
- Patient collection and mail-merge systems
- Health record data capture and retrieval
- Prescription writing
- Report generation

Check Your Understanding 17.2

Instructions: Match the information systems below with the type(s) of information that each is *most likely* to capture.

a. Physician's orders
b. Chest x-ray
c. Applicant's qualifications
d. Employee benefits
e. Drug–drug interactions
f. Laboratory test results
g. Patient admission and discharge dates
h. Inventory of supplies
i. Patient rooms to be cleaned
j. Financial impact of adding a new service
k. Physician office visit note
l. Patient's bill
m. Dose of medication
n. Nursing assessment

1. _____ Clinical decision support system

2. _____ Electronic medical record

3. _____ Facilities management

4. _____ Human resource management

5. _____ Laboratory information system

6. _____ Materials management

7. _____ Nursing information system

8. _____ Computerized provider order entry

9. _____ Medication administration using bar code–enabled point of care

10. _____ Outpatient information systems

11. _____ Patient accounting system

12. _____ Patient registration system

13. _____ Pharmacy information system

14. _____ Payroll system

Strategic Information Systems Planning

Given the size and complexity of healthcare organizations and the number of emerging technologies, strategic information systems planning is an essential first step in adopting new IS technology. **Strategic information systems planning** is the process of identifying and assigning priorities to the various upgrades and changes that might be made in an organization's ISs. Its goal is to ensure that all changes contribute to the achievement of the organization's strategic goals and objectives.

In years past, relatively few healthcare organizations engaged in strategic planning for information systems. If an organization did have an IS plan, it likely had been developed by information services staff without regard to the organization's overall strategic plan.

Today, healthcare leaders understand that effective information management is essential to the success of every organization. Improvements in the organization's ISs must be an integral component of the strategic plan. In addition, the importance of coordinating planning efforts among the various computer users in a healthcare organization is obvious, but the process is not easy.

For example, one of a hospital's strategic goals might be to provide outreach services to rural communities in surrounding counties. If the managers involved in planning the outreach program were unaware of recent advances in telemedical systems, they might not consider the use of information technology to help them achieve the goal. Similarly, without coordinated planning, the **information services department** might go off on its own and acquire new ISs that would not support the outreach program being planned.

The financial and human resources of most healthcare organizations are limited. Different functional areas may want or need to upgrade or replace current ISs with new ones. All the competing requests may be valid and appropriate. For example, the pharmacy director may want to replace an outdated pharmacy IS with state-of-the-art handheld devices designed to prevent and track medication errors. At the same time, the laboratory director may request funds to upgrade the laboratory IS to the latest version. The health information manager may wish to implement a document-imaging system to address space constraints within the **health information services department.** The vice-president for finance may want to install a decision support system on the desktop of every administrator. How can the organization decide which of these requests is the most important to implement?

The IS plan can be thought of as something like a blueprint for remodeling a house. A blueprint that incorporated all the wishes and needs of the family members—enlarged kitchen for mom, new garage for dad, additional bedrooms for the kids, new roof, third bathroom—probably would be too expensive to build and the resulting house might not function well. Family members would need to consider their long-term priorities before deciding how best to invest their limited resources. Similarly, an IS plan should be based on the needs of the organization as a whole and its long-term priorities.

In the earlier example, implementing all the requests for a pharmacy IS, an administrative decision support system, and so on probably would be too expensive and might not support the organization's long-term goals. If the hospital's long-range strategy were to implement a nonproprietary EMR system within two years, each director's request should be considered within the context of how each application would contribute to that goal. Priority would be given to those projects that support the future implementation of an enterprise-wide EMR system.

Adopting new information technology represents an enormous investment in terms of staff time, hardware and software costs, and consulting fees. Establishing enterprise-wide priorities for IS development is not an easy task. Every area of the organization may be able to make a compelling case for why a new IS or new technology is needed and how a new system would help the area contribute to the organization's strategic goals. Many factors come into play. And priorities do change in response to political pressure, patient safety issues, new federal regulations, and other factors.

One approach is to compile a comprehensive list of all of the proposed changes to the organization's ISs. The list would include a description of every proposed change along with information on the new technology's availability and ease of implementation, expected benefits and cost savings, and estimated acquisition and maintenance costs. The list then could be distributed to a broad sample of clinicians, managers, and end users. They would be asked to rank the different systems. The steering committee might oversee such a process under the leadership of the **chief information officer** (CIO) or some other top-level clinician or administrator. For clinical systems, it is critical that the initiative be clinician driven, not IS driven.

The strategic IS plan should serve as a guide to making difficult decisions about where, when, and how an institution should allocate resources for the management of information. The interdisciplinary IS steering committee and its role in setting priorities and managing projects are discussed in more detail later in this chapter.

Systems Development Life Cycle

After a strategic plan for information systems has been established, most healthcare organizations follow a structured process for selecting and implementing new computer-based systems. Such an approach can be extremely beneficial in assessing user needs, identifying various alternatives, gaining user buy-in, selecting a system that meets the needs of users, and implementing the system according to a well-organized, systematic plan. Because the organization's staff may be involved in several IS projects at one time, it is important to follow a consistent process for every IS implementation.

There are many different versions of the **systems development life cycle** (SDLC), but they all include four general phases:

1. Planning and analysis

2. Design

3. Implementation

4. Maintenance and evaluation

The SDLC represents an ongoing process that requires continuous assessment and planning. (Figure 17.2 illustrates the cyclical nature of the SDLC.)

The systems development process involves participation from a wide variety of people with different backgrounds and areas of expertise. Depending on the project's nature and scope, representatives from the key clinical and administrative areas should be involved in the process. For example, if the institution is interested in implementing an enterprise-wide EMR system, representatives from the medical staff, nursing, pharmacy, radiology, laboratory, and other ancillary areas should be included, as well as representatives from HIM services and IS services.

Planning and Analysis

Sometimes it is difficult to tell when systems planning ends and systems analysis begins. This discussion is based on the assumption that the systems planning process resulted in an okay to go ahead with the project. After the decision has been made to explore the need for new information technology further, the feasibility of the system is assessed and the scope of the project defined. The primary focus at the **system planning and analysis** phase is on the business problem, independent of any technology that can or will be used to implement a solution to that problem. That is, emphasis is placed on business issues, not technical or implementation concerns.

During this phase, it is beneficial to examine current systems and problems in order to identify opportunities for improvement or enhancement. Sometimes there is a tendency to

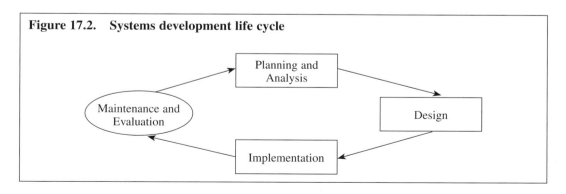

Figure 17.2.   Systems development life cycle

think that implementing new computer technology will solve every information management problem. By examining current systems and problems, the project team may find that current problems are rooted in ineffective procedures rather than technological shortcomings. Communication glitches, inadequate training, and insufficient technical support are examples of procedural problems that can be fixed with nontechnical solutions.

After it is clear that new information technology is needed, the next step is to assess the information needs of users and to define the functional requirements of the system. This process can be very time-consuming. It is helpful to have a formal mechanism for soliciting user information. For example, the organization may ask key representatives from each functional areas to assess the needs within their departments. The assessment might involve administering questionnaires, interviewing staff, or holding interdisciplinary planning sessions. Interdisciplinary planning is a highly structured group process. A series of meetings may be needed to analyze problems and define functional requirements. As part of the needs assessment, it is helpful to collect, organize, and evaluate information about the environment in which the new system is to operate.

Design

The **system design** phase begins after the information needs of the users have been identified. During this phase, it is decided how the new system will be designed or selected. Will the new system be built in house? Will the organization contract with an outside developer to build the system? Will the organization purchase a generic system from a vendor? Because of time, cost, and staffing constraints, most healthcare organizations begin the design process by looking at systems that are already available on the market. The rest of this discussion focuses on the selection of an IS product and vendor. (Chapter 16 discusses the in-house development of information systems.)

Vendor Selection Process

Information about IS vendors and the software and hardware on the market is available from a number of sources. Exhibits at professional association conferences are one source of information. Publications, Web sites, consulting firms, and professional colleagues are others. Often the organization sends a **request for information** (RFI) to a list of vendors known to offer products or systems that may meet its needs. The RFI asks for general product information and is a good tool for prescreening vendors. Responses to the RFI can be used to narrow the list of potential vendors who will receive a **request for proposal** (RFP).

Request for Proposal
The request for proposal (RFP) generally includes a detailed description of the requirements for the system and gives guidelines for vendors to follow in bidding for the contract. For a major system acquisition, Wager, Lee, and Glaser recommend that the RFP include the following elements (2005, 156):

> ***Instructions for vendors.***
>
> - Proposal deadline and contact information: where and when the RFP is due; whom to contact should the vendor have questions.

- Confidentiality statement and instructions: a statement that both the RFP and the responses provided by the vendor are confidential and are proprietary information.

- Specific instructions for completing the RFP and any stipulations with which the vendor must comply in order to be considered.

- Organization objectives: type of system or application being sought; information management needs and plans.

Background of the organization.

- Overview of the facility: size, types of patient services, patient volume, staff composition, strategic goals of organization.

- Application and technical inventory: current systems in use, hardware, software, network infrastructure.

- Systems goals and requirements: goals for the system and functional requirements. Typically this section includes application, technical, and integration requirements.

- Vendor qualifications: general background of vendor, experience, number of installations, financial stability, list of current clients, standard content, and implementation plan.

- Proposed solutions: how vendor believes its product meets the goals and needs of the health care organization. Vendor may include case studies, results from system analysis projects, and other evidence of the benefits of its proposed solution.

- Criteria for evaluating proposals: how the health care organization will make its final decisions on product selection.

- General contractual requirements: such as warranties, payment schedule, penalties for failure to meet schedules specified in contract, vendor responsibilities, and so forth.

- Pricing and support: quote on cost of system, using standardized terms and forms.

There are several ways to approach the evaluation of the vendors' responses to the RFP. For example, the organization may wish to evaluate the extent to which each product meets the functional requirements of the new system. Most organizations look hard at the vendor's track record on previous projects and contact previous clients. The extent to which the vendor's philosophy of systems development aligns with the organization's needs also should be considered.

After the RFP has been distributed to the vendors, the organization may hold a bidders' conference to answer vendors' questions about the RFP. This gives all the vendors the opportunity to receive the same information.

The organization should assess the reliability, cost, and projected benefits of each product. However, evaluation of the vendor and its products may not depend solely on the vendor's response to the RFP. Other formal and informal mechanisms may be used to assess the vendor's fit with the organization and the product's capabilities. For example, it is a good idea to hold vendor presentations, attend user group meetings, and make site visits to other facilities that use the product. The purpose of these activities is to gain as much relevant information as possible. Clinicians and other end users should participate throughout the vendor selection process.

There are times when a healthcare organization might decide that it does not have the IS resources needed to acquire a healthcare information system. Rather than purchasing one, the organization may chose to leverage someone else's infrastructure by contracting with an **application service provider** (ASP). An ASP is a company that deploys, hosts, and manages one or more software packages through centrally located services, often on a fixed per use basis or a subscription basis (Kelly and Legrow 2000). ASPs are a popular option for small community-based physician practices without the IS infrastructure to support a system of their own.

Cost-Benefit Analysis

As part of the selection process, it is important to consider both the anticipated costs and the anticipated benefits of implementing each solution. *Costs* generally include expenditures for hardware, software, network access, and training, as well as operating/maintenance costs, upgrades, technical support, supplies, and additional equipment. Most costs can be identified and measured.

Benefits are often much more difficult to measure. For example, a newly proposed document-scanning system may have both tangible benefits (such as multiple-user access, increased availability, and fewer lost records) and intangible benefits (such as increased physician satisfaction and improved employee morale). Although tangible and intangible benefits are both very important, the intangible benefits can be difficult to quantify. Consequently, it is important to develop a mechanism for evaluating and measuring the costs and benefits of each product.

Describing the different **cost–benefit analysis** methods is beyond the scope of this book. Whitten, Bentley, and Dittman (2005) provide a fairly comprehensive explanation of the different cost–benefit analysis methods.

Contract Negotiations

After the top two or three vendors have been identified, the contract negotiation process can begin. It is generally a good idea to begin contract negotiations with more than one vendor. Competition provides leverage during the negotiation process and gives the organization an alternative when a contract cannot be negotiated successfully with the organization's first choice. The contract generally addresses numerous technical issues, everything from when the system is to be delivered and installed to who is responsible for ensuring that the product works with the organization's other ISs. Internal legal counsel should review the contract carefully before it is signed and binding agreements are made.

Implementation

The **system implementation** phase begins after the contract has been signed. Typically, the organization designates an interdisciplinary implementation team led by a project manager to develop a plan for implementing the new system. The implementation team should include some of the same individuals involved in selecting the new system, as well as other key people.

Selecting an effective project manager is critical to successful system implementation. Ideally, the project manager should be a knowledgeable individual with past experience in similar implementation projects. The project manager should be someone who is highly respected by others in the organization. Finally, he or she should have strong organizational and communication skills and the political influence and authority necessary to get the project done.

However, a well-executed implementation does not guarantee that users will accept a new system. Problems during implementation can lead to user frustration, dissatisfaction, and disillusionment. Indeed, some organizations never recover fully from disastrous system implementations.

The project manager and the implementation team should begin the implementation process by making a list of the tasks to be completed. The scope and complexity of the process depend on the type of system, the number of users, and the complexity of the conversion process. Typical milestones in the implementation process for healthcare information systems include:

- Preparation of the site (for example, remodeling work spaces and installing telephone lines, computer cables, and electrical power lines)

- Installation of hardware and software

- Preparation of data tables

- Construction of system interfaces

- Development of a network infrastructure to support the system

- Training for managers, technical staff, and other end users who will test the new system

- Trial runs of the new system to identify and correct problems

- Preparation of support documentation (for example, procedure manuals)

- Development of backup and disaster recovery procedures

- Training for other end users

- Conversion to the new system

Many implementation activities take place simultaneously. Others need to be completed before other activities can begin. It is generally a good idea for the project manager to use a Gantt chart or another project management tool to schedule and track the milestones in the implementation process. The tool should list the activities to be completed along with the estimated start and completion dates for each, the names of the individuals responsible for each activity, and the resources needed to complete each task. Project management software (for example, Microsoft Project) is useful for creating

Gantt charts and tracking project resources (for example, staff, equipment) and expenditures.

All the implementation tasks are important. However, three are especially critical to the success of the project: testing the new system, training the end users, and converting to the new system.

Testing of the New System

Thorough testing of new systems (hardware and/or software) before the actual conversion date is critical. This means testing, testing, and retesting the system with actual patient data, not sample data the vendor has provided or the organization has created for training purposes. Correcting a problem in the test mode is often easier than correcting it after the system is fully operational. Even though it is nearly impossible to identify and correct every potential problem before a new system goes live, it is essential to identify and correct as many of them as possible.

Training for End Users

It is critical to provide adequate training for the end users of the new system. For any new system to be successful, it must be accepted and used by the staff. When the staff is not thoroughly trained, the result may be low morale and dissatisfaction with the system.

One common approach to staff training is a train-the-trainer program. In this approach, key people in the various functional areas (for example, nursing, laboratory, and billing) are identified and trained first. They then train the other users in their area. This approach is effective because the trainers are still available to help the staff after the system has been installed and the vendor is no longer on-site to answer questions.

It is equally critical to allow adequate time for training. Staff should not have to squeeze in training during their lunch breaks. They will need time to practice using the new system. Just as it is important to use actual data to test the system, it is also important for staff to practice using the new system with actual data on real patients.

Conversion to the New System

Conversion to a new IS often requires significant changes in work flow and organizational structure. The process also demands a lot of staff time and disrupts productivity and business processes if not properly executed and resourced. Adequate technical support staff must be available to assist managers and end users as needed.

Several different approaches may be used to make the conversion from an old IS to a new one. In deciding which approach to use, it is important to consider the nature of the application, the risks and costs associated with each alternative, and the resources available. The most common approaches are parallel, phased, and direct cutover conversion (Wold and Shriver 1994).

The *parallel approach* involves running both the old and the new systems until the managers and staff are confident that the new system works. This approach is costly and can be confusing to staff, but it ensures that a backup system would be available if needed.

One type of *phased approach* involves implementing portions of the new system over time instead of installing the entire system all at once. Another type of phased approach involves implementing systems in selected locations instead of at all locations at the same time. For example, a document-imaging system might be implemented in one clinic as a pilot site, with future plans to deploy the system to other clinics within the facility.

Converting in phased stages helps the staff gain confidence in the new system, helps the implementation team learn from the experience at the pilot site, and ensures that sufficient time is allowed to make the transition smoothly.

Finally, with the *direct cutover approach,* the organization stops using the old system and starts the new one on a specified date. This approach is risky but can work effectively when sufficient testing was done and adequate backup procedures are in place. In fact, it may make more sense to convert via the direct cutover method when the old system is quite different from the new one.

Maintenance and Evaluation

The last phase of the systems development life cycle is **system maintenance and evaluation.** Maintenance and evaluation activities ensure both the short- and long-term success of the information system. Problems inevitably show up after a new IS is put into operation. Adequate IS support staff must be available to identify potential problems and take steps to correct them.

Technical support for critical systems should be available twenty-four hours a day, seven days a week. The patient care IS is probably the most vital system in a healthcare organization. Sufficient technical staff also should be available to oversee the following activities:

- System backups

- Software upgrades

- Equipment maintenance and replacement

- Ongoing user training and assistance

- Disaster recovery

Some IS experts estimate that at least 25 percent of the technical staff's time should be devoted to maintenance activities (Austin and Boxerman 2003). System maintenance can be either performed by full-time employees or contracted out to the system vendor.

Every organization that maintains electronic health information is required by federal law to develop emergency backup procedures and a disaster recovery plan. (See the discussion of the Health Insurance Portability and Accountability Act in chapter 19.) Staff training in emergency procedures also is required. Written backup and emergency procedures should be made readily available to staff.

However, maintaining and supporting new systems is not enough. The effectiveness of every IS should be evaluated on a continuous basis. Continuous evaluation activities ensure that the organization's ISs support its overall mission and goals and meet users' needs.

Healthcare administrators today demand information on the organization's return on investment (ROI) when new technological systems are implemented. The ability to measure ROI is increasingly important as healthcare institutions struggle to manage limited resources more effectively. Consequently, as a part of the system evaluation process, organizations are looking at the organizational, technological, and economic impact of ISs on the enterprise as a whole (Friedman and Wyatt 1997; Anderson and Aydin 2005).

Check Your Understanding 17.3

Instructions: The following is a list of the different tasks or activities that might need to be done to implement an automated coding system. Number the tasks in the order in which they should be carried out. Assign the same number to any tasks that can be done simultaneously.

a. _____ Establish implementation team and develop project time line.

b. _____ Assess the coders' needs.

c. _____ Determine whether the proposed coding program is in line with the organization's strategic plan and mission.

d. _____ Hold bidders' conferences for potential vendors.

e. _____ Prepare a list of users' specifications.

f. _____ Negotiate a contract with the system vendor.

g. _____ Prepare documentation and procedures to support the new system.

h. _____ Determine the date of implementation.

i. _____ Submit an RFI to potential vendors.

j. _____ Train staff on how to use the new system.

k. _____ Test the new system.

l. _____ Submit an RFP to potential vendors.

m. _____ Identify problems with current coding processes and opportunities for improvement.

n. _____ Contact other sites that use the products or systems being considered.

o. _____ Determine conversion plans.

p. _____ Conduct cost–benefit analysis of the different products or systems being considered.

Management of Information Resources

Effectively managing its information resources is just as important to the healthcare organization as keeping its information systems up-to-date. Modern healthcare organizations recognize that information is a critical resource to be managed as carefully as human resources, financial resources, and capital equipment. In large part, the organization's ability to provide high-quality, cost-effective healthcare services depends on the availability of accurate and accessible information.

The concept of **information resource management** (IRM) assumes that information is a valuable resource that must be managed no matter what form it takes or what medium it is stored in. Modern healthcare providers use clinical information for many purposes, including:

- It supports the diagnostic and therapeutic services provided to patients.

- It is used in performance improvement (PI) activities that measure and improve the quality of care.

- It is used to perform medical research and to improve the general health of the public.

Moreover, the reporting of accurate clinical information is the basis of contemporary reimbursement systems.

However, healthcare organizations have not always valued information as an essential resource. The modern notion of managing information resources emerged during the late 1980s. At that time, healthcare organizations were being forced to become more competitive in order to survive in the marketplace. They came to recognize the value of an enterprise-wide perspective on information (Johns 1997) as well as the need to integrate clinical and administrative information. Before that time, most clinical information was managed at the departmental level or stored in paper-based patient records housed in the health record department. The IS departments of this era were chiefly concerned with processing data and played only a minor role in deciding how to use information within the organization.

IRM is a broad concept that encompasses the creation, use, storage, and eventual disposal of all information, whether it is captured and maintained in a paper-based system or a computer-based system. This broad view is congruent with the philosophy of information management adopted by the Joint Commission on Accreditation of Healthcare Organizations (JCAHO). The JCAHO encourages healthcare organizations to develop ISs that support their needs and those of the patients they serve.

In healthcare organizations, the healthcare professionals who provide services to patients in a number of different care settings need information. They also need information to meet the reporting requirements of external accreditation and regulatory agencies and to carry out PI activities. Several categories of information can be captured and used to satisfy these needs, including:

- *Patient-specific information* consists of interpreted data that are linked to individual patients. For example, a blood glucose level for Mr. Smith would be considered patient-specific information.

- *Aggregate information* consists of detailed data sets that are combined to provide a summarization. For instance, adding all the female and male patients for a specific month to arrive at a total number of patients is an example of aggregate information.

- *Expert knowledge-based information* usually refers to expert knowledge bases that are used in expert decision support systems. These automated knowledge bases contain facts about a specific subject area and reasoning processes to evaluate these facts.

- *Comparative information* consists of data sets that have the same attributes but are from different sources and are evaluated or compared against each other. For example, one hospital might want to compare its average length of stay for patients who experienced myocardial infarctions with the average stays of other, similar hospitals.

Each category of information must be managed at multiple points. First, the appropriate sources of data must be identified, and the data must be captured and stored. Data can be defined as noninterpreted facts, images, and sounds that must be analyzed, interpreted, and transformed into information. This information then must be transmitted to the appropriate users for functions such as clinical decision making, administrative decision making, research, performance improvement, and patient education (Clark and Cofer 2000). Thus, information is interpreted data or sets of data whose content is useful to some specific task.

Organizational Models That Support IRM

Managing information at the enterprise level is not an easy task. Healthcare organizations need an organizational structure that facilitates effective information resource management. Figure 17.3 provides an example of an organizational model that supports enterprise-wide IRM.

Role of the Chief Information Officer

The CIO is a senior-level executive. He or she is responsible for leading the strategic IS planning process, for helping the leadership team use ISs in support of strategic planning and management, and for overseeing the organization's IRM functions. These functions are performed by the IS department as well as by the telecommunications, management engineering, and HIM (health record) departments.

The CIO typically reports directly to the organization's chief executive officer (CEO). Through the CIO's efforts as a senior manager, IS activities can be aligned with the organization's mission and strategic priorities.

Role of the Information Systems Steering Committee

The CIO does not determine the strategic vision for information systems or information management alone. Most healthcare organizations establish an IS steering committee. The committee includes clinicians and administrators from key areas throughout the enterprise as well as IS professionals. Working as a team, the IS steering committee assesses the organization's information needs, establishes IS priorities, and oversees IS implementation projects. To be successful, the committee needs senior-level support from the medical staff, nursing, and other clinical areas. All plans for new IS or technology projects should be channeled through the IS steering committee to ensure that they are in line with the organization's strategic vision.

Role of the Chief Information Security Officer

As information management has become more complex and information technology has taken on more strategic importance, a new information management position has emerged: the **chief information security officer** (CISO). The CISO may report directly to the CIO

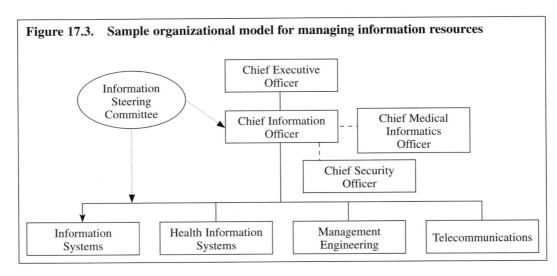

Figure 17.3.   Sample organizational model for managing information resources

or the CEO. The typical CISO is responsible for overseeing the development, implementation, and enforcement of the organization's security policies. He or she manages the security of all patient-identifiable information, whether it is stored in paper-based or computer-based systems.

Recently, the CISO role has become better recognized within healthcare organizations in the context of the new security and confidentiality regulations. Federal agencies developed these regulations in response to passage of the Health Insurance Portability and Accountability Act (HIPAA) of 1996. HIPAA security regulations apply to all patient-identifiable healthcare information created, maintained, or stored in an electronic format. They require administrative, physical, and technical services and mechanisms to safeguard the confidentiality, availability, and integrity of health information. (Information security and privacy issues within the healthcare organization are discussed in detail in chapters 15 and 19.)

Like the CIO, the CISO does not develop policies or make decisions alone. Most healthcare institutions already have or plan to establish information security committees or patient information confidentiality councils. These groups oversee the development and implementation of policies related to the security and confidentiality of patient information. In addition to policy development and enforcement, the committee or council may develop and implement employee education and training programs. The goal of the training programs is to ensure that anyone who creates or uses information understands the importance of protecting it from unauthorized access or disclosure.

Role of the Chief Medical Informatics Officer

The **chief medical informatics officer** (CMIO) is another relatively new position within the information services organizational structure. This position emerged as healthcare organizations recognized the need to have physician leadership in the adoption of clinical ISs. A physician will staff the CMIO position. In some cases, the CMIO is a member of the healthcare organization's medical staff who fulfills this role on a part-time basis. Wager, Lee and, Glaser cite several examples of responsibilities that might be assumed by the CMIO (2005, 288), including:

- Leading the implementation of an EMR system

- Engaging physicians and other healthcare professionals in the development and use of the EMR system

- Leading the clinical informatics steering committee or other designated group that serves as the central governance forum for establishing the organization's clinical IS priorities

- Keeping pulse on the national efforts to develop EHR systems, assuming a leadership role in areas where the national effort and the organization's agenda are synergistic

- Being highly responsible to user needs, such as training, to ensure widespread use and acceptance of clinical ISs

Other IS Leadership Roles

Other leadership roles that have emerged recently within healthcare IS organizational structures are **chief privacy officer,** chief technology officer, and chief nursing informatics officer. The number and type of formal leadership positions will depend on the type and size of the healthcare organization. Because it may be filled by an HIM professional, the role of chief privacy officer is discussed in more detail in the following section. The chief technology officer is generally an IT or network specialist whose focus is on the technical infrastructure of the IS system. The chief nursing informatics officer would fill a similar role as the CMIO, but with a focus on nursing ISs.

Role of the Chief Privacy Officer

In recent years, healthcare organizations have come to recognize the need for a chief privacy officer. In large part, this position has emerged as a result of the HIPAA legislation, but also from growing public concern about privacy in general. Responsibilities include activities related to the development, implementation, and maintenance of, and adherence to, the organization's policies and procedures regarding the privacy of and access to patient-specific information. This position also involves responsibility for ensuring the organization's compliance with all federal, state, and accrediting body rules and regulations concerning the confidentiality and privacy of health-related information (AHIMA 2001).

Role of the Information Services Department

The information services department is generally responsible for ensuring that the organization has the technical infrastructure and staff required to support its healthcare information systems. Common functions of the department include data administration, network administration, network security, database management, systems integration, programming, end-user support, and IS development.

Traditionally, the staff working in the information services department had technical backgrounds in computer science, programming, network administration, and database management. However, managers of information services departments today recognize that technical expertise alone may not be sufficient to support the needs of end users. Consequently, information services managers are hiring healthcare professionals (physicians, nurses, and laboratory technicians) who understand clinical data and patient care processes and also have a background in IS technology (database management, systems analysis and design, or network management). These healthcare professionals often have job titles such as clinical systems analyst.

Role of the Health Information Management Department

The HIM department plays an important role in the management of information and, in particular, the management of patient records. Common functions of the HIM department include record retention and retrieval, diagnostic and procedural coding, medical transcription, release of information, and data management. HITs working in this department have the opportunity to provide leadership in the planning, selection, implementation, and evaluation of enterprise-wide healthcare ISs. HIM professionals bring to the table expertise in classification systems, patient confidentiality, documentation, accreditation standards, and regulations.

Current Issues in the Development of Healthcare Information Systems

Several current issues are influencing the development of healthcare information systems in the United States.

Role of the Internet in Healthcare

The Internet is a network of high-speed networks linked by common protocols and standards. Its unprecedented growth, particularly the World Wide Web and its related technologies, is having a tremendous impact on healthcare and healthcare ISs. A quick search of the Web on the subject of healthcare ISs reveals that many vendors are touting their Internet solutions. Healthcare organizations maintain informational Web pages for patients, providers, and insurers and use Internet technologies to communicate internally and externally with customers and suppliers. Examples of Internet use within healthcare are seemingly endless in today's world. The Web browser has become a familiar tool to healthcare workers, making it possible to search for and quickly find huge amounts of information on virtually any topic, including healthcare.

Most Internet users today equate the Internet with the Web because the Web is the means by which most users interact with the Internet, but the Internet encompasses a great deal more than the Web. The Internet had its beginning in the late 1960s. It was founded to promote national defense and academic research. To a large extent, its use was limited to these two groups until a British scientist created a software protocol named Hypertext Transfer Protocol (HTTP) and introduced the world to a user-friendly multimedia interface with the Internet.

The programming code for displaying files on the Web is called a markup language, and the application that can display the markup language is a Web browser. The most common markup language is hypertext markup language (HTML). HTML defines how text, images, and other content will look when viewed via a Web browser, such as Internet Explorer, Mozilla, or Firefox. Newer markup languages have had an impact on how healthcare and other information is stored. Extensible markup language (XML), for example, is a markup language that goes beyond information display and actually defines the information. XML shows promise as a standard in the development of healthcare applications.

There is no single owner of the Internet. Rather, the backbone of the Internet is owned and maintained by multiple organizations across many countries. Telecommunication companies and Internet service providers (ISPs) control specific segments of the Internet backbone.

Every device or computer that operates within the Internet has a unique identifier, an Internet protocol (IP) address. This address is a four-part number, with the sections divided by periods (or "dots"). IP addresses may be static or dynamic. A *dynamic address* is assigned to a computer, as needed, by a special server that can recognize when the computer or device needs the address. *Static addresses* are permanently assigned to specific computers or devices (Wager, Lee, and Glaser 2005).

Specific Internet protocols allow each computer or device on the Internet to communicate with the others. All computers and devices must adhere to defined protocols in order to work within the Internet environment. This set of Internet protocols is known as Transmission Control Protocol/Internet Protocol (TCP/IP). Hypertext transfer protocol (http) is one of the protocols that make up TCP/IP. HTTP allows the transfer of data coded in the hypertext languages to be transmitted across the Internet. Other common protocols within TCP/IP include e-mail protocols such as Simple Mail Transfer Protocol (SMTP), Post Office Protocol 3 (POP3), and Internet Message Access Protocol (IMAP)(Whatis. com 2002).

Internet standards not only are used to communicate across the Internet, but also have been applied to the computer networks of individual organizations. Following so-called

Internet standards frees individual networks from problems that occur when users work on different types of hardware platforms (IBM versus Macintosh, for example). Compliance with these standards enables different computers and operating systems to access with the same look and feel to the end user. These advances have increased demand among healthcare workers for access to the Web. For example, physicians in many organizations can now access patient information stored in the organization's clinical ISs from any location via a Web interface.

Healthcare workers want to use a single, familiar interface to track lab values, radiology results, patient demographics, and more. The Web browser is rapidly becoming a realistic solution for local as well as remote access. Today, the virtual health record has become a reality. Organizations can achieve the functionality of an EMR without having to invest in a huge data repository or data warehouse. Healthcare information about individual patients or groups of patients can be accessed via Web-based interface engines that bring information from separate databases (such as lab, radiology, health records) to a single workstation. In essence, these interface engines create what appears to be a single health record from multiple databases.

Increased consumer awareness is another outgrowth of the popularity of the Internet. Tens of thousands of Web sites offer information on health topics. Web browser software has made it easy for the average consumer to search and download information from virtually anywhere in the world. By 2000, an estimated 60 million U.S. residents had used the Internet to obtain health information (Fox and Rainie 2000). Consumers can purchase healthcare products, ask questions of health professionals, and engage in discussions with other patients via the Internet. A growing number of healthcare organizations have established Web sites to provide consumers with information on specific diseases and therapies and healthy lifestyles. Many also use their Web sites to promote their healthcare services.

The Internet and its related technologies will continue to play an important role in healthcare in the twenty-first century (NRC 2000). The Internet will be used to improve consumer access to health information and healthcare, to enhance clinical decision making, and to improve health outcomes by making better information available to clinicians on demand.

Concerns about Patient Privacy

The need to balance legitimate access to healthcare information against the patient's right to privacy has been a concern of health information managers and clinicians for a long time. But recent advances in Internet technology as well as other types of communications technology have heightened the public's awareness of potential threats to the confidentiality and security of healthcare information. In response to the public's concerns, Congress passed HIPAA, Public Law 104-191, in 1996. HIPAA was designed to improve the continuity of health insurance coverage, address administrative simplification, and protect data privacy and security.

HIPAA requires that healthcare plans, providers, and information clearinghouses adopt safeguards to protect the integrity and confidentiality of health information. For example, HIPAA regulations require the adoption of standards for the authentication of electronic signatures. Although the HIPAA security regulations apply specifically to patient-identifiable information that is maintained or transmitted electronically, the information does not lose its protection simply because it was printed out on paper. It is the information that is protected, not the medium in which the information appears (Gilbert 2000). Failure to comply with HIPAA regulations can result in substantial civil and criminal penalties.

Check Your Understanding 17.4

Instructions: Indicate whether the following statements are true or false (T or F).

1. _____ The concept of information resource management assumes that information is a valuable resource that must be managed in computer-based patient records.

2. _____ Before the 1980s, most clinical information was managed at the enterprise-wide level.

3. _____ The CIO is responsible for overseeing the healthcare organization's information resource management functions.

4. _____ The CISO is responsible for managing the security of all patient-identifiable information in the healthcare organization.

5. _____ The CISO role has become better recognized within healthcare organizations since passage of the HIPAA regulations.

6. _____ Managers of IS departments today recognize that technical expertise alone is sufficient to support the needs of end users.

7. _____ Web browsers make it possible to search for and quickly locate huge amounts of information on almost any health-related topic.

8. _____ Because Web technology is expensive, it is limited to large facilities with extensive IS budgets.

Real-World Case

This case is based on an article in the *Journal of American Health Information Management Association* (Wager et al. 1999).

The Spring Garden Family Practice in York, Pennsylvania, converted its paper-based health record system to an electronic medical record system in 1995. Before the conversion, Spring Garden's staff was buried in paper. They hoped that the implementation of an electronic system would improve office efficiency by automating the tedious tasks of filing and retrieving paper records. They also hoped that the new computer-based system would reduce stress levels, improve job satisfaction, make communication and documentation easier, and promote the quality of patient care.

Today, Spring Garden's staff members all agree that the goals they set for the project have been achieved. They attribute much of the project's success to the selection of an appropriate EMR product developed by a reputable vendor. They also credit the process they used to implement the system, the practice's strong leadership, and the training and evaluation process they developed as part of the project. In addition, the staff's commitment to the project's success was essential.

The practice's medical director led the decision to implement a computer-based system. Before the system was implemented, staff members had few computer skills. The medical director was trained first, and he worked directly with the vendor to learn how to use the software efficiently. After the medical director was confident in his new skills, he introduced the rest of the staff to the features of the new system a little at a time. The office administrator and the support staff tested and refined the proposed changes in procedures. This allowed them to gain confidence in their new skills at the same time they were actively involved in implementing the new system.

The whole project took about six months to complete. The staff spent the first three months converting paper-based patient records to the new EMR format. To save time, they converted only active records. The clinicians learned to dictate medical notes and information about allergies, medications, and immunizations directly into the system. Information captured during patient visits and information provided by other facilities were entered electronically or scanned into the record. During the conversion process, the staff continued to refer to the paper records until all the active electronic records were complete.

Today, all the clinical and support staff members use the EMR in their everyday work. They report that communication and productivity have improved significantly. Indeed, they have experienced no significant disadvantages to using the new system.

Summary

Early computer systems were introduced to healthcare in the 1960s. These systems were predominately mainframe systems used to support financial and/or administrative functions. The 1970s saw the introduction of turnkey systems. These systems also ran on large mainframe systems that often were not flexible enough to address the information needs of individual departments. By the 1980s, personal computers were being used in healthcare and smaller-scale, stand-alone systems for department applications had been introduced. This put information in the hands of the users but led to the development of many separate systems throughout the organization that could not talk to each other. In the 1990s, integrated healthcare information systems that support clinical, administrative, and decision support functions evolved. These systems use advanced network technologies such as the Internet to ensure seamless operations across the healthcare enterprise.

Healthcare information system (IS) applications can be categorized as clinical, administrative, and management support. To be used to their full potential, these systems should be integrated into an enterprise-wide IS that supports the organization's mission.

Strategic IS planning establishes a blueprint for meeting users' different needs. During the planning process, user needs are assessed, priorities established, and decisions made. The interdisciplinary planning process should include key representatives from upper management to ensure alignment with the organization's overall strategic plan.

One of the best-known models for selecting and implementing new ISs is the systems development life cycle (SDLC). The SDLC includes four phases performed as an ongoing process: planning and analysis, design, implementation, and maintenance and evaluation.

Healthcare organizations today recognize that information is an essential resource that must be managed just as other valuable resources are. This recognition has led to new organizational structures that support information resource management. Some of the key positions in these new structures include the chief information officer (CIO), the IS steering committee, the chief security officer, and the chief privacy officer. In many organizations, the health information management and IS departments report directly to the CIO.

Use of the Internet in developing healthcare ISs is booming. The Internet is having a tremendous impact on healthcare because it encourages consumers to actively participate in their own healthcare. Increased use of the Internet and other communications technologies has led to a focus on the need for legislation to protect patient privacy and confidentiality. Portions of the Health Insurance Portability and Accountability Act passed in 1996 address data privacy and security concerns.

References

American Health Information Management Association. 2001. Sample chief privacy officer job description. Available online from www.ahima.org/search/index.html.

Anderson, J.G., and C. Aydin. 2005. *Evaluating the Organizational Impact of Health Care Information Systems,* 2nd ed. New York: Springer.

Austin, C.J., and S.B. Boxerman. 2003. *Information Systems for Health Services Administration,* 6th ed. Chicago: Health Administration Press.

Barlas, S. 2002 (September). Report from the FDA's bar coding initiative. *Healthcare Informatics,* pp. 17–18.

Bates, D.W. 2005. Physicians and ambulatory electronic health records. *Health Affairs* 24(5):1180–89.

Bates, D.W., and Gawande, A. 2003. Improving safety with information technology. *New England Journal of Medicine* 348:2526–34.

Bauer, D.W., and J. Cree. 1995. Results from the use of a 3-year computer competency curriculum in a family practice residency. *Family Medicine* 27:20–27.

Bockle, G., et al. 1996 (June). Structured evaluation of computer systems. *Computer* 29:45–51.

Clark, J.S., and J. Cofer. 2000. *Information Management: The Compliance Guide to the JCAHO Standards,* 3rd ed. Marblehead, MA: Opus Communications.

Dick, R.S., and E.B. Steen, eds. 1991. *The Computer-Based Patient Record: An Essential Technology for Health Care.* Washington, DC: National Academy Press for the Institute of Medicine.

Fox, S., and L. Rainie. 2000. *The Online Health Care Revolution: How the Web Helps Americans Take Better Care of Themselves.* Washington, DC: Pew Charitable Trusts.

Friedman, C.P., and J.C. Wyatt. 1997. *Evaluation Methods in Medical Informatics.* New York: Springer.

Garets, D., and M. Davis. 2005. EMRS and EHRs: Concepts as different as apples and oranges at least deserve separate names. *Healthcare Informatics* 22(10):53–54.

Gilbert, F.E. 2000 (Sept. 16). Demystifying HIPAA. Presentation to Association of Pathology Chairs West and Midwest Regional Meeting. Available online from ecgmc.com.

Hillestad, R., et al. 2005. Can electronic medical record systems transform health care? Potential health benefits, savings, and costs. *Health Affairs* 24(5):1103–17.

Hunter, R.L. 1999. The past and future of laboratory information systems. *Annals of Clinical and Laboratory Science* 29(3):176–84.

Institute of Medicine, Committee on Data Standards for Patient Safety 2003. *Key Capabilities of an Electronic Health Record System.* Washington, DC: National Academies Press.

Institute of Medicine. 2001. *Crossing the Chasm: A New Health System for the 21st Century.* Washington, DC: National Academies Press.

Institute of Medicine. 2000. *To Err Is Human: Building a Safer Health System.* Washington, DC: National Academies Press.

Johns, M.L. 1997. *Information Management for Health Professions.* Albany, NY: Delmar.

Kelly, P., and G. Legrow. 2000. *Medicaid Health Plans: Are Application Service Providers Right for You? A Market Segment Report.* Oakland, CA: California Healthcare Foundation.

Kennedy, O.G., G.M. Davis, and S. Heda. 1992. Clinical information systems: 25-year history and the future. *Journal of the Society for Health Systems* 3(4):49–60.

Malec, B.T. 1998. Administrative applications. In *Information Systems for Health Services Administration,* edited by C.J. Austin and S.B. Boxerman. Chicago: Health Administration Press.

National Research Council. 2000. Networking health: Prescriptions for the Internet. Available online from nas.edu/nrc/nrc.

Office of the National Coordinator. 2005 (Oct. 7). American health information community potential break-throughs. Available online from hhs.gov/healthit/breakthrough.html.

Teich, J.M. and M.M. Wrinn. 2000 (Jan./Feb.). Clinical decision support systems come of age. *MD Computing* 17(1):43–6.

Wager, K.A., et al. 2000. Impact of an electronic medical record system on community-based primary care practices. *Journal of the American Board of Family Practice* 13(5):338–48.

Wager, K.A., F.W. Lee, and J.P. Glaser. 2005. *Managing Health Care Information Systems: A Practical Approach for Health Care Executives.* San Francisco: Jossey Bass.

Wager, K.A., F.W. Lee, and A.W. White. 2001. Life after a disastrous electronic medical record implementation: One clinic's experience. *Annals of Cases on Information Technology* 3:153–68.

Wager, K.A., F.W. Lee, R. Glorioso, and L. Bergstrom. 1999. Working smarter, not harder. *Journal of American Health Information Management Association* 70(6):44–46.

Whatis.com. 2002. *The Whatis.com Encyclopedia of Technology Terms.* Indianapolis: Que.

Whitten, J.L., L.D. Bentley, and K.C. Dittman. 2005. *Systems Analysis and Design Methods,* 6th ed. New York: McGraw-Hill.

Wold, G. H., and R.F. Shriver. 1994. *The Healthcare Systems Planning Manual: Evaluating, Selecting, and Implementing Information Systems throughout the Organization.* Chicago: Probus Publishing Company.

Chapter 18

Information Systems for Managerial and Clinical Support

Merida L. Johns, PhD, RHIA

Learning Objectives

- To differentiate among strategic, tactical, and operational decision making

- To understand the difference between structured and unstructured decisions

- To identify the types of information needed by different healthcare organization decision makers

- To define and give an example of a management information system

- To define and give an example of a decision support system

- To define and give an example of an executive information system

- To identify types of information technologies that can be used to support the physician–patient relationship and decision making

Key Terms

Computer telephony

Computer–telephone integration (CTI)

Consumer informatics

Data mining

Data warehousing

Decision support system

Executive information system

Expert system

Fax on demand

Groupware

Information kiosk

Internet browsers

IP telephony

Knowledge management system (KMS)

Management information system (MIS)

Operational decision making

Private branch exchange (PBX)

Push technology

Speech recognition

Strategic decision making

Structured decision

Tactical decision making

Unified messaging

Unstructured decision

Videoconferencing

Introduction

Information and associated technologies are vital components of any healthcare organization. However, to be useful, information must be relevant, timely, accurate, and available in a way that supports the needs of the organization's decision makers.

Healthcare organizations have many different decision makers. Executive managers, such as chief executive officers (CEOs) and organizational vice presidents, need certain types of information to make strategic and long-range decisions. Managers, such as department directors, also need information to make decisions. However, the decisions a manager makes are more tactical in nature than the strategic decisions made by senior executives.

As discussed in chapter 4, **decision support systems** are a component of electronic health record systems. Physicians and other clinicians need information to make decisions. However, the information they need is very different from the information that managers need. Thus, the healthcare organization's different decision makers need distinctly different information to support their individual work tasks.

This chapter builds on information presented in chapters 16 and 17 and discusses in greater depth how information systems can provide support for the different decision makers in the healthcare organization. Such decision makers include executives, managers, supervisors, and clinicians. Understanding how information needs to be set up is important because some of the health information technician's work may involve preparing or extracting data to help the organization's decision makers do their jobs.

Theory into Practice

Decision support systems that deliver important data to clinicians have traditionally been passive systems. What this means is that physicians have to rely on actively seeking data by reading paper printouts or by looking at a computer terminal that displays reminders that data fall outside a normal range of values.

At the University of Utah Medical Center, an information system (IS) called the Clinical Event Manager (CEM) helps physicians with clinical decision making by using **push technology.** Push technology is an active technology that "pushes" information directly to the end user when the information is available.

CEM automatically monitors electronic patient data and examines it for critical items such as abnormal laboratory values and therapeutic drug levels. When the system identifies an abnormal laboratory value, a potential drug–drug interaction, or an adverse drug event, it sends a message to the physician via a text pager or to an e-mail account. In one study that evaluated the system, 93 percent of the physicians said the alerts provided useful or new information that might otherwise have been missed. Examples of messages sent to clinicians include the following:

- Notification of laboratory results (for example, when hemoglobin is less than 8.0 or has dropped by 1 gram since the last laboratory result)

- Potential drug–drug interactions (for example, when a drug, such as Septra, has been prescribed that may interact with a current medication, such as warfarin)

- Adverse drug event monitoring (for example, when a patient on a nonsteroidal antiinflammatory drug has developed a low platelet count) (Warner et al. 1998)

- Antibiotic assistance (for example, when a positive organism is not treated or a cheaper antibiotic is available)

Key Concepts and Decision Support Systems

Information is useful only if it can be applied to support the tasks of end users. Thus, information useful to the CEO of a facility may not be useful to a supervisor in a clinical department. The reverse also is true. Information useful to a first-line supervisor may be inadequate for the decision-making purposes of a senior manager. Thus, different levels of decision making require different types of information.

Decision-Making Levels

Traditionally, organizational decision making has been divided into three levels: strategic, tactical, and operational (O'Brien 1999).

Strategic Decision Making

Strategic decision making is usually limited to boards of directors, CEOs, and top executives. These are the individuals who make decisions about the organization's strategic direction. They are interested in broad-based information that helps to explain the political, economic, and competitive business environment.

Strategic and long-range planning decisions are often referred to as **unstructured decisions.** These are decisions that are made without following a prescribed method, formula, or pattern.

In contrast, a **structured decision** is made by following a formula or a step-by-step process. An example of a structured decision in a healthcare organization would be how to assign a principal diagnosis. A coder faced with this problem must follow specific rules in every case. However, an executive doing long-range planning has no rules or formulas to follow in determining how to solve a problem.

Tactical Decision Making

Tactical decision making is usually done by department or business unit directors. Tactical decisions include short- and medium-range plans, schedules, budgets, and so on. They also may include development of policies and procedures for the business unit. These types of management decisions are often referred to as semistructured decisions. In other words, the department or business directors follow certain rules of thumb in making their decisions.

Operational Decision Making

Operational decision making involves the day-to-day operation of a business unit or the day-to-day execution of a job task. Operational decisions include developing short-range plans and schedules. For example, a transcription supervisor who makes up a weekly schedule for transcription support is making an operational decision. He or she knows from past experience and data how many reports must be transcribed on specific days of the week and schedules this support task accordingly.

Operational decisions are very structured. Inventory management is another type of operational decision. For example, when the inventory of central supply items reaches a certain point, the items are reordered automatically.

Figure 18.1 shows the classic decision-making pyramid. Operational decisions provide the foundation of the pyramid. Semistructured, or tactical, decisions are in the middle, followed by strategic decisions, which are the most unstructured.

Information Requirements for Decision Levels

Because there are different levels of decision making within an organization and because the decisions range from very structured to very unstructured, the type of information required for each level is very different. Table 18.1 shows the kinds of decisions that organizational decision makers make and the type of information they need to make them.

Executive Decision Makers

Executives make strategic and unstructured decisions and usually need information that is both internal and external to the organization. The CEO is concerned with what is going on both within the organization and outside the organization. In other words, the CEO is concerned with the total environment.

Internal information relates to how the organization is operating. Executives use internal information to identify problems within the organization and to identify their causes. Top executives use external information to help identify potential opportunities in the general business marketplace. In addition to internal and external information, top executives need information that is summarized and wide in scope. They also use information that is analyzed using a variety of models and statistical methods so that they can evaluate different alternatives.

Tactical Decision Makers

Managers who make tactical decisions are more likely to use internal information about the organization than external data. They need summarized data that keep them informed and help them to identify problems. After problems are identified, the managers usually need more detailed information to help explain why the problems occurred and to help them decide how to address them.

Figure 18.1. Decision-making pyramid

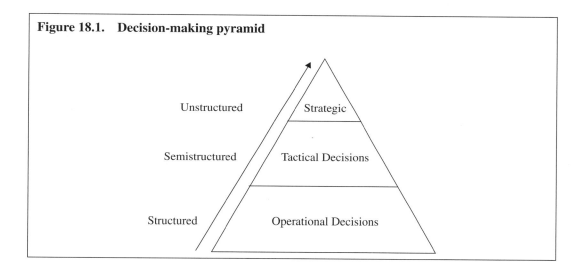

Table 18.1. Examples of decisions and information characteristics

Organization Level	Decision Type	Information Characteristics
Executive management	Unstructured decisions	• Summarized data • Internal and external data • Background data • Ad hoc reports
Middle management	Semistructured decisions	• Summarized data • Internal data • Monitoring data • Deviations from expected performance • Scheduled reports • Exception reports
Supervisory management and end users	Structured decisions	• Detailed, operational data • Scheduled reports • Structured reports • Regular reports

Operational Decision Makers

Managers who make operational decisions need only internal information. They make decisions about the day-to-day operation of a unit. These managers include supervisors over coding, transcription, release of information, and so on. Usually, the information that managers need to make operational decisions must be detailed, rather than summarized. Frequently, such information provides data on production or signals inconsistencies or errors that require the supervisor's attention. Usually, decisions made on the basis of such data are routine and based on predetermined rules.

Check Your Understanding 18.1

Instructions: Complete the following statements with the most appropriate answer.

1. _____ Information is useful only if it _____.
   a. Can be applied to support tasks of end users
   b. Is in the form of numbers
   c. Can be translated to paper
   d. Is in a computer system

2. _____ Strategic decision making is typically performed by _____.
   a. Clinicians
   b. Executives
   c. Managers
   d. Supervisors

3. _____ Structured decisions are generally made at the _____ level.
   a. Managerial
   b. Operational
   c. Strategic
   d. Tactical

4. _____ Executives are usually faced with solving problems that are _____.
   a. Day to day
   b. Tactical
   c. Structured
   d. Unstructured

5. _____ Medium-range plans, schedules, and budgets are considered _____ decisions.
   a. Operational
   b. Tactical
   c. Strategic
   d. Unstructured

6. _____ Developing a three-year strategic plan for an entire organization would be considered _____ decision making.
   a. Operational
   b. Structured
   c. Tactical
   d. Unstructured

7. _____ Organization executives need external information to _____.
   a. Identify problems within the organization
   b. Make day-to-day decisions
   c. Identify potential opportunities in the general marketplace
   d. Explain why problems are occurring within the organization

8. ____ Information that is wide in scope and highly summarized is usually used by ____.
    a. Executives
    b. Frontline end users
    c. Managers
    d. Supervisors

9. ____ Reviewing a hospital census report each day would be most useful to ____.
    a. Clinicians
    b. Executive management
    c. Middle management
    d. Operational management

10. ____ Summarized information about coding errors would be most useful for ____ decision making.
    a. Executive
    b. Operational
    c. Strategic
    d. Unstructured

Information Systems That Support Decision Making

Because the operation of any healthcare organization involves a variety of decisions and different decision makers, no one IS can provide decision support adequately. Thus, different types of information systems are needed to help executives, managers, supervisors, and clinicians make decisions. This section discusses four types of information systems. (See table 18.2.) These information systems were briefly introduced in chapter 16.

Management Information System

The **management information system** (MIS) was the first type of automated IS geared specifically to providing decision support to managers. Today, MISs typically support a variety of day-to-day activities. They provide routine and scheduled reports, displays, and responses specified in advance by managers. One example of an MIS is a daily report of incomplete health records with a detailed listing of days incomplete and responsible physicians.

Another type of MIS report is an activity-based costing report for the finance department. This report shows the cost and variance from predicted costs of different services.

MISs are used primarily in monitoring performance and providing background information about the organization's overall activity. Traditional MIS support takes the form of periodic, scheduled reports such as daily staffing reports, monthly budget reports, and daily census reports.

Management information reports also produce exception reports. These reports are produced only when exceptional or out-of-range conditions occur. One example of an exception report would be a report listing all accounts receivable over thirty days. Another example would be a utilization management report listing all patients who had exceeded the normal length of stay (LOS) in the hospital.

In addition to scheduled routine and exception reports, some MISs produce demand reports. These are reports where the manager can use a report generator to obtain a customized report when and where he or she needs it. An example of a report generator is the Microsoft Access™ database management system.

Table 18.2. Decision support information systems and their characteristics		
Information System	**Type of Support**	**Typical Users**
Management information system	• Periodic, exception, and demand reports • Measures performance and compares to predetermined threshold levels • Monitors performance	• Managers • Supervisors • End users who receive feedback about their own performance
Executive information system	• Provides immediate access to information relating to the organization's key success factors • Provides forms and reports tailored to a specific executive	• Executives • High-level managers
Decision support system	• Provides information in various formats • Provides interactive models • Provides analytical tools and statistical methods to analyze data • Allows what-if analysis • Allows "how-can" analysis	• Analysts • Managers
Expert system	• Has a specific knowledge base • Is used to solve problems in a narrowly focused knowledge area	• Users who need access to an expert knowledge base

Decision Support System

A decision support system (DSS) is a type of management information system. However, the DSS goes further in providing decision support to managers, analysts, and executives. An MIS provides reports such as lists of patients, variance reports, and exception reports produced in a standard format and on a scheduled basis. Essentially, MISs are static, meaning that they provide information that cannot be manipulated. In contrast, DDSs are interactive systems that allow managers and analysts to manipulate data using analytical models and statistical techniques.

With a DSS, a manager can ask what-if questions. For example, if the manager of the emergency department wanted to determine the best staffing pattern to ensure that patients are seen as quickly as possible, he or she might enter the number of patient visits, the type of visit (emergency, urgent), and the top waiting period in minutes. Using a mathematical or statistical model, the DSS could calculate the optimal number and mix of employees (physicians, nurses, and technicians) needed to staff the emergency department.

Executive Information System

An **executive information system** (EIS) combines many of the features of the management information and decision support systems. It can produce standard, scheduled, and periodic reports but is not limited to producing them. An EIS can provide top executives with the information they need whenever they need it and in whatever form they want it (Alter 1992).

Executive information systems are easier to use than decision support systems. For example, they allow executives to choose from among numerous tabular or graphical formats. Another important feature of an EIS is a capability called drill down. Drill down enables the user to find even more detailed information. For example, a CEO reading a computer management report showing a decline in average daily census over the past month might decide to investigate why the decline has occurred. With drill-down capabilities, the CEO would immediately be able to look at more specific details to determine whether all or only certain hospitals are contributing to the decline.

Expert System

An **expert system** (ES) is somewhat different from the other information management systems. It supports the work of professionals engaged in the design, diagnosis, or evaluation of complex situations requiring expert knowledge in a well-defined and usually limited area (Alter 1992). An ES uses artificial intelligence techniques to capture the knowledge of human experts and to translate and store it in a database or knowledge base.

ESs can be used in addition to other information systems, particularly in situations where answers to questions or problems are difficult to determine. For example, expert systems are used to diagnose and troubleshoot equipment malfunctions. However, they also are used in making recommendations on loan portfolios, performing insurance underwriting, and making demographic forecasts. In healthcare, ESs sometimes are used to aid clinicians in making diagnoses or selecting the best treatment regimen for a patient.

Knowledge Management System

As noted in chapter 16, a **knowledge management system** (KMS) is a type of system that supports the creation, organization, and dissemination of business or clinical knowledge and expertise to providers, employees, and managers throughout a healthcare enterprise.

A KMS is usually composed of an electronic library or central repository of best practices that offers enhanced search capabilities. Information is organized by specific business domain in the electronic library. Employees can access the electronic library through the Internet or an extranet to search for information. KMSs also use special software that allows employees to collaborate in teams to use or add to the knowledge in the electronic library.

An example of a KMS is one developed at Partners Healthcare in Boston. This system integrates the clinical database and patient electronic records and embeds drug information into the physician order-entry process. Using this type of system the physician is alerted to potential drug interactions before an order is processed. This system reportedly has reduced medication errors by 55 percent (Davenport and Glaser 2002).

Research System

Data warehousing and **data mining** are types of systems used to analyze data for decision-making purposes. Raghupathi defines data warehousing as "setting up large stores of data for strategic decision support and analysis" (2000, 18). In a data warehouse, selected data are extracted from multiple sources in the organization's IS. A data warehouse, therefore, is a consolidated database maintained separately from the organization's operational systems. Data in such a warehouse are updated periodically and are essentially a "snapshot in time" of the organization's data. Such warehouses are used primarily for managerial decision support purposes.

Data warehousing is gaining in popularity. This is particularly true in healthcare, where decision makers rely on accurate and timely information, both financial and clinical. Pharmaceutical manufacturers are using data warehousing for marketing and research. Insurance companies are using it to form clinical repositories, merging their members' claims and clinical data. Such information can provide a better understanding of cost-effectiveness and quality of care. Futures studies performed by AHIMA indicate that HIM professionals will have jobs that encompass roles in developing data warehouses.

Check Your Understanding 18.2

Instructions: Match the descriptions with the appropriate terms.

1. _____ Was the first type of automated IS to provide decision support to managers
2. _____ Primarily provides static, scheduled reports
3. _____ Supports the creation or dissemination of business or clinical knowledge
4. _____ Uses models and statistical analysis to help decision makers solve problems
5. _____ Supports the work of professionals engaged in the design, diagnosis, or evaluation of complex situations
6. _____ Aids clinicians in making diagnoses or selecting the best treatment regimen for a patient
7. _____ Is an automated daily report of incomplete health records
8. _____ Is used primarily for monitoring purposes
9. _____ Reports out-of-range conditions
10. _____ Is able to ask what-if questions

a. Decision support system
b. Exception report
c. Executive information system
d. Expert system
e. Knowledge management system
f. Management information system

Examples of Managerial and Clinical Decision Support Systems

As stated earlier, many types of information systems are used to help support decision making in healthcare institutions. The following examples represent only a few of them.

Managerial EIS Example

The Veterans Health Administration of the Department of Veterans Affairs is implementing a decision support system (DSS) in all its medical centers. The DSS is designed to give cost and quality assessment information for managing the medical centers' business and clinical processes. The way the system works is that patient encounter information is collected from all the medical centers and entered into a large database. Using the DSS, managers can access the database to determine (1) the utilization of resources by groups of patients and (2) the cost of that utilization at each medical center and at the national level.

For example, managers can group patients by ICD-9-CM codes, major diagnostic categories, and diagnosis-related groups (DRGs). The managers then can drill down and get more detailed information by applying any variable, such as patient age, gender, or LOS. Costs and other utilization patterns can be compared among various patient groups as well as various VA medical centers (Green and McSherry 1998, 413–20).

This example describes the implementation of a DSS that primarily supports management decision making. The system analyzes patient clinical data in terms of resource utilization. Managers can use this information to determine how to better distribute and manage resources. In addition, they can use it to produce ad hoc reports and can use drill-down features to obtain more specific data or to manipulate the different variables mentioned in the example. Given the description, this system would be classified as an EIS.

Clinical MIS Example

The Michigan Childhood Immunization Registry (MCIR) is a statewide, regionally coordinated database that stores information on all children who received immunizations in the state of Michigan. It reveals whether a child is due to receive any immunizations and makes recommendations for the next set of immunizations. Moreover, it produces a reminder to parents of children who are due to receive immunizations and recalls parents whose children are overdue (DeMars and Hardings 1998, 451–62). Because reports on immunization status are periodic, scheduled reports, this type of support fits the definition of an MIS.

Clinical DSS Example

A sophisticated online order-entry system at Meridian Health Systems is providing allergy checks, duplicate-order checks, generic and therapeutic checks, and drug–drug interaction checks. Some of the specific therapeutic checks include:

- Prothrombin times and partial thromboplastin times display on the order-entry screens for warfarin and heparin.

- Glucose levels and the most recent insulin sliding-scale order information display on sliding-scale insulin order-entry screens.

- Heparin guidelines appear when intravenous heparin orders are entered (Jenders, Quinn, and Scherpbier 1998, 573–79).

Management DSS Example

A special type of DSS called a simulation was developed to perform a bed need analysis for obstetrical units. Its purpose was to determine the optimal staffing and bed resources for specific situations. The analysis considered variables such as patient type (scheduled patient, C-section patient, induction patient, and so on) and room type (waiting room, triage room, early labor room, C-section prep room, and so on). It also looked at how the different rooms can be used, the effect of current patient scheduling practices, and how an increase in patient volume would affect staffing and bed need. The hospital can use this information to determine how best to change current scheduling practices or, alternatively, what new bed and room resources it needs to add (Hager et al. 1998, 199–214).

In the case above, the system is interactive, allows the end user to manipulate the data, and uses simulation models to help determine optimal resource utilization. End users can ask what-if questions and can manipulate any of the variables, such as patient volume and number of beds, to determine their effect on current resources. Because of these features, this system falls into the DSS category.

Other Technologies That Support Decision Making

Besides the information systems discussed, other types of information technologies support executives, managers, supervisors, and clinicians in their decision making. Some of these technologies are emerging. This means that the knowledge base of the technology is expanding and its application in the marketplace is just being tapped. Emerging technologies have the potential to create a new industry or transform an existing one. Consider the cell phone. This technology was only emerging at the end of the 1990s. Most people in the late 1990s did not own a cell phone. In just a few years, this "emerging technology" has totally transformed the communications industry.

As you read the following sections, think about how each of these technologies can be used to support tactical, operational, or strategic decision making.

Technologies for Virtual Teamwork

In a diverse healthcare delivery market, where the need for specialized services may be great, but the availability is in short supply, technology can provide new collaborative opportunities that help managers or clinicians make decisions. For example, a heart specialist is unlikely to set up practice in a small, rural community for fear of professional isolation and a lower-income potential. Obviously, access to such a resource would be of great benefit to the rural general practice physician, particularly in an emergency situation where a patient may not survive a lengthy trip to an urban hospital. Fortunately, technology has advanced sufficiently to provide multiple, stable technology solutions.

The popularity and availability of the Internet and related technologies have brought ease of use and made long-distance hookups more affordable. Physician collaboration via conferencing, e-mail, and remote diagnostic imaging, coupled with remote home monitoring and the advent of computer-based patient records, provides the physician with tremendous medical tools and connectivity. **Videoconferencing** solutions no longer need to cost thousands of dollars and require specialized, expensive equipment. Today's **Internet browsers** offer tools that give physicians a substantial collaborative advantage.

Specialized Videoconferencing Systems
In the early days of videoconferencing, healthcare facilities usually needed dedicated communication networks in order to broadcast images and sound. This presented a number of problems. For example, the bandwidth required to transmit group discussions successfully among several locations required expensive leased lines. In addition, the facilities needed specialized equipment to capture and display the images. Moreover, providers sometimes

needed the ability to examine patient data or review diagnostic images while in conference. But this was awkward, particularly when the videoconferencing equipment was located in a public area such as a conference room. Finally, computer equipment often would not interface with the videoconferencing software.

Today, specialized videoconferencing systems can provide video, audio, computer, and imaging system connectivity. Such systems allow several physicians to collaborate while providing access to network resources. Information from a computer-based patient record (CPR) can be viewed on the same screen with a physician's image and diagnostic imagery. Audio and information updates occur in real time. Physicians can annotate on-screen data by drawing or typing additional information while conferencing with each other.

Today, the availability of small digital cameras and notebook computer systems has helped lower the cost of videoconferencing systems. Currently, an individual using a PC notebook can attach a small camera, connect the video and audio output jacks to the appropriate system connectors, connect to the videoconferencing system with the appropriate software client, and participate in a group consult with a minimal investment of time and money.

As mentioned above, traditional videoconferencing required dedicated networks or expensive leased telephone lines to carry the volumes of data needed by collaborating physicians. However, advances in compression algorithms have greatly reduced the amount of data to be passed across a public communication network, thus making the data available more easily and efficiently for collaborative sessions.

In addition, Internet technologies now blur the lines between public telephone networks and private communication systems. Web clients now include conferencing software that enables users to take part in discussions. With the integration of the Internet and telephone systems, patients can have voice discussions with physicians and simultaneously examine information on a corresponding Web site. In fact, Web pages now provide "hot buttons" to initiate a one-on-one voice conversation with medical staff. Such systems depend on the tight integration of Web technologies and private telephone exchanges. However, as discussed later in this chapter, computer technology, telephone technology, and the Web are converging.

Groupware

Another important emerging tool for the medical staff is **groupware.** Groupware applications can combine different document types with the corresponding work process into a tightly integrated work flow. For example, a physician who wants to check a particular patient's status can call up the patient's health record on the computer. The computer document will include diagnostic images, lab information, transcribed reports, and additional information such as histories and prescribed drugs. The physician can review any recent transcriptions and note any needed changes to the document. After the document is closed, the changes are routed back to transcription for annotation. Noting laboratory results, a physician can prescribe a new drug and automatically dispatch the information to the pharmacy.

Moreover, after reviewing the patient's condition, the physician may decide to consult with a specialist. The system then checks to see whether the specialist is available and, if not, sends the specialist an e-mail. The information is confirmed and now can continue through additional work flows in accounting, health information management, and other care areas.

Check Your Understanding 18.3

Instructions: Indicate whether the following statements are true or false (T or F).

1. _____ Emerging technologies are "science-based" innovations that have the potential to create a new industry or transform an existing one.

2. _____ Genetic engineering could be classified as an emerging technology.

3. _____ Videoconferencing and groupware are technologies that help facilitate the integration of teamwork.

4. _____ Integrated applications are easy to develop.

5. _____ Groupware applications can combine different document types with the corresponding work process into a tightly integrated work flow.

6. _____ Today, the availability of small digital cameras and notebook computer systems has helped lower the cost of videoconferencing systems.

7. _____ Specialized videoconferencing systems are able to provide video, audio, computer, and imaging system connectivity.

Technologies to Improve Patient–Physician Contact

One of the primary steps in providing healthcare is to establish the patient–physician relationship. Any technology that improves and enhances this relationship will provide better and more efficient patient care and decision making. When patients can communicate information to their physicians in a timely and confidential manner, they are more likely to confide sensitive information. The more information a physician can collect during an encounter, the more accurate the diagnosis and treatment.

Increasingly, patients are becoming more involved in their own healthcare decisions. Searching for and accessing information about diseases, treatment options, or pharmaceuticals through the Internet has become commonplace. The movement toward more consumer-centric healthcare information systems is commonly referred to as **consumer informatics.** The personal health record (PHR) is an example of a consumer-centric IS. The PHR is a concept that encourages patients to take an active role in collecting and maintaining their health information and help them make better healthcare decisions. Information technologies that can help support joint decision making between clinicians and patients are discussed below.

Information Kiosks

With the advent of managed care, the formation of integrated delivery systems, and the many new services available, patients sometimes find it difficult to find their way through the care system. Most healthcare organizations assist patients by setting up **information kiosks** in strategic locations. An information kiosk is a computer station that patients and families can use to access information on a variety of subjects. For example, they can locate offices and services within the facility, find information on physicians and physician resources, and access patient educational materials.

To access information from a kiosk, the patient uses a touch-screen monitor. This type of monitor allows the patient to make a selection on the screen simply by touching it. The newest kiosks are using **speech recognition.** These systems allow people with physical challenges to interact with the kiosks using their voice. (Additional advances in speech and voice recognition are discussed later in this chapter.)

When a patient is in a care delivery system and using its resources, communication with caregivers is of prime concern. A patient undergoing complex diagnostic procedures or treatment may need to communicate with his or her physician rapidly and dependably. Advances in communication technologies will enhance communications within healthcare systems. Such technologies include the integration of private and public telephone services and their connection with database systems.

Telephone Interface Systems

How many of us have been in the situation where we need to get information fast or reach someone's office to schedule an appointment? How often are we put on hold or transferred to the wrong office? A rapidly emerging technology is starting to make it possible to reduce these types of errors and ensure more efficient client interactions. Such systems offer not only improved call handling, but also access to more resources than just call routing. The technology that makes this possible is called **computer telephony.**

In the past, clinics and hospitals realized significant financial savings by operating their own telephone systems. Privately owned telephone systems are known as **private branch exchanges** (PBXs). The public telephone system will connect several incoming lines to this private exchange. The organization's private exchange then is programmed with features that either are not offered by the public telephone system or would be too expensive.

Computer–telephone integration (CTI) gives healthcare organizations the ability to improve the efficiency and effectiveness of patient communications. Inbound and outbound calls can be fully integrated with business application processes and database information. These applications may reside throughout an organization on different computer host platforms and local-area networks (LANs). The combination of caller and database information enables appropriate resources to be located and brought together quickly. This produces faster, more effective responses to callers, thus reducing call-handling time and effort while minimizing errors.

For example, a physician may need rapid access to a patient's lab results. Rather than calling someone and having the information retrieved manually (which takes time and can introduce error or misinterpretation), the physician can call an automated system. The call system may identify the physician by telephone number. After retrieving the physician's identity information, the system would request pass code verification (usually a PIN number). When the physician has been verified, the system presents a list of options, including one to retrieve lab results. The physician then enters the patient's identifier. The identifier is forwarded to the lab results retrieval application, and the physician is given a list of available labs. Using the telephone keypad or interactive voice response (IVR) system, the physician selects a particular lab event. The application may then verbally respond with the lab result.

A few years ago, this would have been considered science fiction. Today, the integration of telephone and computer technology makes it routine.

Computer–Telephone Applications and Caller Assistance

The issues of CTI relate primarily to call control, caller identification, collection of call event data, and caller interaction using technologies such as speech-to-text and speech recognition. After a caller is identified, the intelligence for call processing comes from enterprise applications and database systems.

It is expensive to upgrade older information systems to support LAN client–server systems. Internal workgroup communications and information exchange also must rely on this type of multimedia communication.

However, CTI has its limitations. The integration of CTI technology and its applications must be designed carefully. With CTI, the desktop PC can replace the telephone console to provide simpler, easier-to-use interfaces. However, callers may still have to use a twelve-button keypad. This type of keypad is awkward to use and can be error prone during call processing. Even with technologies such as speech recognition and text-to-speech, sequential call flow logic can be confusing and time-consuming. The organization must provide options for live person interaction.

IP Telephony

The rapid expansion of the Internet has provided additional opportunities. One such opportunity is Internet protocol (IP) telephony. **IP telephony** allows real-time calls to be initiated through the Internet instead of the public telephone system. In addition to telephone-to-telephone connections, IP telephony can include PC-to-PC connections and PC-to-telephone connections. It can provide access to applications such as toll bypass, international calling, real-time and store-and-forward fax, unified messaging, Web-based call centers, and IP videoconferencing.

Web Centers

Web centers provide telephone support for the facility's Web site. Web callers can access the organization from their PCs and a Web page on the Internet. Web browsers can access healthcare functions, information retrieval, data entry, e-mail, and real-time voice/video. Such services allow callers to use screen-based interfaces controlled by the enterprise Web server.

The potential benefits to healthcare customers and providers are enormous. With a live connection to a facility, patient and physician can share information on the same Web page simultaneously.

Unified Messaging

Unified messaging is the ability for an individual to receive and/or retrieve various forms of messaging at a single access point, including voice, e-mail, fax, and video mail. This is especially important for users such as physicians and clinical staff who move around a lot. Single-session access to all forms of incoming and outgoing messages while using a single-transport infrastructure can save on equipment, implementation, and management costs.

Fax on Demand

Fax-on-demand services will benefit greatly from computer–telephone integration. A user may select from a list of available fax sources by keying the corresponding number of a fax title or from multiple fax messages via the twelve-digit telephone keypad. When the call has ended, the faxes are sent to the number indicated during the call session. In addition, such systems can send information from database systems based on caller ID. A physician can use such a system to request lab results, review orders from an order-entry system, or retrieve transcription reports.

Check Your Understanding 18.4

Instructions: Match the descriptions with the appropriate terms.

a. Kiosk
b. CTI
c. IP telephony
d. Web centers
e. Unified messaging

1. ____ Relates primarily to call control, caller ID, collection of call event data, and caller interaction using technologies such as speech-to-text and speech recognition

2. ____ Provide telephone support for the facility Web site

3. ____ Ability for an individual to receive and/or retrieve various forms of messaging at a single-access point, including voice, e-mail, fax, and video mail

4. ____ Computer station dedicated to providing information on a variety of subjects

5. ____ Enables real-time calls to be initiated through the Internet instead of the public telephone system

---

Role of the Health Information Technician in Decision Supporting Information Technologies

Why is a knowledge of decision support important to the health information technician (HIT)? In 1996, the American Health Information Management Association (AHIMA) identified several new roles for the health information management (HIM) professional and created an action plan to help the profession assume leadership in filling these new jobs. The action plan was titled Vision 2006. One of the new roles that AHIMA identified was that of decision support specialist.

Today, HIM professionals are becoming the preferred experts to assume these new career opportunities. Some of the specific job tasks that HIM professionals may perform in the development and utilization of decision support systems include data collection, data entry, and data extraction.

Real-World Case

The following case study is adapted from an article by Hohmann, Buff, and Wietecha (1998).

One of the top forces driving data automation in healthcare today is the need for comparative performance measurement databases. The adoption of such databases is based on the industrywide need for methods to perform quantitative assessment of clinical data. These data can be analyzed and tracked through the integrated use of decision support systems.

In the case of one cardiac surgery team in an acute care facility in the Northeast, the system is not a single entity. The team draws on a number of information resources, including the Summit National Cardiac Databases.

The team uses the data for decision support in three ways. First, the data are used to track trends and identify variations in care. Second, the data provide the basis for making decisions for performance improvement initiatives as well as a system for ongoing performance feedback. Third, the data within the decision support system are used for comparing internal data with external benchmarks.

The team initially established a series of targets for monitoring its patients' clinical outcomes. The targets were based on internal and external data as well as the professional judgment of the team. Outcome indicators then were developed for several aspects of surgical cardiac care.

The team also documented baseline performance and began to monitor the facility's progress toward meeting the targets. After an initial period of stabilization, the team identified a trend in which increasing mortality correlated with increasing cost and length of stay. At first, it seemed that the trend was the result of postoperative complications. After the team drilled farther into the data, however, they decided to concentrate on analyzing the primary cause of death.

They selected mortality rate, primary cause of death, direct cost per case, and average length of stay as the primary measures of clinical outcome. Ultimately, as a result of the information the system provided, the team was able to revamp the preoperative risk estimation process and develop protocols for management of its patients' primary cause of death. By documenting and tracking primary cause of death, the team was able to demonstrate changes in the distribution of primary cause of death after implementation of the new postoperative protocols.

Using clinically integrated decision support systems in departmental performance improvement has many implications, which focus on clinical, financial, and marketing concerns. In this case, the system's most important outcome is improved patient care.

Summary

Healthcare organizations have many levels of decision makers—executive managers, department supervisors, clinicians, and so on. Generally, the decision making done in healthcare organizations falls into three categories: strategic decision making, tactical decision making, and operational decision making.

Each category of decision making, and each level of decision maker, has specific information requirements. For example, because they are concerned with the overall organization, executive decision makers generally need information from both within and outside the facility. On the other hand, because they focus on identifying and solving problems within the facility, tactical decision makers primarily need internal information. Finally, because they are more concerned with the day-to-day operations of a unit, operational decision makers need only internal information.

Basically, the different levels of decision makers in healthcare organizations can use four types of information systems to support their decision-making needs—a management information system, a decision support system, an executive support system, and an expert system. Data-warehousing and data-mining technologies can support many of these decision-making applications. These information systems can be as effective in helping to make clinical decisions as they are in making managerial decisions and are considered essential for a fully functional electronic health record system.

Other information technologies also can support managerial and clinical decision making. For example, technologies that provide collaborative opportunities, such as video-conferencing and groupware, can help managers or clinicians make decisions. Knowledge management systems that organize, catalog, and disseminate business or clinical knowledge is a new type of application that supports both managerial and clinical decision making. Decision making, however, is not limited to managers and clinicians. Increasingly, patients are becoming more involved in making decisions about their own healthcare. Many technologies can help patients to access healthcare information and increase timely and efficient communication with healthcare providers.

The growth of decision support systems and consumer health informatics has opened up a number of career opportunities for health information management professionals. Moreover, these opportunities are likely to expand as technology evolves to make information available to healthcare decision makers in new and more effective ways.

References

Alter, S. 1992. *Information Systems: A Management Perspective.* Reading, MA: Benjamin Cummings Publishing Company.

Davenport, T.H., and Glaser, J. 2002 (July). Just in time delivery comes to knowledge management. *Harvard Business Review* pp. 107–111.

DeMars, C.L., and K.B. Hardings. 1998. Developing a successful statewide immunization registry. *Proceedings of the 1998 Annual HIMSS Conference and Exhibition.* Chicago: HIMSS.

Green, H., and E. McSherry. 1998. Decision support system multiple hospital rollup. *Proceedings of the 1998 Annual HIMSS Conference and Exhibition.* Chicago: HIMSS.

Hager, J., R. Archer, K. Baho, N. LaVine, and J. Smith. 1998. The next generation of simulation: Obstetric bed need/staffing projections. *Proceedings of the 1998 Annual HIMSS Conference and Exhibition.* Chicago: HIMSS.

Hohmann, S., E.L. Buff, and G. Wietecha. 1998. Monitoring performance improvement using decision support systems. *Journal of American Health Information Management Association* 69(10):36–39.

Jenders, R.A., M.M. Quinn, and H.J. Scherpbier. 1998. Clinical decision support: Implementation strategies, case studies, and Arden Syntax Tutorial. *Proceedings of the 1998 Annual HIMSS Conference and Exhibition.* Chicago: HIMSS.

O'Brien, J.A. 1999. *Management Information Systems: Managing Information Technology in the Internet-Worked Enterprise.* Boston: Irwin/McGraw-Hill.

Raghupathi, Wullianallur. 2000. Information technology in healthcare: A review of key applications. In *Healthcare Information Systems,* edited by P.L. Davidson. Boca Raton, FL: Auerbach.

Warner, H.R., S. Miller, K. Jennings, H. Lundsgaarde, P. Pincetl, E. Roginson, J. Sommers, and C. Childress. 1998. *Clinical Event Management Using Push Technology: Implementation and Evaluation at Two Health Care Centers. AMIA 1998 Annual Symposium.* Philadelphia: Hanley & Belfus.

Chapter 19
Information Security

Merida L. Johns, PhD, RHIA

Learning Objectives

- To understand the differences among the terms *confidentiality, privacy,* and *security*

- To describe the elements of a data security program

- To identify the greatest threats to the security of health information

- To discuss methods for minimizing threats to data security

- To describe the primary components of the security provisions of the Health Insurance Portability and Accountability Act

- To understand the roles and responsibilities of health information technicians with regard to data security

Key Terms

Access control

Administrative controls

Administrative provisions

Application controls

Audit controls

Business continuity plan

Contingency and disaster planning

Data availability

Data integrity

Data security

Encryption

Flexibility of approach

General Rules

Implementation specifications

Network controls

Physical access controls

Physical safeguards

Public Law 104-191

Risk analysis

Risk management

Security breach

Security program

Security threat

Technical safeguard provisions

Introduction

In the past twenty-five years, there has been significant growth in the collection and use of personal healthcare data. In part, this growth has occurred because the data are being used in the delivery of patient care. But it also has occurred because a growing number of companies and agencies such as third-party payers, employer healthcare benefit plans, government programs, research programs, and public health interests are using the data for reasons not directly related to patient care.

Computers also have contributed to the growth in the collection and use of patient data. Because today's computers are faster and can store greater amounts of data, it is much easier to collect, maintain, aggregate, and disseminate personal healthcare data today than it was even a decade ago.

Who is actually collecting and seeing all these data on patients? Accounts of the number of individuals who have access to patient health information vary widely. It is estimated that anywhere between 150 and 400 people may have the opportunity to see the sensitive data maintained in a patient's health record (U.S. Congress 1993; Gorman 1996; IOM 1991). Many of these people are the healthcare professionals who deliver direct patient care, such as nurses, physicians, and therapists.

However, many secondary users also collect information kept in the patient's health record. These users include researchers, pharmaceutical companies, health and life insurance companies, credit card agencies, banking companies, and the civil and criminal justice systems (U.S. Congress 1993). Indeed, some secondary users and other private companies have "begun to act on the commercial incentive" to gather and sell aggregate healthcare data without the patients' knowledge. Even vendors of healthcare information systems have been known to collect patient data through contractual arrangements with healthcare providers (U.S. Congress 1993, 11).

Recently, the National Research Council (NRC) issued a report that identified new entrants into the information-sharing market. The NRC report noted that the new users of health information typically are companies that have significant business interests in the collection of individually identifiable health information. In the main, they provide products and services to the healthcare industry. Examples of such companies are medical and surgical suppliers, pharmaceutical companies, reference laboratories, and businesses that offer information technology services.

Until recently, no uniform national standard was in place to protect the confidentiality and security of patient information. However, in 1996, the Health Insurance Portability and Accountability Act (HIPAA) contained provisions that would lead to the development of **data security** standards on a national level. The standards that grew out of this legislation are based on sound data security practices that should be implemented in every healthcare facility, regardless of size. Every organization is subject to security breaches by people from both inside and outside the organization. It is essential to recognize the scope of the data security problem and to develop a systematic and comprehensive program to deal with it.

This chapter examines the basic elements of a data security program. It explains why each element is important for ensuring the integrity and availability of patient data and for protecting patient data from unauthorized access. The chapter also offers examples of the disastrous consequences of not instituting effective security practices.

Theory into Practice

The following real-life case illustrates what can happen to data security when technical errors occur and there is an insufficient change in the procedures currently in place. The case appeared in an article titled "Emails Violate Privacy of Health Plan Members," which was published in the *San Francisco Chronicle* on August 10, 2000.

> A major health plan violated the patient confidentiality of hundreds of members when e-mails containing sensitive medical information, names, and home phone numbers were mistakenly sent to the wrong people. In a glitch that raised privacy concerns, a programming error occurred at a Maryland web site server facility that the health plan uses for its online service. The online service lets members ask for medical and pharmaceutical advice and schedule appointments.
>
> The error affected 858 members before the online support crew caught the mistake and shut down the program. Had the technical workers not spotted the problem, it could have affected more than 8,000 members who were receiving e-mail responses at the time.
>
> The programming error was executed when the health plan was performing a routine upgrade to its online system. The online system attracts over 20,000 people per month, and so the consequences of the error could have been a lot greater had it not been spotted early.
>
> Privacy experts say that the incident raises concerns about the safety of online medical services, particularly when the healthcare industry is pushing digital medical care as the "new frontier" to cut costs and improve access.

The **security breach** in this case resulted from a technical glitch and poor practices in the course of upgrading a computer system. However, security breaches also can occur when an intruder hacks into the system. More often, however, they occur when an employee of the organization either performs an unauthorized access of information or deliberately alters or destroys information. Statistics from the Federal Bureau of Investigation (FBI) show that 70 percent of all security problems begin inside the organization (Balwin 1999).

Therefore, the organization's security program must have protections in place to keep its employees honest as well as to keep outsiders from harming or accessing information resources. Good data security does not just happen. It requires planning and the implementation of realistic policies and procedures that address both internal and external threats.

Confidentiality, Privacy, and Security

Confusion about the meanings of the terms *privacy, confidentiality,* and *security* frequently result in their misuse. As discussed in chapter 7, in the healthcare context, *privacy* is usually understood to mean the right of individuals to limit access to information about their person. This is also called informational privacy (Gostin et al. 1995). Confidentiality, on the other hand, refers to the expectation that information shared by an individual with a healthcare provider during the course of care will be used only for its intended purpose. Thus, disclosure of information beyond its intended purpose without the patient's knowledge and consent is a violation of confidentiality.

What, then, is data security? Security can be defined as the protection measures and tools for safeguarding information and information systems. NRC (2000) defines security as:

- The protection of information systems against unauthorized access to, or modification of, information

- The denial of service to unauthorized users

- The provision of service to authorized users

Data security includes a variety of protection measures that safeguard data and computer programs from undesired occurrences and exposures. These measures include:

- *Management practices,* such as prohibiting employees from sharing their passwords

- ***Physical safeguards,*** such as ensuring that doors to areas that house major computer systems are locked to keep out unauthorized persons

- *Technical measures* (or those controlled by the computer software), such as ensuring that only certain passwords allow an individual access to patient data

Thus, a healthcare data security system is concerned with implementing security measures that safeguard both the data and the systems that collect, maintain, and store the data. Table 19.1 provides a description of the differences among privacy, confidentiality, and security as stated by the Computer-based Patient Record Institute (CPRI).

Table 19.1.	Descriptions of privacy, confidentiality, and security
Informational privacy	The right of individuals to keep information about themselves from being disclosed to anyone
Confidentiality	The act of limiting disclosure of private matters
Security	Means to control access and protect information from accidental or intentional disclosure to unauthorized persons and from alteration, destruction, or loss
Source: CPRI 1996.	

Elements of a Security Program

What elements of a **security program** could help prevent an error from occurring, such as the one discussed in the e-mail example earlier in this chapter? Data security embodies three basic concepts:

- Protecting the privacy of data
- Ensuring the integrity of data
- Ensuring the availability of data

Protecting the Privacy of Data

Within the context of data security, protecting data privacy basically means defending or safeguarding access to information. In other words, only those individuals who need to know information should be authorized to access it.

Also, protecting informational privacy usually refers primarily to patient-related data. However, the privacy of other information in the healthcare organization should be protected as well. For example, certain information about providers (physicians, nurses, therapists, and so on), employees, and the organization itself should be considered confidential. Information leaked to unauthorized individuals about providers, employees, or the organization can have as devastating an effect as information leaked about patients.

Ensuring the Integrity of Data

Data integrity means that data should be complete, accurate, consistent, and up-to-date. Ensuring the integrity of healthcare data is important because providers use them in making decisions about patient care. For example, an error made in recording a drug dosage that caused the wrong amount of medication to be given to a patient could result in significant injury or even loss of life. Thus, one important aspect of any security program is to put in place measures that protect the integrity of data.

The issue of data integrity should not be taken lightly. Studies on data accuracy in healthcare indicate that it is a major issue of concern (IOM 1991). Thus, a security program is as much about ensuring data quality and accuracy as it is about maintaining informational privacy.

Ensuring the Availability of Data

Ensuring **data availability** means making sure the organization can depend on the system to perform exactly as expected, without error, and to provide information when and where it is needed. Some studies have indicated that information required for patient care is unavailable in up to 30 percent of patient visits (IOM 1991).

One problem lies in the retrieval of information in both paper and computer formats. Another problem occurs when the computer system operation is unreliable. For example, sometimes the system experiences unscheduled downtime and is unable to process or provide access to information. A good security program will ensure that data are available seven days a week, twenty-four hours a day.

Given these principles, a data security program must cover many things. It must:

- Protect informational privacy by ensuring that data cannot be accessed by unauthorized persons

- Build in safeguards to ensure that data are not altered or destroyed in an unauthorized manner

- Have mechanisms in place to ensure that computer systems operate effectively and can provide information when and where it is needed

Check Your Understanding 19.1

Instructions: Indicate whether the following statements are true or false (T or F).

1. ____ In the past twenty-five years, there has been a lot of growth in the collection and use of health information.

2. ____ It is estimated that between 150 and 400 people may see sensitive data collected about a patient.

3. ____ One of the most important jobs of the health information technician is to ensure that health data are protected from unauthorized use.

4. ____ According to an FBI study, 70 percent of all security breaches are made by company employees.

5. ____ Confidentiality is the right of individuals to limit access to information about their person.

6. ____ Data security includes all the protection measures and tools for safeguarding information.

7. ____ Prohibiting an employee from sharing his or her computer password is an example of a physical safeguard.

8. ____ Protection of informational privacy may be defined as the safeguard of information from unauthorized access.

9. ____ Data integrity means that data are available when and where they are needed.

10. ____ Informational privacy only relates to patient information.

Security Threats

Before implementing a security program, it is important to understand the potential threats to data security. Any number of things can happen to cause the loss of informational privacy or to impair data integrity or availability.

Threats from People

Basically, threats to data security from people can be classified into five categories. (See figure 19.1.) These include:

- *Threats from insiders who make unintentional mistakes:* Such threats could be employees who accidentally make a typographical error, inadvertently delete files on a computer disk, or unknowingly give out confidential information. Unintentional error is one of the major causes of security breaches.

- *Threats from insiders who abuse their access privileges to information:* Such threats could be employees who knowingly disclose information about a patient to individuals who do not have proper authorization. They also could be employees with access to computer files who purposefully snoop for information they do not need to perform their job.

- *Threats from insiders who access information or computer systems for spite or profit:* Generally, such employees seek information for the purpose of committing fraud or theft. For example, an employee may use a computer system to skim money from the organization. Another may change files or data in time and attendance records, inventory systems, or long-distance telephone systems.

- *Threats from intruders who attempt to access information or steal physical resources:* Individuals may physically come onto the organization's property to access information or steal equipment such as laptop computers or printers. They also may hang around the organization's buildings hoping to access information from unprotected computer terminals or to read or take paper documents, computer disks, or other information.

- *Threats from vengeful employees or outsiders who mount attacks on the organization's information systems:* Disgruntled employees might destroy computer hardware or software, delete or change data, or enter data incorrectly into the computer system. Outsiders might mount attacks that can harm the organization's information

---

Figure 19.1.   Categories of people-oriented security threats

- Insiders who make innocent mistakes
- Insiders who abuse their privileges
- Insiders who access or alter data for spite or profit
- Physical intruders who steal or otherwise harm systems
- Vengeful employees or outsiders who mount attacks

resources. For example, malicious hackers could plant viruses in the computer system or break into telecommunications systems to degrade or disrupt system availability.

Three of the five types of threats listed above involve the organization's employees. Although surveys of computer professionals show that about half the attacks on computer systems come from outside the organization, an FBI study revealed that disgruntled employees are responsible for nearly 90 percent of computer crimes that result in financial loss to the organization (CSI/FBI 1997).

Threats Caused by Environmental and Hardware or Software Factors

People are not the only threats to data security. Natural disasters such as earthquakes, tornadoes, floods, and hurricanes can demolish physical facilities and electrical utilities. According to the Federal Emergency Management Agency (FEMA), there has been a yearly average of thirty-three declared disasters in the United States over the past two decades. There were seventy-five declared emergencies in 1996 and sixty-five in 1998. To recover from the devastation that natural disasters can cause, organizations must have good backup and recovery procedures in place.

Other causes of security breaches are utility, software, and hardware failures. These include hardware breakdowns and software failures that cause information systems to shut down or malfunction unexpectedly. Examples would be a hard-disk crash that destroys or corrupts data or a program code that does not execute properly and alters or destroys information.

Electrical outages and power surges also can cause problems. When an electrical outage occurs, for example, information is unavailable to the end user. In addition, data might be corrupted or even lost. Power surges also can destroy or corrupt information. Thus, organizations must have the appropriate equipment to protect information systems from power surges and backup equipment to keep them running during an outage.

Yet another type of threat is a hardware or software malfunction. Security breaches may be introduced when new software or hardware is added to the system. One well-publicized case occurred when a health maintenance organization (HMO) was upgrading the software on its Web site. During the upgrade, hundreds of e-mails containing sensitive medical information and the names and home phone numbers of patients were sent to the wrong people by mistake. Basically, the security breach was caused by a programming error that was not caught before the system upgrade (*San Francisco Chronicle* 2000). Thus, organizations must follow good configuration management procedures to ensure that software and hardware malfunctions do not seriously affect data security.

Strategies for Minimizing Security Threats

What strategies should organizations use to protect their information systems? Figure 19.2 lists the most common approaches. Taken together, they form a data security program.

Establish a Security Organization
The first and most fundamental strategy is to establish a security organization that is responsible for managing all aspects of computer security. This usually involves

---

Figure 19.2. Common approaches to protecting information systems

- Establishing a security organization
- Implementing an employee security awareness program
- Conducting a risk analysis and assessment
- Establishing access controls
- Implementing physical and management controls
- Implementing software application controls
- Developing a disaster recovery and business continuity plan
- Implementing network controls

---

appointing someone in the organization to coordinate the development of security policies and to ensure that they are followed. Generally, this individual is called the chief security officer (CSO).

In addition to appointing someone to the CSO position, the security organization should appoint an advisory or policy-making group. This group is often called the Information Security Committee. This committee usually works with the CSO to evaluate the organization's security needs, to establish security policy, and to ensure that all organizational policies are followed.

Implement an Employee Security Awareness Program

A second strategy in developing a good security program is to implement an employee security awareness program. As discussed above, employees are often responsible for threats to data security. Consequently, employee awareness is a particularly important tool in reducing security breaches.

The organization should offer a formal program that educates every new employee on the confidential nature of patient and organization-related data. The program should inform employees about the organization's security policies and the consequences of failing to comply with them. Ordinarily, the organization should give each employee a copy of its security policies as they relate to his or her job function. It also should require every employee to sign a yearly confidentiality statement. Finally, because data security is such an important part of everyone's job, employees should receive periodic security reminders.

Establish a Risk Management Program

Another strategy in protecting the organization's data is to establish a risk management program. **Risk management** encompasses the identification, management, and control of untoward events. It begins by conducting a **risk analysis.** Identifying **security threats** or risks, determining how likely it is that any given threat may occur, and estimating the impact of an untoward event are all parts of a risk assessment (Johns 2001). Among the threats to security are human error, such as a data-entry mistake, unauthorized physical access to data, sabotage, power failures, and malfunction of software or hardware (Johns 2001).

It makes no sense to implement security solutions without first identifying the organization's weaknesses. For example, if the organization is unlikely to experience a catastrophic event such as a tornado, it makes no sense to implement an expensive security solution to protect against such an event. On the other hand, if the facility's employees are connected to the Internet, it makes sense to implement security solutions that will keep hackers out of the facility's computer systems.

When risks have been identified, it is important to estimate their likelihood of occurring and what their impact on information assets might be. Not all information is of equal importance, so it is essential to determine the value of information to the organization when establishing a risk management program. For example, what impact would a security breach have on quality of care, revenue, service, or organizational image? Several different methodologies can be used to carry out a risk analysis. Calculations of risks based on unintentional occurrences such as power failures or data-entry error are usually based on the probability of the specific event occurring. Calculations of risk for intentional risk such as fraud or theft are usually based on such factors as the attractiveness of a system to a perpetrator and the degree of system vulnerability (Johns 2001).

A sample threat assessment matrix is included in figure 19.3 (Johns 2002). This matrix lists various possible security threats and the things that should be considered for assessing each threat. For example, if the number of users was high, the volume of transactions was high, and the information system was complex, the threat of possible human unintentional error would be high. Risk procedures to manage a threat of unintentional human error should be implemented, such as increased employee training and increased auditing of output for errors.

Establish Access Controls

Establishing **access controls** is a fundamental security strategy. Basically, the term *access control* means being able to identify which employees should have access to what data. The rule of thumb is that employees should have access only to data they need to do their jobs. For example, an admitting clerk and a healthcare provider would not have access to the same kinds of data.

Determining what data to make available to an employee usually involves identifying classes of information based on the employee's role in the organization. Thus, the organization would determine what information an admitting clerk, for example, would need to know to do his or her job. Thereafter, every individual who works as an admitting clerk would have access to the same information.

Every job role in the organization would be identified along with the type of information required to perform it. This is often referred to as role-based access. Although there are other types of access control strategies, role-based access is probably the one used most often in healthcare organizations.

Implement Physical and Administrative Controls

Physical access controls are safeguards that protect physical equipment, media, or facilities. For example, doors leading to the areas that house mainframes and other principal computing equipment should have locks on them. In addition, locks should be installed on personal computers and terminals to help guard against theft. Other physical controls might include positioning computer terminal screens so that confidential data are not exposed to public view.

Administrative controls include policies and procedures that address the management of computer resources. For example, one such policy might direct users to log off

Figure 19.3.   Sample threat assessment matrix

This tool should be used with the Valuation Matrix to determine priority for assignment of security safeguards.

Application/System					
Threat	**Considerations**	**High**	**Med**	**Low**
Unintentional human error	• Number of users • Daily transactions • Complexity of system use • Level of employee system training			
Programming development	In-house development • Level of SAD methodology • Quality control procedures • Implemented testing procedures • Complexity of system • Number of interfaces • Level of security features Proprietary development • Years in the market • Evaluation reviews • Complexity of system • Vendor reputation • Number of interfaces • Level of security features			
Fraud or theft Employee sabotage	• Contains patient-related data • Contains financial data • Contains proprietary business data • Electronic commerce • Level of security features • Employee satisfaction level • Dial-up lines • Open network			
Loss of physical facilities or infrastructure	• Likelihood of natural disaster • Condition of physical plant • Age and condition of equipment • Maintenance schedule • Reliability of utilities • Level of system redundancy			
Malicious hackers	• Level of company visibility • Patient-related data • Financial data • Electronic commerce • Buffer overflows • Dial-up lines • Use of open network			
Industrial espionage	• Financial/strategic data • Patient-related data • Risk management/legal data			

the computer system when they are not using it. Another policy might prohibit employees from accessing the Internet for purposes that are not work related.

Implement Software Application Controls

Another security strategy is to implement **application controls.** These are controls contained in the application software or computer programs. One common application control is password management. It involves keeping a record of end users' identifications and passwords and then matching the passwords to each end user's privileges. Password management ensures that end users can access only the information they have permission to access.

Another type of application control is the edit check. Edit checks help to ensure data integrity by allowing only reasonable and predetermined values to be entered into the computer.

Yet another application control is the audit trail. The audit trail is a software program that tracks every single access to data in the computer system. It logs the name of the individual who accessed the data, the date and time, and the action taken (for example, modifying, reading, or deleting data). Depending on the organization's policy, audit trails are reviewed periodically or on predetermined schedules. Audit trails document when data have been accessed and by whom. Review of audit trails can help detect whether a breach of security has occurred.

Application controls are important because they are automatic checks that help preserve data confidentiality and integrity.

Develop a Business Continuity Plan

What happens when an organization's computer systems are damaged or destroyed by an intentional or unintentional event or a natural disaster such as a flood, tornado, or hurricane? Even though such an event may be unlikely to occur, organizations must be prepared in the event that one does.

Organizations develop a **business continuity plan** (BCP) to handle an unexpected computer shutdown caused by an intentional or unintentional event or during a natural disaster. An example of a computer shutdown caused by hackers would be considered an intentional event. A shutdown due to a software error would likely be classified as an unintentional event. Examples of natural disasters include floods, hurricanes, and tornadoes.

Sometimes BCP is also called **contingency and disaster planning.** The BCP typically includes policies and procedures to help the business continue operation during the unexpected shutdown or disaster. It also includes procedures the business can implement to restore its computer systems and resume normal operation after the disaster.

The BCP is based on information gathered during the risk assessment and analysis discussed above. The risk assessment includes the probability that an unexpected shutdown will occur. Using this information, the BCP is developed based on the following steps (Johns, 2001):

1. Identifying the minimum allowable time for system disruption

2. Identifying alternatives for system continuation

3. Evaluating cost and feasibility of each alternative

4. Developing procedures required for activating the plan

An important part of the BCP is planning how the computer system can be returned to normal operation and ensuring the availability and accuracy of data after a disaster. Restoring system integrity and ensuring that all data are recovered requires that all parts of the system be verified after the disaster has occurred. Usually one system or one component of a system is brought up at a time and processes are verified that they are working correctly.

The typical contents of a BCP include:

- *Assigning responsibility for development and implementation of the plan:* This includes identifying the responsibilities of the security management team, the emergency operation team, and the damage assessment team and how all teams are coordinated.

- *Determining how a disaster is identified:* This includes the definition of disaster and its identification; notification procedures; identification of disaster cause; and communication procedures.

- *Putting in place a recovery plan:* For example, outlining the recovery organization and staffing, having in place vendor contracts and backup plans, having plans to recover data affected by the disaster, and having alternate-site contracts in place.

- *Testing the plan:* A plan is only as good as its implementation. The BCP must be tested periodically to ensure that all parts of the plan, from disaster identification to recovery work, run smoothly (Johns 2001).

Implement Network Controls

A final strategy that can be used to guard against security breaches is to implement **network controls.** All kinds of networks are used to transmit healthcare data today, and the data must be protected from intruders and corruption during transmission. With the widespread use of the Internet, network controls also are important to prevent the threat of hackers.

Implement Data Quality Control Processes

Ensuring data quality is an essential part of any data security program. The various dimensions of data quality are addressed in chapter 2. Among these dimensions are: accuracy, accessibility, comprehensiveness, consistency, currency, definition, granularity, precision, relevancy, and timeliness.

Responsibility for ensuring data quality is shared by many organization stakeholders. For example, data item definition may be the responsibility of the data administrator or those in charge of the data dictionary. Depending on the type of data, determining data granularity may be the responsibility of various department heads or clinical managers. Data accuracy begins with any individual who enters or documents data.

Monitoring and tracking systems that ensure data quality are part of a data security program. All the dimensions of data quality should be addressed in a formal data quality management program. Aspects of such a program are discussed in chapter 2.

Data accessibility, consistency, and definition are three data quality dimensions that are often addressed using computer tools. Data accessibility means that the data are easily obtainable. Computer tools are used to monitor unscheduled computer downtime, determine why failures occurred, and provide data to help minimize future problems.

Data consistency means that data do not change no matter how often or in how many ways they are stored, processed, or displayed. Data values are consistent when the value of any given data element is the same across applications and systems. Procedures are usually developed to monitor data periodically to ensure that they are consistent as they move through computer processes or from one system to another.

Data definition means that data are defined. Every data element should have a clear definition and a range of acceptable values. Data definitions and their values are usually stored in a data dictionary.

Components of a Security Program

How can the different threats to data security be managed in a coordinated security program? First and most important, someone from inside the organization must be given responsibility for data security. This individual should be someone at the middle or senior management level. As mentioned earlier, he or she is frequently called the chief security officer (CSO). Figure 19.4 lists some of the CSO's functions.

In addition, the organization should form a data security committee. This committee would work with the CSO to set security policies and procedures for the entire organization. Frequently, the data security committee also monitors implementation of the organization's security policy. Finally, the committee often reviews employee violations of security policy and makes recommendations for disciplinary action.

Besides the CSO and the data security committee, every employee in the organization who handles information should have assigned responsibilities with regard to security. This includes senior management, department directors and supervisors, and end users. Figure 19.5 provides a sample employee accountability policy.

When the data security policies and procedures are in place, the CSO is responsible for ensuring that everyone follows them. This is done using monitoring and evaluation systems, usually on an annual basis. Many organizations use outside information systems auditing firms to do their security policy evaluations. In addition to the yearly audit, the CSO might establish procedures to audit and evaluate current processes randomly.

All data security policies and procedures should be reviewed and evaluated at least every year to make sure they are up-to-date and still relevant to the organization.

Check Your Understanding 19.2

Instructions: Match the terms with their definitions. Some terms may be used more than once.

1. _____ Employee who makes a typographical mistake

2. _____ Earthquake

3. _____ Computer disc crash

4. _____ Power surge

5. _____ Chief security officer

6. _____ Employee confidentiality agreement

7. _____ Data security committee

8. ____ Identification of most likely security threats

9. ____ Identification of the information that employees need to perform their job functions

10. ____ Locks on computer room doors

11. ____ Controls contained in software or computer programs

12. ____ Edit check

13. ____ Implemented during a disaster

14. ____ Prevents hacking into a computer system

15. ____ Computer terminals do not face public areas

a. Access control
b. Application control(s)
c. Business continuity plan
d. Employee training
e. Environmental threat
f. Hardware failure
g. Network controls
h. People threat
i. Physical control
j. Risk analysis
k. Security organization

Status of Data Security

How vulnerable is health information, and what is the status of data security in healthcare organizations? The National Research Council (NRC) examined both these issues in its landmark report titled *For the Record*. In it, the NRC indicated that "health care organizations will have to work individually, collectively, and with relevant government entities to address the broad scope of concerns regarding privacy and security" (NRC 2000).

The NRC also made five overriding recommendations for improving the privacy and security of electronic health information at the level of the individual healthcare organization as well as the system as a whole:

- All organizations that handle patient-identifiable healthcare information, regardless of size, should adopt the set of technical and organizational policies, practices, and procedures as outlined in the NRC report.

- The federal government and the healthcare industry should take action to create the infrastructure necessary to support the privacy and security of electronic health information.

- The federal government should work with industry to promote and encourage an informed public debate. The purpose of the debate would be to determine an appropriate balance between the privacy concerns of patients and the information needs of the different users of health information.

Figure 19.4.   Common functions of the chief security officer

- Conducting strategic planning for information system security
- Developing a data and information systems security policy
- Developing data security and information systems procedures
- Managing confidentiality agreements for employees and contractors
- Setting up mechanisms to ensure that data security policies and procedures are followed
- Coordinating employee security training
- Monitoring audit trails to identify security violations
- Conducting risk assessment of enterprise information systems
- Developing a business continuity plan

Figure 19.5.   Employee accountability policy

Senior Management
- Ensures that the security program supports the strategic information systems plan of the organization
- Provides management support and resources to maintain the security program
- Mediates the resolution of disputes regarding data policies and procedures

Data Security Manager
- Works with data security committee to establish and implement policies, standards, and guidelines
- Develops and administers information security program
- Communicates security program requirements, security standards, and security concerns to senior management

Department Managers and Supervisors
- Ensure that employees under their supervision are aware of and observe all data security and legal requirements
- Ensure that all employees under their jurisdiction receive appropriate security training for their job level
- Ensure that appropriate procedures are in place to protect privacy and confidentiality of information under their jurisdiction

End Users
- Respect the privacy and confidentiality of information and others and ensure that confidential or sensitive information is protected from improper disclosure
- Respect the integrity of information under their control and not intentionally develop or use any unauthorized mechanisms to alter or destroy information
- Abide by restrictions to security access and do not attempt to subvert or bypass any installed security mechanisms
- Follow incident response procedures and report any security breaches or potential breaches to the appropriate authority

- Any effort to develop a universal patient identifier should weigh its presumed advantages against potential privacy concerns.

- The federal government should take steps to improve information security technologies for healthcare applications.

HIPAA Security Provisions

As mentioned in the introduction to this chapter, the Health Insurance Portability and Accountability Act (HIPAA) was passed in 1996. The act, also called **Public Law 104-191,** includes provisions for insurance reform and administrative simplification. Included in the administrative simplification provisions was a requirement about setting standards to protect health information. Later, the Department of Health and Human Services established security and privacy standards that every healthcare provider, healthcare clearinghouse, or health plan that electronically maintains or transmits patient health information must meet.

The HIPAA security standards evolved directly from the first and third recommendations set forth in the NRC report mentioned earlier. Thus, HIPAA represents an attempt to establish best practices and standards for health information security.

The HIPAA data security provisions are divided into several provisions. These include:

- **General Rules**

- Administrative safeguards

- Physical safeguards

- Organizational requirements and policies

- Procedures and documentation requirements

The content of each section closely parallels the mechanisms for minimizing security threats discussed earlier in this chapter. Essentially, the HIPAA security provisions follow what has already been established in the information systems field as best practices for the development and implementation of good security policy. Because health information technicians (HITs) should be involved with many aspects of HIPAA security implementation, all these sections are discussed below.

The following discussion of HIPAA Security is based upon the Security Standards Final Rule (Department of Health and Human Services, 2003) and adapted from *HIPAA Security: Computer Based Training Modules* (Johns, 2003).

General Rules

The **General Rules** provide the objective and scope for the HIPAA security rule as a whole. They specify that covered entities must develop a security program that includes a range of security safeguards that protect individually identifiable health information maintained or transmitted in electronic form. The General Rules include the following):

- *General requirements:* These are requirements that all covered entities must follow in their security program. For example, these include:

  —Ensuring the confidentiality, integrity, and availability of all electronic protected health information (ePHI) that is created, received, maintained, or transmitted by the covered entity

  —Protecting PHI against any reasonably anticipated threats or hazards to the security or integrity of PHI

  —Protecting PHI against any reasonably or anticipated uses or disclosure that are not permitted under the HIPAA Privacy Rule

  —Ensuring compliance with HIPAA security rules by workforce members

- **Flexibility of approach:** HIPAA allows a covered entity to adopt security protection measures that are appropriate for its organization. For example, security mechanisms will be different in complex organizations than in small organizations. Security protections in a large medical facility will be more complex than those implemented in a small group practice. In determining which security measures to use, the following must be taken into account:

  —Size, complexity, and capabilities of the covered entity

  —Technical infrastructure, hardware, and software capabilities

  —Security measure costs

  —Probability and criticality of the potential risks to electronic PHI

  HIPAA requires that covered entities conduct and document organizational and risk assessments in making the determination of which security measures are appropriate in their specific situations. Examples of risk assessment measures were discussed at the beginning of this chapter.

- *Standards:* Standards that covered entities must comply with include those in sections 164.308, 164.310, 164.12, 164.314, and 164.316 of the HIPAA Security Rule. This means that covered entities must comply with the standards in any of these subparts.

- ***Implementation specifications:*** Implementation specifications define how standards are to be implemented. Implementation specifications are either "required" or "addressable." Covered entities must implement all implementation specifications that are "required." For those implementation specifications that are labeled "addressable," the covered entity must conduct a risk assessment and evaluate whether the specification is appropriate to its environment.

- *Maintenance:* HIPAA requires covered entities to maintain their security measures. Maintenance requires review and modification, as needed, to comply with the provision of reasonable and appropriate protection of electronic PHI.

Administrative Provisions

Administrative provisions are documented, formal practices to manage data security measures throughout the organization. Basically, they require the facility to establish a security management process similar to the concepts discussed earlier in this chapter.

The administrative provisions detail how the security program should be managed from the organization's perspective. Policies and procedures should be written and formalized in a policy manual. The organization should issue a statement of its philosophy on data security. Further, it should make a chart outlining data security authority and responsibilities throughout the organization. Figure 19.6 shows what an organization's general policy on data security might look like.

The administrative provisions include the following nine standards that must be implemented by covered entities:

- *Security management process:* An organization must have a defined security management process. This means that there is a process in place for creating, maintaining, and overseeing the development of security policies and procedures and conducting risk analysis, risk management, development of a sanction policy, and review of information system activity.

- *Assigned security responsibility:* Each covered entity must identify a security official who has been assigned security responsibility for the development and implementation of the policies and procedures required by the HIPAA Security Rule. Frequently, this individual is given the title of chief security officer (CSO).

- *Workforce security:* The covered entity must ensure appropriate access to individually identifiable information to workforce members who need to use electronic PHI to perform their job duties. Likewise, covered entities must prevent access to information to those who do not need it.

- *Information access management:* The fourth standard requires covered entities to implement a program of information access management. This includes specific policies and procedures to determine who should have access to what information.

- *Workforce security awareness and training:* This is one of the most important safeguards in a security program. HIPAA requires that employees and other workforce members have formal training in proper data security handling.

- *Security incident procedures:* HIPAA requires that organizations establish security incident procedures so that management and employees know what to do in the event of a security breach.

- *Contingency plan:* The seventh provision requires that a contingency plan be developed and tested. This is to ensure that procedures are in place to handle an emergency response in the event of an untoward event such as a power outage.

- *Evaluation:* A periodic technical and nontechnical evaluation must be performed in response to environmental or operational changes affecting the security of electronic PHI.

Figure 19.6.   Sample organizational policy on data security

Policy Statement

Background

The State University relies heavily on computers to meet its operational, financial, and information requirements. These computer systems, related data files, and the information derived from them are important assets of the university. A system of internal controls exists to safeguard these assets. Information is processed in a secure environment, and all computer account owners share responsibility for the security, integrity, and confidentiality of information. This policy covers both accidental and intentional disclosure of, or damage to, university information.

Scope

This policy statement applies to the security, integrity, and confidentiality of information obtained, created, or maintained by university employees. The definition of information includes paper documents and all computer-related activities involving mainframes, micro- and minicomputers, and service bureaus.

Definitions

Owner/Program Manager: The owner of a collection of information is the person responsible for the business results of that system or the business use of the information. Where appropriate, ownership may be shared by managers of different departments. Ownership of corporate systems is assigned and monitored via the "Profile" system.

Custodian: The custodian is responsible for the processing and storage of the information. For mainframe, micro, and mini applications, the owner or user may retain custodial responsibilities.

User: The user is any person authorized to read, enter, or update information by the owner of the information.

Data: Information stored in any form by the university that is used as a basis for official reasoning, discussion, presentation, or calculation.

Information: Source documents, electronic data files, and any data or reports derived from them.

Responsibilities

Owner: Information processed by a computerized system must have an identified owner, and this assignment must be formally documented. The owner may delegate ownership responsibilities to another individual. The owner of information has the authority and responsibility:
- To judge the value of the information and classify it
- To authorize access and assign custody of information
- To specify controls and communicate the control requirements to the custodian and users of the information
- To determine the statutory requirements regarding retention and privacy of the information, and communicate this information to the custodian

Custodian: The custodian is responsible for the administration of controls as specified by the owner. This includes the responsibility:
- To provide physical and technical safeguards
- To provide procedural guidelines for the users
- To administer access to information
- To evaluate the cost-effectiveness of controls

User: A user of information has the responsibility:
- To use the information only for the purpose intended by the owner
- To comply with all controls established by the owner and the custodian
- To ensure that classified or sensitive information is not disclosed to anyone without permission of the owner
- To ensure that his or her individual passwords are not disclosed to, or used by, others
- To become familiar with and abide by the Computing Facilities User Guidelines

Enforcement: A violation of standards, procedures, or guidelines established pursuant to this policy shall be presented to management for appropriate action and could result in disciplinary action, including expulsion, dismissal, and/or legal prosecution.

- *Business associate agreement:* A business associate agreement is required whenever electronic PHI is handled or exchanged through a third party who is not a covered entity. Essentially, the agreement is a written contract whereby the business associate agrees to handle data in a secure manner that meets HIPAA stipulations.

Physical Safeguards

Physical safeguards include the protection of computer systems from natural and environmental hazards and intrusion. This provision consists of the following (Johns 2003):

- *Facility access controls:* This includes establishing safeguards to prohibit the physical hardware and computer system itself from unauthorized access while ensuring that proper authorized access is allowed. Safeguards are also required to protect the computer system from untoward physical events (for example, fire, flooding, electrical malfunctions).

- *Workstation use:* Provisions under workstation use require that policies and procedures be in place that document the proper functions to be performed on workstations. For example, workforce members who use workstations that access PHI are required to log off the computer system when they leave their workstation. Covered entities also are required to document the physical attributes of the surroundings of a workstation or a class of workstations that can access electronic PHI. Figure 19.7 offers an example of a policy on terminal use.

- *Workstation security:* Physical safeguards must be implemented to ensure workstation security. This means that there must be safeguards in place to protect any workstations that access PHI from unauthorized access. For example, automatic logoffs may be required after a workstation has been idle for a set period of time.

- *Devices and media:* HIPAA requires the devices and media on which data are stored be protected. This requires policies and procedures that ensure that disks, tapes, and videos are physically protected from harm or intrusion. Essentially, the organization must have controls for tracking the access, removal, and disposal of hardware and software. For example, sign-out logs must be used when anyone removes media from the secured computer location. In addition, monitoring procedures must be in place to review sign-out logs and to check and evaluate audit trains. Further, the organization must have procedures to follow for data backup as well as for the disposal of disks and other media, including paper reports and records.

Technical Safeguards

The **technical safeguard provisions** consist of five broad categories. Essentially, the provisions include those things that can be implemented from a technical standpoint using computer software. These provisions include:

- *Access controls:* The access controls standard requires implementation of technical procedures to control access to health information. The procedures would be executed through some type of software program. Essentially, this requirement ensures that individuals are given access to only the data they need to perform their jobs. The regulations state that access should be determined by one of three techniques: context-based, role-based, and user-based access schemes. Having procedures in place that determine what data an individual can have access to based on their job duties is an example of an access control.

- *Audit controls:* The audit controls standard requires that audit controls be established so that system activities can be monitored. This means that organizations must keep documented logs of system access and access attempts. The logs should document who accessed the system, when the access occurred, and what type of activity took place. Audit trails are an example of an audit control.

- *Data integrity:* The data integrity standard requires covered entities to implement policies and procedures to protect electronic PHI from improper alteration or destruction. In other words, this standard requires organizations to provide corroboration that their data have not been altered in an unauthorized manner. Data authentication can be substantiated through audit trails and system logs that track users who have accessed and/or modified data via unique identifiers.

Figure 19.7.   Sample policy on terminal use

Policy on Terminal Controls

Purpose: To prevent unauthorized access to State University data by providing terminal controls

Scope: University terminals

Standard: Proper physical and software control mechanisms shall be in place to control access to and use of devices connected to university computer systems

Guidelines:

- *Hardware terminal locking:* In areas that are not physically secured, terminals should be equipped with locking devices to prevent their use during unattended periods. The locks should be installed in addition to programmed restrictions, such as automatic disconnect after a given period of inactivity.

- *Operating system identification of terminals:* All terminal activity should be controlled by the operating system, which should be able to identify terminals, whether they are hardwired or connected through communications lines. The operating system should inspect log-on requests to determine which application the terminal user desires. The user should identify an existing application and supply a valid user ID and password combination. If the log-on request is valid, the operating system should make a logical connection between the user and the application.

- *Limitation of log-on attempts:* Limit system log-on attempts from remote terminal devices. More than three unsuccessful attempts should result in termination of the session, generation of a real-time security violation message to the operator and/or the ISO (and log of said message in an audit file), and purging of the input queue of messages from the terminal.

- *Time-out feature:* Ensure that the operating system provides the timing services required to support a secure operational environment. Inactive processes or terminals (in an interactive environment) should be terminated after a predetermined period.

- *Dial-up control:* The communications software should ensure a clean end of connection in all cases, especially in the event of abnormal disconnection.

- *Person or entity authentication:* This standard requires covered entities to implement procedures that verify that a person or entity seeking access to electronic PHI is the one claimed. For example, an entity can be a human user of a system or another machine that has access to or transmits electronic PHI. Assignment of a unique identifier (such as a password) to workforce members is an example of person authentication.

- *Transmission security:* The Internet and communications networks of many types have become an integral part of most business information systems. Because these networks transmit large amounts of data, there is a good potential for security breaches. Essentially, the controls applicable in transmission security are similar to those discussed already. HIPAA requires organizations to have integrity and access controls in place as well as entity authentication and audit trails. For example:

  —Access controls provide protection of sensitive communication transmissions over open or private networks so that the data cannot be easily intercepted and interpreted by parties other than the intended recipient.

  —Access controls ensure that a user has access to what information is needed to do his or her job and nothing else.

In addition, the standard requires the use of **encryption,** when deemed appropriate, for data transmitted over public networks or communication systems. Encryption is a process that encodes textual material, converting it to scrambled data that must be decoded in order to be understood. This means that the message is a jumble of unreadable characters and symbols as it is transmitted through the telecommunication network. When the message is received, it is changed to a readable form. Data encryption that goes across transmission lines is important because someone can easily eavesdrop using devices called sniffers. Sniffers can be attached to networks for the purpose of diverting transmitted data. Protecting data during transmission is only one role of encryption. Passwords stored in a database also may be encrypted. Thus, if a hacker breaks into the password database, the data will be unusable.

Organizational Requirements

This section includes just two standards; one addresses business associates and the other addresses requirements for group health plans.

- *Business associate contracts:* Covered entities must obtain a written contract with business associates who handle electronic PHI. The written contract must stipulate that the business associate will implement administrative, physical, and technical safeguards that reasonably and appropriately safeguard the confidentiality, integrity, and availability of the electronic PHI that it creates, receives, maintains or transmits on behalf of the covered entity. The contract must ensure that any agent, including a subcontractor, agrees to implement reasonable and appropriate safeguards. Specifically, HIPAA requires a business associate to report to the covered entity any security incident of which it becomes aware. The covered entity must authorize termination of the contract if it determines that the business associate has violated a material term of the contract.

- *Group health plans:* Requirements for group health plans specify that plan sponsors must reasonably and appropriately safeguard electronic PHI that they create, receive, maintain, or transmit.

- The Privacy Rule limits the health information that health plans, health insurance companies, and HMOS can disclose to plan sponsors. For example, this information is limited to summary health information for the purposes of obtaining premium bids from health plans for health insurance coverage or modifying, amending or terminating the plan or for providing information on whether or not an individual is participating, enrolled or disenrolled in the plan.

- Health plan documents must include requirements for a plan sponsor to:

  —Implement the same security measures required by the HIPAA Privacy Standard for information it creates, receives, maintains, or transmits on behalf of the health plan

  —Ensure that the sponsor's employees' duties are adequately separated to ensure that PHI is not being used for employment or other employee-benefit decisions

  —Require agents of the sponsor to provide reasonable and appropriate protection of health information provided to them by the plan sponsor

  —Report any security incident of which it becomes aware to the health plan

Policies and Procedures and Documentation Requirements

HIPAA requires that covered entities have security policies and procedures and that they be documented in written format. Other information about any actions, assessments, or activities associated with the HIPAA Security Rule also must be in a written format.

- *Policies and procedures:* Covered entities must implement reasonable and appropriate policies and procedures to comply with the HIPAA security standards, implementation specifications, and other requirements. Policies and procedures should be developed and implemented, taking into account the section on flexibility outlined in the rule.

- *Documentation:* Covered entities must maintain their security policies and procedures in written form. This includes formats that may be electronic. Any actions, assessments, or activities of the HIPAA Security Rule also must be documented in a written format.

  Documentation must be retained for six years from the date of its creation or the date when it last was in effect, whichever is later. It must be made available to those individuals responsible for implementing security procedures. Further, it must be reviewed periodically and updated, as needed, in response to environmental or organizational changes that affect the security of electronic PHI.

Check Your Understanding 19.3

Instructions: Complete each statement with the best choice.

1. _____ provide the objective and scope for the HIPAA Security Rule as a whole.
   a. Administrative safeguards
   b. Documentation requirements
   c. General rules
   d. Physical safeguards

2. _____ ensures that procedures are in place to handle an emergency response in the event of an untoward event such as a power outage.
   a. An audit control
   b. A contingency plan
   c. Employee training
   d. Password protection

3. _____ ensure that a user has only the information needed to perform his or her job.
   a. Audit controls
   b. Access controls
   c. Person identification forms
   d. Workstation safeguards

4. _____ A visitor sign-in sheet to a computer area is an example of _____ control.
   a. Administrative
   b. Audit
   c. Facility access
   d. Workstation

5. _____ The process that encodes textual material, converting it to scrambled data that must be decoded, is _____.
   a. An audit trail
   b. An encryption
   c. A password
   d. A physical safeguard

6. _____ According to HIPPA standards, the designated individual responsible for data security _____.
   a. Must be identified by every covered entity
   b. Is only required in large facilities
   c. Is only required in hospitals
   d. Is not required in small physician office practices

7. _____ Written business associate agreements are required with _____.
   a. Any company where work is outsourced
   b. Any outside company that handles electronic data
   c. Any outside company that handles electronic PHI
   d. Every outside company

8. _____ Covered entities must retain documentation of their security policies for at least _____.
   a. Six years
   b. Six years from the date of origination
   c. Six years from the date when last in effect
   d. Six years from the date of the last incident

9. ____ Security policies ____.
   a. Must be maintained in written format
   b. May be oral agreements between supervisors and employees
   c. May be written or oral
   d. May not be in an electronic form

10. ____ Workforce security awareness and training is required ____.
   a. For all workforce members
   b. Only for workforce members who handle PHI
   c. Only for workforce members who handle electronic data
   d. Only for workforce members who handle electronic PHI

Roles and Responsibilities of the Health Information Technician

Why should health information professionals be concerned with data security? As custodians of patient information, they are responsible for ensuring that it is adequately protected from unauthorized use. In addition, they are responsible for ensuring that the data are correct and available when needed. After all, if data are incorrect or unavailable when needed, they essentially are useless for patient care.

The HIT's role with regard to data security includes being knowledgeable about security threats and measures that protect healthcare data. This role also may include implementing or monitoring compliance with the healthcare organization's security policy and procedures. As a user of health information, the HIT must:

- Respect the privacy and confidentiality of information and ensure that confidential or sensitive information is protected from improper disclosure

- Respect the integrity of information under his or her control and not intentionally develop or use any unauthorized mechanisms to alter or destroy information

- Comply with the legal protection provided by copyright and license to programs and data

- Respect the intended usage for which access to computing resources was granted

- Abide by restrictions to security access and not attempt to subvert or bypass any installed security mechanisms

- Follow incident response procedures and report any security breaches or potential breaches to the appropriate authority

- Ensure that critical data are appropriately backed up

Real-World Case

On October 10, 1996, *USA Today* reported that a public healthcare worker removed some computer disks from the public health clinic that contained HIV patient–related data. The stolen information was then sent to two newspapers.

The *Boston Globe* reported that a temporary employee stole personal patient information from the Dana Farber Cancer Institute. The employee allegedly used information from one patient and ran up $2,500 worth of telephone charges.

Summary

Every healthcare organization must make the protection of healthcare information a top priority. The cost of security breaches reaches into the billions of dollars every year for American industry in general. For the healthcare industry, these costs include not only potential monetary losses, but also jeopardy to patient privacy.

Health information can be protected through a total security program that combines administrative, technical, and physical controls. Each of these controls is equally important in providing a safety net for information. When any one control is lacking, the security program is vulnerable to many potential threats from both within and outside the healthcare organization.

The Health Insurance Portability and Accountability Act contains standards that have become the basis for national security standards. The HIPAA data security provisions are divided into four categories: administrative provisions, physical safeguards, technical safeguards, and network and communication safeguards.

Health information management professionals are the custodians of patient information. As such, they have a responsibility to protect the integrity and confidentiality of patient information and to monitor the healthcare facility's compliance with its own data security policies and procedures.

References

Balwin, Gary. 1999 (October). Information age requires strategic plans. *Health Data Management*. Available online from healthdatamanagement.com.

Computer-based Patient Record Institute. 1996. *Glossary of Terms Related to Information Security*. Schaumburg, IL: CPRI.

CSI/FBI Computer Crime and Security Survey. 1997 (spring). *Computer Security Issues and Trends*.

Department of Health and Human Services. 2003. 45 CFR Parts 160, 162, and 164. *Federal Register*. Vol 68. No 34. February 20, 2003.

Emails violate privacy of health plan members, *San Francisco Chronicle,* August 10, 2000.

Gorman, P. 1996. Who's looking at your files? *Time,* May 6, p. 60.

Gostin, L., O.J. Turek-Brezina, M. Powers, and R. Kozloff. 1995. Privacy and security of health information in the emerging health system. *Health Matrix: Journal of Law-Medicine* 3:18.

Institute of Medicine. 1991. *The Computer-Based Patient Record: An Essential Technology for Health Care,* edited by Richard S. Dick and Elaine B. Steen. Washington, DC: National Academy Press.

Johns, M.L. 2003. *HIPAA Security: Computer Based Training Modules.* Chicago: Holistic Training Solutions.

Johns, M.L. 2002. *HIPAA Security Tool Kit.* Chicago: Holistic Training Solutions.

Johns, M.L. 2001. Security and confidentiality. In *Evaluating and Implementing Electronic Medical Records Systems,* edited by Jerome Carter. Philadelphia: American College of Physicians.

National Research Council, System Security Study Committee, Computer Science and Telecommunications Board, Commission on Physical Sciences, Mathematics, and Applications. 2000. *Computers at Risk: Safe Computing in the Information Age.* Washington, DC: National Academy Press.

University of Houston Security Manual. Available online from uh.edu/infotech/pnp/security/policy.html.

U. S. Congress, Office of Technology Assessment. 1993. *Protecting Privacy in Computerized Medical Information,* OTA-TCT-576. Washington, DC: U.S. Government Printing Office.

Part V
Organizational Resources

Chapter 20
Principles of Work Planning and Organization

Sandra Fuller, MA, RHIA

Learning Objectives

- To identify organizational tools used for communication, including mission, vision, and values

- To understand the role of committees and teams

- To identify the steps in the strategic planning process

- To understand how position descriptions, performance standards, and staff schedules are used as tools in human resource management

- To understand the importance of policy statements and how they relate to procedures

- To understand how job descriptions are used in recruitment and hiring

- To identify effective steps in conducting an interview

- To understand the benefits of teamwork in an organization and to identify the steps in creating an effective team

- To understand the relationship among performance standards, performance review, and performance counseling

- To identify the key steps the supervisor should take in performance counseling or in taking disciplinary action

- To describe the quality improvement cycle and the steps for change

- To understand the budget process and how it relates to organizational and department goals and assumptions

- To identify the methods for supply management

Key Terms

Action steps

Assets

Board of governors

Board of trustees

Budget assumptions

Bureaucracy

Career planning

Chain of command

Change management

Conflict management

Delegation of authority

Disciplinary action

Employee orientation

Environmental assessment

Executive management

Executive managers

Executive sponsor

Fixed costs

Grievance management

Hierarchy

Human resources

Inventory control

Job redesign

Middle management

Middle managers

Operational plan

Organizational chart

Performance counseling

Performance evaluations

Performance standards

Position descriptions

Process redesign

Quality improvement process

Recruitment

Revenues

Staff retention

Standing committees

Supervisory management

Supervisory managers

Supply management

Systems thinking

Values statement

Variable costs

Vision statement

Introduction

Work planning and organization are critical elements in implementing the mission of an organization and achieving its long-term strategic goals and short-term operational goals. These goals are achieved through application of the organization's resources, including its human, financial, and physical **assets.** Supervisors and team leaders contribute directly to managing the organization's resources effectively and efficiently. In other words, they are responsible for ensuring that the organization performs the right activities in the best ways possible to achieve its mission.

In addition to modern management theories, there is the fundamental principle that people accomplish more working collectively than they do working individually. Along with planning tools and methods to monitor resources, team leaders and supervisors can add value on a daily basis to the organizations where they work and the people with whom they work.

Over the past twenty years, a number of industrial management theories have been adapted for use in healthcare organizations, including continuous performance improvement and total quality management (discussed in detail in chapters 11 and 12). Generally, the overarching philosophy of modern management emphasizes the needs of customers as the focus of every organization's value system. And customer is being defined in the broadest sense to include everyone who receives some sort of service from someone else.

In healthcare organizations, team leaders work on many levels, from supervisors of small functional teams to leaders of cross-functional quality improvement teams. For many supervisors, their leadership role is only one aspect of their job. In contrast, the work of executive-level administrators is entirely managerial. Just as every experienced specialty physician starts out as a lowly medical student, supervisors in healthcare organizations begin their careers by practicing the basics.

This chapter discusses the nature of organizations and the basic elements of team leadership. In addition, it describes management of the organization's **human resources** and the supervisor's role in the organization's recruitment and retention efforts. The fundamentals of work planning and elements of expense management and budgeting also are addressed. Finally, quality improvement within a health information management function is examined.

Theory into Practice

As healthcare organizations were challenged to move from a paper-based medical record to an electronic health record (EHR). Without the financial resources to undertake a full-scale EHR implementation, the leadership of one hospital's health information management (HIM) department had to come up with a plan to migrate from the existing paper system in a way that would add value, but temper the investment. Based on input from other departments, it was decided to begin with implementation of an EHR in the emergency department. A cross-functional team was established to ensure that the information collected in the EHR would provide all the required information for patient care and administrative requirements such as reporting sexually transmitted disease cases to the state department of health and billing.

Data collected on paper forms were identified and categorized as required, important, or unnecessary. The cross-functional team then mapped those data elements to the data dictionary in the new EHR system. Additional fields were identified to ensure that all necessary data would be collected. Work flows were determined for all the functions, but the HIM supervisor led the team in mapping the work flows for administrative reporting and billing. The purpose was to ensure that all data would be collected and available on system-generated reports and to coders for code validation.

When the work flows and data systems had been finalized across all teams and all changes had been made to the EHR, the HIM supervisor was one of the key individuals working with another team to design and implement training for physicians, nurses, and clerical staff in use of the system. Post implementation, the HIM supervisor performed routine audits of record completion and suggested system changes and reinforced training.

Principles of Organization

Organization is the planned coordination of the activities of more than one person for the achievement of a common purpose or goal. It is accomplished through the division of labor and function and is based on a **hierarchy** of authority and responsibility (Schein 1980). Like other types of businesses, healthcare facilities are a type of formal organization. That is, they have established goals and a specific purpose for existing.

Jobs and the people who perform them are structured in a way that accomplishes the goals of an organization. Some organizational tools are used to communicate the structure, the purpose, and the methods used to accomplish the shared work of the organization's members. Organizations are like sports teams in that they have specific positions, a pre-defined set of rules, and a goal of winning. Organizations also use communications tools that are similar to a players roster (position descriptions), a rule or play book (policies and procedures), and a record of wins and losses (a budget and financial records). Although the purpose, structure, and methods vary widely, all healthcare organizations use common systems and tools to achieve their goals.

Nature of Organization

By nature, humans are social creatures. They are biologically designed to live within groups of their own kind. Moreover, they continuously form and reform informal and formal groups of various sizes (two members to billions) and longevity (a few seconds to a few centuries). No two groups have identical purposes, membership, or rules. Therefore, every human group is unique.

There is an endless variety of groups. Groups range from relatively informal friend-ships, families, and social clubs to extremely formal businesses, educational institutions, and national governments. They can be loose, unstructured, and temporary. An example of an extremely loose, short-term group might be that of a dozen people who planned last year's holiday party. But even the most informal groups have a purpose and a set of more or less well-communicated rules. In this example, the group's purpose was to get from point A to point B. The rules required that the bus driver follow a preestablished route and that the riders pay a preestablished fare.

Although every group of humans is unique, interactions among humans follow pre-dictable patterns. Human behavior has been studied for untold centuries. Theories on organizational behavior have been offered ever since humans learned how to communi-cate with each other. Although few principles of organizational behavior go unchallenged, centuries of observation have produced some basic rules. For example, one unchanging principle of organizational behavior seems to be that the group's structure affects the way its members interact with each other. And the structural effects can have both positive and negative consequences for the group as a whole as well as for its individual members.

Organizational Structure

At least until recent decades, formal organizations such as healthcare and manufacturing institutions have tended to be structured as relatively inflexible hierarchies. In a hierarchy, every member of the organization is assigned a specific rank. Each rank, in turn, carries a specific level of decision-making authority as well as specific responsibilities within the institution. Hierarchies are authoritarian in nature. In other words, they are strictly con-trolled by a powerful elite working "at the top" of the organization. These few individuals make almost every significant decision on behalf of the entire organization.

Historically, large government institutions have tended to be organized as rigid bureau-cratic structures. In a **bureaucracy,** as in a hierarchy, positions within the formal organiza-tion are assigned specific ranks. Hierarchical ranks are based on levels of decision-making authority. In contrast, bureaucratic ranks are based on levels of technical expertise.

The purpose of bureaucratic organizations is to conduct highly complex and regulated processes. The structure of the bureaucratic organization reflects the processes it was designed to carry out. Therefore, bureaucracies operate according to well-established and often inflexible rules. Each individual within the bureaucracy is responsible for carrying out only a small, well-defined element of the larger process. The Social Security Administration is a good example of a government bureaucracy. It was created in 1935 with the sole purpose of implementing the Social Security Act.

Both hierarchies and bureaucracies depend on authoritarian **chains of command.** In a traditional chain-of-command structure, one manager oversees the work of many employees, but each employee is accountable to only one boss. The structures of military organizations, for example, are organized around extremely rigid chains of command.

Obviously, management systems and organizational structures have been used by humans working in groups since the beginning of civilization. There is little historical documentation of the management systems in use during ancient times, but the achievements of ancient civilizations reflect their effectiveness. The desert pyramids of Egypt, the Roman aqueducts of Western Europe, and the mountain temples of Peru could not have been realized without systematic planning and organization.

In modern times, organizational structure has been studied systematically since the early twentieth century. In the following decades, a number of new management theories were suggested and each seems to have required innovations in organizational structure. The period of economic rebuilding after the Second World War ushered in the current era of business thinking. Business and management theorists W. Edwards Deming and Joseph M. Juran began developing *modern* management systems in the early 1950s. (See chapter 12.)

Today's management systems are modern in that they are moving away from the traditional authoritarian models that have prevailed since the Industrial Revolution. Most of all, they are modern in that they recognize the potential value of change and treat it as an opportunity rather than as a threat.

Modern management systems are based on the objective statistical analysis of data and information. They emphasize the benefits of sharing authority among employees and managers. They also favor interdisciplinary and cross-functional cooperation and teamwork over bureaucratic regulation and authoritarian control. Modern management systems value continual learning and demand systems thinking (Senge 1990, 6–8). (**Systems thinking** is an objective way of looking at work-related ideas and processes. Its goal is to allow people to uncover ineffective patterns of behavior and thinking and then find ways to make lasting improvements.)

In large part, modern management systems represent a rejection of the traditional authoritarian, hierarchical, and bureaucratic approaches to organization and management. However, because the traditional systems have been the accepted norm since the Industrial Revolution, they have proved difficult to displace.

Today, management theorists such as Peter Senge continue to lead the movement to establish information-based management systems and team-based organizational structures in all types of business endeavors. Modern quality management philosophies such as continuous quality improvement are based in modern management thinking. Avedis Donabedian, Steven Shortell, and Donald Berwick, among others, are leading the movement to apply modern quality management concepts to healthcare organizations. (Quality management is discussed in detail in chapters 11 and 12.)

Supervisory Management

Managers at all levels of the organization are held directly responsible for handling its resources effectively and efficiently. However, the scope of managerial accountability among supervisors and managers varies considerably. It depends on the size and organization of the facility they work in, the nature of their responsibilities, and their position within their facility.

Small healthcare organizations such as physician group practices employ many fewer people than large organizations such as hospitals. They also have much simpler organizational, operational, and reporting structures. Moreover, unlike large organizations, they are often owned by a single physician or a group of physicians. However, the fundamental management functions for both large and small healthcare organizations are similar.

Organizations with more than a few employees (for example, twenty or more) usually have three basic levels of management: **supervisory management, middle management,** and **executive management.** In general, supervisory-level managers perform the organization's daily work, middle-level managers monitor and coordinate its ongoing activities, and executive-level managers focus on its future.

Supervisory management oversees the organization's efforts at the staff level and monitors the effectiveness of everyday operations and individual performance against preestablished standards. Further, it ensures that the organization's human assets are used effectively and that its policies and procedures are carried out consistently.

Supervisory managers work in small (two- to ten-person) functional workgroups or teams. They often perform hands-on functions in addition to supervisory functions. They also play an important role in staff training and recruitment/retention efforts. Supervisory managers direct daily work, create work schedules, and monitor the quality of the work and the productivity of the staff. They are important resources in revising procedures and conducting performance reviews because they are familiar with the work of the unit and the performance of individual staff members. Supervisory managers usually have advanced technical skills that allow them to perform the most complex functions of the work team. However, most supervisors have limited financial authority and must seek approval from higher-level managers before spending money or hiring staff. Depending on the size and structure of the organization, HIM supervisors report to another supervisory-level manager or to a department-level manager or assistant manager.

Effective supervisory managers are extremely important in healthcare, where the greatest part of the organization's resources is expended at the operational level. Labor costs represent the greatest investment the organization makes. Staff and supervisory healthcare workers include nurses, clinical therapists, diagnostic technicians, dietary workers, laboratory workers, environmental support staff, and administrative support staff. Health information technicians (HITs) provide vital administrative services and support patient care by protecting the accuracy and confidentiality of clinical databases and health records. Among other responsibilities, they also ensure the financial health and future of their organizations by providing high-quality clinical coding services.

To lead effectively, every supervisor should have an understanding of the principles and tools used to manage the human resource. Many of these tools, such as **position descriptions, performance standards,** and job procedures are discussed later in the chapter.

Middle Management

Middle management is concerned primarily with facilitating the work performed by super-visory- and staff-level personnel as well as by executive leaders. The responsibilities of middle management include:

- Developing, implementing, and revising the organization's policies and proce-dures under the direction of executive managers

- Executing the organizational plans developed at the board and executive levels

- Providing the operational information that executives need to develop meaningful plans for the organization's future

Middle managers oversee operations of a broader scope in their work as managers or assistant managers of departments or disciplinary functions. For example, they direct health information management, nursing, risk management, and facilities management functions.

Typically, middle managers are responsible for performing a limited number of hands-on analytical and/or decision-making functions related directly to the departments they manage. In an HIM department, for example, an assistant director's responsibilities might include tracking the quality of clinical databases and overseeing coding compliance programs. HIM managers participate on a number of permanent and temporary interdisciplinary committees dealing with subjects that relate to the organization's information resources. They also initi-ate interdepartmental efforts to address issues that go beyond department-level operations. In small healthcare organizations, the HIM director may play additional managerial roles in risk management, quality management, and/or utilization management.

Depending on the size and structure of the organization, middle managers in HIM report to a department-level director or an executive manager (vice-president) on the organization's senior management team. In a multifacility healthcare delivery network, the director of HIM services might report to the vice-president of operations (sometimes referred to as the chief operating officer, or COO) or the vice-president of information services (sometimes called the chief information officer, or CIO). In a small community hospital, the HIM director might report to the CEO (chief executive officer), the CFO (chief financial officer), or the COO.

Executive Management and Governance

The highest managerial level of the healthcare organization may be divided into two entities: executive management and the governing board. (The word *governance* means government.) **Executive managers** are employees of the organization. They are hired either by the board or by the organization's CEO with board approval. In publicly owned organizations, board members are elected to their positions by the owners or stockholders. In privately owned organizations, board members are appointed.

Role of Executive Managers

Executive management is primarily responsible for setting the organization's future direc-tion and establishing its strategic plan. To that end, executive management works to ensure that the organization uses its assets wisely, fulfills its current mission, and works toward achieving a meaningful vision for the future. Executive managers oversee broad functions, departments, or groups of departments. Additionally, they are responsible for establishing the policies of healthcare organizations and leading their quality improvement and compliance initiatives. Executive managers also work with other community leaders to make sure that healthcare organizations contribute to the well-being of the communities they serve.

Depending on the complexity of the organization, the titles of executive managers vary. The different titles include CEO, president, executive vice-president, senior vice-president, vice-president, and director. Executive managers may report to other executive managers, to higher-level vice-presidents, or to the CEO.

In most organizations, the CEO is the highest-ranking manager. (CEOs sometimes hold more than one title. For example, the head of an organization might have the title president and CEO.) The CEO and/or president reports directly to the board of directors.

Role of the Governing Board

Healthcare organizations such as hospitals, for-profit healthcare businesses, and multifacility healthcare delivery networks are organized as legal entities, or corporations. Every state has laws that dictate how corporations are to be structured and run within its jurisdiction. However, all state incorporation laws are consistent in one area: responsibility for the operation of every healthcare organization ultimately lies with its **board of governors, board of trustees,** or board of directors. (The name and structure of the board depend on the profit-making status of the organization, among other factors.) Thus, the board is the final authority in setting the organization's strategic direction, mission and vision, and general philosophy and ethical base.

Typically, the board consists of a chairperson and ten to twenty board members. It represents the interests of the organization's owners. Any number of different entities may own large healthcare organizations, including federal, state, and local governments; investor groups; educational institutions; and religious organizations. Moreover, healthcare organizations may be owned privately or publicly. In publicly owned entities, investors purchase stock on national and international stock exchanges and receive a share of the profits in the form of dividends.

Roles of Teams and Committees

Like other complex organizations, healthcare facilities often confront problems that cross traditional department lines. At those times, committees or teams may be created to identify issues, set policy, or solve problems. In larger facilities, **standing committees** may exist, such as the medical staff committee, a quality improvement committee, or an infection control committee. Standing committees are put in place to oversee ongoing and cross-functional issues. They are given a broader charge, and committee members are normally appointed for a term that may last one to three years to ensure continuity. Some facilities may have a health information committee or a medical record committee; in other organizations oversight of the information resources may be assigned to one of the other standing committees.

Teams are created to address a more specific issue and generally disband when their work is complete. Teams may be cross-departmental or may be formed within a single department. They should be composed of people who are in the best position to contribute to the charge and communicate the outcome. In the formation of teams, the charge should be carefully considered to ensure clarity of purpose and appropriate results. The charge should consider the amount of authority the team is being given. For instance, a cross-departmental team might be given the charge of investigating alternative sick leave policies but would rarely be given ultimate authority to establish the policy when the decision could have a significant financial impact on the organization. Committees and teams are ways to involve more people in decision making, enrich jobs, and develop leadership skills.

Organizational Tools

In today's healthcare organizations, effective management demands that virtually every member of the organization understand its overall purpose. In addition, each member must be prepared to support and foster achievement of that purpose. Mission statements, vision statements, and values statements are all effective tools in communicating this information throughout the organization.

Policies and procedures also can be considered organizational tools. *Policies* are written descriptions of the organization's formal positions. *Procedures* are the approved methods for implementing those positions. Together, they spell out what the organization expects employees to do and how they are expected to do it. (Policies and procedures are explained in more detail in the section on human resources management later in this chapter.)

Organizational Charts

An **organizational chart** is a graphic representation of the organization's formal structure. It shows the organization's various activities and the specific members or categories of members assigned to carry them out. The chart for a very small organization might list the actual names of employees or individual position titles. The chart for a very large organization would list the various functional groups or departments responsible for each area of operations.

Traditionally, the reporting relationships between individuals and groups also are indicated according to accepted labeling conventions. For example, a solid line between two elements on a chart indicates a direct reporting relationship and a broken line indicates an indirect reporting relationship. (See figures 20.1, 20.2, and 20.3 for examples of organizational charts developed for different types of healthcare organizations.)

Today's healthcare organizations are somewhat less concerned with official lines of authority. Rather, they are concerned with the interrelationships of workgroups and functions. Individual departments and interdepartmental workgroups sometimes develop detailed organizational charts as a first step in redesigning work processes. The charts then can be used as the basis for creating work-flow diagrams and flowcharts. The purpose of these graphic tools is to help work teams visualize current and proposed processes and then suggest and implement improvements.

Some organizations also include organizational charts in their official position (job) descriptions. In this context, the charts put the work of a specific position or employee into the larger context of how the whole organization works as a system of interdependent processes.

Mission, Vision, and Values Statements

A mission statement is a short description of the general purpose of an organization or group. For healthcare organizations, the mission statement usually includes a broad definition of the services the organization provides and the communities/customers it serves. A **vision statement** is a short description of the organization's ideal future state. One way

Figure 20.1.   Sample organizational chart for an acute care hospital with outpatient services

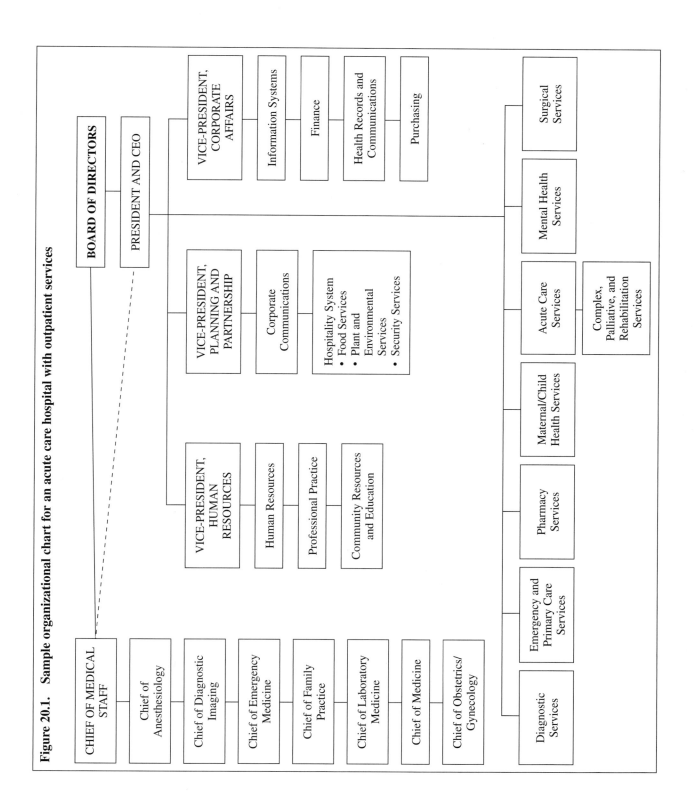

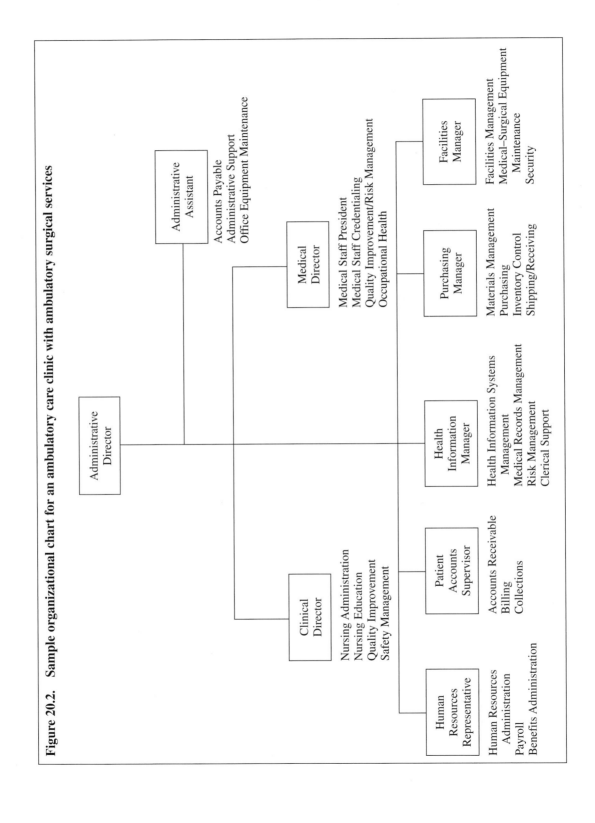

Figure 20.2. Sample organizational chart for an ambulatory care clinic with ambulatory surgical services

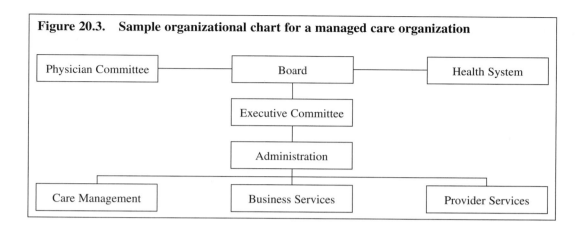

Figure 20.3.   Sample organizational chart for a managed care organization

to make the distinction between an organization's mission and its vision is to think of the concepts in the following way:

- The mission is a *realistic* expression of what the organization actually does at the current time.

- The vision is an *idealistic* portrayal of what the organization would like to become sometime in the future.

Most healthcare organizations update their mission and vision statements regularly as part of the strategic planning process. (Strategic planning is discussed later in this chapter.) The facility shares these statements internally with its employees and medical staff and externally with its customers and the community it serves. The statements are meant to inform, guide, and inspire. Figure 20.4 provides examples of vision and mission statements from healthcare organizations.

Healthcare organizations use mission and vision statements at many different levels. An individual organization usually develops statements for the enterprise as a whole. A multifacility healthcare system usually develops statements for the system as a whole as well as for each individual facility within it. Departments, work teams, and even temporary task forces also often develop vision and mission statements. These groups use the statements to express and communicate their specific purpose and goals.

Many healthcare organizations also develop statements that communicate their social and cultural belief system, or their values. The **values statement** provides a way to support the type of behavior the organization wishes to encourage among its members. For example, the American Health Information Management Association (AHIMA) has established the following list of values. According to the list, last updated in 2001, the association supports:

- A code of ethical health information management practices

- The public's right to private and high-quality health information

- The celebration and promotion of diversity

Figure 20.4.   Sample mission and vision statements

General Hospital Affiliated with a Larger Healthcare System

Lutheran Hospital's **mission** is to improve the health of the communities we serve by providing high-quality services in a responsible and caring way.

Our **vision** is to become the leader in promoting healthy life-styles in an atmosphere of spiritual support, dignity, compassion, and mutual respect for all.

Community General Hospital

Anytown General Hospital's **mission** is to provide quality health services and technology to meet the changing healthcare needs of the people of southwestern Minnesota.

Anytown General Hospital's **vision** is to become the hospital of choice for residents of Polk, Sunny Isle, and Spring counties, a position we strive to strengthen by our long-term commitment to:

• Teamwork
• Service excellence
• Compassionate care
• Cost consciousness
• Continuous improvement

Academic Medical Center

Prairie University Hospital's **mission** is to provide the most up-to-date medical and surgical services available in the three-state area and to train medical students and graduate physicians to meet current and future challenges in healthcare.

Our **vision** is the achievement of healthy communities and progress toward the future of healthcare for Montana, western North Dakota, and northwestern South Dakota.

Specialty Hospital

The **mission** of Women's Hospital of Somewhereville is to meet the healthcare needs of our patients and to exceed their service expectations.

Our **vision** is of a hospital:

• Providing services with compassion and kindness
• Striving for performance improvement
• Fostering pride and integrity
• Aiming for increased cost-effectiveness and productivity

Specialty Clinic within an Academic Medical Center

The **mission** of the Midwest Asthma Center is to:

• Provide optimal medical care for persons with asthma and related illnesses
• Develop new knowledge about asthma and its management through medical research
• Promote improved understanding about asthma and related illnesses through providing educational programs and materials for our patients, for other healthcare providers, and for the community

The **vision** of the Midwest Asthma Center is to provide the highest quality of integrated comprehensive care for persons with asthma and related illnesses and to be one of the centers of excellence in the world for asthma treatment, research, and education.

Primary Care Physicians' Practice

The **mission** of Coastal Shores Primary Care Associates is to serve the unique needs of individuals and families by providing high-quality, coordinated, primary care medical services through an efficient, accessible, and responsive network of caring providers.

Our **vision** is to be the primary care medical group of choice in the Atlantic County area by delivering high-quality, individualized, and efficient patient care.

Check Your Understanding 20.1

Instructions: Indicate whether the following statements are true or false (T or F).

1. ____ Continuous performance improvement and total quality management are examples of industrial management theories.

2. ____ Systems thinking is a subjective way to look at work-related ideas and processes.

3. ____ Ultimate responsibility for the organization's operation lies with its chief executive officer.

4. ____ Today's healthcare organizations are increasingly concerned with official lines of authority.

5. ____ Supervisory management sets the organization's future direction and establishes its goals.

Human Resources

The most important asset of any healthcare organization is its employees. Staff salaries and benefits usually make up most of the organization's operating budget. More critically, however, staff represents the organization to the patients and to other individuals the organization serves. Effective team leadership and supervision of employees leads to improved performance, increased productivity, and reduced expenses. Becoming an effective team leader requires more than developing and using supervisory tools; it requires nurturing a productive working relationship with staff and colleagues.

Effective management of human resources includes team leadership, selecting the right team members, ensuring ongoing performance, and developing people for the future. People work in a variety of configurations within any organization. From a traditional department configuration, where a supervisor or team leader works with a group of employees, to cross-functional teams, committees, and workgroups, performance can be heightened by effective leadership.

Fundamentals of Team Leadership

The term *leadership* has been defined as the "art of mobilizing others to want to struggle for shared aspirations" (Kouzes and Posner 1995, 30). The words want to are key to this definition. Leaders inspire and motivate others to choose to follow them instead of using their positions to force compliance. Because of this, leaders can work at any level of an organization. Although some people are more natural leaders than others, leadership can be practiced and learned. According to Kouzes and Posner (1995), leaders:

- Search for opportunities, [challenging] the status quo to improve their organization and realize the vision

- Experiment and take risks, ensuring that they learn from previous mistakes

- Envision the future, imagining new scenarios and developing vision

- Enlist others, attracting others to join them in their pursuit of the future

- Foster collaboration, promoting trust and a shared vision for the future

- Strengthen others by sharing information and power
- Set an example by role-modeling behaviors that make everyone successful
- Achieve small wins, demonstrating success and building commitment to action
- Recognize contributions, linking rewards with performance
- Celebrate accomplishments, taking the time to acknowledge success

Team leadership is a critical factor in the success of any team. Whether the team is charged with a specific short-term task or a standing team within a department, an effective leader can make a big difference in its outcome. Additionally, team leadership is a great opportunity to improve skills, provide professional development, and make a contribution to the organization. Good team leaders not only have a vision, but they also are able to communicate that vision to the other members of the team. They create an atmosphere of challenge, commitment, and determination that excites individuals and inspires performance.

A successful team facilitator provides leadership by (Bennett-Woods 1997):

- Creating a purpose and general framework for the project prior to the first meeting
- Encouraging the team to fully discuss the opportunities and potential pitfalls of the task
- Ensuring that all members of the team participate and reach consensus on the purpose
- Establishing specific goals and measurable objectives around which planning can occur and progress can be measured
- Making sure all decisions and plans are consistent with the purpose and goals
- Building trust among team members by emphasizing the unique role and importance of each team member
- Functioning as a cheerleader, reminding team members of the purpose and goals, celebrating achievements, and recognizing the efforts of individual team members

Teams do not work in a vacuum, so in addition to creating an effective team, the team leader must work to ensure that the organization supports the team by providing appropriate resources and commitment. Key to this job is to identify and communicate with all the stakeholders. The team leader may do this directly or may enlist the aid of an **executive sponsor.** An executive sponsor ensures that the team stays on track and communicates its progress to other key leaders. An executive sponsor also may ensure that the team obtains the organizational support, normally time and information, required to accomplish its goal. A key role for the team leader is regular communication with the executive sponsor, manager, or director.

The biggest advantage of a team over an individual is the team's ability to bring a variety of perspectives and expertise to the issue. The team leader's responsibility is to ensure that each member has the opportunity to contribute. One way to accomplish this is to provide the team with structured tools to assist in their discussion. Developing flowcharts for each technical area being considered can clarify the process and document several perspectives. This activity often identifies unnecessary complexity and miscommunication in any process. Revised flowcharts can be used describe changes and communicate new work flows. Facilitated brainstorming is another method to engage all members of a team in problem solving, by allowing them to be creative in a safe and nonjudgmental exercise.

To ensure participation, a team leader must demonstrate good interpersonal skills, act as a role model for the team, and build a climate of productive work behaviors. Effective teams set ground rules. For instance, team members might decide that all meetings will start on time, minutes will be recorded, decisions must be reached by consensus, and everyone will participate in discussions. The early establishment of rules can reduce conflict as the team moves forward.

However, not all teams are effective and the causes for problems vary. For example, a team without a clear purpose could create a product that does not accomplish the work for which it was designed. A leader who dominates the team could reduce its effectiveness and frustrate its members. Members who do not participate, have insufficient expertise, or are unconcerned with success could cause the team to fail. And members who work outside the team or do not support its decisions to others can create dissension and reduce support for the outcome.

Leading teams is an important part of managing human resources. Careful consideration should be given to creating the team's purpose and composition. Team members need to feel that their work is important and that their contribution makes a difference. A well-run team can be an effective and productive force. A poorly run team can waste time and frustrate and demoralize staff.

Selecting the Right Team

Whether selecting a permanent staff team or members of a team for a short-term project, making the right choice is fundamental to the team's success. Putting together a team involves understanding the challenge to be faced and considering all of the perspectives, experience, and knowledge that will be needed. The stakes are higher if a hiring decision is involved, so additional care should be taken when making a hiring decision.

Recruitment and Retention

Recruitment is the process of finding, soliciting, and attracting employees. Retention is the ability to keep valuable employees from seeking employment elsewhere.

Staff Recruitment

Understanding the organization's recruitment and hiring policies or seeking the assistance of human resources is necessary before announcing the vacancy.

There are several ways to advertise a staff opening, both internally and externally. The first thing to consider is whether to promote someone from inside or to look for candidates outside the organization. The advantage to promoting from within is that the act often motivates employees to do well, learn new skills, and work toward advancement. To advertise a vacancy internally, the organization might post it on facility bulletin boards or list it in the organization's newsletter or Web site. The supervisor or department manager may announce an opening at a routine staff meeting or use any other communication channels available. Management must communicate a promotional opportunity to all staff rather than to the employee who is the most likely candidate. Broad posting is seen as fair and strengthens communication of the underlying message that, whenever possible, internal candidates are considered first.

However, if the position cannot be filled from within, there are several ways to advertise it externally. For example, the organization might run an ad in a newspaper, post the job on recruitment Web sites, announce the opportunity at professional meetings, contact people who have previously applied or expressed interest in working at the organization, or work through a recruiter.

In most cases, the approach used depends on the position. For example, the facility might run an ad for a file room position in a local newspaper, but not in a professional journal. On the other hand, the facility might turn to a professional recruiter when trying to fill a department director or experienced coding position.

As in every industry, job seekers looking for professional-level positions in healthcare submit resumes. A resume describes the candidate's educational background and work experience and usually includes information on personal and professional achievements. Candidates also often submit a cover letter describing the type of position in which they are interested. Finally, today, it is common for candidates and organizations to conduct the preliminary screening process through electronic mail.

Most organizations ask every candidate to complete a formal job application. People seeking entry-level positions may be asked to complete an application, but not necessarily to submit a resume.

Interviewing is the most important skill that supervisors use in hiring new staff. However, many supervisors receive little formal training in interviewing techniques and/or have little practical experience. Even supervisors and managers with many years of experience sometimes dread the interviewing process.

Shortcomings in training and experience are common problems, but they can be overcome through self-education and mentoring. However, failure to adequately prepare for conducting the interview has consequences that are just as serious as having inadequate interviewing skills. Some supervisors and managers even begin the interview without having read the applicant's resume or thought about the questions they need to ask. And too often, updating the position description is the last step in the selection process instead of the first.

The interview itself has four basic purposes:

- To obtain information from the applicant about his or her past work history and future goals

- To give information to the applicant about the organization's mission and goals and the nature of the employment opportunity

- To evaluate the applicant's work experience, attitudes, and personality as a potential fit for the organization

- To give the applicant an opportunity to evaluate the organization as a potential fit for his or her current and future employment goals

A key part of the interview will deal with whether the candidate's education and experience provide a good fit for the job. Competency-based questions may be asked and a test of their technical skills may be administered.

If the candidate has had previous supervisory experience, ask how he or she would handle a situation where two employees have a disagreement about a work assignment. This may provide insight into how the candidate listens, empowers employees, or approaches conflict. For a candidate without supervisory experience, change the question to how he or she thinks it should be handled or how he or she has seen it handled effectively.

Here are some examples of interview questions that can be added to specific questions about a candidate's resume or qualifications for a particular job:

- Why are you looking for a job?

  Beware of candidates who talk negatively about a previous employer, this may signal a lack of responsibility for their own actions and may indicate how they will talk about your organization in the future.

- Because not everyone in a company is well liked by everyone, what would someone who did not like you have to say?

  The answer may provide insight into how this person gets along with others.

- What has been your biggest mistake at work, and what did you learn from it?

  If the candidate cannot describe a mistake, he or she may lack self-reflection and may not consider mistakes as learning opportunities.

- What criticisms would your previous manager have about you?

  This answer may provide insight into work habits or performance.

The final step in selecting a new member for your team is to check references. Even though most companies do not provide a lot of information, you can confirm the accuracy of the information the candidate has provided you, including work history and education. Candidates can lie on their resumes and applications, so checking references is a relatively easy way to verify that the facts are true.

Staff Retention

It is normal to have a certain level of staff turnover. Employees move, retire, or seek other careers. A supervisor can do little to prevent turnover caused by personal change. However, the supervisor and organizational policies can have an impact on **staff retention.** The following questions should be considered:

- Do organizational policies support continued education either financially or through flexible work schedules?

- Do employees have the opportunity to advance their careers within the organization?

- Are salaries and benefits competitive?

- Do working conditions provide a comfortable and safe environment?

Although a supervisor may have limited influence on these elements of employment, he or she may be able to address other concerns that often cause employees to seek other jobs. For example, employees can become dissatisfied if they feel that their work is not appreciated or they are being treated unfairly. In some cases, they become dissatisfied because they do not understand how their job contributes to the organization's goals or perhaps they feel overworked or underutilized. In other cases, employees may resent being too carefully supervised or working in a constant state of chaos. The challenge to the supervisor is to find a balance that appeals to each employee and is seen as fair by all. This is no small task.

Staff turnover is expensive in terms of both lost productivity and recruitment and training costs. To ensure effective management, turnover should be monitored across time and benchmarked with the rest of the organization and/or other organizations in the community or area. Routine satisfaction surveys can help provide information on how employees are feeling about their jobs and insights into how the facility might improve working conditions. The exit interview is another way to obtain information on how employees feel about their jobs and what issues cause them to leave.

Orientation and Training

One of the key ingredients in employee satisfaction is feeling knowledgeable and competent. This begins with an effective orientation and training program for new employees. Just as the supervisor prepared for the interview and selection of a new employee, he or she must plan how the new employee will learn about the organization, the department, and the job.

Most large organizations have a formal new **employee orientation** process. This process may involve a one-on-one session with human resources, group training with new employees from all over the organization, or some form of computer-based training.

Generally, the orientation session addresses the organization's mission and vision, goals, and structure; general employment policies; employee conduct; communication; and confidentiality. It also may include a tour of the facility and cover computer access and responsibilities. If the organization provides this type of orientation, the supervisor must know the material covered and feel comfortable answering any questions or directing the new employee to the appropriate resource for follow-up.

After orientation to the organization, the employee should be oriented to the department or area in which he or she will work. A departmental orientation checklist might include:

- Mission and vision
- Goals
- Structure
- Communication policies
- Procedure for requesting time off
- Person to notify in case of absence
- Tour
- Introductions
- Confidentiality policies
- Evaluation process
- Schedules

The departmental orientation should clarify the rules to follow and provide a context for job performance.

After the new employee has been oriented to the organization and the department, he or she is ready for specific job training. The position description is a good place to begin. This document is usually shared in the interview process, but it takes on new meaning when the employee actually begins work.

The supervisor should first explain why each task in the position description is performed and then review the policies and procedure for the task. This gives the employee information about work flow and available resources. Next, the supervisor should demonstrate how to do the task using the procedure for it. Having observed the supervisor perform the task, the employee should feel comfortable enough to try it. The supervisor now should observe the employee's work, correcting any errors and answering questions. Finally, the employee should be allowed time to work on his or her own. The supervisor should check the new employee's work periodically to ensure that the employee understands the training and the product is error free.

The supervisor must be very patient during the first days and schedule adequate time to spend with the new hire. Everyone learns differently and at a different pace. The first days not only establish how the employee will do the job, but they also contribute to ongoing relationships.

Delegation of Authority and Empowerment

Yet another important part of the team leader's function is that of empowering employees and team members through the **delegation of authority.** The level of authority an employee is given and the types of decisions he or she is empowered to make should be considered when setting the salary for the position and determining its educational and experiential requirements. The responsibilities of the position should be clearly described in the job description. The supervisor can then use the job description in setting performance expectations with individual employees.

Delegating responsibilities and projects to other people on the staff can benefit managers and supervisors in a number of ways. For example, delegating authority:

- Frees the team leader to perform more important or complex tasks
- Increases the leader's capacity and productivity
- Reduces delays in decision making
- Develops the staff's capacity and abilities

As a rule, employees should be given as much control over their jobs and the work of teams as possible. One reason for this is that they usually have the most information about how to improve the processes and productivity in their own areas or address the challenge they have been given. The team leader's role is to establish expectations and provide a reason for employees to want to do a better job. This may be accomplished through recognition, promotion, or other types of motivation.

When delegating authority, team leaders should prepare staff members to succeed by:

- Explaining exactly what needs to be done
- Describing clear expectations

- Setting clear deadlines
- Granting authority to make relevant decisions
- Ensuring appropriate communication and reporting
- Providing the resources needed to complete the task

Performance Management

In most organizations, **performance evaluations** are used to structure discussions regarding individual performance. Routinely done on an annual basis, performance reviews include:

- Assessment of the employee's performance compared to performance standards or previously set goals
- Development of goals for the future year
- Development of a plan for professional development

Reviews also may include an employee's self-assessment. In some organizations, other employees may contribute information to the review. In the case of a supervisor, his or her staff may participate in the evaluation. This form of evaluation in which supervisor, peers, and staff contribute is called a 360-degree evaluation.

Many organizations base pay increases on the results of an annual performance review. Whether or not the evaluation affects salary, the annual review is an opportunity to formally discuss accomplishments, development, and new expectations.

Periodic Performance Reviews

Performance management is an ongoing challenge. Information about performance should be collected regularly and shared with the employee, whether the job is coding records or directing a department. Good performance results should be shared to encourage and reward ongoing success.

Performance issues are rarely resolved by ignoring them. Understanding the cause of problems and working with employees to resolve them is an important supervisory task. Actions that can be taken to improve performance include retraining, streamlining responsibilities, reestablishing expectations, and monitoring progress.

Performance Counseling and Disciplinary Action

When actions taken to improve performance are unsuccessful, more formal counseling and even **disciplinary action** may be required. Most organizations have formal processes in place to ensure that all staff are treated fairly and that employment laws are considered. Supervisors should consult with the human resources department to ensure that any disciplinary actions comply with approved procedures.

The steps described in establishing performance standards, hiring and training employees, and conducting routine performance reviews are all necessary before doing performance counseling or taking disciplinary action. Moreover, steps to improve performance should be taken in all cases.

Performance counseling usually begins with informal counseling or a verbal warning. No record is kept in the employee's file.

Progressive discipline begins with formal documentation of the problem and the steps taken to correct it. Employees may be required to submit an action plan of steps they are committed to take to resolve issues and improve their performance. Execution of the action plan may be binding on the employee, and failure to comply could result in termination.

In other environments, disciplinary actions include suspension from employment without pay, demotion to a job with lower expectations and less pay, or termination. In some cases, more than one of these actions may be taken. Generally, however, suspension and demotion are less popular than the use of binding performance improvement plans because suspension and demotion create a punitive atmosphere. Such punitive actions also affect the morale of other employees and staff. Empowering employees to create a plan of action places the responsibility for performance improvement in their own hands.

Regardless of the counseling or disciplinary actions mandated by the organization, supervisors should take some key steps of their own. They should:

- Be clear and direct with the employee about problems and consequences

- Support the employee's efforts to improve or resolve issues

- Document the steps taken to improve performance

- Follow all organizational policies

- Consult with human resources

- Keep performance issues confidential

- Be consistent with all employees

Conflict Management

Sometimes problems arise because of conflicts between employees. It is not unusual for people to disagree. Indeed, sometimes a difference of opinion can increase creativity. However, conflict can waste time, reduce productivity, and decrease morale. When taken to the extreme, it can threaten the safety of employees and cause damage to property.

Conflict management focuses on working with individuals to find a mutually acceptable solution. There are three ways to address conflict:

- *Compromise:* In this method, both parties must be willing to lose or give up a piece of their position.

- *Control:* In this method, interaction may be prohibited until the employees' emotions are under control. The supervisor also may structure their interactions. For example, he or she can set ground rules for communicating or dealing with specific issues. Another form of controlling is personal counseling. Personal counseling focuses on how people deal with conflict rather than on the cause of disagreements.

- *Constructive confrontation:* In this method, both parties meet with an objective third party to explore their perceptions and feelings. The desired outcome is to produce a mutual understanding of the issues and to create a win–win situation.

Grievance Management

Grievance management includes the policies and procedures used to handle employee complaints. Employees have the right to disagree with management and can express their opinions in a variety of ways. They should be encouraged to bring problems and concerns directly to their supervisor. If they do not achieve satisfaction at that level, the supervisor should explain their options. For example, dissatisfied employees should understand that they can either take their issues to the next management level or discuss them with human resources.

Employees who belong to a union should follow the grievance procedures set by their union. Union contracts usually specify the types of actions employees can take and the time frames for filing grievances. The contracts usually specify time frames for responses and define the formal process for elevating the consideration or resolution of a grievance. Grievances taken to the highest levels will likely have to be resolved through mediation or arbitration.

Each of these steps takes time and can cost money. Therefore, supervisors should try to avoid grievances by maintaining open and effective communication with their staff.

Staff Development

Staff development is extremely important. It is driven by three conditions:

- The rate of change in healthcare

- The introduction of new technology into the workplace

- The increased demand on maximizing productivity

Supervisors are responsible for creating an environment that develops the skills of their staff. No one can make another person learn something, but providing the opportunity for development is critical to creating a successful learner. Following are the three main approaches to training:

- *On-the-job training* provides direct, realistic training in the specific tasks required by the position. The employee's supervisor and peers are available for immediate feedback because they are involved in the training process. On-the-job training can be used with individuals who do not do well in traditional classroom training but can easily handle the work.

- *Information presentation* resembles the traditional classroom approach to education. This approach may include lectures, small group discussions, case studies, audiovisual techniques, and computer-assisted instruction. The training may be offered by the employer, a college or university, professional associations, or for-profit training centers. Information presentation methods range in scope from one-day courses to for-credit college programs. They vary in effectiveness based on the skill being taught, the match of teaching style to learner, and how well the information learned can be applied directly to the job.

- *Action-based methods* of training involve simulations, role-playing, and case studies. Role-playing and simulations give learners the ability to practice new behaviors in a safe environment. Conducted in small group settings, a situation is described and individuals are given roles to act out. In a simulation, in addition to playing a role, learners normally use a defined set of resources to solve a problem. Case studies are a more passive form of training. Instead of actually participating in a situation, the learners study how an individual or organization responded to a real-life situation and what the outcomes were.

Regardless of the form of training used, a commitment to ongoing training is critical to maintain and enhance skills, to prepare people for new and higher-level jobs, and to create an interesting and rewarding work environment.

Job Redesign

One way a supervisor can create a positive and rewarding work environment is through **job redesign.** Creatively aligning the needs of the organization with the skills and interests of the employee and then designing the job to meet those needs is job redesign at its best. The reasons to redesign a job may be to introduce new tools or technology, improve a process, use employee skills more effectively, or provide better customer service. Generally, all these outcomes can be addressed through job redesign.

The best way to begin the process of job redesign is to discuss the job with the employee. The supervisor should identify barriers to the employee's current work and areas of frustration. Perhaps the employee feels that he or she is wasting time performing a task at a lower skill level than the rest of the work. Perhaps he or she would like to take on more complex work.

The supervisor should examine the work-flow process that includes the employee's job. Does the process involve other tasks the employee could assume? Are there functions in related processes that could be combined into the employee's job? If several people perform similar work, a test or pilot of a new job design might be done with one or two individuals to work out unanticipated problems.

It is important to ensure that training is provided for any new work. Job redesign is one way to initiate or manage change in the workplace, but managing change is an ongoing challenge.

Career Planning and Lifelong Learning

Finding a job is different from planning a career. Although **career planning** may include getting a job, a career extends beyond current job requirements and positions the employee for more challenging and diverse work. When assisting an employee in career planning, supervisors should take the following actions:

- *Lead by example:* Their commitment to lifelong learning should be evident in their actions. They should show how they have enhanced their careers by accepting risk, new challenges, and added responsibilities.

- *Create a supportive environment:* Supervisors should allow time for training and allocate money, whenever possible, to advance the skills of employees. Scheduling must be flexible to allow employees to pursue advanced degrees or continuing education.

- *Provide career counseling:* When possible, supervisors should provide staff with career counseling resources within the organization or connect with community college or university training counselors.

- *Create a partnership:* Supervisors should expect employees to fulfill their commitments when it comes to training and education.

Career planning and lifelong learning are personal. No supervisor can accept responsibility for planning someone else's career. However, through effective leadership, employees can be encouraged and rewarded to see beyond their current job.

Check Your Understanding 20.2

Instructions: Indicate whether the following statements are true or false (T or F).

1. _____ Contemporary performance and quality improvement theories are based on the idea that systems are at the root of most performance problems, not people.

2. _____ Staff turnover is expensive in terms of lost productivity and recruitment and training costs.

3. _____ Supervisory-level management responsibilities include new employee orientation and training.

4. _____ One thing that teams have in common is that their members are usually from the same department.

5. _____ When redesigning a job, the supervisor should not discuss potential changes with the employee.

Fundamentals of Work Planning

In healthcare organizations, the planning function includes strategic and operational planning. Strategic planning generally deals with the organization's long-term approach to the future. Most healthcare organizations' strategic plans apply to activities over at least a five-year period. Operational planning generally deals with the organization's short-term activities. Most healthcare organizations' **operational plans** apply chiefly to the next calendar year.

Strategic Planning

Strategic planning is concerned primarily with how the organization will respond to changes in its external environment in the foreseeable future, usually the next five to ten years. Environmental factors include changes in the organization's external business climate, its competitive status, and/or the broader social and political climate in which it operates.

Strategic planning is an ongoing activity. The output of the strategic planning process is a yearly update and revision of the organization's written strategic plan. The updates focus on action planning for the upcoming year and project plans over several subsequent years.

As noted earlier, primary responsibility for strategic planning lies with the organization's board of directors. However, the board works closely with the executive management team throughout the strategic planning process. In large part, the board depends on the executive staff to provide the information on which the process is based. In turn, the executive team gathers and formulates strategic planning information that was originally collected and analyzed by middle-level managers. As part of their regular management duties, middle-level managers collect a great deal of detailed operational information from the records and databases created by supervisors and staff-level employees.

The strategic planning process is not the same for every organization. Its details vary significantly depending on the type of services the organization provides and its size and structure, corporate structure (for example, for profit versus not for profit), and competitive status. In most healthcare organizations, however, strategic planning involves the following general steps:

1. *Conducting an environmental assessment:* An **environmental assessment** is a collection of information about changes that have occurred in the organization's internal and external environment since the previous year. They may have potentially positive or negative effects on the organization that can be considered threats and/or opportunities for the future. An example of an internal change might include an increased movement toward employee unionization. An external change might be a merger between two of the organization's biggest competitors.

2. *Developing and/or revising the mission and vision statements in response to the environmental assessment:* The organization's mission and vision statements represent broad expressions of its current and future purpose. When the results of the environmental assessment point to a need for fundamental change within the organization, these public statements represent the organization's first acknowledgment and response to that need.

3. *Developing and/or revising the values statements:* The beliefs and values of healthcare organizations usually are rooted in a fundamental respect for the rights and uniqueness of individuals. As such, they do not change significantly from year to year. Changes in the wording or direction of the organization's mission and vision, however, sometimes require a minor rewording of its values statements.

4. *Developing and/or revising the strategic plan for the upcoming year:* In most healthcare organizations, the board's strategic planning committee revises and updates the strategic plan. It works directly with key members of the organization's executive management team to analyze information and trends. Specific strategies for the future are developed on the basis of these trends. The strategic planning committee and executive leaders also work together to make plans for succeeding years. Together, they develop of list of specific recommendations for action.

5. *Revising the strategic plan for the succeeding years in light of the changes made to the plan for the upcoming year:* In addition to devising strategies for the upcoming year, the future strategic plan may need revision. Revisions may be needed to address changes in strategic direction, new regulations that require a long-term response, or economic or technical changes that affect the organization. Frequently, changes in the coming year's plan have a ripple effect on future years.

6. *Developing specific action steps for the upcoming year:* Strategic plans often include a list of specific **action steps** (or plans) the organization should take in the near future. The plans describe projects to be undertaken by board-designated committees or managerial action teams to address threats or opportunities. For example, the strategic planning committee of a private urban hospital might recommend that the hospital initiate a plan to close its emergency department within the next five years. Such a recommendation might be made if the hospital's environmental assessment revealed significant financial losses as a result of providing uncompensated care to uninsured emergency patients.

7. *Discussing the proposed strategic plan with the board of directors and making changes as a result:* In the next step of the strategic planning process, the strategic planning committee communicates its draft plan to the board for comments and reactions. Such discussions are conducted during private meetings of the full board officiated by the board chairman.

8. *Officially documenting the board's approval of the plan:* For the strategic plan to become official, the board must approve it through a legal voting process. The board's actions are then documented in the meeting minutes and become a part of the organization's official records.

9. *Communicating the strategic plan to the administrators and managers:* After the new plan has been accepted by a majority of the board, the executive leadership team communicates it to other executive managers of the organization. In turn, the executive managers provide relevant details of the plan to the departmental or functional managers responsible for carrying out its provisions. Under the leadership of executive and middle managers, project teams are created to develop specific design and implementation plans. These plans bring the board's strategic ideas to reality.

10. *Developing operational plans for the upcoming year on the basis of the action steps and future direction documented in the final strategic plan:* Most organizations develop their time lines for operational planning and budgeting to coincide with the board's strategic planning decisions. Successful implementation of the strategic plan requires investments reflected in the budget and incremental achievement of operational objectives.

Operational Planning

After the strategic plan is in place and has been communicated to managers and staff, an annual operational plan is established to meet the objectives of the strategic plan. The operational plan has a much more defined time frame, usually one or two years. The organization as a whole may have an operational plan, but certainly each department within the organization creates an annual plan that states its goals and objectives. Operational plans are tied to budget planning because resources are usually required to meet operational plans.

Departmental planning can be approached in several ways. Information is usually gathered to assess the department's strengths and weaknesses and to identify and prioritize initiatives for the coming year. Customer satisfaction surveys can be developed and the results used in planning. Department supervisors may identify recurrent service or production problems that should be addressed in the operational plan. Reviewing the organization's plans to ensure that the department has the resources to contribute to overall success is an essential step. In addition, opportunities may exist for improving productivity through the replacement of equipment or the streamlining of processes.

Department managers play the key role in assembling the operational plan for a department. Other members of the staff, however, may have a role in compiling information or suggesting process changes within a department and within the framework of the operational plan and priorities.

Supervisors organize the work of their teams by setting short-term (usually daily or weekly) goals. These goals must take into account the overall productivity requirements of both the immediate workgroup and the larger functional workgroup (or department) within which the team operates.

The goal-setting process is relatively straightforward. The supervisor's own manager usually provides information on how much work must be accomplished over the upcoming period of time or which operational improvements need to be implemented. The supervisor then determines how much work each team member must accomplish for the team to keep up with its workload.

Obviously, the team's performance depends on the aggregate performance of its members. The challenge for the supervisor is to ensure that each team member has the training and knowledge to carry out the duties assigned. Therefore, a vital component of organization at the supervisory level is organizing the individual tasks in such a way that the employee assigned to perform each task is qualified to do so.

Expense Budgets

An important part of operational planning is planning for and then managing the expenses of the department or section. Financial control is an ongoing process that begins with a budget or financial plan and continues with ongoing monitoring. Effective financial control creates opportunities for improvements in the use of the organization's resources.

The budget is the primary tool for financial control. It represents the organization's financial plan for the coming time period, in most cases a year. The budget year or fiscal year covers twelve months but may not run from January through December. Different companies use different fiscal years for a variety of reasons. Budgeting is also a process. It is laying out a plan and then routinely checking actual results against the plan and making adjustments as necessary.

Budgeting is part of the overall planning process. A budget should support the goals of the organization, not establish them. However, the reality of available resources may alter the approach or time taken in reaching those goals.

Budgets can be broken down into several parts. First, there are **revenues** and expenses. *Revenues* are monies that will be paid to the organization or income that will be earned by the organization. *Expenses* are monies that will be spent by the organization.

Expenses can be further broken down into fixed and variable costs. **Fixed costs** are costs that remain the same regardless of how much work is done. For instance, depreciation, space costs or rent, managers' salaries, and general office expenses are all fixed costs. **Variable costs** include employee salaries, materials, and other expenses related to how much work is done. For example, the amount of work to be done in a transcription department determines how many staff members are needed, how much paper will be used, and how many computer supplies will be consumed. There probably will be only one manager regardless of the number of transcriptionists employed. However, the number of supervisors may be semivariable depending on whether other shifts are required or whether the supervisor-to-employee ratio becomes too high.

All these items involve the operating budget. In addition to operating expense is capital expense. Capital budgets include those items the organization will purchase whose value extends beyond one year. Examples include buildings, equipment, and computers.

Budgeting Process

At the department level, budgeting usually begins with developing a clear statement of the goals the department wants to achieve in the coming year. Information about the overall organization's budget planning is frequently contained in **budget assumptions.** These assumptions may include an estimation of how revenues will increase or decrease and what limits will be placed on expenses.

HIM functions are largely expense based, with limited revenue in areas such as photocopying records for release to outside parties. In some cases, revenue is generated through charging other departments for services (for example, transcription services). The department manager must understand the budget assumptions before starting the department's budget. Anticipating increased volume within the department is related to the organization's assumptions of volume, although there may not be a direct relationship. Also, any plans to increase or decrease work or any changes in regulations that will affect the operation should be considered at budget time.

Several approaches can be taken to develop a budget. Historical projections are based on looking at prior budgets and actual expense reports and then projecting a percentage increase. This might be useful in cases where there is no anticipated increase in staff, but there is an expected salary increase of 4 percent overall. Another method is called zero-based budgeting. In this approach, each cost is built from scratch without reference to historical information. Each cost is developed based on the number of units required and the price per unit. This works well in areas where costs are highly variable and can be directly related to how much work will be produced in the coming year.

Typically, departments use a combination of approaches. Although salaries and benefits may be increased based on a percentage, the projected cost of certain supplies such as chart folders would be based on actual anticipated usage and price per folder. It is important to verify prices with suppliers prior to budgeting to anticipate any increases. Regardless of the approach taken, managers must thoroughly understand the prior year's budget and year-to-date variations in actual performance before beginning the budget.

Usually, a budget review process is part of developing the overall budget. This may include a formal presentation of the budget to senior management. The department manager should understand the entire budget process and be aware of deadlines for submission of the budget.

Financial Control

Financial control does not end with successful budget presentation. Monitoring ongoing expenses and revenues is an important management responsibility. The budget is a plan. When the actual does not match the plan, a variety of actions can be taken. In most organizations, monthly reports detailing revenues and expenses are provided. In addition, reports are generated that compare monthly and year-to-date actual results with the budget. These reports should be reviewed each month to ensure that there are no errors in assigning revenues or expenses to the correct budgets and to monitor actual results from the plan. The manager should:

1. Understand what caused the variation or variance from the budget

2. Determine whether the variance will continue or whether it was a one-time occurrence

3. Determine what actions are necessary to modify future results in order to achieve the overall targets

Staying within the budget is only half the equation. Equally important is completing the objectives set out for the year. Meeting the operational goals is as important as meeting the financial ones. Successful managers keep both in mind as they work to implement the plan.

Supply Management

There is little more frustrating for a supervisor than work coming to a stop because of a shortage of supplies. Imagine a release of information function, still heavily reliant on paper copies when there is no copy paper. Backlogs build, staff members have to be redeployed, and supplies purchased on short notice are frequently more expensive. **Supply management** can therefore be an extremely important element of controlling overall costs.

Effective Purchasing

The first step in supply management is an effective purchasing process. This may be as straightforward as sitting down with an office supply catalog or as complex as issuing a formal request for proposal (RFP). Matching the right purchasing process to the supply is key in getting the right product at the best price. Standardized general office supplies usually assist in both purchasing and inventory control. Items such as pens, note pads, paper, and all general office supplies should be a compromise between meeting the needs of different staff members and cost. This usually requires a purchasing policy that centralizes ordering authority. The organization as a whole may have contracts or other requirements regarding where supplies are purchased and what supplies are authorized.

In larger types of purchases or customized purchases, an RFP is frequently done to ensure that the required products are purchased at the best price. RFPs are almost always required for other types of purchases such as services or software and contain elements such as requirements, cost, service, and information about the supplying company. Additionally, an RFP may contain a request for references. In the area of supplies, file folders may be purchased through an RFP or some other formal purchase process. The requirements would include specifications for paper weight and color, dividers, fasteners, and so on. As health information moves to new technologies, the types of supplies will require change (for example, electronic storage media may replace file folders).

Inventory Control

One of the key elements of supply management is **inventory control.** Inventory control is the balance between purchasing and storing the supplies needed and not wasting money or space should the requirements for that supply change or the space available for storage be limited. Centralized purchasing allows better record keeping of how much of an individual supply is used within a given time frame. This information allows the purchaser to better estimate the required on-hand inventory and the amount of time from order placement to order fulfillment. A spreadsheet with all the inventory items, suppliers, current stock, distribution schedule, and cost can be extremely valuable in inventory control. One final purpose for tracking inventory is to identify possible theft of supplies when normal usage rates change for unexplained reasons.

Supplier Relationships

Finally, maintaining a productive relationship with suppliers can help control costs and improve efficiency. Spend time with sales representatives discussing current purchases and suggested alternatives. Encourage representatives to discuss new products or services the company offers. Discuss issues that concern purchasing behavior. For example, taking advantage of volume discounts may not be available due to storage limitations, but some suppliers can assist by providing storage or offering other solutions. Compare products across suppliers, for both quality and price. Although it may be more convenient to use a single supplier, cost and quality advantages may outweigh the convenience. In addition to communicating with suppliers, discuss product choice and satisfaction with other professional colleagues.

To execute an operational plan, a sound budget and strong supply management are critical, but the biggest factor in success is staffing. Tools are available to help with understanding staffing requirements and planning work that can be adopted by anyone responsible for executing an operational plan.

Staffing

In most healthcare organizations, payroll and benefits consume the most resources. Therefore, adequate time and attention must be paid to the management of human resources. Beyond the financial reason, employees' attitudes and morale affect their ability to perform any task effectively. This becomes even more important when their work involves caring for patients directly or supporting the caregivers.

Large entities such as hospitals, large physician groups, and managed care organizations commonly have a human resources department that acts as a reference and support for supervisors. However, any supervisor must have some understanding of the principles of human resources management to lead effectively.

Staffing Tools

Several tools may be used to plan and manage staff resources. For example, position descriptions outline the work and qualifications required by the job. Performance standards establish expectations for how well the job will be done and how much work will be accomplished.

In addition to these basics, supervisors must use work schedules to ensure that there is adequate coverage and staff to complete the required work. Schedules are developed first to provide adequate coverage during the hours the organization or department is open for business.

In hospitals, it is not uncommon to find some part of the HIM department open twenty-four hours a day, seven days a week. This enables HIM staff to provide information for admissions to the hospital or emergency department, support discharges and transfers, or handle other tasks requiring full-time coverage. In some organizations, the demand for those services is small enough that business office staff, nursing staff, or emergency department personnel can be cross-trained to perform basic HIM tasks.

Another scheduling consideration is space. Space limitations for workstations or workers in the file room may require scheduling staff to other shifts or days. In addition, staff preferences need to be considered in creating the schedule. Balancing the demands of the organization with individual requests for alternate or flexible start times makes scheduling an important part of the supervisor's responsibility.

When there is an understanding of what the coverage needs are, and any space limitations are considered, the next factor to be considered is work flow. Work-flow analysis ensures that tasks are done in the most efficient order by considering all the steps in a process and then understanding and documenting how they relate to each other. A work-flow diagram is often used as a method of documentation because it clearly depicts each step in the process and can point out dependencies and redundancies.

When an optimal work flow is determined, the amount of work and the staff required to complete it must be considered. In a following section on performance and practice standards, the approach described to determine the performance standard is applied to determine the time required to complete a task. That time is then translated into numbers of full-time equivalents (FTEs) and then staffing assignments can be made.

Written policies and procedures explaining staffing requirements and scheduling assist the supervisor in being fair and objective and help the staff understand the rules. The amount of personal time off, as sick leave or vacation, also factors into development of a staff schedule and the overall assessment of staff required. The general rule of thumb is that each staff member will produce 1,080 hours of work in the course of a year.

An example taken from a physician office practice may be useful. One job that must be done each day is pulling charts on existing patients for upcoming appointments. Space limitations allow only one day to pull the charts and store them outside the main file area. A work-flow analysis shows that this task is best done when all the charts are returned to the file at the close of each business day because it is more efficient to pull charts from the main file than to waste time looking for them throughout the clinic. Moreover, until an electronic health record is in place, staff must check for the latest lab reports and update the record prior to the appointment. When this step is done after all the charts are pulled, any missing reports can be printed and attached to the record. Chart filing, pulling, and checking for laboratory work can be done by staff with the same skill level, but the work flow suggests that this function is best performed as operations slow from midafternoon into the evening. Based on volume and time, one person should be able to perform this function routinely each day. However, what happens when that person is on vacation or out for an unanticipated leave? Are other people in the office during the evening? Working alone may create a security concern. Perhaps current staff are unwilling to work evening hours. A variety of possible solutions might be considered. Two part-time employees willing to cover for each other when either was out of the office could share the job. If no other workers currently work evening hours, a group of off-hours tasks could be created (coding, transcription, and so on). The work could be combined into other people's existing tasks and spread at both ends of the day so that some tasks are completed in the afternoon and extended to early evening and others are completed by an early morning shift. There is probably no one right solution, but considering all the elements of staffing is required to create a best solution for a given situation.

Frequently, organizations have some type of position classification system that combines jobs with similar levels of responsibility and qualifications into fair wage ranges and benefit packages. For instance, all supervisors may be classified into one wage and benefit category but have unique job descriptions. These classifications also may determine whether an employee belongs to a union.

Position Descriptions

A position, or job, description outlines the work an individual does. It generally consists of three parts: a summary of the position, including its purpose; a list of duties; and the qualifications for the job. Position descriptions also contain the title of the job.

Position descriptions are used in the recruitment and interviewing phase to explain the work to prospective candidates. They also enable supervisors or human resources personnel to set appropriate wages for positions. Moreover, they may be used to resolve performance problems. The supervisor can use the position description to clarify the tasks the employee is expected to perform.

Generally, job descriptions are needed when:

- An entirely new kind of work is required.
- Jobs change and the old description no longer fits the work.
- A change in technology or processes dramatically affects the work to be done.

Sometimes top performers outgrow their current descriptions. They may find more efficient ways of doing part of their assigned tasks and/or seek new, more interesting or more meaningful work. Sometimes employees seek a new or updated job description to support an increase in salary, benefits, or a change in title.

When writing new position descriptions, supervisors may use existing descriptions of other, related jobs or interview staff members who are currently performing some of the tasks intended for the new job. They also might ask staff members to keep a diary of how they spend their time for a period that reflects a comprehensive cycle of their work. Staff members with more repetitive daily activities may only need to record their activities for a week. In contrast, staff members with more diverse tasks may need a month to document the scope of their duties.

Performance/Practice Standards

In addition to a position description, performance standards are developed for the key functions of the job. These standards indicate each function's level of acceptable execution. Normally, performance standards are set for both quantity and quality and should be as objective and measurable as possible.

Each organization may have a unique approach to the structure of performance standards, such as in the number of levels of measurement. For example, one function of the coder's job would be to code a certain number of charts per day. Some organizations might have only one level of expected performance (for example, no fewer than twenty charts per day). Others might have several levels of expected performance. For example:

30–35 charts per day	Outstanding
25–29 charts per day	Exceeds expectations
20–24 charts per day	Meets expectations
15–19 charts per day	Needs improvement
Fewer than 14 charts per day	Unsatisfactory

The following example shows how a quality standard might be used as a performance indicator of coding accuracy. For example:

91–95 percent accuracy	Outstanding
86–90 percent accuracy	Exceeds Expectations
81–85 percent accuracy	Meets Expectations
76–80 percent accuracy	Needs improvement
80 percent or less	Unsatisfactory

In this example, a definition for coding accuracy might be helpful. For example, accurate coding includes capturing accurate codes and sequencing them appropriately for all diagnoses and procedures that affect reimbursement.

Standards that are measurable and relevant to an employee's overall performance are helpful in setting clear expectations. They also are helpful in providing useful feedback. Standard setting may be accomplished in a variety of ways. For example, the supervisor might do one of the following:

1. *Check industry benchmarks or standards:* If the supervisor finds that industry benchmarks or standards are available for the task, he or she should evaluate their relevancy to the work in his or her environment.

2. *Collect data on current performance:* When more than one person is performing a task, the data could be collected over time and averaged. The experience and overall performance of each person must be considered in setting the standard. If there are not enough employees to capture data internally, the supervisor might contact other facilities to establish a standard as long as work conditions are comparable.

3. *Share the standards with any employee who performs that task:* Employees must understand the standards and how information about their performance will be collected.

4. *Determine a collection process:* Quantitative measures can be relatively easy to evaluate. In the preceding coding example, the abstracting system may record how many health charts each staff person codes daily. The average then could be generated over all the charts coded every day. If no automated method of data capture is available, actual work could be tracked manually either daily or for selected periods of time throughout the year. Data on the quality level may be harder to aggregate. Supervisors can check a random sample of work over time or discuss the work with a colleague. Findings from external reviews of work such as audits can be used. Whatever the method, the findings should be reported to staff members on a regular basis so that they clearly understand what is expected of them throughout the year.

Policies and Procedures

Policies and procedures also are critical tools that may be used to ensure consistent quality performance. A *policy* is a statement about what an organization or department does. For example, a policy might state that patients are allowed to review their health records upon request with a care provider or in the HIM department. Policies should be clearly stated and comprehensive. They must be developed in accordance with applicable laws and reflect actual practice. Because they may be used as documentation of intended practice in a lawsuit, policies should be developed very carefully.

A *procedure* describes how work is done and how policies are carried out. Procedures are instructions that ensure high-quality, consistent outcomes for tasks done, especially when more than one person is involved.

One of the benefits of developing a procedure is that time is taken to analyze the best possible method of completing a process. This analysis may begin by developing a flowchart to document work flow, decision points, and the flow required to complete a procedure. (Flowcharts are discussed in detail in chapter 12.)

After a flowchart is completed, the steps in the process are written down in order. When more than one person is involved in completing a procedure, each person who performs a task is documented. Anyone generally competent to perform a task should be able to complete it after reading a well-written procedure. This usually takes several drafts that have been reviewed by people who actually perform the work. Moreover, it might be useful to ask someone unfamiliar with the job to try to complete it using the written procedure.

Writing a procedure also offers a great opportunity to identify ways to streamline the process. Are supplies available and organized in a way that makes work efficient? Would it be faster to complete one type of task for all the work, or should each job be completed before the next task is begun? A procedure for the process of logging in requests for information might be as follows:

1. The receptionist opens all incoming mail daily before 10 a.m. He or she then confirms that the date on the date stamp is accurate and stamps all mail in the upper right-hand corner.

2. The receptionist sorts requests for medical information into three categories: legal, medical, or insurance. He or she then counts the requests in each category, clips or binds the requests for each category together, writes the count on a Post-it™ note, and places the note on the top request of each bundle. The bundles are then delivered to the release of information (ROI) inbox. (The inbox is located on the ROI supervisor's desk.)

3. The ROI coordinator picks up medical requests for information from the ROI inbox each morning after 10 a.m. He or she enters the number of requests on a daily work log (an Excel™ spreadsheet stored on G:roi/requests/medical).

It would be inefficient for the receptionist to open, date stamp, and deliver each piece of mail individually. This procedure would continue through the logging process. However, this example shows how a detailed procedure would be useful in training a new receptionist or ROI coordinator or in providing instructions to anyone needed to perform this task in the regular employee's absence. It also highlights that the receptionist would need to be trained to identify different types of information requestors.

Several tools may be used to effectively communicate the purpose, scope, and details of the work done by employees in the organization. The supervisor is responsible for developing and maintaining these tools. However, the supervisor's role does not end here. Given the tools just described, he or she is ready to hire, train, and interact with employees.

Check Your Understanding 20.3

Instructions: Complete the following sentences with the most appropriate word or words.

1. _____ Strategic planning is concerned primarily with how the organization will respond to changes in its _____ in the foreseeable future.
   - a. Long-range goals
   - b. Mission statement
   - c. External environment
   - d. Vision statement

2. _____ In developing the organization's strategic plan for the coming year, the board's strategic planning committee works with the _____.
   - a. Supervisory-level managers
   - b. Executive management team
   - c. Board of governors
   - d. Middle managers

3. _____ Strategic plans often include specific _____ steps that the organization should take in the near future.
   - a. Revision
   - b. Administrative
   - c. Action
   - d. Implementation

4. _____ Team leaders organize the work of their teams by setting _____ goals
   - a. Long-term
   - b. Short-term
   - c. Action
   - d. Future

5. _____ Inventory control, supplier relationships, and _____ are all elements of supply management.
   - a. Effective purchasing
   - b. Position descriptions
   - c. Requests for proposal
   - d. Job enrichment

6. _____ A new job description is not required when _____.
   - a. The job has changed to include new work not in the previous description.
   - b. The employee wants a raise.
   - c. Technology has substantially changed the job.
   - d. A new job is being performed.

7. _____ The focus of conflict management is that of _____.
   - a. Getting personal counseling for the parties involved
   - b. Separating the parties involved so that they do not have to work together
   - c. Working with the parties involved to find a mutually acceptable solution
   - d. Bringing disciplinary action against one party or the other

8. _____ The ultimate goal of constructive confrontation is to _____.
   - a. Encourage employees to file grievances
   - b. Prevent interaction between the two parties
   - c. Provide one-on-one personal counseling
   - d. Create a win–win situation

Performance and Quality Improvement for HIM Functions

The purpose of efficient health information management is to provide high-quality information for decision making at all levels. Whether it is access to patient-specific information at the point of care or trended data to make planning decisions, information is a key resource to improving care and healthcare delivery. An ongoing performance improvement system for HIM should be in place to ensure that the information service meets the needs of all users.

A Model for Quality Improvement

Most healthcare organizations have an established approach to quality improvement. The HIM function may report in some key indicators to that effort. For instance, the number of incomplete records may be reported as it is an outcome reported to the Joint Commission on Accreditation of Healthcare Organizations (JCAHO). Training and other resources for departmental quality improvement efforts may be available from this organizational program.

A departmental or functional **quality improvement process** would include these steps:

- Problem identification
    1. Identify key performance measures.
    2. Measure current performance.
    3. Create a flowchart of the current process.
    4. Brainstorm problem areas within the current process.
    5. Research all regulatory requirements related to the current process.
    6. Compare the current process to the organization's performance standards and/or nationally recognized standards.
    7. Conduct a survey to gather customer input on their needs and expectations.
    8. Prioritize problem areas for focused improvement.
- Process redesign
    1. Incorporate findings or changes identified in the research phase of the improvement process.
    2. Collect focused data from the prioritized problem areas.
    3. Create a flowchart of the redesigned process.
    4. Develop policies and procedures that support the redesigned process.
    5. Educate involved staff on the new process.

Problem Identification

To understand the steps of problem identification or improvement opportunity, consider each one separately.

The first step is to identify key performance measures. These are the ongoing outcomes of the principal activities that affect the overall delivery of HIM services to customers (physicians, the operating room, revenue cycle management team, nursing units, regulatory agencies, or others). Key performance measures may include transcription turnaround, availability of paper or electronic information for admissions or clinic visits, days in accounts receivables, and so on.

Ongoing measuring and monitoring of the key performance measures would signal an interruption or degradation of service that may need to be addressed and is step two in the problem identification process. In most cases, there is an acceptable range of variation that would not signal further investigation or a result may be affected by a known and temporary event (for example, turnaround times could rise because a power outage delayed transcription).

Where monitoring demonstrates a significant variation from internal or external benchmarks, further investigation may be warranted. Creating a flowchart of the current process is a good way to document the process. This should be done with involvement of the staff most directly involved in the process. Also, it is important to document the process as it really occurs, not as it should happen.

Discussion of the flowchart may uncover redundancies or points of failure in the process. Brainstorming the possible problems with each step in the process (particularly where handoffs are made from one step to another) is useful in collecting a variety of opinions on where the flaws exist. Documenting the current process and then brainstorming potential problems reduce the likelihood of making assumptions of what should be fixed without adequate study.

Consideration should be given to all regulatory requirements of a process. Sometimes deleting a step that seems to be a perfect way to improve efficiency is actually required. Omission of this step could create a new set of problems in the future. By contrast, sometimes review of a regulation finds that a process you thought was required is actually just an artifact of history and can be easily eliminated.

Next, compare the current process with the organization's performance standards or other national benchmarks or best practices. This is where a literature review is very helpful in supplying current information. If no national benchmarks are available, using networking tools to collect information from other organizations about their process and outcomes can add to the analysis.

Conducting a survey of customer expectations and needs can assist quality improvement activities in at least two important ways. First, it provides direct input into the problem or issue under study. Second, it signals the user community that their concerns are important and will help drive the solution.

Finally, prioritize the problem areas for focused improvement. This is necessary in cases where study has determined that there is more than one opportunity for improvement, a not uncommon occurrence. Determine which area of focus appears to have the most impact on customer outcomes or improved efficiency that may indirectly best meet the customer needs.

When the factors that contribute to a process and the opportunities to improve sustained performance are identified and understood, the next focus is process redesign.

Process Redesign

The work of **process redesign** begins with a specific target for improvement activities. The research done during problem identification becomes the basis for considering new approaches to the process. Where best practice information exists in the literature or was identified from other forms of data gathering, it should be applied to the new process.

Additional data may need to be collected about the specific process identified for improvement. Time studies, observations, or other data collection activities may be required to completely understand the reasons for delay, error, or variation.

The next step is to create a new flowchart of the revised process. Again, a flowchart documents each step in the process and clearly communicates the new process to everyone involved. This step helps facilitate the last step in the process, which is to educate staff on the new process.

With the new process in place, the cycle returns to the beginning and data again are routinely collected and monitored. Additional actions still may be necessary to meet the requirements or expectations of the user community. The original process identified additional actions that may be considered for adjustment, and those changes could be put into place when the new process is stabilized. The process of managing the change in any process should not be underestimated as it is critical to the ongoing success of any new system.

Change Management

The real work begins at the point of completing the redesign. A flowchart is only a piece of paper until the process that it describes is adopted and fully utilized. In quality improvement activities, **change management** is the key to making improvements happen.

- *Becoming a change agent:* Team leaders should demonstrate a willingness to investigate new ideas, learn new skills, and solve new problems. Only by engaging change will they have the credibility to lead others to accept change.

- *Being available to listen to staff:* Leaders should ask questions to understand staff's anxieties and concerns. This can be done through team meetings and informal discussions. Clearing the air and raising and answering questions can reduce fear of, and resistance to, change.

- *Holding on to the vision:* In times of change and stress, it may seem easier, or maybe even more prudent, to step back from the organization's vision or goal. However, it is during change that leaders must be even more dedicated to achieving their vision. They must demonstrate commitment through actions and then campaign for support of the vision. They should encourage and clarify the vision to others and let their commitment show.

- *Continuing to delegate:* Part of demonstrating commitment and risk taking is to let others share the risk. Only with true ownership of the problem will team members feel they own the solution.

- *Measuring and celebrating success:* When the vision of the future state is clear, it is easy to measure progress toward reaching it. And being able to measure progress is key to maintaining enthusiasm for the journey.

Change can be challenging, energizing, and overwhelming. Preparing to manage change includes making a commitment to quality improvement that is recognized by the entire team.

Check your Understanding 20.4

Instructions: Indicate whether the following statements are true or false (T or F).

1. _____ Quality improvement activities only apply to direct patient care.

2. _____ When leading change, a supervisor should not ask staff questions.

3. _____ Opportunities for improving processes should be prioritized before they are implemented.

4. _____ A customer survey helps communicate the value of the customer's input.

5. _____ Intermittent, focused monitoring is the only way to identify potential improvement opportunities

Real-World Case

Figure 20.5 shows the resume of one of the numerous candidates applying for a coding specialist position. The staff position is being added to the HIM department of a large metropolitan medical center where you have worked for the past seven years. The purpose of the new position is to help the current staff to handle its increased workload since implementation of the outpatient prospective payment system for Medicare patients earlier in the year. You are a registered health information technologist with almost ten years of coding experience. Recently, you were promoted to supervisor for the department's five-person outpatient services team. You have never been responsible for interviewing employment candidates before.

Your own manager (the assistant director of the HIM department) has already developed a detailed job description for the new position. (See figure 20.6, pp. 919–20.) She has promised to help you to get ready for the interviews. Still, you are more than a little nervous about taking on this part of your new job. Look at the resume and think about the steps you will need to take before interviewing the candidate.

Summary

Organizations are complex and ever changing, whether they are multihospital systems or small group practices. Whether the structure is hierarchical or team based, planning and organizing are important functions in maximizing the organization's assets. Included among those assets are the people who carry out the mission as staff, the teams that come together to solve problems and the resources they use to perform their work.

As the most critical and costly resource in any healthcare organization, staff members should be organized and led to maximize their contribution. Before the hiring process takes place, effective people management begins with appropriate job design and position description development. Job descriptions, along with effective hiring practices, assist in selecting the best candidates. When hired, ensuring that employees are well oriented and trained begins a working relationship that is fostered through the use of teams, employee empowerment, and staff development planning.

Improving the performance of any organization begins with regular measuring and monitoring. Most improvement activities are incremental and do not create sweeping change on their own, but in combination with other steps and over time, these small steps can have a large impact on the work of the organization. These positive changes create an environment that engages people in their work and allows them to make meaningful contributions.

Figure 20.5.   Resume for the real-world case

RESUME

Stephen Jeremy Johnsen, RHIT

222 Brickpath Way	**Born 1/23/1971**
Chicago, ILL 60622	**Height 5 ft 9 in**
773/222-2222	**Weight 180 lb**

Goal: Looking for a job that lets me use my education and my knowledge of hospital coding and billing

Salary: $30,000+, opportunity for advancement

2000–2001	Coder Lincoln Valley Community Hospital
	I left to move to Chicago to be with my girlfriend
1999	Billing specialist University Medical Center, Chapaigne, Illinois
	Was here for almost a year; disliked manager; needed more money
1996–1999	Coder Medical Record Temporary Specialists, Urbana, IL
	Worked on and off for temporary agency while I finished my computer programming degree
1994–1999	School Oakwood Community College
	Worked as a orderly to earn money for classes, majored in health information technology (graduated 1996) and computer programming
1989–1992	Army Stationed in South Carolina, Germany, trained as medical corpsman
1989	School, majored in business but dropped out to join Army and earn money for school
1989	Graduated Glenview high school, Computer club, Music Camp, Varsity football, worked in father's landscape business during summers

*References available

Figure 20.6.   Job description for the real-world case

Position Description

Position Title: APC Coordinator

**Immediate
Supervisor:**   Director of Health Information Management

General Purpose: The purpose of this position is to create consistency and efficiency in outpatient claims processing and data collection to optimize APC reimbursement and facilitate data quality in outpatient services.

Responsibilities:

- Performs data quality reviews on outpatient encounters to validate the ICD-9-CM, CPT, and HCPCS Level II code and modifier assignments, APC group appropriateness, missed secondary diagnoses and/or procedures, and compliance with all APC mandates and outpatient reporting requirements.

- Monitors medical visit code selection by departments against facility-specific criteria for appropriateness. Assists in the development of such criteria as needed.

- Monitors outpatient service mix reports and the leading medical visit, surgical service, significant procedure, and ancillary APCs assigned in the facility to identify patterns, trends, and variations in the facility's frequently assigned APC groups. Once identified, evaluates the causes of the change, and takes appropriate steps in collaboration with the right department to effect resolution or explanation of the variance.

- Continuously evaluates the quality of clinical documentation to spot incomplete or inconsistent documentation for outpatient encounters that impact the code selection and resulting APC groups and payment. Brings identified concerns to medical staff committee or department managers for resolution.

- Provides and/or arranges for training to facility healthcare professionals on the use of coding guidelines and practices, proper documentation techniques, medical terminology, and disease processes appropriate to the job description and function as it relates to the APC and other outpatient data quality management factors.

- Maintains knowledge of current professional coding certification requirements and promotes recruitment and retention of certified staff in coding positions when possible.

- Reports to the facility Compliance Committee each quarter.

- Abides by the Standards of Ethical Coding as set forth by the American Health Information Management Association and monitors coding staff for violations and reports to the HIM Director when areas of concern are identified. Concerns involving compliance issues are forwarded to the Compliance Committee for action.

(Continued on next page)

Figure 20.6. *(Continued)*

Position Description—APC Coordiinator—Page 2

Responsibilities: *(continued)*	• Develops reports and collects and prepares data for studies involving outpatient encounter data for clinical evaluation purposes and/or financial impact and profitability.

• Serves as the facility representative for APCs by attending outpatient coding and reimbursement workshops and bringing back information to the appropriate departments. Communicates any APC updates published in third-party payer newsletters/bulletins and provider manuals to all facility staff that need this information.

• Keeps abreast of new technology in coding and abstracting software and other forms of automation and stays informed about transaction code sets, HIPAA requirements, and other future issues impacting the coding function.

• Demonstrates competency in the use of computer applications and APC Grouper Software, OCE edits and all coding, software and hardware currently in use in the HIM department.

• Performs periodic claim form reviews to check code transfer accuracy from the abstracting system and the chargemaster.

• Evaluates, records, and responds to the Peer Review Organization APC change and/or denial notices. Provides appropriate documentation from required source to the PRO when appealing a PRO decision.

• Monitors outpatient unbilled accounts report for outstanding and/or uncoded outpatient encounters to reduce Accounts Receivable days for outpatients.

• Serves on the Chargemaster maintenance committee.

Qualifications:

• Minimum of associate's degree in a health services discipline. Formal HIM education with national certification, RHIA or RHIT preferred.

• Coding certification required from the American Health Information Management Association or the American Academy of Professional Coders.

• Minimum of five years progressive coding or coding review experience in ICD-9-CM, CPT, and HCPCS with claims processing and/or data management responsibilities a plus.

• Good oral and written communication skills and comprehensive knowledge of the APC structure and regulatory requirements.

• Prefer someone with past auditing experience or strong training background in coding and reimbursement.

References

Armstrong, M. 1999. *How to Be an Even Better Manager,* 5th ed. London: Kogan Page Ltd.

Bennett-Woods, D. 1997. Team facilitation skills: A step beyond running a good meeting. *Journal of American Health Information Management Association* 68 (1):20–23.

Cooke, R.A. 1993. *The McGraw-Hill 36-Hour Course in Finance for Nonfinancial Managers.* San Francisco: McGraw-Hill.

Daley, D.M. 2002. *Strategic Human Resource Management.* Upper Saddle River, NJ: Prentice-Hall.

Duncan, W.J., and P.M. Ginter. 2000. Principles of management. In *Health Information: Management of a Strategic Resource,* 2nd ed., edited by M. Abdelhak et al. Philadelphia: W. B. Saunders Company.

Gift, R.G., and C.F. Kinney, eds. 1996. *Today's Management Methods: A Guide for the Health Care Executive.* Chicago: American Hospital Publishing.

Haiman, T. 1984. *Supervisory Management for Health Care Organizations,* 3rd ed. St. Louis: Catholic Health Association of the United States.

Kouzes, J.M., and B.Z. Posner. 1995. *The Leadership Challenge.* San Francisco: Jossey-Bass.

Martin, D. 1993. *Teamthink: Using the Sports Connection of Develop, Motivate, and Manage a Winning Business Team.* New York. Penguin Group.

Peters, T. 1987. *Thriving on Chaos.* New York: Alfred A. Knopf.

Rosner, B., A. Halcrow, and A. Levins. 2001. *The Boss's Survival Guide.* New York: McGraw-Hill.

Schein, E.H. 1980. *Organizational Psychology,* 3rd ed. Englewood Cliffs, NJ: Prentice-Hall.

Senge, P.M. 1990. *The Fifth Discipline.* New York: Doubleday Currency.

Shaw, P., C. Elliott, P. Isaacson, and Elizabeth Murphy. 2003. *Quality and Performance Improvement in Healthcare.* Chicago. AHIMA.

Weston, J.F., and T.E. Copeland. 1989. *Managerial Finance,* 8th ed. Chicago: Dryden Press.

Appendices, Glossary, and Index

Appendix A
Sample HIM Position Descriptions

The following position descriptions and related articles may be found in the AHIMA Web site at ahima.org. In some cases, access is restricted to AHIMA members. (Some descriptions are included in more than one category.) The Web site is regularly updated to reflect current and emerging practice areas.

Role	Job Title
Compliance	Compliance and Privacy Officer—eHealth Compliance Director Compliance Officer Compliance Specialist HIPAA Compliance Coordinator
Consulting	*See: Starting a consulting business*
Data management	APC Coordinator Cancer Registrar Clinical Coding Specialist Clinical Data Specialist Data Quality Manager Data Resource Administrator Decision Support Specialist DRG Coordinator HIM Clerk Information Security Manager Information Services Manager MPI Manager Patient Information Coordinator Research Data Analyst

Role	Job Title
EHR	Clinical Analyst Clinical Applications Coordinator Clinical Project Manager, Senior Project Manager Clinical Research Associate Clinical Vocabulary Manager Compliance and Privacy Officer—eHealth Enterprise Applications Specialist Health Systems Specialist Health Information Services Department Technician Information Privacy Coordinator Integration Architect (Implementation) Optical Imaging Coordinator Process Improvement Engineer Records and Information Coordinator Risk Management Specialist Senior Document Coordinator Solution Analyst Solution Consultant Systems Analyst *See: EHR career opportunities: Sample HIM job descriptions*
Emerging roles	Clinical Data Specialist Data Quality Manager Data Resource Administrator Health Information Manager for Integrated Systems Information Security Manager Patient Information Coordinator Research and Decision Support Specialist *See: Evolving HIM careers: Seven roles for the future*
General	Educator Health Information Management Director HIM Domain Manager Medical Staff Coordinator Patient Information Coordinator Risk Manager Utilization Management Director
Privacy & security	Compliance and Privacy Officer—eHealth Compliance and Regulatory Management Officer Compliance Manager, Director, Officer Copy Service Manager Corporate Compliance Director Disclosure Coordinator Information Officer, Chief Information Officer Information Security Manager Information Services Manager Medical Records Manager Patient Accounts Manager Privacy Officer, Chief Privacy Officer Release of Information Coordinator Security Manager, Director, Officer *See: Success at every level: A career ladder for privacy officers*
Quality	Quality Improvement Director

Appendix B
Sample Notice of Health Information Practices

This notice describes how information about you may be used and disclosed and how you can get access to this information. Please review it carefully.

Understanding Your Health Record/Information

Each time you visit a hospital, physician, or other healthcare provider, a record of your visit is made. Typically, this record contains your symptoms, examination and test results, diagnoses, treatment, and a plan for future care or treatment. This information, often referred to as your health or medical record, serves as a:

- basis for planning your care and treatment;
- means of communication among the many health professionals who contribute to your care;
- legal document describing the care you received;
- means by which you or a third-party payer can verify that services billed were actually provided;
- tool in educating health professionals;
- source of data for medical research;
- source of information for public health officials charged with improving the health of the nation;
- source of data for facility planning and marketing; and
- tool with which we can assess and continually work to improve the care we render and the outcomes we achieve.

Understanding what is in your record and how your health information is used helps you to:

- ensure its accuracy;
- better understand who, what, when, where and why others may access your health information; and
- make more informed decisions when authorizing disclosure to others.

Your Health Information Rights

Although your health record is the physical property of the healthcare practitioner or facility that compiled it, the information belongs to you. You have the right to:

- request a restriction on certain uses and disclosures of your information as provided by 45 CFR 164.522;

- obtain a paper copy of the notice of information practices upon request;

- inspect and copy your health record as provided for in 45 CFR 164.524;

- amend your health record as provided in 45 CFR 164.528;

- obtain an accounting of disclosures of your health information as provided in 45 CFR 164.528;

- request communications of your health information by alternative means or at alternative locations; and

- revoke your authorization to use or disclose health information except to the extent that action has already been taken.

Our Responsibilities

This organization is required to:

- maintain the privacy of your health information;

- provide you with a notice as to our legal duties and privacy practices with respect to information we collect and maintain about you;

- abide by the terms of this notice;

- notify you if we are unable to agree to a requested restriction; and

- accommodate reasonable requests you may have to communicate health information by alternative means or at alternative locations.

We reserve the right to change our practices and to make the new provisions effective for all protected health information we maintain. Should our information practices change, we will mail a revised notice to the address you've supplied us.

We will not use or disclose your health information without your authorization, except as described in this notice.

For More Information or to Report a Problem

If have questions and would like additional information, you may contact the Director of Health Information Management at (444) 111-1111.

If you believe your privacy rights have been violated, you can file a complaint with the Director of Health Information Management or with the Secretary of Health and Human Services. There will be no retaliation for filing a complaint.

Examples of Disclosures for Treatment, Payment, and Health Operations

We will use your health information for treatment. For example: Information obtained by a nurse, physician, or other member of your healthcare team will be recorded in your record and used to determine the course of treatment that should work best for you. Your physician will document in your record his/her expectations of the members of your healthcare team. Members of your healthcare team will then record the actions they took and their observations. In that way the physician will know how you are responding to treatment.

We will also provide your physician or a subsequent healthcare provider with copies of various reports that should assist him/her in treating you once you're discharged from this hospital.

We will use your health information for payment. For example: A bill may be sent to you or a third party payer. The information on or accompanying the bill may include information that identifies you, as well as your diagnosis, procedures and supplies used.

We will use your health information for regular health operations. For example: Members of the medical staff, the risk or quality improvement manager, or members of the quality improvement team may use information in your health record to assess the care and outcomes in your case and others like it. This information will then be used in an effort to continually improve the quality and effectiveness of the healthcare and service we provide.

Other Uses or Disclosures

Business Associates: There are some services provided in our organization through contacts with business associates. Examples include physician services in the Emergency Department and Radiology, certain laboratory tests, and a copy service we use when making copies of your health record. When these services are contracted, we may disclose your health information to our business associates so that they can perform the job we've asked them to do and bill you or your third-party payer for services rendered. So that your health information is protected, however, we require the business associate to appropriately safeguard your information.

Directory: Unless you notify us that you object, we will use your name, location in the facility, general condition, and religious affiliation for directory purposes. This information may be provided to members of the clergy and, except for religious affiliation to other people who ask for you by name.

Notification: We may use or disclose information to notify or assist in notifying a family member, personal representative, or another person responsible for your care, your location, and general condition.

Communication with Family: Health professionals, using their best judgment, may disclose to a family member, other relative, close personal friend, or any other person you identify health information relevant to that person's involvement in your care or payment related to your care.

Research: We may disclose information to researchers when their research has been approved by an Institutional Review Board that has reviewed the research proposal and established protocols to ensure the privacy of your health information.

Funeral Directors: We may disclose health information to funeral directors consistent with applicable law to carry out their duties.

Organ Procurement Organizations: Consistent with applicable law, we may disclose health information to organ procurement organizations or other entities engaged in the procurement, banking, or transplantation of organs for the purpose of tissue donation and transplant.

Marketing: We may contact you to provide appointment reminders or information about treatment alternatives or other health-related benefits and services that may be of interest to you.

Fund Raising: We may contact you as part of a fund-raising effort.

Food and Drug Administration (FDA): We may disclose to the FDA health information relative to adverse events with respect to food, supplements, product and product defects, or post marketing surveillance information to enable product recalls, repairs, or replacement.

Workers' Compensation: We may disclose health information to the extent authorized by, and to the extent necessary to comply with, laws relating to workers' compensation or other similar programs established by law.

Public Health: As required by law, we may disclose your health information to public health or legal authorities charged with preventing or controlling disease, injury, or disability.

Correctional Institution: Should you be an inmate of a correctional institution, we may disclose to the institution or agents thereof, health information necessary for your health, and the health and safety of other individuals.

Law Enforcement: We may disclose health information for law enforcement purposes as required by law, or in response to a valid subpoena.

Federal law makes provision for your health information to be released to an appropriate health oversight agency, public health authority or attorney, provided that a workforce member or business associate believes in good faith that we have engaged in unlawful conduct or have otherwise violated professional or clinical standards and are potentially endangering one or more patients, workers, or the public.

My signature below indicates that I have been provided with a copy of the notice of privacy practices.

_____
Signature of Patient or Legal Representative

Date:

If signed by legal representative, relationship to patient_____

Effective Date:

Distribution: Original to provider; copy to patient

The above form is not meant to encompass all the various ways in which any particular facility may use health information. For example, those who use protected health information for fundraising or marketing will want to add those types of disclosures. It is intended to get readers started insofar as developing their own notices. As with any form of this nature, the document should be reviewed and approved by legal counsel prior to implementation.

Source: AHIMA. 2002 (November). Practice brief (updated): Notice of information practices. *Journal of American Health Information Management Association.* Available online from ahima.org.

Appendix C
Check Your Understanding

Chapter 1

Check Your Understanding 1.1.
1. b
2. b
3. b
4. a
5. a

Check Your Understanding 1.2
1. c
2. d
3. a
4. d
5. b

Chapter 2

Check Your Understanding 2.1
1. T
2. F
3. F
4. T
5. T
6. F
7. F
8. T
9. F
10. F

Check Your Understanding 2.2
1. F
2. T
3. F
4. T
5. F
6. T
7. F
8. T
9. F
10. T

Check Your Understanding 2.3
1. d
2. h
3. a
4. i
5. b
6. c
7. g
8. e

Chapter 3

Check Your Understanding 3.1
1. b
2. d
3. b
4. a
5. c
6. a
7. c
8. b
9. d
10. a

Check Your Understanding 3.2
1. b
2. a
3. c
4. c
5. d
6. b
7. c
8. d

Check Your Understanding 3.3
1. d
2. b
3. b
4. a
5. b

Check Your Understanding 3.4
1. a
2. d
3. c
4. a
5. b
6. a
7. d
8. b
9. c
10. b

Chapter 4

Check Your Understanding 4.1
1. a
2. b
3. d
4. b
5. a
6. a
7. a

Check Your Understanding 4.2
1. b
2. a
3. c
4. e
5. d

Check Your Understanding 4.3
1. F
2. T
3. F
4. F
5. F

Check Your Understanding 4.4
1. A CDR is optimized to process transactions. A CDW is optimized to perform data analysis.

2. Data exchange standards ensure that data can be sent from one system to another. Data comparability standards ensure that the meaning of the data is the same in both systems.

3. A data dictionary is a set of tables holding the metadata for each term in a database table. Metadata are data about data.

4. A controlled vocabulary is a set of terms allowed to be used in an application. A standard vocabulary is a set of terms developed through a formal group process accredited by ANSI.

5. Vocabulary is a set of terms used in a language. Classification is a grouping of the terms into categories.

6. Discrete data represent encoded values that can be processed by the computer. Digital images are pictures of data which cannot be interpreted by computer processing.

7. Speech recognition is a process where the computer recognizes patterns of speech and is able to convert it to text. Natural language processing converts unstructured text into discrete data.

8. DBMS is software that helps organize and manage data in a database. CDSS is software that evaluates discrete data in logical structures and rules to produce reminders, alerts, and context-sensitive templates.

9. LAN is a set of hardware and software to transmit data from one computer to another in a small geographic area. An intranet is a LAN based on Internet technology.

10. RFID uses radio waves to transmit data across relative short distances. T1 lines are telephone services that provide for high-speed secure transmission of data across long distances.

Matching:
1. i
2. j
3. h
4. g
5. b
6. a
7. f
8. c
9. d
10. e

Check Your Understanding 4.5
Correct sequence:
1. Integration test
2. Migration path
3. Turnover strategy
4. Training
5. Issues management
6. Change control
7. Due diligence
8. Request for proposal
9. Chart conversion
10. System build

Check Your Understanding 4.6
1. Risk analysis
2. Contingency planning
3. Business associate agreement
4. Authentication
5. Access controls
6. Digital signature
7. Admissibility
8. Virtual private network
9. Data quality management

Chapter 5

Check Your Understanding 5.1
1. b
2. d
3. d
4. b
5. a
6. c
7. b
8. b
9. d
10. d

Check Your Understanding 5.2
1. c
2. b
3. a
4. b
5. d
6. d
7. c
8. c

Chapter 6

Check Your Understanding 6.1
1. Bacillary, Bacilluria, Bacillus, Back
2. abortus infection, anthracis infection, coli, Flexner's
3. a. P
   b. D
   c. D
   d. P
   e. D
   f. P

Check Your Understanding 6.2
1. benign
2. malignant metastatic site
3. malignant primary site
4. carcinoma in situ

Check Your Understanding 6.3
1. 99311
2. 90807
3. 33470
4. 01200
5. 87551
6. 77295
7. 0071T

Check Your Understanding 6.4
1. e
2. a
3. b

Check Your Understanding 6.5
1. T
2. T
3. F
4. F
5. T

Check Your Understanding 6.6
1. F
2. T
3. T
4. T
5. T

Check Your Understanding 6.7
1. T
2. F
3. T
4. T
5. F

Check Your Understanding 6.8
1. T
2. F
3. T
4. F
5. T

Chapter 7

Check Your Understanding 7.1
1. d
2. b
3. b
4. c
5. b

Check Your Understanding 7.2
1. a
2. d
3. d
4. b
5. b
6. d
7. d
8. c

Check Your Understanding 7.3
1. a
2. c
3. d
4. a
5. c

Check Your Understanding 7.4
1. d
2. b
3. b
4. c
5. d
6. c

Check Your Understanding 7.5
1. b
2. d
3. c
4. a
5. d
6. d
7. c
8. b
9. c
10. c

Check Your Understanding 7.6
1. c
2. a
3. d
4. c
5. d
6. b
7. a
8. b
9. c
10. c

Check Your Understanding 7.7
1. c
2. a
3. b
4. d
5. a
6. a
7. c
8. a
9. a

10. a
11. b
12. d
13. b
14. a
15. c

Check Your Understanding 7.8
1. T
2. F
3. F
4. F
5. T
6. T
7. F
8. T
9. T
10. F

Check Your Understanding 7.9
1. a
2. b
3. a
4. d
5. a
6. a
7. c
8. d

Chapter 8

Check Your Understanding 8.1
1. b
2. d
3. b
4. d
5. d
6. c
7. c
8. b
9. c
10. b
11. c
12. b
13. b
14. d
15. a

Check Your Understanding 8.2

1. a
2. c
3. b
4. b
5. a

Check Your Understanding 8.3

1. c
2. d
3. b
4. d
5. a
6. d

Check Your Understanding 8.4

1. a
2. c
3. a
4. b
5. b

Check Your Understanding 8.5

1. a
2. b
3. b
4. b
5. c
6. d
7. d

Chapter 9

Check Your Understanding 9.1

1. T
2. F
3. T
4. T
5. F

Check Your Understanding 9.2

1. b
2. d
3. a
4. a

5. c
6. d
7. b
8. a
9. b
10. c

Check Your Understanding 9.3

1. F
2. T
3. F
4. F
5. T

Chapter 10

Check Your Understanding 10.1

1. b
2. c
3. a

Check Your Understanding 10.2

1. 2,418
2. 2,540
3. 2,540
4. 1,095
5. 139,617.1
6. 373.7

Calculation of variance:

$$s^2 = \sum_{i}^{n} (X_i - \overline{X})^2 / N - 1$$

$$= 1,954,640/15 - 1$$

$$= 139,617.1$$

Calculation of standard deviation:

$$s = \sqrt{\sum_{i}^{n} (X_i - \overline{X})^2 / N - 1}$$

$$= \sqrt{1,954,640/15 - 1}$$

$$= 373.3$$

Weight (X)	(XX)	(XX)²
1,720	−698	487,204
1,735	−683	466,489
1,800	−618	381,924
2,300	−18	13,924
2,400	−8	324
2,450	32	1,024
2,485	67	4,489
2,540	122	14,884
2,540	122	14,884
2,600	182	33,124
2,640	222	49,284
2,715	297	88,209
2,750	332	110,224
2,780	362	131,044
2,815	397	157,609
36,270		1,954,640

Check Your Understanding 10.3
1. d
2. e
3. b
4. c
5. a

Check Your Understanding 10.4
1. a. 275
   b. 277
   c. 277
   d. 547
2. a. 8
   b. 10
3. a. 17
   b. 15
   c. 22

4. 1,536
5. a. 16.2
   b. 13.5
   c. 19.9

Check Your Understanding 10.5
1. a. 91.9%
   b. 93.7%
   c. 90.8%
   d. 90.0%
   e. 87.7%
   f. 93.9%
   g. 91.7%
2. a. 183.9
   b. 13.3
   c. 83.6%
   d. 60.4%

Check Your Understanding 10.6
1. a. 91
   b. 4
2. a. 96
   b. 31
   c. 187
   d. 30
   e. 1
   f. 1
   g. 346
   h. 57.7

Check Your Understanding 10.7
1. 1.9%
2. 1.1%
3. 2.1%
4. 2.5%
5. 1.9%
6. 1.5%

Check Your Understanding 10.8
1. 47.7%
2. 48.8%

Check Your Understanding 10.9
1. $(8 \times 100)/30 = 26.7\%$
2. $(122 \times 100)/822 = 14.8\%$

Check Your Understanding 10.10
1. $(10,464 \times 10,000)/141,655,135 =$ 7.39 per 100,000
2. $(3,627 \times 100,000)/146,701,578 =$ 2.47 per 100,000
3. $(14,091 \times 100,000)/288,356,713 =$ 4.89 per 100,000
4. $(4,198 \times 10,000)/22,366,506 =$ 1.88 per 10,000
5. $(1,509 \times 10,000)/22,550,100 =$ 0.67 per 10,000

Check Your Understanding 10.11
1. Incidence is the number of **new** cases of a particular disease in a population for a given time period Prevalence is the number of cases of a particular disease in a population for a given time period
2. a. White women: $(1,595 \times 10,000)/5,035,239 =$ 3.2 per 10,000
        Black women: $(179 \times 10,000)/720,544 =$ 2.5 per 10,000
    b. $(1,774 \times 10,000)/5,755,783 =$ 3.1 per 10,000

Check Your Understanding 10.12
1. a. 38,220,659
    b. $19,729
    c. 4.6 days
    d. 2.2%
    e. 48
    f. $753,648,903,686

Check Your Understanding 10.13
1. F
2. F
3. T
4. T
5. T

Chapter 11

Check Your Understanding 11.1
1. a
2. d
3. b
4. d
5. d
6. d
7. a
8. b
9. d
10. a

Check Your Understanding 11.2
1. e
2. h
3. b
4. i
5. c
6. g
7. j
8. f
9. a
10. d

Check Your Understanding 11.3
1. b
2. d
3. c
4. c
5. b
6. c
7. d
8. c
9. e
10. b

Chapter 12

Check Your Understanding 12.1

1. F
2. T
3. F
4. T
5. F
6. T
7. T
8. T
9. T
10. F
11. F
12. T

Check Your Understanding 12.2

Part 1

1. T
2. T
3. F (The manager's job is to REDUCE all inherent variation from processes, rather than REMOVE.)
4. T
5. T
6. F (the patient is an example of an EXTERNAL customer of a healthcare organization, rather than INTERNAL.)
7. T

Part 2

1. f, b
2. b
3. a
4. b, e
5. c
6. d

Check Your Understanding 12.3

Part 1

1. d
2. a
3. c
4. g
5. f

6. b
7. e

Part 2

1. T
2. F (Most people resist change because it produces fear.)
3. F (An organization that promotes learning in all its employees is MORE likely (rather than less likely) to embrace the philosophy of continual performance improvement.)
4. T
5. T

Check Your Understanding 12.4

Part 1

1. a
2. d
3. d
4. a
5. a
6. b
7. d
8. b
9. d
10. c
11. e
12. a
13. a
14. b, d
15. e

Part 2

1. F (Healthcare information systems are much LESS state-of-the-art than information systems in the financial and insurance industries, rather than much MORE.)
2. T
3. T
4. T
5. F (Data and information are NOT the same. Information requires analysis and interpretation of raw data.)

Chapter 13

Check Your Understanding 13.1

1. b
2. d
3. d
4. a
5. c
6. c
7. a
8. d

Check Your Understanding 13.2

1. b
2. g
3. a
4. d
5. h
6. c
7. e
8. f

Check Your Understanding 13.3

1. a
2. b
3. f
4. e
5. d
6. c

Check Your Understanding 13.4

1. F
2. T
3. T
4. T
5. T
6. T
7. T
8. F
9. T
10. T

Check Your Understanding 13.5

1. c
2. d
3. a
4. c
5. a
6. b
7. d
8. b

Check Your Understanding 13.6

1. c
2. e
3. a
4. h
5. j
6. f
7. d
8. g
9. i
10. b

Check Your Understanding 13.7

1. F
2. T
3. T
4. F
5. T
6. T
7. F
8. T

Chapter 14

Check Your Understanding 14.1

1. e
2. d
3. g
4. h
5. a
6. b
7. c
8. f
9. j
10. i

Check Your Understanding 14.2

1. b
2. c
3. a
4. d
5. d
6. a
7. d
8. b
9. d
10. b
11. a
12. d
13. a
14. a
15. d
16. b
17. c
18. c
19. a
20. d
21. b
22. a

Check Your Understanding 14.3

1. e
2. b
3. d
4. a
5. f
6. g
7. c

Chapter 15

Check Your Understanding 15.1

1. d
2. b
3. c
4. b
5. a

Check Your Understanding 15.2

1. a
2. b
3. d
4. d
5. c
6. b
7. d
8. d
9. d
10. a

Check Your Understanding 15.3

1. d
2. a
3. a
4. d
5. b

Check Your Understanding 15.4

1. c
2. a
3. c
4. a
5. b
6. d
7. d
8. a
9. b
10. d
11. b
12. b
13. c
14. d
15. d
16. d
17. d
18. a
19. c
20. a
21. d
22. d
23. b
24. d
25. d
26. b
27. b
28. c
29. d
30. d
31. d

Check Your Understanding 15.5

1. c
2. c
3. b
4. a
5. c
6. b
7. d

Chapter 16

Check Your Understanding 16.1

1. b
2. c
3. b

Check Your Understanding 16.2

1. e
2. b
3. e
4. a

Check Your Understanding 16.3

1. a
2. b
3. b
4. d
5. c

Check Your Understanding 16.4

1. F
2. T
3. F
4. F
5. T
6. F
7. T
8. F
9. T
10. T

Check Your Understanding 16.5

1. c
2. e
3. g
4. d

5. j
6. b
7. i
8. h
9. a
10. f

Check Your Understanding 16.6

1. T
2. F
3. F
4. T
5. F

Chapter 17

Check Your Understanding 17.1

1. a
2. a
3. a
4. c
5. b
6. a
7. b
8. b
9. c
10. c

Check Your Understanding 17.2

1. e
2. e
3. i
4. c, d
5. f
6. h
7. n
8. a
9. m
10. k
11. l
12. g
13. e
14. d

Check Your Understanding 17.3

a. 11
b. 3
c. 1
d. 7
e. 4
f. 10
g. 13
h. 11
i. 5
j. 13
k. 12
l. 6
m. 2
n. 8
o. 14
p. 9

Check Your Understanding 17.4

1. F
2. F
3. T
4. T
5. T
6. F
7. T
8. F

Chapter 18

Check Your Understanding 18.1

1. a
2. b
3. b
4. d
5. b
6. d
7. c
8. a
9. d
10. b

Check Your Understanding 18.2

1. f
2. f
3. e
4. a
5. d
6. d
7. b
8. f
9. b
10. a

Check Your Understanding 18.3

1. T
2. T
3. T
4. F
5. T
6. T
7. T

Check Your Understanding 18.4

1. b
2. d
3. e
4. a
5. c

Chapter 19

Check Your Understanding 19.1

1. T
2. T
3. T
4. T
5. F
6. T
7. F
8. T
9. F
10. F

Check Your Understanding 19.2

1. h
2. e
3. f
4. f
5. k
6. d
7. k
8. j
9. a
10. i
11. b
12. b
13. c
14. g
15. i

Check Your Understanding 19.3

1. c
2. b
3. b
4. c
5. b
6. a
7. c
8. c
9. a
10. a

Chapter 20

Check Your Understanding 20.1

1. T
2. F
3. F
4. F
5. F

Check Your Understanding 20.2

1. T
2. T
3. T
4. F
5. F

Check Your Understanding 20.3

1. c
2. b
3. c
4. b
5. a
6. b
7. c
8. d

Check Your Understanding 20.4

1. F
2. F
3. T
4. T
5. F

Glossary

Abbreviated Injury Scale (AIS): A set of numbers used in a trauma registry to indicate the nature and severity of injuries by body system

Abstracting: 1. The process of extracting information from a document to create a brief summary of a patient's illness, treatment, and outcome 2. The process of extracting elements of data from a source document or database and entering them into an automated system

Accept assignment: A term used to refer to a provider's or a supplier's acceptance of the allowed charges (from a fee schedule) as payment in full for services or materials provided

Acceptance testing: Final review during EHR implementation to ensure that all tests have been performed and all issues have been resolved, usually triggers the final payment for the system and when a maintenance contract becomes effective

Access control: 1. A computer software program designed to prevent unauthorized use of an information resource 2. The process of designing, implementing, and monitoring a system for guaranteeing that only individuals with a legitimate need are allowed to view or amend specific data sets

Accession number: A number assigned to each case as it is entered in a cancer registry

Accession registry: A list of cases in a cancer registry in the order in which they were entered

Accounts receivable (A/R): Records of the payments owed to the organization by outside entities such as third-party payers and patients

Accreditation: 1. A voluntary process of institutional or organizational review in which a quasi independent body created for this purpose periodically evaluates the quality of the entity's work against preestablished written criteria 2. A determination by an accrediting body that an eligible organization, network, program, group, or individual complies with applicable standards

Accreditation Association for Ambulatory Health Care (AAAHC): A professional organization that offers accreditation programs for ambulatory and outpatient organizations such as single- and multispecialty group practices, ambulatory surgery centers, college/university health services, and community health centers

Accreditation organization: A professional organization that establishes the standards against which healthcare organizations are measured and conducts periodic assessments of the performance of individual healthcare organizations

Accreditation standards: Preestablished statements of the criteria against which the performance of participating healthcare organizations will be assessed during a voluntary accreditation process

Accredited Standards Committee X12N (ASC X12N): A committee of the National Standards Institute that develops and maintains standards for the electronic exchange of business transactions, such as 837—Health Care Claim, 835—Health Care Claim Payment/Advice, and others

Action steps: Specific plans an organization intends to accomplish in the near future as an effort toward achieving its long-term strategic plan

Activities of daily living (ADL): The basic activities of self-care, including grooming, bathing, ambulating, toileting, and eating

Actor: The role a user plays in a system

Acute care prospective payment system (PPS): The reimbursement system for inpatient hospital services provided to Medicare and Medicaid beneficiaries that is based on the use of diagnosis-related groups as a classification tool

Administrative controls: Policies and procedures that address the management of computer resources

Administrative information systems: A category of healthcare information systems that supports human resources management, financial management, executive decision support, and other business-related functions

Administrative law: A body of rules and regulations developed by various administrative entities empowered by Congress; falls under the umbrella of public law

Administrative provisions: Documented, formal practices to manage data security measures throughout the healthcare organization

Administrative services only (ASO) contract: An agreement between an employer and an insurance organization to administer the employer's self-insured health plan

Administrative simplification: A term referring to HIPAA's attempt to streamline and standardize the healthcare industry's nonuniform and seemingly chaotic business practices, such as billing

Admissibility: The condition of being admitted into evidence in a court of law

Admission utilization review: A review of planned services (intensity of service) and/or a patient's condition (severity of illness) to determine whether care must be delivered in an acute care setting

Advance Beneficiary Notice (ABN): A statement signed by the patient when he or she is notified by the provider, prior to a service or procedure being done, that Medicare may not reimburse the provider for the service, wherein the patient indicates that he will be responsible for any charges

Advance directive: A legal, written document that describes the patient's preferences regarding future healthcare or stipulates the person who is authorized to make medical decisions in the event the patient is incapable of communicating his or her preferences

Affinity grouping: A technique for organizing similar ideas together in natural groupings

Age Discrimination in Employment Act: Federal legislation that prohibits employment discrimination against persons between the ages of forty and seventy and restricts mandatory retirement requirements except where age is a bona fide occupational qualification

Agency for Healthcare Research and Quality (AHRQ): The branch of the United States Public Health Service that supports general health research and distributes research findings and treatment guidelines with the goal of improving the quality, appropriateness, and effectiveness of healthcare services

Aggregate data: Data extracted from individual health records and combined to form de-identified information about groups of patients that can be compared and analyzed

All patient DRGs (AP-DRGs): A case-mix system developed by 3M and used in a number of state reimbursement systems to classify non-Medicare discharges for reimbursement purposes

Allied health professional: A credentialed healthcare worker who is not a physician, nurse, psychologist, or pharmacist (for example, a physical therapist, dietitian, social worker, or occupational therapist)

Alphabetic filing system: A system of health record identification and storage that uses the patient's last name as the first component of identification and his or her first name and middle name or initial for further definition

Alphanumeric filing system: A system of health record identification and storage that uses a combination of alphabetic letters (usually the first two letters of the patient's last name) and numbers to identify individual records

Ambulatory payment classification (APC) system: The prospective payment system used since 2000 for reimbursement of hospitals for outpatient services provided to Medicare and Medicaid beneficiaries

Ambulatory surgery center (ASC): Under Medicare, an outpatient surgical facility that has its own national identifier; is a separate entity with respect to its licensure, accreditation, governance, professional supervision, administrative functions, clinical services, record keeping, and financial and accounting systems; has as its sole purpose the provision of services in connection with surgical procedures that do not require inpatient hospitalization; and meets the conditions and requirements set forth in the Medicare Conditions of Participation

American Association of Health Plans (AAHP): The trade organization for health maintenance organizations, preferred provider organizations, and other network-based health plans created by the merger of the Group Health Association of America and the American Managed Care and Review Association

American Association of Medial Record Librarians (AAMRL): The name adopted by the Association of Record Librarians of North America in 1944; precursor of the **American Health Information Management Association**

American Association of Medical Colleges (AAMC): The organization established in 1876 to standardize the curriculum for medical schools in the United States and to promote the licensure of physicians

American College of Healthcare Executives (ACHE): The national professional organization of healthcare administrators that provides certification services for its members and promotes excellence in the field

American College of Radiology-National Electrical Manufacturers Association (ACR-NEMA): The professional organizations (ACR) and trade associations (NEMA) that work collaboratively to develop digital imaging standards

American College of Surgeons (ACS): The scientific and educational association of surgeons formed to improve the quality of surgical care by setting high standards for surgical education and practice

American College of Surgeons Commission on Cancer: The organization that approves cancer-related programs, including cancer registries and trauma centers

American Health Information Management Association (AHIMA): The professional membership organization for managers of health record services and healthcare information systems as well as coding services; provides accreditation, certification, and educational services

American Hospital Association (AHA): The national trade organization that provides education, conducts research, and represents the hospital industry's interests in national legislative matters; membership includes individual healthcare organizations as well as individual healthcare professionals working in specialized areas of hospitals, such as risk management

American Medical Association (AMA): The national professional membership organization for physicians that distributes scientific information to its members and the public, informs members of legislation related to health and medicine, and represents the medical profession's interests in national legislative matters

American Medical Record Association (AMRA): The name adopted by the American Association of Medical Record Librarians in 1970; precursor of the **American Health Information Management Association**

American National Standards Institute (ANSI): The organization that accredits all U.S. standards development organizations to ensure that they are following due process in promulgating standards

American Nurses Association (ANA): The national professional membership association of nurses that works for the improvement of health standards and the availability of health-care services, fosters high professional standards for the nursing profession, and advances the economic and general welfare of nurses

American Osteopathic Association (AOA): The professional association of osteopathic physicians, surgeons, and graduates of approved colleges of osteopathic medicine that inspects and accredits osteopathic colleges and hospitals

American Society for Healthcare Risk Management (ASHRM): The professional society for healthcare risk management professionals that is affiliated with the American Hospital Association and provides educational tools and networking opportunities for its members

American Society for Testing and Materials (ASTM): A national organization whose purpose is to establish standards on materials, products, systems, and services

Americans with Disabilities Act of 1990: Federal legislation that makes it illegal to discriminate against individuals with disabilities in employment, public accommodations, public services, transportation, and telecommunications

Ancillary systems: Electronic systems that generate clinical information (such as laboratory information systems, radiology information systems, pharmacy information systems, and so on)

Anesthesia report: The report that notes any preoperative medication and response to it, the anesthesia administered with dose and method of administration, the duration of administration, the patient's vital signs while under anesthesia, and any additional products given the patient during a procedure

APC grouper: Software programs that help coders determine the appropriate ambulatory payment classification for an outpatient encounter

Appeal: A request for reconsideration of a negative claim decision

Appellate court: In a state court system, the court that hears appeals of final judgments from state trial courts

Application controls: Security strategies, such as password management, included in application software and computer programs

Application service provider (ASP): A third-party service company that delivers, manages, and remotely hosts standardized applications software via a network through an outsourcing contract based on fixed, monthly usage or transaction-based pricing

Arbitration: A proceeding in which disputes are submitted to a third party or a panel of experts outside the judicial trial system

Architecture: The configuration, structure, and relationships of hardware (the machinery of the computer including input/output devices, storage devices, and so on) in an information system

Artificial intelligence: High-level information technologies used in developing machines that imitate human qualities such as learning and reasoning

Assembler: A computer program that translates assembly-language instructions into machine language

Assembly language: A second-generation computer programming language that uses simple phrases rather than the complex series of switches used in machine language

Assets: The human, financial, and physical resources of an organization

Association of Record Librarians of North America (ARLNA): Organization formed ten years after the beginning of the hospital standardization movement whose original objective was to elevate the standards of clinical record keeping in hospitals, dispensaries, and other healthcare facilities; precursor of the **American Health Information Management Association**

ASTM International: Formerly known as the American Society for Testing and Materials, a system of standards developed primarily for various EHR management processes

ASTM Standard E1384-02a: Standard that identifies the content and structure for EHRs, covering all types of healthcare services, including acute care hospitals, ambulatory care, skilled nursing facilities, home healthcare, and specialty environments

Audit controls: A method for monitoring attempts to gain access to a computer information system

Audit trail: A chronological set of computerized records that provides evidence of information system activity (log-ins and log-outs, file accesses) that is used to determine security violations

Auditing: The performance of internal and/or external reviews (audits) to identify variations from established baselines (for example, review of outpatient coding as compared with CMS outpatient coding guidelines).

Authenticate: Confirm by signing

Authentication: 1. The process of identifying the source of health record entries by attaching a handwritten signature, the author's initials, or an electronic signature 2. Proof of authorship that ensures, as much as possible, that log-ins and messages from a user originate from an authorized source

Authorization: The granting of permission to disclose confidential information; as defined in terms of the HIPAA privacy rule, an individual's formal, written permission to use or disclose his or her personally identifiable health information for purposes other than treatment, payment, or healthcare operations

Authorization to disclose information: An authorization that allows the healthcare facility to verbally disclose or send health information to other organizations; *See* **Authorization**

Autodialing system: A method used to automatically call and remind patients of upcoming appointments

Autonomy: A core ethical principle centered on the individual's right to self-determination that includes respect for the individual; in clinical applications, the patient's right to determine what does or does not happen to him or her in terms of healthcare

Autopsy report: Written documentation of the findings from a postmortem pathological examination

Average daily census: The mean number of hospital inpatients present in the hospital each day for a given period of time

Average length of stay (ALOS): The mean length of stay for hospital inpatients discharged during a given period of time

Balance billing: A reimbursement method that allows providers to bill patients for charges in excess of the amount paid by the patients' health plan or other third-party payer (not allowed under Medicare or Medicaid)

Balanced Budget Refinement Act (BBRA) of 1999: The amended version of the Balanced Budget Act of 1997 that authorizes implementation of a per-discharge prospective payment system for care provided to Medicare beneficiaries by inpatient rehabilitation facilities

Bar chart: A graphic technique used to display frequency distributions of nominal or ordinal data that fall into categories

Bed count (complement): The number of inpatient beds set up and staffed for use on a given day

Bed count day: A unit of measure that denotes the presence of one inpatient bed (either occupied or vacant) set up and staffed for use in one twenty-four-hour period

Benchmarking: An analysis process that is based on comparison

Beneficence: A legal term that means promoting good for others or providing services that benefit others, such as releasing health information that will help a patient receive care or will ensure payment for services received

Best of breed: A vendor strategy used when purchasing an EHR that refers to system applications that are considered the best in their class

Best of fit: A vendor strategy used when purchasing an EHR in which all the systems required by the healthcare facility are available from one vendor

Bioethics: A field of study that applies ethical principles to decisions that affect the lives of humans, such as whether to approve or deny access to health information

Blue Cross and Blue Shield (BC/BS): The first prepaid healthcare plans in the United States; Blue Shield plans traditionally cover hospital care and Blue Cross plans cover physicians' services

Board of governors (Board of trustees): The elected or appointed group of officials who bear ultimate responsibility for the successful operation of a healthcare organization

Brainstorming: A group problem-solving technique that involves the spontaneous contribution of ideas from all members of the group

Breach: A violation of the law

Budget assumptions: Information about the overall organization's budget planning that sometimes includes an estimation of how revenues will increase or decrease and what limits will be placed on expenses

Bugs: Problems in software that prevent the smooth application of a function

Bundled payments: A category of payments made as lump sums to providers for all healthcare services delivered to a patient for a specific illness and/or over a specified time period; they include multiple services and may include multiple providers of care

Bureaucracy: A formal organizational structure based on a rigid hierarchy of decision making and inflexible rules and procedures

Business associate: According to the HIPAA privacy rule, an individual (or group) who is not a member of a covered entity's workforce but who helps the covered entity in the performance of various functions involving the use or disclosure of patient-identifiable health information

Business continuity plan: A program that incorporates policies and procedures for continuing business operations during a computer system shutdown; sometimes called **contingency and disaster planning**

Business process: A set of related policies and procedures that are performed step by step to accomplish a business-related function

Capitation: A method of healthcare reimbursement in which an insurance carrier prepays a physician, hospital, or other healthcare provider a fixed amount for a given population without regard to the actual number or nature of healthcare services provided to the population

Care plan: The specific goals in the treatment of an individual patient, amended as the patient's condition requires, and the assessment of the outcomes of care; serves as the primary source for ongoing documentation of the resident's care, condition, and needs

Career planning: Looking beyond simply getting a job to position oneself for more challenging and diverse work in the long term

Case definition: A method of determining criteria for cases that should be included in a registry

Case fatality rate: The total number of deaths due to a specific illness during a given time period divided by the total number of cases during the same period

Case finding: A method of identifying patients who have been seen and/or treated in a healthcare facility for the particular disease or condition of interest to the registry

Case management: 1. The ongoing, concurrent review performed by clinical professionals to ensure the necessity and effectiveness of the clinical services being provided to a patient 2. A process that integrates and coordinates patient care over time and across multiple sites and providers, especially in complex and high-cost cases 3. The process of developing a specific care plan for a patient that serves as a communication tool to improve quality of care and reduce cost

Case-mix group (CMGs): The ninety-seven function-related groups into which inpatient rehabilitation facility discharges are classified on the basis of the patient's level of impairment, age, comorbidities, and functional ability and other factors

Case-mix group (CMG) relative weights: Factors that account for the variance in cost per discharge and resource utilization among case-mix groups

Case-mix index (CMI): The average relative weight of all cases treated at a given facility or by a given physician, which reflects the resource intensity or clinical severity of a specific group in relation to the other groups in the classification system; calculated by dividing the sum of the weights of diagnosis-related groups for patients discharged during a given period divided by the total number of patients discharged

Categorically needy eligibility groups: Categories of individuals to whom states must provide coverage under the federal Medicaid program

Causation: In law, a relationship between the defendant's conduct and the harm that was suffered

Cause-and-effect diagram: *See* **fishbone diagram**

Cause-specific death rate: The total number of deaths due to a specific illness during a given time period divided by the estimated population for the same time period

Census: The number of inpatients present in a healthcare facility at any given time

Centers for Medicare and Medicaid Services (CMS): The division of the Department of Health and Human Services that is responsible for developing healthcare policy in the United States and for administering the Medicare program and the federal portion of the Medicaid program; called the Health Care Financing Administration (HCFA) prior to 2001

Certification: 1. The process by which a duly authorized body evaluates and recognizes an individual, institution, or educational program as meeting predetermined requirements 2. An evaluation performed to establish the extent to which a particular computer system, network design, or application implementation meets a prespecified set of requirements

Certification Commission on Health Information Technology (CHHIT): An effort initiated by the private sector to evaluate and potentially test EHR products against specific criteria, drawn from the HL7 standard EHR system functionality

Chain of command: A hierarchical reporting structure within an organization

Change agent: An individual within an organization whose primary responsibility is to facilitate change

Change management: The formal process of introducing change, getting it adopted, and diffusing it throughout the organization

Chargemaster: A financial management form that contains information about the organization's charges for the healthcare services it provides to patients

Chart conversion: An EHR implementation activity in which data from the paper chart are converted into electronic form

Checksheet: A tool that permits the systematic recording of observations of a particular phenomenon so that trends or patterns can be identified

Chief executive officer (CEO): The senior manager appointed by a governing board to direct an organization's overall management

Chief financial officer (CFO): The senior manager responsible for the fiscal management of an organization

Chief information officer (CIO): The senior manager responsible for the overall management of information resources in an organization

Chief information security officer (CISO): A recently created position that is responsible for overseeing the development, implementation, and enforcement of a healthcare organization's security policies, managing the security of all patient-identifiable information, whether stored in paper-based or computer-based systems

Chief medical informatics officer (CMIO): A relatively new position within the information services organizational structure, typically held by a member of the medical staff and responsible for, among other things, leading EMR system implementation, engaging healthcare professionals in the system's development and use, and leading the group designated to serve as the central governance forum for establishing the healthcare organization's clinical IS priorities

Chief nursing officer (CNO): The senior manager (usually a registered nurse with advanced education and extensive experience) responsible for administering patient care services

Chief operating officer (COO): Individual who oversees the healthcare organization's internal operations, usually including direct patient care services, but not financial or information-related services

Chief privacy officer: A position that (1) oversees activities related to the development, implementation, and maintenance of, and adherence to, organizational policies and procedures regarding the privacy of and access to patient-specific information and (2) ensures compliance with federal, state, and accrediting body rules and regulations concerning the confidentiality and privacy of health-related information

Civilian Health and Medical Program of the Uniformed Services (CHAMPUS): A federal program providing supplementary civilian-sector hospital and medical services beyond that which is available in military treatment facilities to military dependents, retirees and their dependents, and certain others

Civilian Health and Medical Program-Veterans Affairs (CHAMPVA): The federal healthcare benefits program for dependents of veterans rated by the Veterans Administration as having a total and permanent disability, for survivors of veterans who died from VA-rated service-connected conditions or who were rated permanently and totally disabled at the time of death from a VA-rated service-connected condition, and for survivors of persons who died in the line of duty

Claim: Itemized statement of healthcare services and their costs provided by a hospital, physician's office, or other healthcare provider; submitted for reimbursement to the healthcare insurance plan by either the insured party or by the provider

Claims management: A function related to risk management that enables an organization to track descriptive claims information (incidents, claimants, insurance, demands, dates, and so on), along with data on investigation, litigation, settlement, defendants, and subrogation

Class: The higher-level abstraction of an object that defines its properties and operations

Classification system: 1. A system for grouping similar diseases and procedures and organizing related information for easy retrieval 2. A system for assigning numeric or alphanumeric code numbers to represent specific diseases and/or procedures

Client: A patient who receives behavioral or mental health services

Client/server architecture: A computer architecture in which multiple computers (clients) are connected to other computers (servers) that store and distribute large amounts of shared data

Clinical coding: The process of assigning numeric or alphanumeric classifications to diagnostic and procedural statements

Clinical data repository (CDR): A central database that focuses on clinical information

Clinical data warehouse (CDW): A database that makes it possible to access data from multiple databases and combine the results into a single query and reporting interface; also called a **data warehouse**

Clinical decision support (CDS): The process in which individual data elements are represented in the computer by a special code to be used in making comparisons, trending results, and supplying clinical reminders and alerts

Clinical information system (CIS): A category of a healthcare information system that includes systems that directly support patient care

Clinical pathway: A tool designed to coordinate multidisciplinary care planning for specific diagnoses and treatments

Clinical practice guideline: A detailed, step-by-step guide used by healthcare practitioners to make knowledge-based decisions related to patient care and issued by an authoritative organization such as a medical society or government agency; *See* **clinical protocol**

Clinical privileges: The authorization granted by a healthcare organization's governing board to a member of the medical staff that enables the physician to provide patient services in the organization within specific practice limits

Clinical protocol: Specific instructions for performing clinical procedures established by authoritative bodies, such as medical staff committees, and intended to be applied literally and universally; *See* **clinical practice guideline**

Clinical quality assessment: The process for determining whether the services provided to patients meet predetermined standards of care

Clinical trial: A controlled research study involving human subjects that is designed to evaluate prospectively the safety and effectiveness of new drugs, tests, devices, or interventions

Clinical vocabulary: A formally recognized list of preferred medical terms

CMS-1500: The universal insurance claim form developed and approved by the American Medical Association and the Centers for Medicare and Medicaid Services. Physicians use it to bill Medicare, Medicaid, and private insurers for services provided.

Coding specialist: The healthcare worker responsible for assigning numeric or alphanumeric codes to diagnostic or procedural statements

Coinsurance: Cost-sharing in which the policy or certificate holder pays a pre-established percentage of eligible expenses after the deductible has been met

Collaborative Stage Data Set: A new standardized neoplasm staging system developed by the American Joint Commission on Cancer

Collective bargaining: The negotiating process between an employer and a labor union, usually regarding working conditions, wages, and so on

Column/field: A basic fact within a table, such as LAST_NAME, FIRST_NAME, and date of birth

Commission on Accreditation for Health Informatics and Information Management Education (CAHIIM): The accrediting organization for educational programs in health informatics and information management

Commission on Accreditation of Rehabilitation Facilities (CARF): A private, not-for-profit organization that develops customer-focused standards for behavioral healthcare and medical rehabilitation programs and accredits such programs on the basis of its standards

Common-cause variation: The source of variation in a process that is inherent within the process

Communications technology: Computer networks in an information system

Communities of Practice (CoP): A Web-based electronic network for communication among members of the American Health Information Management Association

Community Health Dimension (CHD): One aspect of a national health information network infrastructure that acknowledges the importance of population-based health data and resources that are necessary to improve public health

Community-acquired infection: An infectious disease contracted as the result of exposure before or after a patient's period of hospitalization

Comorbidity: A medical condition that coexists with the primary cause for hospitalization and affects the patient's treatment and length of stay

Compiler: 1. A type of software that looks at an entire high-level program before translating it into machine language 2. A third-generation programming language

Complaint: A written legal statement from a plaintiff that initiates a civil lawsuit

Compliance: 1. The process of establishing an organizational culture that promotes the prevention, detection, and resolution of instances of conduct that do not conform to federal, state, or private payer healthcare program requirements or the healthcare organization's ethical and business policies 2. The act of adhering to official requirements

Compliance program guidance: The information provided by the Office of the Inspector General of the Department of Health and Human Services to help healthcare organizations develop internal controls that promote adherence to applicable federal and state guidelines

Complication: A medical condition that arises during an inpatient hospitalization (for example, a postoperative wound infection)

Computer output to laser disk/enterprise report management (COLD/ERM): Technology that electronically stores documents and distributes them with fax, e-mail, Web, and traditional hard-copy print processes

Computer telephony: A combination of computer and telephone technologies that allows people to use a telephone handset to access information stored in a computer system or to use computer technology to place calls within the public telephone network

Computer virus: A software program that attacks computer systems and sometimes damages or destroys files

Computer-based patient record (CPR): An electronic patient record housed in a system designed to provide users with access to complete and accurate data, practitioner alerts and reminders, clinical decision support systems, and links to medical knowledge; *See* **electronic health record**

Computerized provider order entry (CPOE): Systems that allow physicians to enter medication or other orders and receive clinical advice about drug dosages, contraindications, or other clinical decision support; sometimes called **computerized physician order entry**

Computers on wheels (COWs): Term affectionately used to refer to notebook computers mounted on carts and moved with the users

Computer–telephone integration (CTI): An integration of computer technology and public telephone services that allows people to access common computer functions such as database queries via telephone handsets or interactive voice technology

Concurrent review: A review of the health record while the patient is still hospitalized or under treatment

Concurrent utilization review: An evaluation of the medical necessity, quality, and cost-effectiveness of a hospital admission and ongoing patient care at or during the time that services are rendered

Conditions for Coverage: Standards applied to facilities that choose to participate in federal government reimbursement programs such as Medicare and Medicaid; *See* **Conditions of Participation**

Conditions of Participation: The administrative and operational guidelines and regulations under which facilities are allowed to take part in the Medicare and Medicaid programs; published by the Centers for Medicare and Medicaid Services, a federal agency under the Department of Health and Human Services; also called **Conditions for Coverage**

Confidentiality: A legal and ethical concept that establishes the healthcare provider's responsibility for protecting health records and other personal and private information from unauthorized use or disclosure

Conflict management: A problem-solving technique that focuses on working with individuals to find a mutually acceptable solution

Consent: A means for residents to convey to healthcare providers their implied or expressed permission to administer care or treatment or to perform surgery or other medical procedures

Consent to treatment: Legal permission given by a patient or a patient's legal representative to a healthcare provider that allows the provider to administer care and/or treatment or to perform surgery and/or other medical procedures

Consolidated Health Informatics (CHI) initiative: The effort to achieve CHI through federal agencies spearheaded by the Office of National Coordinator for Health Information Technology

Constitutional law: The body of law that deals with the amount and types of power and authority that governments are given

Consultation report: Health record documentation that describes the findings and recommendations of consulting physicians

Consumer informatics: The field of information science concerned with the management of data and information used to support consumers by consumers (the general public) through the application of computers and computer technologies

Contextual: The condition of depending on the parts of a written or spoken statement that precede or follow a specified word or phrase and can influence its meaning or effect

Contingency and disaster planning: *See* **business continuity plan**

Continued-stay utilization review: A periodic review conducted during a hospital stay to determine whether the patient continues to need acute care services

Continuity of care record (CCR): Documentation of care delivery from one healthcare experience to another

Continuous quality improvement (CQI): 1. A management philosophy that emphasizes the importance of knowing and meeting customer expectations, reducing variation within processes, and relying on data to build knowledge for process improvement 2. A continuous cycle of planning, measuring, and monitoring performance and making knowledge-based improvements

Continuum of care: The range of healthcare services provided to patients, from routine ambulatory care to intensive acute care

Controlled vocabulary: A predefined set of terms and their meanings that may be used in structured data entry or natural language processing to represent expressions

Coordination of benefits (COB) transaction: The electronic transmission of claims and/or payment information from a healthcare provider to a health plan for the purpose of determining relative payment responsibilities

Core data elements/core content: A small set of data elements with standardized definitions often considered to be the core of data collection efforts

Core measure: Standardized performance measures developed to improve the safety and quality of healthcare (for example, core measures are used in the Joint Commission on Accreditation's ORYX initiative)

Corporate negligence: The failure of an organization to exercise the degree of care considered reasonable under the circumstances that resulted in an unintended injury to another party

Cost outlier: Exceptionally high costs associated with inpatient care when compared with other cases in the same diagnosis-related group

Cost outlier adjustment: Additional reimbursement for certain high-cost home care cases based on the loss-sharing ratio of costs in excess of a threshold amount for each home health resource group

Cost–benefit analysis: A process that uses quantitative techniques to evaluate and measure the benefit of providing products or services compared to the cost of providing them

Council on Certification: An arm of AHIMA that today fulfills the role of the Board of Registration, a certification board instituted in 1933 to provide a baseline by which to measure qualified medical record librarians

Counterclaim: In a court of law, a countersuit

Court order: An official direction issued by a court judge and requiring or forbidding specific parties to perform specific actions

Courts of appeal: A branch of the federal court system that has the power to hear appeals on the final judgments of district courts

Covered entity: According to the HIPAA privacy rule, any health plan, healthcare clearinghouse, or healthcare provider that transmits specific healthcare transactions in electronic form

Credentialing: The process of reviewing and validating the qualifications (degrees, licenses, and other credentials), of physicians and other licensed independent practitioners, for granting medical staff membership to provide patient care services

Critical pathway: The sequence of tasks that determine the project finish date

Cross-claim: In law, a complaint filed against a codefendant

Crude death rate: The total number of deaths in a given population for a given period of time divided by the estimated population for the same period of time

Current Procedural Terminology **(CPT):** A comprehensive, descriptive list of terms and numeric codes used for reporting diagnostic and therapeutic procedures and other medical services performed by physicians; published and updated annually by the American Medical Association

Curriculum: A prescribed course of study in an educational program

Customer: An internal or external recipient of services, products, or information

Daily inpatient census: The number of inpatients present at census-taking time each day, plus any inpatients who were both admitted and discharged after the census-taking time the previous day

Dashboards: Reports of process measures to help leaders know what is currently going on so that they can plan strategically where they want to go next; sometimes called **scorecards**

Data: The dates, numbers, images, symbols, letters, and words that represent basic facts and observations about people, processes, measurements, and conditions

Data accessibility: The extent to which healthcare data are obtainable

Data accuracy: The extent to which data are free of identifiable errors

Data availability: The extent to which healthcare data are accessible whenever and wherever they are needed

Data comparability: The standardization of vocabulary such that the meaning of a single term is the same each time the term is used in order to produce consistency in information derived from the data

Data comprehensiveness: The extent to which healthcare data are complete

Data confidentiality: The extent to which personal health information is kept private

Data consistency: The extent to which healthcare data are reliable

Data conversion: The task of moving data from one data structure to another, usually at the time of a new system installation

Data currency: The extent to which data are up-to-date; *See* **data timeliness**

Data definition: The specific meaning of a healthcare-related data element

Data dictionary: A descriptive list of the data elements to be collected in an information system or database whose purpose is to ensure consistency of terminology

Data element: An individual fact or measurement that is the smallest unique subset of a database

Data Elements for Emergency Department Systems (DEEDS): A data set designed to support the uniform collection of information in hospital-based emergency departments

Data exchange standards: Protocols that help ensure that data transmitted from one system to another remain comparable

Data granularity: The level of detail at which the attributes and values of healthcare data are described

Data integrity: 1. The extent to which healthcare data are complete, accurate, consistent, and timely 2. A security principle that keeps information from being modified or otherwise corrupted either maliciously or accidentally

Data mining: The process of extracting information from a database and then quantifying and filtering discrete, structured data

Data precision: The extent to which data have the values they are expected to have

Data quality management: A managerial process that ensures the integrity (accuracy and completeness) of an organization's data during data collection, application, warehousing, and analysis

Data relevancy: The extent to which healthcare-related data are useful for the purpose for which they were collected

Data security: The process of keeping data safe from unauthorized alteration or destruction

Data set: A list of recommended data elements with uniform definitions that are relevant for a particular use

Data timeliness: *See* **data currency**

Data type: A technical category of data (text, numbers, currency, date, memo, and link data) that a field in a database can contain

Data warehouse: A database that makes it possible to access data from multiple databases and combine the results into a single query and reporting interface

Data warehousing: A type of system used to analyze data for decision-making purposes

Database: An organized collection of data, text, references, or pictures in a standardized format, typically stored in a computer system for multiple applications

Database management system (DBMS): Computer software that enables the user to create, modify, delete, and view the data in a database

Decision support system (DSS): A computer-based system that gathers data from a variety of sources and assists in providing structure to the data by using various analytical models and visual tools in order to facilitate and improve the ultimate outcome in decision-making tasks associated with nonroutine and nonrepetitive problems

Deemed status: An official designation indicating that a healthcare facility is in compliance with the Medicare *Conditions of Participation;* to qualify for deemed status, facilities must be accredited by the Joint Commission on Accreditation of Healthcare Organizations or the American Osteopathic Association

Defendant: In civil cases, an individual or entity against whom a civil complaint has been filed; in criminal cases, an individual who has been accused of a crime

Deficiency slip: A device for tracking information (for example, reports) missing from a paper-based health record

De-identified information: Health information from which all names and other identifying descriptors have been removed to protect the privacy of the patients, family members, and healthcare providers who were involved in the case

Delegation of authority: The assignment of authority or responsibility

Delinquent record: An incomplete record not finished or made complete within the time frame determined by the medical staff of the facility

Demographic information: Information used to identify an individual, such as name, address, gender, age, and other information linked to a specific person

Department of Health and Human Services (HHS): The cabinet-level federal agency that oversees all of the health- and human-services–related activities of the federal government and administers federal regulations

Deposition: A method of gathering information to be used in a litigation process

Descriptive statistics: A set of statistical techniques used to describe data such as means, frequency distributions, and standard deviations; statistical information that describes the characteristics of a specific group or a population

Designated record set: A group of records maintained by or for a covered entity that may include patient medical and billing records; the enrollment, payment, claims adjudication, and cases or medical management record systems maintained by or for a health plan; or information used, in whole or in part, to make patient care-related decisions

Diagnosis-related groups (DRGs): A unit of case-mix classification adopted by the federal government and some other payers as a prospective payment mechanism for hospital inpatients in which diseases are placed into groups because related diseases and treatments tend to consume similar amounts of healthcare resources and incur similar amounts of cost; in the Medicare and Medicaid programs, one of more than 500 diagnostic classifications in which cases demonstrate similar resource consumption and length-of-stay patterns

***Diagnostic and Statistical Manual of Mental Disorders, Fourth Revision, Text Revision* (DSM-IV-TR):** The 2004 text revision of the *Diagnostic and Statistical Manual of Mental Disorders, Fourth Revision,* with updated clinical terms, but very few coding changes

Diagnostic codes: Numeric or alphanumeric characters used to classify and report diseases, conditions, and injuries

Digital dictation: A process in which vocal sounds are converted to bits and stored on computer for random access

Digital images: Data provided in a computer-readable format

Digital Imaging and Communication in Medicine (DICOM): A standard that promotes a digital image communications format and picture archive and communications systems for use with digital images

Discharge abstract system: A data repository (usually electronic) used for collecting information on demographics, clinical conditions, and services in which data are condensed from hospital health records into coded data for the purpose of producing summary statistics about discharged patients

Discharge planning: The process of coordinating the activities related to the release of a patient when inpatient hospital care is no longer needed

Discharge summary: A summary of the resident's stay at the long-term care facility that is used along with the postdischarge plan of care to provide continuity of care for the resident upon discharge from the facility

Discharge utilization review: A process for assessing a patient's readiness to leave the hospital

Disciplinary action: Action taken to improve unsatisfactory work performance or behavior on the job

Discounting: The application of lower rates of payment to multiple surgical procedures performed during the same operative session under the outpatient prospective payment system; the application of adjusted rates of payment by preferred provider organizations

Discovery: *See* **discovery process**

Discovery process: The pretrial stage in the litigation process during which both parties to a suit use various strategies to identify information about the case, the primary focus of which is to determine the strength of the opposing party's case

Discrete data: Data that represent separate and distinct values or observations; that is, data that contain only finite numbers and have only specified values

Disease index: A list of diseases and conditions of patients sequenced according to the code numbers of the classification system in use

Disease management (DM): 1. A more expansive view of case management in which patients with the highest risk of incurring high-cost interventions are targeted for standardizing and managing care throughout integrated delivery systems 2. A program focused on preventing exacerbation of chronic diseases and on promoting healthier life styles for patients and clients with chronic diseases

Disease registry: A centralized collection of data used to improve the quality of care and measure the effectiveness of a particular aspect of healthcare delivery

District court: The lowest tier in the federal court system, which hears cases involving felonies and misdemeanors that fall under federal statute and suits in which a citizen of one state sues a citizen of another state

Diversity jurisdiction: Refers to district court cases that involve suits where a citizen of one state sues a citizen of another state and the amount in dispute exceeds $75,000

Document imaging: The practice of electronically scanning written or printed paper documents into an optical or electronic system for later retrieval of the document or parts of the document if parts have been indexed

DRG grouper: A computer program that assigns inpatient cases to diagnosis-related groups and determines the Medicare reimbursement rate

Dual core (vendor strategy): A vendor strategy in which one vendor primarily supplies the financial and administrative applications and another vendor primarily supplies the clinical applications

Duty: Obligation

E codes (external cause of injury code): A supplementary ICD-9-CM classification used to identify the external causes of injuries, poisonings, and adverse effects of pharmaceuticals

Edit: A condition that must be satisfied before a computer system can accept data

Electronic data interchange (EDI): A standard transmission format using strings of data for business information communicated among the computer systems of independent organizations

Electronic document management system (EDMS): A storage solution based on digital scanning technology in which source documents are scanned to create digital images of the documents that can be stored electronically on optical disks

Electronic document/content management (ED/CM): A type of electronic document management system that uses methods such as bar coding on the forms to identify specific content

Electronic health record (EHR): A computerized record of health information and associated processes; *See* **computer-based patient record** and **computer-based health record**

Electronic medical record (EMR): A form of computer-based health record in which information is stored in whole files instead of by individual data elements

Electronic medication administration record (EMAR): A system designed to prevent medication errors by checking a patient's medication information against his or her barcoded wristband

Electronic prescribing (e-Rx): When a prescription is written from the personal digital assistant and an electronic fax or when an actual electronic data interchange transaction is generated that transmits the prescription directly to the retail pharmacy's information system

Electronic remittance advice (ERA): A classification of payment information from third-party payers that is communicated electronically

Electronic signature authentication (ESA): A system that requires the author of a document to sign onto a patient record using a user ID and password, reviews the document to be signed, and indicates approval

Emergency Maternal and Infant Care Program (EMIC): The federal medical program that provides obstetrical and infant care to dependents of active-duty military personnel in the four lowest pay grades

Employee orientation: The process in which employees are introduced to an organization and a new job

Employer-based self-insurance: An umbrella term used to describe health plans that are funded directly by employers to provide coverage for their employees exclusively in which employers establish accounts to cover their employees' medical expenses and retain control over the funds but bear the risk of paying claims greater than their estimates

Encoded: Converted into code

Encoder: Specialty software used to facilitate the assignment of diagnostic and procedural codes according to the rules of the coding system

Encryption: The process of transforming text into an unintelligible string of characters that can be transmitted via communications media with a high degree of security and then decrypted when it reaches a secure destination

Environmental assessment: External—a collection of information about changes that have occurred in the healthcare industry as well as the broader U.S. economy during a specified time period; internal—a collection of information about changes that have occurred within an organization during a specified time period

Episode-of-care (EOC) reimbursement: A category of payments made as lump sums to providers for all healthcare services delivered to a patient for a specific illness and/or over a specified time period; also called **bundled payments** because they include multiple services and may include multiple providers of care

Equal Employment Opportunity Act: The 1972 amendment to the Civil Rights Act of 1964 prohibiting discrimination in employment on the basis of age, race, color, religion, sex, or national origin

Equal Pay Act of 1963 (EPA): The federal legislation that requires equal pay for men and women who perform substantially the same work

Essential Medical Data Set (EMDS): A recommended data set designed to create a health history for an individual patient treated in an emergency service

Ethernet: A popular protocol (format) for transmitting data in local area networks

Ethicist: An individual trained in the application of ethical theories and principles to problems that cannot be easily solved because of conflicting values, perspectives, and options for action

Ethics: A field of study that deals with moral principles, theories, and values; in healthcare, a formal decision-making process for dealing with the competing perspectives and obligations of the people who have an interest in a common problem

Evidence-based medicine: Healthcare services based on clinical methods that have thoroughly tested through controlled, peer-reviewed biomedical studies

Exclusive provider organization (EPO): Hybrid managed care organization that provides benefits to subscribers only when healthcare services are performed by network providers; sponsored by self-insured (self-funded) employers or associations and exhibits characteristics of both health maintenance organizations and preferred provider organizations

Executive information system (EIS): An information system designed to combine financial and clinical information for use in the management of business affairs of a healthcare organization

Executive management: The managerial level of an organization that is primarily responsible for setting the organization's future direction and establishing its strategic plan

Executive manager: A senior manager who oversees a broad functional area or group of departments or services, sets the organization's future direction, and monitors the organization's operations

Executive sponsor: An individual who helps a team leader keep the team on track and sometimes ensures that the team obtains the organizational support required to accomplish its goal

Expert system: A type of information system that supports the work of professionals engaged in the development or evaluation of complex activities that require high-level knowledge in a well-defined and usually limited area

Explanation of Benefits (EOB): A statement issued to the insured and the healthcare provider by an insurer to explain the services provided, amounts billed, and payments made by a health plan

Expressed consent: The spoken or written permission granted by a patient to a healthcare provider that allows the provider to perform medical or surgical services

Extended care facility: A healthcare facility licensed by applicable state or local law to offer room and board, skilled nursing by a full-time registered nurse, intermediate care, or a combination of levels on a twenty-four-hour basis over a long period of time

Extensible markup language (XML): A standardized computer language that allows the interchange of data as structured text

External reviews (audits): A performance or quality review conducted by a third-party payer or consultant hired for the purpose

Extranet: A system of connections of private Internet networks outside an organization's firewall that uses Internet technology to enable collaborative applications among enterprises

Facilities management: The functional oversight of a healthcare organization's physical plant to ensure operational efficiency in an environment that is safe for patients, staff, and visitors

Facility-based registry: A registry that includes only cases from a particular type of healthcare facility, such as a hospital or clinic

Facility-specific system: A computer information system developed exclusively to meet the needs of one healthcare organization

Fair Labor Standards Act of 1938 (FLSA): The federal legislation that sets the minimum wage and overtime payment regulations

False Claims Act: Federal legislation stipulating that an individual may file claim (for example, against a hospital) for up to ten years after an incident has occurred

Fax on demand: A service in which a user may select from a list of available fax sources by keying the corresponding number of a fax title or from multiple fax messages via a twelve-digit telephone keypad

Federal Employees' Compensation Act (FECA): The legislation enacted in 1916 to mandate workers' compensation for civilian federal employees, whose coverage includes lost wages, medical expenses, and survivors' benefits

Fee schedule: A list of healthcare services and procedures (usually CPT/HCPCS codes) and the charges associated with them developed by a third-party payer to represent the approved payment levels for a given insurance plan; also called table of allowances

Fee-for-service basis: A method of reimbursement through which providers retrospectively receive payment based on either billed charges for services provided or on annually updated fee schedules; also called **fee-for-service reimbursement**

Fetal autopsy rate: The number of autopsies performed on intermediate and late fetal deaths for a given time period divided by the total number of intermediate and late fetal deaths for the same time period

Fetal death (stillborn): The death of a product of human conception before its complete expulsion or extraction from the mother regardless of the duration of the pregnancy

Fetal death rate: A proportion that compares the number of intermediate and/or late fetal deaths to the total number of live births and intermediate or late fetal deaths during the same period of time

Fiscal intermediary (FI): An organization that contracts with the Centers for Medicare and Medicaid Services to serve as the financial agent between providers and the federal government in the local administration of Medicare Part B claims

Fishbone diagram: A performance improvement tool used to identify or classify the root causes of a problem or condition and to display the root causes graphically; also called **cause-and-effect diagram**

Fixed costs: Resources expended that do not vary with the activity of the organization, for example, mortgage expense do not vary with patient volume

Flexibility of approach: Condition under HIPAA in which a covered entity can adopt security protection measures that are appropriate for its organization

Flowchart: A graphic tool that uses standard symbols to visually display detailed information, including time and distance, of the sequential flow of work of an individual or a product as it progresses through a process

Food and Drug Administration (FDA): The federal agency responsible for controlling the sale and use of pharmaceuticals, biological products, medical devices, food, cosmetics, and products that emit radiation, including the licensing of medications for human use

Force-field analysis: A performance improvement tool used to identify specific drivers of, and barriers to, an organizational change so that positive factors can be reinforced and negative factors reduced

Foreign key: A key attribute used to link one entity/table to another

Frequency distribution: A table or graph that displays the number of times (frequency) a particular observation occurs

Frequency polygon: A type of line graph that represents a frequency distribution

General Rules: HIPAA data security provisions that provide the objective and scope for the HIPAA security rule as a whole

Geographic practice cost index (GPCI): An index developed by the Centers for Medicare and Medicaid Services to measure the differences in resource costs among fee schedule areas compared to the national average in the three components of the relative value unit: physician work, practice expenses, and malpractice coverage

Global payment: A form of reimbursement used for radiological and other procedures that combines the professional and technical components of the procedures and disperses payments as lump sums to be distributed between the physician and the healthcare facility

Global surgery payment: A payment made for surgical procedures that includes the provision of all healthcare services, from the treatment decision through postoperative patient care

Graphical user interface (GUI): A style of computer interface in which typed commands are replaced by images that represent tasks, for example, small pictures (icons) that represent the tasks, functions, and programs performed by a software program

Grievance management: The policies and procedures used to handle employee complaints

Gross autopsy rate: The number of inpatient autopsies conducted during a given time period divided by the total number of inpatient deaths for the same time period

Gross death rate: The number of inpatient deaths that occurred during a given time period divided by the total number of inpatient discharges, including deaths, for the same time period

Group health insurance: A prepaid medical plan that covers the healthcare expenses of an organization's full-time employees

Group model health maintenance organization: A type of health plan in which an HMO contracts with an independent multispecialty physician group to provide medical services to members of the plan

Group practice without walls (GPWW): A type of managed care contract that allows physicians to maintain their own offices and share administrative services

Groupware: An Internet technology that consolidates documents from different information systems within an organization into a tightly integrated workflow

Hard-coding: The process of attaching a CPT/HCPCS code to a procedure located on the facility's chargemaster so that the code will automatically be included on the patient's bill

Hardware: The machines and media used in an information system

Health Care Quality Improvement Program (HCQIP): A quality initiative begun in 1992 by the Health Care Financing Administration and implemented by peer review organizations that uses patterns of care analysis and collaboration with practitioners, beneficiaries, providers, plans, and other purchasers of healthcare services to develop scientifically based quality indicators and to identify and implement opportunities for healthcare improvement

Health information exchange (HIE): A plan in which health information is shared among providers

Health information management (HIM): An allied health profession that is responsible for ensuring the availability, accuracy, and protection of the clinical information that is needed to deliver healthcare services and to make appropriate healthcare-related decisions

Health information services department: The department in a healthcare organization that is responsible for maintaining patient care records in accordance with external and internal rules and regulations

Health information technology (HIT): The technical aspects of processing health data and records, including classification and coding, abstracting, registry development, storage, and so on

Health Insurance Portability and Accountability Act of 1996 (HIPAA): The federal legislation enacted to provide continuity of health coverage, control fraud and abuse in healthcare, reduce healthcare costs, and guarantee the security and privacy of health information. The act limits exclusion for preexisting medical conditions, prohibits discrimination against employees and dependents based on health status, guarantees availability of health insurance to small employers, and guarantees renewability of insurance to all employees regardless of size. Public Law 104-191, also known as the Kassebaum-Kennedy Law.

Health Level Seven (HL7): A standards development organization accredited by the American National Standards Institute that addresses issues at the seventh, or application, level of healthcare systems interconnections

Health maintenance organization (HMO): Entity that combines the provision of health-care insurance and the delivery of healthcare services, characterized by: (1) organized healthcare delivery system to a geographic area, (2) set of basic and supplemental health maintenance and treatment services, (3) voluntarily enrolled members, and (4) predetermined fixed, periodic prepayments for members' coverage

Health Plan Employer Data and Information Set (HEDIS): A set of performance measures developed by the National Commission for Quality Assurance that are designed to provide purchasers and consumers of healthcare with the information they need to compare the performance of managed care plans

Health record: A paper- or computer-based tool for collecting and storing information about the healthcare services provided to a patient in a single healthcare facility; also called a patient record, medical record, resident record, or client record, depending on the healthcare setting

Health record number: A unique numeric or alphanumeric identifier assigned to each patient's record upon admission to a healthcare facility

Health savings accounts (HSAs): Savings accounts designed to help people save for future medical and retiree health costs on a tax-fee basis, part of the 2003 Medicare bill; also called **medical savings accounts**

Health services research: Research conducted on the subject of healthcare delivery that examines organizational structures and systems as well as the effectiveness and efficiency of healthcare services

Health systems agency (HSA): A type of organization called for by the Health Planning and Resources Development Act of 1974 to have broad representation of healthcare providers and consumers on governing boards and committees

Healthcare claims and payment/advice transaction: An electronic transmission sent by a health plan to a provider's financial representative for the purpose of providing information about payments and/or payment processing and information about the transfer of funds

Healthcare Common Procedure Coding System (HCPCS): An alphanumeric classification system that identifies healthcare procedures, equipment, and supplies for claim submission purposes; the three levels are as follows: I, *Current Procedural Terminology* codes, developed by the AMA; II, codes for equipment, supplies, and services not covered by *Current Procedural Terminology* codes as well as modifiers that can be used with all levels of codes, developed by CMS; and III (eliminated December 31, 2003 to comply with HIPAA), local codes developed by regional Medicare Part B carriers and used to report physicians' services and supplies to Medicare for reimbursement

Healthcare information standards: Guidelines developed to standardize data throughout the healthcare industry (for example, developing uniform terminologies and vocabularies)

Healthcare Integrity and Protection Data Bank: A database maintained by the federal government to provide information on fraud-and-abuse findings against U.S. healthcare providers

Healthcare provider: A provider of diagnostic, medical, and surgical care as well as the services or supplies related to the health of an individual and any other person or organization that issues reimbursement claims or is paid for healthcare in the normal course of business

Healthcare provider dimension (HPD): One of the three dimensions of a national health information network that includes information obtained during the patient care process and integrates it with clinical guidelines, protocols, and selected information the provider is authorized to access from the personal health record, as well as information relevant to the patient's care from the community health dimension

Hierarchy: An authoritarian organizational structure in which each member is assigned a specific rank that reflects his or her level of decision-making authority within the organization

Hill-Burton Act: The federal legislation enacted in 1946 as the Hospital Survey and Construction Act to authorize grants for states to construct new hospitals and, later, to modernize old ones

Histocompatibility: The immunologic similarity between an organ donor and a transplant recipient

Histogram: A graphic technique used to display the frequency distribution of continuous data (interval or ratio data) as either numbers or percentages in a series of bars

Home Assessment Validation and Entry (HAVEN): A type of data-entry software used to collect Outcome and Assessment Information Set (OASIS) data and then transmit them to state databases; imports and exports data in standard OASIS record format, maintains agency/patient/employee information, enforces data integrity through rigorous edit checks, and provides comprehensive online help

Home health agency (HHA): A program or organization that provides a blend of home-based medical and social services to homebound patients and their families for the purpose of promoting, maintaining, or restoring health or of minimizing the effects of illness, injury, or disability

Home healthcare: The medical and/or personal care provided to individuals and families in their place of residence with the goal of promoting, maintaining, or restoring health or minimizing the effects of disabilities and illnesses, including terminal illnesses

Home health prospective payment system (HH PPS): The reimbursement system developed by the Centers for Medicare and Medicaid Services to cover home health services provided to Medicare beneficiaries

Home health resource group (HHRG): A classification system with eighty home health episode rates established to support the prospective reimbursement of covered home care and rehabilitation services provided to Medicare beneficiaries during sixty-day episodes of care

Hospice: An interdisciplinary program of palliative care and supportive services that addresses the physical, spiritual, social, and economic needs of terminally ill patients and their families

Hospice care: The medical care provided to persons with life expectancies of six months or less who elect to forgo standard treatment of their illness and to receive only palliative care

Hospital-acquired infection: An infection acquired by a patient while receiving care or services in a healthcare organization

Hospital autopsy rate: The total number of autopsies performed by a hospital pathologist for a given time period divided by the number of deaths of hospital patients (inpatients and outpatients) whose bodies were available for autopsy for the same time period

Hospital discharge abstract system: A group of databases compiled from aggregate data on all patients discharged from a hospital

Hospital (nosocomial) infection rate: The number of infections that occur in a hospital's various patient care units on a continuous basis

Hospital information system (HIS): The comprehensive database containing all the clinical, administrative, financial, and demographic information about each patient served by a hospital

Hospital Standardization Program: An early twentieth-century survey mechanism instituted by the American College of Surgeons and aimed at identifying quality-of-care problems and improving patient care; precursor to the survey program offered by the Joint Commission on Accreditation of Healthcare Organizations

Hospitalist: Physicians employed by teaching hospitals to play the role that admitting physicians fulfill in hospitals that are not affiliated with medical training programs

Hospitalization insurance (Medicare Part A): A federal program that covers the costs associated with inpatient hospitalization as well as other healthcare services provided to Medicare beneficiaries

House of Delegates: An important component of the volunteer structure of the American Health Information Management Association that conducts the official business of the organization and functions as its legislative body

Human–computer interface: The device used by humans to access and enter data into a computer system, such as a keyboard on a PC, personal digital assistant, voice recognition system, and so on

Human resources: The employees of an organization

Hybrid health record: A health record that is includes both paper and electronic elements

Identifier standards: Recommended methods for assigning unique identifiers to individuals (patients and clinical providers), corporate providers, and healthcare vendors and suppliers

Imaging technology: Computer software designed to combine health record text files with diagnostic imaging files

Implementation specifications: Descriptions that define how HIPAA standards are to be implemented

Implied consent: The type of permission that is inferred when a patient voluntarily submits to treatment

Incidence: The number of new cases of a specific disease

Incidence rate: A computation that compares the number of new cases of a specific disease for a given time period to the population at risk for the disease during the same time period

Incident report: A quality/performance management tool used to collect data and information about potentially compensable events (events that may result in death or serious injury)

Indemnity plans: Health insurance coverage provided in the form of cash payments to patients or providers

Independent practice association (IPA): An open-panel health maintenance organization that provides contract healthcare services to subscribers through independent physicians who treat patients in their own offices; the HMO reimburses the IPA on a capitated basis; the IPA may reimburse the physicians on a fee-for-service or a capitated basis

Index: An organized (usually alphabetical) list of specific data that serves to guide, indicate, or otherwise facilitate reference to the data

Indian Health Service (IHS): The federal agency within the Department of Health and Human Services that is responsible for providing federal healthcare services to American Indians and Alaska natives

Individually identifiable health information: According to HIPAA privacy provisions, that information that specifically identifies the patient to whom the information relates

Infection control: A system for the prevention of communicable diseases that concentrates on protecting healthcare workers and patients against exposure to disease-causing organisms and promotes compliance with applicable legal requirements through early identification of potential sources of contamination and implementation of policies and procedures that limit the spread of disease

Information: Factual data that have been collected, combined, analyzed, interpreted, and/or converted into a form that can be used for a specific purpose

Information kiosk: A computer station located within a healthcare facility that patients and families can use to access information

Information resource management: A concept that assumes that information is a valuable resource that must be managed, regardless of the form it takes or the medium in which it is stored

Information services department: *See* **health information services department**

Information system (IS): An automated system that uses computer hardware and software to record, manipulate, store, recover, and disseminate data (that is, a system that receives and processes input and provides output); often used interchangeably with **information technology (IT)**

Information technology (IT): Computer technology (hardware and software) combined with telecommunications technology (data, image, and voice networks); often used interchangeably with **information system (IS)**

Injury (harm): In a negligence lawsuit, one of four elements, which may be economic (hospital expenses and loss of wages) and noneconomic (pain and suffering), that must be proved to be successful

Injury Severity Score (ISS): An overall severity measurement maintained in the trauma registry and calculated from the abbreviated injury scores for the three most severe injuries of each patient

Inpatient: A patient who is provided with room, board, and continuous general nursing services in an area of an acute care facility where patients generally stay at least overnight

Inpatient bed occupancy rate (percentage of occupancy): The total number of inpatient service days for a given time period divided by the total number of inpatient bed count days for the same time period

Inpatient psychiatric facility (IPF): A healthcare facility that offers psychiatric medical care on an inpatient basis; CMS established a prospective payment system for reimbursing these types of facilities using the current DRGs for inpatient hospitals

Inpatient rehabilitation facility (IRF): A healthcare facility that specializes in providing services to patients who have suffered a disabling illness or injury in an effort to help them achieve or maintain their optimal level of functioning, self-care, and independence

Inpatient Rehabilitation Validation and Entry (IRVEN): A computerized data-entry system used by inpatient rehabilitation facilities

Inpatient service day: A unit of measure equivalent to the services received by one inpatient during one twenty-four-hour period

Inputs: Data entered into a hospital system (for example, the patient's knowledge of his or her condition, the admitting clerk's knowledge of the admission process, and the computer with its admitting template are all inputs for the hospital's admitting system)

Institute of Electrical and Electronics Engineers (IEEE): A national organization that develops standards for hospital system interface transactions, including links between critical care bedside instruments and clinical information systems

Institute of Medicine (IOM): A branch of the National Academy of Sciences whose goal is to advance and distribute scientific knowledge with the mission of improving human health

Institutional Review Board: An administrative body that provides oversight for the research studies conducted within a healthcare institution

Insured: A holder of a health insurance policy

Insurer: An organization that pays healthcare expenses on behalf of its enrollees

Integrated delivery network (IDN): *See* **integrated delivery system**

Integrated delivery system (IDS): A system that combines the financial and clinical aspects of healthcare and uses a group of healthcare providers, selected on the basis of quality and cost management criteria, to furnish comprehensive health services across the continuum of care; *See* **integrated provider organization** and **integrated delivery system**

Integrated health record format: A system of health record organization in which all the paper forms are arranged in strict chronological order and mixed with forms created by different departments

Integrated health records: *See* **integrated health record format**

Integrated provider organization (IPO): An organization that manages the delivery of health-care services provided by hospitals, physicians (employees of the IPO), and other healthcare organizations (for example, nursing facilities); *See* **integrated delivery system**

Integration testing: A form of testing during EHR implementation performed to ensure that the interfaces between applications and systems work

Integrity: The state of being whole or unimpaired

Intensity-of-service screening criteria: Preestablished standards used to determine the most efficient healthcare setting in which to safely provide needed services

Intentional tort: A circumstance where a healthcare provider purposely commits a wrongful act that results in injury

Interface: The zone between different computer systems across which users want to pass information (for example, a computer program written to exchange information between systems or the graphic display of an application program designed to make the program easier to use)

International Classification of Diseases for Oncology, Third Edition **(ICD-O-3):** A system used for classifying incidences of malignant disease

International Classification of Diseases, Ninth Revision, Clinical Modification (ICD-9-CM): A classification system used in the United States to report morbidity and mortality information

International Classification of Diseases, Tenth Revision, Clinical Modification (ICD-10-CM): The planned replacement for ICD-9-CM, volumes 1 and 2, developed to contain more codes and allow greater specificity

International Classification of Diseases, Tenth Revision, Procedure Coding System (ICD-10-PCS): A separate procedure coding system that would replace ICD-9-CM, volume 3, intended to improve coding accuracy and efficiency, reduce training effort, and improve communication with physicians

Internet: An international network of computer servers that provides individual users with communications channels and access to software and information repositories worldwide

Internet browsers: A type of client software that facilitates communications among World Wide Web information servers

Internet protocol (IP) telephony: A type of communications technology that allows people to initiate real-time calls through the Internet instead of the public telephone system

Interoperability: The ability, generally by adoption of standards, of systems to work together

Interpreter: A type of communications technology that converts high-level language statements into machine language one at a time

Interrater reliability: A measure of a research instrument's consistency in data collection when used by different abstractors

Intranet: A private information network that is similar to the Internet and whose servers are located inside a firewall or security barrier so that the general public cannot gain access to information housed within the network

Inventory control: The balance between purchasing and storing needed supplies and not wasting money or space should the requirements for those supplies change or the space available for storage be limited

Investor-owned hospital chain: Group of for-profit healthcare facilities owned by stockholders

Issues management: The process of resolving unexpected occurrences (for example, the late delivery of needed supplies or an uncorrected system problem)

Job redesign: The process of realigning the needs of the organization with the skills and interests of the employee and then designing the job to meet those needs (for example, in order to introduce new tools or technology or provide better customer service)

Joinder: In a countersuit, a third party against whom the defendant files a complaint

Joint Commission on Accreditation of Healthcare Organizations (JCAHO): A private, not-for-profit organization that evaluates and accredits hospitals and other healthcare organizations on the basis of predefined performance standards

Judicial law: The body of law created as a result of court (judicial) decisions

Jurisdiction: The power and authority of a court to hear and decide specific types of cases

Justice: The impartial administration of policies or laws that takes into consideration the competing interests and limited resources of the individuals or groups involved

Key field: An explanatory notation that uniquely identifies each row in a database table; *See* **primary key**

Knowledge management system (KMS): A type of system that supports the creation, organization, and dissemination of business or clinical knowledge and expertise to providers, employees, and managers throughout a healthcare enterprise

Language translator: A software system that translates a program written in a particular computer language into a language that other types of computers can understand

Length of stay (LOS): The total number of patient days for an inpatient episode, calculated by subtracting the date of admission from the date of discharge

Liability: 1. A legal obligation or responsibility that may have financial repercussions if not fulfilled 2. An amount owed by an individual or organization to another individual or organization

Licensure: The legal authority or formal permission from authorities to carry on certain activities that by law or regulation require such permission (applicable to institutions as well as individuals)

Line graph: A graphic technique used to illustrate the relationship between continuous measurements; consists of a line drawn to connect a series of points on an arithmetic scale; often used to display time trends

Litigation: A civil lawsuit or contest in court

Local area network (LAN): A network that connects multiple computer devices via continuous cable within a relatively small geographic area

Long-term care hospital (LTCH): A hospital with an average length of stay of twenty-five days or more

Low-utilization payment adjustment (LUPA): An alternative (reduced) payment made to home health agencies instead of the home health resource group reimbursement rate when a patient receives fewer than four home care visits during a sixty-day episode

Machine language: Binary codes made up of zeroes and ones that computers use directly to represent precise storage locations and operations

Mainframe: A computer architecture built with a single central processing unit to which dumb terminals and/or personal computers are connected

Mainframe architecture: The term used to refer to the configuration of a mainframe computer

Major diagnostic category (MDC): Under diagnosis-related groups (DRGs), one of twenty-five categories based on single or multiple organ systems into which all diseases and disorders relating to that system are classified

Major medical insurance: Prepaid healthcare benefits that include a high limit for most types of medical expenses and usually require a large deductible and sometimes place limits on coverage and charges (for example, room and board)

Malfeasance: A wrong or improper act

Managed care: 1. Payment method in which the third party payer has implemented some provisions to control the costs of healthcare while maintaining quality care 2. Systematic merger of clinical, financial, and administrative processes to manage access, cost, and quality of healthcare

Managed care organization (MCO): A type of healthcare organization that delivers medical care and manages all aspects of the care or the payment for care by limiting providers of care, discounting payment to providers of care, and/or limiting access to care

Management information system (MIS): A computer-based system that provides information to a healthcare organization's managers for use in making decisions that affect a variety of day-to-day activities

Management service organization (MSO): An organization, usually owned by a group of physicians or a hospital, that provides administrative and support services to one or more physician group practices or small hospitals

Management support information systems: Systems that provide information primarily to support manager decision making

Master patient index (MPI): A list or database created and maintained by a healthcare facility to record the name and identification number of every patient who has ever been admitted or treated in the facility;

Maternal death rate: For a hospital, the total number of maternal deaths directly related to pregnancy for a given time period divided by the total number of obstetrical discharges for the same time period; for a community, the total number of deaths attributed to maternal conditions during a given time period in a specific geographic area divided by the total number of live births for the same time period in the same area

Maternal mortality rate: The rate that measures deaths associated with pregnancy for a community for a specific period of time

Mean: A measure of central tendency that is determined by calculating the arithmetic average of the observations in a frequency distribution

Median: A measure of central tendency that shows the midpoint of a frequency distribution when the observations have been arranged in order from lowest to highest

Mediation: In law, when a dispute is submitted to a third party to facilitate agreement between the disputing parties

Medicaid: An entitlement program that oversees medical assistance for individuals and families with low incomes and limited resources; jointly funded between state and federal governments

Medical foundation: Multi-purpose, non-profit service organization for physicians and other healthcare providers at the local and county level; as managed care organizations, medical foundations have established preferred provider organization, exclusive provider organizations, and management service organizations, with emphases on freedom of choice and preservation of the physician-patient relationship

Medical Group Management Association (MGMA): A national organization composed of individuals actively engaged in the business management of medical groups consisting of three or more physicians in medical practice

Medical history: A record of the information provided by a patient to his or her physician to explain the patient's chief complaint, present and past illnesses, and personal and family medical problems; includes a description of the physician's review of systems

Medical Literature, Analysis, and Retrieval System Online (MEDLINE): A computerized, online database in the bibliographic Medical Literature Analysis and Retrieval System (MEDLARS) of the National Library of Medicine

Medical malpractice: The professional liability of healthcare providers in the delivery of patient care

Medical staff bylaws: A collection of guidelines adopted by a hospital's medical staff to govern its business conduct and the rights and responsibilities of its members

Medical staff classifications: Categories of clinical practice privileges assigned to individual practitioners on the basis of their qualifications

Medical staff privileges: Categories of clinical practice privileges assigned to individual practitioners on the basis of their qualifications

Medical transcription: The conversion of verbal medical reports dictated by healthcare providers into written form for inclusion in patients' health records

Medically needy option: An option in the Medicaid program that allows states to extend eligibility to persons who would be eligible for Medicaid under one of the mandatory or optional groups but whose income and/or resources fall above the eligibility level set by their state

Medicare: A federally funded health program established in 1965 to assist with the medical care costs of Americans sixty-five years of age and older as well as other individuals entitled to Social Security benefits owing to their disabilities

Medicare Advantage (Medicare Part C): Optional managed care plan for Medicare beneficiaries who are entitled to Part A, enrolled in Part B, and live in an area with a plan; types include health maintenance organization, point-of-service plan, preferred provider organization, and provider-sponsored organization; formerly **Medicare+Choice**

Medicare carrier: A health plan that processes Part B claims for services by physicians and medical suppliers (for example, the Blue Shield plan in a state)

Medicare Conditions of Participation or Conditions for Coverage: A publication that describes the requirements that institutional providers (such as hospitals, skilled nursing facilities, and home health agencies) must meet to receive reimbursement for services provided to Medicare beneficiaries

Medicare fee schedule (MFS): A feature of the resource-based relative value system that includes a complete list of the payments Medicare makes to physicians and other providers

Medicare Modernization Act of 2003 (MMA): Legislation passed in 2003 designed to expand healthcare services for seniors, with a major focus on prescription drug benefits

Medicare prospective payment system: *See* **acute care prospective payment system, home health prospective payment system,** and **skilled nursing facility prospective payment system**

Medicare Summary Notice (MSN): A summary sent to the patient from Medicare that summarizes all services provided over a period of time with an explanation of benefits provided

Medigap: A private insurance policy that supplements Medicare coverage

Message format standards: Protocols that help ensure that data transmitted from one system to another remain comparable

Microcomputer: A personal computer characterized by its relatively small size and fast processing speed

Middle management: The management level in an organization that is concerned primarily with facilitating the work performed by supervisory- and staff-level personnel as well as by executive leaders

Middle managers: The individuals in an organization who oversee the operation of a broad scope of functions at the departmental level or who oversee defined product or service lines

Migration path: A series of steps required to move from one situation to another

Minicomputer: A small, mainframe computer

Minimum Data Set (MDS) for Long-Term Care: The instrument specified by the Centers for Medicare and Medicaid Services that requires nursing facilities (both Medicare certified and/or Medicaid certified) to conduct a comprehensive, accurate, standardized, reproducible assessment of each resident's functional capacity

Minimum Data Set Version 2.0 (MDS 2.0): A federally mandated standard assessment form that Medicare- and/or Medicaid-certified nursing facilities must use to collect demographic and clinical data on nursing home residents

Minimum necessary standard: A stipulation of the HIPAA privacy rule that requires healthcare facilities and other covered entities to make reasonable efforts to limit the patient-identifiable information they disclose to the least amount required to accomplish the intended purpose for which the information was requested

Mirrored processing: The act of entering data into a primary and a secondary server simultaneously so that the second server can continue to process the data in the event the primary server crashes

Misfeasance: Relating to negligence, improper performance during an otherwise correct act

Mission (statement): A short description of an organization's or group's general purpose for existing

Mode: A measure of central tendency that consists of the most frequent observation in a frequency distribution

Morality: A composite of the personal values concerning what is considered right or wrong in a specific cultural group

Morbidity: A term referring to the state of being diseased (including illness, injury, or deviation from normal health); the number of sick persons or cases of disease in relationship to a specific population

Mortality: 1. A term referring to the incidence of death in a specific population 2. The loss of subjects during the course of a clinical research study

Multivoting technique: A decision-making method for determining group consensus on the prioritization of issues or solutions

National Alliance for Health Information Technology (NAHIT): A partnership of government and private sector leaders from various healthcare organizations working to use technology to achieve improvements in patient safety, quality of care and operating performance; founded in 2002

National Center for Health Statistics (NCHS): The federal agency responsible for collecting and disseminating information on health services utilization and the health status of the population in the United States

National Committee for Quality Assurance (NCQA): A private not-for-profit accreditation organization whose mission is to evaluate and report on the quality of managed care organizations in the United States

National Committee on Vital and Health Statistics (NCVHS): A public policy advisory board that recommends policy to the National Center for Health Statistics and other health-related federal programs

National conversion factor (CF): A mathematical factor used to convert relative value units into monetary payments for services provided to Medicare beneficiaries

National Correct Coding Initiative (NCCI): A series of code edits on Medicare Part B claims

National Council for Prescription Drug Programs (NCPDP): An organization that develops standards for exchanging prescription and payment information

National Drug Codes (NDC): Codes that serve as product identifiers for human drugs, currently limited to prescription drugs and a few selected over-the-counter products

National Guideline Clearinghouse (NGC): A partnership among the Agency for Healthcare Research and Quality, the American Medical Association, and the American Association of Health Plans that allows free online access to its clinical guidelines

National health information infrastructure (NHII): An infrastructure proposed by the National Committee on Vital and Health Statistics in 2002 that would be a set of technologies, standards, applications, systems, values, and laws that support all facets of provider healthcare, individual health, and public health; also called a **national health information network**

National health information network (NHIN): System that links various healthcare information systems together, allowing patients, physicians, healthcare institutions, and other entities nationwide to share clinical information privately and securely

National Information Infrastructure-Health Information Network Program (NII-HIN): A national quasi-governmental organization that provides oversight of all healthcare information standards in the United States

National Institutes of Health (NIH): Federal agency of the Department of Health and Human Services comprising a number of institutes that carry out research and programs related to certain types of diseases, such as cancer

National Labor Relations Act: Federal legislation that provides, among other things, procedures for union representation and prohibits unfair labor practices by unions, such as coercing nonstriking employees, and by employers, such as interference with the union selection process and discrimination against employees who support a union

National Library of Medicine (NLM): The world's largest medical library and a branch of the National Institutes of Health

National patient safety goals (NPSGs): Goals issued by the Joint Commission on Accreditation of Healthcare Organizations to improve patient safety in healthcare organizations nationwide

National Practitioner Data Bank (NPBD): A data bank established by the federal government through the 1986 Health Care Quality Improvement Act that contains information on professional review actions taken against physicians and other licensed healthcare practitioners, which healthcare organizations are required to check as part of the credentialing process

National provider identifier (NPI): An eight-character alphanumeric identifier used to identify individual healthcare providers for Medicare billing purposes

National Uniform Claim Committee (NUCC): The national group that replaced the Uniform Claim Form Task Force in 1995 and developed a standard data set to be used in the transmission of noninstitutional provider claims to and from third-party payers

National Vaccine Advisory Committee (NVAC): A national advisory group that supports the director of the National Vaccine Program

Natural language: A fifth-generation computer programming language that uses human language to give people a more natural connection with computers

Natural language processing (NLP): The extraction of unstructured or structured medical word data, which are then translated into diagnostic or procedural codes for clinical and administrative applications

Negligence: A legal term that refers to the result of an action by an individual who does not act the way a reasonably prudent person would act under the same circumstances

Net autopsy rate: The ratio of inpatient autopsies compared to inpatient deaths calculated by dividing the total number of inpatient autopsies performed by the hospital pathologist for a given time period by the total number of inpatient deaths minus unautopsied coroners' or medical examiners' cases for the same time period

Net death rate: The total number of inpatient deaths minus the number of deaths that occurred less than forty-eight hours after admission for a given time period divided by the total number of inpatient discharges minus the number of deaths that occurred less than forty-eight hours after admission for the same time period

Network: 1. A type of information technology that connects different computers and computer systems so that they can share information 2. Physicians, hospitals, and other providers who provide healthcare services to members of a managed care organization; providers may be associated through formal or informal contracts and agreements

Network controls: A method of protecting data from unauthorized change and corruption during transmission among information systems

Network model health maintenance program: Program in which participating HMOs contract for services with one or more multispecialty group practices

Network protocol: A set of conventions that governs the exchange of data between hardware and/or software components in a communications network

Network provider: A physician or another healthcare professional who is a member of a managed care network

Newborn: An inpatient who was born in a hospital at the beginning of the current inpatient hospitalization

Newborn autopsy rate: The number of autopsies performed on newborns who died during a given time period divided by the total number of newborns who died during the same time period

Nomenclature: A recognized system of terms used in a science or art that follows pre-established naming conventions; a disease nomenclature is a listing of the proper name for each disease entity with its specific code number

Nominal group technique: A group process technique that involves the steps of silent listing, recording each participant's list, discussing, and rank ordering the priority or importance of items

Nonfeasance: A type of negligence meaning failure to act

Nonmaleficence: A legal principle that means "do no harm"

Nonparticipating providers: A healthcare provider who did not sign a participation agreement with Medicare and so is not obligated to accept assignment on Medicare claims

Normal distribution: A theoretical family of continuous frequency distributions characterized by a symmetric bell-shaped curve, with an equal mean, median, and mode, any standard deviation, and with half of the observations above the mean and half below it

North American Association of Central Cancer Registries (NAACCR): A national organization that certifies state, population-based cancer registries

Nosology: The branch of medical science that deals with classification systems

Notice of privacy practices: A statement (mandated by the HIPAA privacy rule) issued by a healthcare organization that informs individuals of the uses and disclosures of patient-identifiable health information that may be made by the organization, as well as the individual's rights and the organization's legal duties with respect to that information

Notifiable disease: A disease that must be reported to a government agency so that regular, frequent, and timely information on individual cases can be used to prevent and control future cases of the disease

Numeric filing system: A system of health record identification and storage in which records are arranged consecutively in ascending numerical order according to the health record number

Nursing vocabularies: A classification system used to capture documentation on nursing care

Object: The basic component in an object-oriented database that includes both data and their relationships within a single structure

Object-oriented database (OODB): A type of database that uses commands that act as small, self-contained instructional units (objects) that may be combined in various ways

Object-relational database: A type of database (both object oriented and relational) that stores both objects and traditional tables

Occupational Safety and Health Act (OSHA) of 1970: The federal legislation that established comprehensive safety and health guidelines for employers

Occurrence screening: A risk management technique in which the risk manager reviews the health records of current and discharged hospital inpatients with the goal of identifying potentially compensable events

Office of the National Coordinator of Health Information Technology (ONC): Office that provides leadership for the development and implementation of an interoperable health information technology infrastructure nationwide to improve healthcare quality and delivery

Omnibus Budget Reconciliation Act (OBRA): Federal legislation passed in 1987 that required the Health Care Financing Administration (now renamed the Centers for Medicare and Medicaid Services) to develop an assessment instrument (called the resident assessment instrument) to standardize the collection of patient data from skilled nursing facilities

Operating system: Processes that are affected by what is going on around them and must adjust as the environment changes

Operational decision making: A process for addressing problems that come up in the day-to-day operation of a business unit or the day-to-day execution of a work task

Operational plan: The short-term objectives set by an organization to improve its methods of doing business and achieve its planned outcomes

Operation index: A list of the operations and surgical procedures performed in a healthcare facility that is sequenced according to the code numbers of the classification system in use

Operation support systems (OSS): An information system that facilitates the operational management of a healthcare organization

Operative report: A formal document that describes the events surrounding a surgical procedure or operation and identifies the principal participants in the surgery

Organizational chart: A graphic representation of an organization's formal structure

ORYX initiative: A Joint Commission on Accreditation of Healthcare Organizations initiative that supports the integration of outcomes data and other performance measurement data into the accreditation process

Outcome indicators: A measurement of the end results of a clinical process (for example, complications, adverse effects, patient satisfaction) for an individual patient or a group of patients within a specific diagnostic category; *See* **outcome measure**

Outcome measure: *See* **outcome indicator**

Outcomes and Assessment Information Set (OASIS): A standard core assessment data tool developed to measure the outcomes of adult patients receiving home health services under the Medicare and Medicaid programs

Outguide: A device used in paper-based health record systems to track the location of records removed from the file storage area

Out-of-pocket expenses: Healthcare costs paid by the insured (for example, deductibles, copayments, and coinsurance) after which the insurer pays a percentage (often 80 or 100 percent) of covered expenses

Outpatient: A patient who receives ambulatory care services in a hospital-based clinic or department

Outpatient code editor (OCE): A software program linked to the Correct Coding Initiative that applies a set of logical rules to determine whether various combinations of codes are correct and appropriately represent the services provided

Outpatient prospective payment system (OPPS): The Medicare prospective payment system used for hospital-based outpatient services and procedures that is predicated on the assignment of ambulatory payment classifications

Outputs: The outcomes of inputs into a system (for example, the output of the admitting process is the patient's admission to the hospital)

Packaging: A payment under the Medicare outpatient prospective payment system that includes items such as anesthesia, supplies, certain drugs, and the use of recovery and observation rooms

Palliative care: A type of medical care designed to relieve the patient's pain and suffering without attempting to cure the underlying disease

Pareto chart: A bar graph that includes bars arranged in order of descending size to show decisions on the prioritization of issues, problems, or solutions

Partial hospitalization: A term that refers to limited patients stays in the hospital setting, typically as part of a transitional program to a less intense level of service; for example, psychiatric and drug and alcohol treatment facilities that offer services to help patients reenter the community, return to work, and assume family responsibilities

Pathology report: A type of health record or documentation that describes the results of a microscopic and macroscopic evaluation of a specimen removed or expelled during a surgical procedure

Patient account number: A number used assigned by a healthcare facility for billing purposes that is unique to a particular episode of care; a new account number is assigned each time the patient receives care or services at the facility

Patient advocacy: The function performed by patient representatives (sometimes called ombudsmen) who respond personally to complaints from patients and/or their families

Patient assessment instrument (PAI): A standardized tool used to evaluate the patient's condition after admission to, and at discharge from, the healthcare facility

Patient care charting system: A system in which caregivers enter data into health records

Patient history questionnaire: A series of structured questions to be answered by patients to provide information to clinicians about their current health status

Patient safety: The condition of a patient being safe from harm or injury

Patient's bill of rights: The protections afforded to individuals who are undergoing medical procedures in hospitals or other healthcare facilities; also referred to as **patient rights**

Patient Self-Determination Act (PSDA): The federal legislation that requires healthcare facilities to provide written information on the patient's right to issue advance directives and to accept or refuse medical treatment

Patient-specific/identifiable data: Personal information that can be linked to a specific patient, such as age, gender, date of birth, and address

Payer of last resort: A Medicaid term that means that Medicare pays for the services provided to individuals enrolled in both Medicare and Medicaid until Medicare benefits are exhausted and Medicaid benefits begin

Pay for performance (P4P): A type of incentive to improve clinical performance using the electronic health record that could result in additional reimbursement or eligibility for grants or other subsidies to support further HIT efforts

Pay for quality (P4Q): A type of incentive to improve the quality of clinical outcomes using the electronic health record that could result in additional reimbursement or eligibility for grants or other subsidies to support further HIT efforts

Payment status indicator (PSI): An alphabetic code assigned to CPT/HCPCS codes to indicate whether a service or procedure is to be reimbursed under the Medicare outpatient prospective payment system

Peer review organization (PRO): Until 2002, a medical organization that performs a professional review of medical necessity, quality, and appropriateness of healthcare services provided to Medicare beneficiaries; now called quality improvement organization (QIO)

Performance counseling: Guidance provided to an individual in an attempt to improve his or her work performance

Performance evaluations: Reviews of employee job performance

Performance indicators: A measure used by healthcare facilities to assess the quality, effectiveness, and efficiency of their services

Performance standards: The stated expectations for acceptable quality and productivity associated with a job function

Peripheral: Any hardware device connected to a computer (for example, a keyboard, mouse, or printer)

Per member per month (PMPM): *See* **per patient per month**

Per patient per month (PPPM): A type of managed care arrangement by which providers are paid a fixed fee in exchange for supplying all of the healthcare services an enrollee needs for a specified period of time (usually one month but sometimes one year)

Personal digital assistant (PDA): A hand-held microcomputer, without a hard drive, that is capable of running applications such as e-mail and providing access to data and information, such as notes, phone lists, schedules, and laboratory results, primarily through a pen device

Personal health dimension (PHD): One of three dimensions of the national health information network privacy concept that supports individuals in managing their own wellness and healthcare decision making

Personal health record (PHR): An electronic or paper health record maintained and updated by an individual for himself or herself

Pharmacy benefits manager (PBM): The vendor selected by the Bureau of Workers' Compensation to process outpatient medication bills submitted electronically

Physical access controls: 1. Security mechanisms designed to protect an organization's equipment, media, and facilities from physical damage or intrusion 2. Security mechanisms designed to prevent unauthorized physical access to health records and health record storage areas

Physical examination report: Documentation of a physician's assessment of a patient's body systems

Physical safeguards: Measures such as locking doors to safeguard data and computer programs from undesired occurrences and exposures

Physician-hospital organization (PHO): An integrated delivery system formed by hospitals and physicians (usually through managed care contracts) that allows for cooperative activity but permits participants to retain some level of independence

Physician index: A list of patients and their physicians that is usually arranged according to the physician code numbers assigned by the healthcare facility

Physician's orders: A physician's written or verbal instructions to the other caregivers involved in a patient's care

Picture archiving and communications system (PACS): An integrated computer system that obtains, stores, retrieves, and displays digital images (in healthcare, radiological images)

Pie chart: A graphic technique in which the proportions of a category are displayed as portions of a circle (like pieces of a pie)

Plaintiff: The group or person who initiates a civil lawsuit

Plan-do-study-act (PDSA) cycle: A performance improvement model designed specifically for healthcare organizations

Point of care (POC): The place or location where the physician administers services to the patient

Point-of-service (POS) plan: A type of managed care plan in which enrollees are encouraged to select healthcare providers from a network of providers under contract with the plan but are also allowed to select providers outside the network and pay a larger share of the cost

Policies: 1. Governing principles that describe how a department or an organization is supposed to handle a specific situation 2. Binding contracts issued by a healthcare insurance company to an individual or group in which the company promises to pay for healthcare to treat illness or injury

Policyholder: An individual or entity that purchases healthcare insurance coverage

Population-based registry: A type of registry that includes information from more than one facility in a specific geopolitical area, such as a state or region

Portals: Special Web pages that offer secure access and entry of data upon authorization of the owner of the page

Position descriptions: A document that outlines the work responsibilities associated with a job

Postoperative infection rate: The number of infections that occur in clean surgical cases for a given time period divided by the total number of operations within the same time period

Potentially compensable event: An event that may result in financial liability for a healthcare organization, for example, an injury, accident, or medical error

Practice management system (PMS): Software designed to help medical practices run more smoothly and efficiently

Preadmission utilization review: A type of review conducted before a patient's admission to an acute care facility to determine whether the planned service (intensity of service) or the patient's condition (severity of illness) warrants care in an inpatient setting

Preemption: In law, the principle that a statute at one level supercedes or is applied over the same or similar statute at a lower level, for example, the federal HIPAA privacy provisions trump the same or similar state law with certain exceptions

Preferred provider organization (PPO): A managed care arrangement based on a contractual agreement between healthcare providers (professional and/or institutional) and employers, insurance carriers, or third-party administrators to provide healthcare services to a defined population of enrollees at established fees that may or may not be a discount from usual and customary or reasonable charges

Premium: Amount of money that a policyholder or certificate holder must periodically pay an insurer in return for healthcare coverage

Prevalence rate: The proportion of people in a population who have a particular disease at a specific point in time or over a specified period of time

Primary care manager (PCM): The healthcare provider assigned to a TRICARE enrollee

Primary care physician (PCP): 1. Physician who provides, supervises, and coordinates the healthcare of a member and who manages referrals to other healthcare providers and utilization of healthcare services both inside and outside a managed care plan 2. The physician who makes the initial diagnosis of a patient's medical condition

Primary data source: A record developed by healthcare professionals in the process of providing patient care

Primary key: *See* **key field**

Principal diagnosis: The disease or condition that was present on admission, was the principal reason for admission, and received treatment or evaluation during the hospital stay or visit

Principal procedure: The procedure performed for the definitive treatment of a condition (as opposed to a procedure performed for diagnostic or exploratory purposes) or for care of a complication

Privacy: The quality or state of being hidden from, or undisturbed by, the observation or activities of other persons or freedom from unauthorized intrusion; in healthcare-related contexts, the right of a patient to control disclosure of personal information

Privacy officer: The individual responsible for the development and implementation of an organization's privacy policies and procedures

Privacy standards: Rules, conditions, or requirements developed to ensure the privacy of patient information

Private branch exchange (PBX): A switching system for telephones on private extension lines that allows access to the public telephone network

Private law: The collective rules and principles that define the rights and duties of people and private businesses

Problem list: A list of illnesses, injuries, and other factors that affect the health of an individual patient, usually identifying the time of occurrence or identification and resolution

Problem-oriented health record format: A health record documentation approach in which the physician defines each clinical problem individually

Problem-oriented health records: Patient records in which clinical problems are defined and documented individually

Procedural codes: The numeric or alphanumeric characters used to classify and report the medical procedures and services performed for patients

Procedures: The steps taken to implement a policy

Process: A systematic series of actions taken to create a product or service

Process indicators: Specific measures that enable the assessment of the steps taken in rendering a service

Process redesign: The second step in a quality improvement process in which the findings in the research phase are identified, focused data from the prioritized problem areas are collected, a flowchart of the redesigned process is created, policies and procedures are developed, and staff are educated on the new process

Productivity software: A type of computer software used for word-processing, spreadsheet, and database management applications

Professional component (PC): 1. The portion of a healthcare procedure performed by a physician 2. A term generally used in reference to the elements of radiological procedures performed by a physician

Professional standards review organization (PSRO): An organization responsible for determining whether the care and services provided to hospital inpatients were medically necessary and met professional standards in the context of eligibility for reimbursement under the Medicare and Medicaid programs

Programming language: A set of words and symbols that allows programmers to tell the computer what operations to follow

Programs of All-Inclusive Care for the Elderly (PACE): A state option legislated by the Balanced Budget Act of 1997 that provides an alternative to institutional care for individuals fifty-five years old or older who require the level of care provided by nursing facilities

Progress notes: The documentation of a patient's care, treatment, and therapeutic response that is entered into the health record by each of the clinical professionals involved in a patient's care, including nurses, physicians, therapists, and social workers

Proportion: A type of ratio in which the elements included in the numerator also must be included in the denominator

Proportionate mortality ratio (PMR): The total number of deaths due to a specific cause during a given time period divided by the total number of deaths due to all causes

Prospective utilization review: A review of a patient's health records before admission to determine the necessity of admission to an acute care facility and to determine or satisfy benefit coverage requirements

Protected health information (PHI): Under HIPAA, all individually identifiable information, whether oral or recorded in any form or medium, that is created or received by a healthcare provider or any other entity subject to HIPAA requirements

Protocol: In healthcare, a detailed plan of care for a specific medical condition based on investigative studies; in medical research, a rule or procedure to be followed in a clinical trial; in a computer network, a protocol used to address and ensure delivery of data

Public assistance: A monetary subsidy provided to financially needy individuals

Public health: An area of healthcare that deals with the health of populations in geopolitical areas, such as states and counties

Public health services: Services concerned primarily with the health of entire communities and population groups

Public law: A type of legislation that involves the government and its relations with individuals and business organizations

Public Law 104-191: The alternate name for the Health Insurance Portability and Accountability Act (HIPAA) passed in 1996; *See* **Health Insurance Portability and Accountability Act of 1996**

Purged records: Patient health records that have been removed from the active file area

Push technology: A type of active computer technology that sends information directly to the end user as the information becomes available

Quality: The degree or grade of excellence of goods or services, including, in healthcare, meeting expectations for outcomes of care

Quality improvement organization (QIO): An organization that performs medical peer review of Medicare and Medicaid claims, including review of validity of hospital diagnosis and procedure coding information; completeness, adequacy, and quality of care; and appropriateness of prospective payments for outlier cases and nonemergent use of the emergency room; until 2002, called peer review organization

Quality improvement process: An approach undertaken to improve healthcare delivery that involves two principal steps: problem identification and process redesign

Quality indicator: A standard against which actual care may be measured to identify a level of performance for that standard

Quantitative analysis: A review of the health record to determine its completeness and accuracy

Range: A measure of variability between the smallest and largest observations in a frequency distribution

Rate: A measure used to compare an event over time; a comparison of the number of times an event did happen (numerator) with the number of times an event could have happened (denominator)

Ratio: 1. A calculation found by dividing one quantity by another 2. A general term that can include a number of specific measures such as proportion, percentage, and rate

Read Codes: The former name of the United Kingdom's CTV3 codes; named for James Read, the physician who originally devised the system to organize computer-based patient data in his primary care practice

Record locator service (RLS): A service that indicates where a given patient may have health information using probability equations

Recovery room report: A type of health record documentation used by nurses to document the patient's reaction to anesthesia and condition after surgery; also called **recovery room record**

Recruitment: The process of finding, soliciting, and attracting employees

Redundant arrays of independent (or inexpensive) disks (RAID): A method of ensuring data security

Reengineering: Fundamental rethinking and radical redesign of business processes to achieve significant performance improvements

Regional health information organization (RHIO): An organization that manages the local deployment of systems promoting and facilitating the exchange of healthcare data within a national health information network

Registration: The act of enrolling

Rehabilitation Act: Federal legislation passed in 1973 to protect handicapped employees against discrimination

Rehabilitation services: Health services provided to assist patients in achieving and maintaining their optimal level of function, self-care, and independence after some type of disability

Reimbursement: Compensation or repayment for healthcare services

Relational database: A type of database that stores data in predefined tables made up of rows and columns

Relative value unit (RVU): A number assigned to a procedure that describes its difficulty and expense in relationship to other procedures.

Release of information (ROI): The process of disclosing patient-identifiable information from the health record to another party

Remittance advice (RA): An explanation of payments (for example, claim denials) made by third-party payers

Request for information (RFI): A written communication often sent to a comprehensive list of vendors during the design phase of the systems development life cycle to ask for general product information

Request for proposal (RFP): A type of business correspondence asking for very specific product and contract information that is often sent to a narrow list of vendors that have been preselected after a review of requests for information during the design phase of the systems development life cycle

Requisition: A request from an authorized health record user to gain access to a medical record

Resident assessment instrument (RAI): A uniform assessment instrument developed by the Centers for Medicare and Medicaid Services to standardize the collection of skilled nursing facility patient data; includes the Minimum Data Set 2.0, triggers, and resident assessment protocols

Resident assessment protocol (RAP): A summary of a long-term care resident's medical condition and care requirements

Resident Assessment Validation and Entry (RAVEN): A type of data-entry software developed by the Centers for Medicare and Medicaid Services for long-term care facilities and used to collect Minimum Data Set assessments and to transmit data to state databases

Resource Utilization Groups, Version III (RUG-III): A case-mix–adjusted classification system based on Minimum Data Set assessments and used by skilled nursing facilities

Resource-based relative value scale (RBRVS): A Medicare reimbursement system implemented in 1992 to compensate physicians according to a fee schedule predicated on weights assigned on the basis of the resources required to provide the services

Respite care: A type of short-term care provided during the day or overnight to individuals in the home or institution to temporarily relieve the family home caregiver

Retrospective payment system: Type of fee-for-service reimbursement in which providers receive recompense after health services have been rendered

Retrospective review: The part of the utilization review process that concentrates on a review of clinical information following patient discharge

Retrospective utilization review: A review of records some time after the patient's discharge to determine any of several issues, including the quality or appropriateness of the care provided

Revenue codes: A three- or four-digit number in the chargemaster that totals all items and their charges for printing on the form used for Medicare billing

Revenues: The charges generated from providing healthcare services; earned and measurable income

Right-to-work laws: Federal legislation dealing with labor rights (examples include workers' compensation, child labor, and minimum wage laws)

Risk analysis: An assessment of possible security threats to the organization's data

Risk management (RM): A comprehensive program of activities intended to minimize the potential for injuries to occur in a facility and to anticipate and respond to ensuing liabilities for those injuries that do occur

Root-cause analysis: A technique used in performance improvement initiatives to discover the underlying causes of a problem

Row/record: A set of columns or a collection of related data items in a table

Rules and regulations: Operating documents that describe the rules and regulations under which a healthcare organization operates

Run chart: A type of graph that shows data points collected over time and identifies emerging trends or patterns

Safety management: A system for providing a risk-free environment for patients, visitors, and employees

Scatter diagram: A graph that visually displays the linear relationships among factors

Scorecards: Reports of outcomes measures to help leaders know what they have accomplished; sometimes called **dashboards**

Screen prototype: A sketch of the user interface of each screen that is anticipated in a project

Secondary data source: Data derived from the primary patient record, such as an index or a database

Secondary storage: The permanent storage of data and programs on disks or tapes

Security: 1. The means to control access and protect information from accidental or intentional disclosure to unauthorized persons and from unauthorized alteration, destruction, or loss 2. The physical protection of facilities and equipment from theft, damage, or unauthorized access; collectively, the policies, procedures, and safeguards designed to protect the confidentiality of information, maintain the integrity and availability of information systems, and control access to the content of these systems

Security breach: A violation of the policies or standards developed to ensure security

Security management: The oversight of facilities, equipment, and other resources, including human resources and technology, to reduce the possibility of harm to or theft of these assets of an organization

Security program: A plan outlining the policies and procedures created to protect healthcare information

Security standards: Statements that describe the processes and procedures meant to ensure that patient-identifiable health information remains confidential and protected from unauthorized disclosure, alteration, and destruction

Security threat: A situation that has the potential to damage a healthcare organization's information system

Sentinel event: According to the JCAHO, an unexpected occurrence involving death or serious physical or psychological injury, or the risk thereof

Sequence diagram: A systems analysis tool for documenting the interaction between an actor and the information system

Serial numbering system: A type of health record identification and filing system in which patients are assigned a different but unique numerical identifier for every admission

Serial–unit numbering system: A health record identification system in which patient numbers are assigned in a serial manner but records are brought forward and filed under the last number assigned

Server: A type of computer that makes it possible to share information resources across a network of client computers

Server redundancy: Situation where two servers are duplicating effort

Severity-of-illness screening criteria: Standards used to determine the most appropriate setting of care based on the level of clinical signs and symptoms that a patient shows upon presentation to a healthcare facility

Shared systems: Systems developed by data-processing companies in the 1960s and 1970s to address the computing needs of healthcare organizations that could not afford, or chose not to purchase, their own mainframe computing systems

Skilled nursing facility (SNF): A long-term care facility with an organized professional staff and permanent facilities (including inpatient beds) that provides continuous nursing and other health-related, psychosocial, and personal services to patients who are not in an acute phase of illness but who primarily require continued care on an inpatient basis

Skilled nursing facility prospective payment system (SNF PPS): A per-diem reimbursement system implemented in July 1998 for costs (routine, ancillary, and capital) associated with covered skilled nursing facility services furnished to Medicare Part A beneficiaries

Social Security Act of 1935: The federal legislation that originally established the Social Security program as well as unemployment compensation, and support for mothers and children; amended in 1965 to create the Medicare and Medicaid programs

Social Security number (SSN): A unique numerical identifier assigned to every U.S. citizen

Software: A program that directs the hardware components of a computer system to perform the tasks required

Source-oriented health record format: A system of health record organization in which information is arranged according to the patient care department that provided the care

Special-cause variation: An unusual source of variation that occurs outside a process but affects it

Specialty software: A type of applications software that performs specialized, niche functions such as encoding or drawing and painting

Speech recognition: Situation where speech is converted to text on a screen

Staff model health maintenance organization: A type of health maintenance that employs physicians to provide healthcare services to subscribers

Staff retention: The process of keeping valued employees on the job and reducing turnover

Stage of the neoplasm: A classification of malignancies (cancers) according to the anatomic extent of the tumor, such as primary neoplasm, regional lymph nodes, and metastases

Standard: 1. A scientifically based statement of expected behavior against which structures, processes, and outcomes can be measured 2. A model or example established by authority, custom, or general consent or a rule established by an authority as a measure of quantity, weight, extent, value, or quality

Standard deviation: A measure of variability that describes the deviation from the mean of a frequency distribution in the original units of measurement; the square root of the variance

Standard vocabulary: A vocabulary that is accepted throughout the healthcare industry

Standards development organizations (SDOs): Private or government agencies involved in the development of healthcare informatics standards at a national or international level

Standing committees: Committees that are put in place to oversee ongoing and cross-functional issues (examples include the medical staff committee, a quality improvement committee, or an infection control committee)

State Children's Health Insurance Program (SCHIP): The children's healthcare program implemented as part of the Balanced Budget Act of 1997; sometimes referred to as the Children's Health Insurance Program, or CHIP

State workers' compensation insurance funds: Funds that provide a stable source of insurance coverage for work-related illnesses and injuries and serve to protect employers from underwriting uncertainties by making it possible to have continuing availability of workers' compensation coverage

Statistical process control chart: A type of run chart that includes both upper and lower control limits and indicates whether a process is stable or unstable

Statutory law: Written law established by federal and state legislatures

Storage area network (SAN): Storage devices organized into a network so that they can be accessible from any server in the network.

Storage management software: Software used to manage the SAN, keep track of where data are stored, and move older data to less expensive, but still accessible, storage locations

Storyboard: A type of poster that includes text and graphics to describe and illustrate the activities of a performance improvement project

Straight numeric filing system: A health record filing system in which health records are arranged in ascending numerical order

Strategic decision making: A type of decision making that is usually limited to individuals, such as boards of directors, chief executive officers, and top-level executives, who make decisions about the healthcare organization's strategic direction

Strategic information systems planning: A process for setting IS priorities within an organization; the process of identifying and prioritizing IS needs based on the organization's strategic goals with the intent of ensuring that all IS technology initiatives are integrated and aligned with the organization's overall strategic plan

Stress testing: Testing performed toward the end of EHR implementation to ensure that the actual number, or load, of transactions that would be performed during peak hours can be performed

Structure and content standards: Common data elements and definitions of the data elements to be included in an electronic patient record

Structured decision: A decision made by following a formula or a step-by-step process

Structured query language (SQL): A fourth-generation computer language that includes both DDL and DML components and is used to create and manipulate relational databases

Structure indicators: Quality indicators that measure the attributes of an organizational setting, such as number and qualifications of staff, adequacy of equipment and facilities, and adequacy of organizational policies and procedures

Subacute care: A type of step-down care provided after a patient is released from an acute care hospital (including nursing homes and other facilities that provide medical care, but not surgical or emergency care)

Subject matter jurisdiction: Pertaining to district courts, jurisdiction to hear cases involving felonies and misdemeanors that fall under federal statutes

Subpoena ad testificandum: A command to appear at a certain time and place to give testimony on a certain matter

Subpoena duces tecum: A written document directing individuals or organizations to furnish relevant documents and records

Summons: An instrument used to begin a civil action or special proceeding and is a means of acquiring jurisdiction over a party

Supercomputer: The largest, fastest, and most expensive type of computer that exists today

Supervisory management: Management level that oversees the organization's efforts at the staff level and monitors the effectiveness of everyday operations and individual performance against preestablished standards

Supervisory managers: Managers who oversee small (two- to ten-person) functional workgroups or teams and often perform hands-on functions in addition to supervisory functions

Supplemental medical insurance (Medicare Part B): A voluntary medical insurance program that helps pay for physicians' services, medical services, and supplies not covered by Medicare Part A

Supply management: Management and control of the supplies used within an organization

Supreme Court: The highest court in the U.S. legal system; hears cases from the U.S. Courts of Appeals and the highest state courts when federal statutes, treaties, or the U.S. Constitution is involved

System build: The creation of data dictionaries, tables, decision support rules, templates for data entry, screen layouts, and reports used in a system

System design: The second phase of the systems development life cycle

System implementation: The third phase of the systems development life cycle

Systemized Nomenclature of Medicine Clinical Terminology (SNOMED CT): A concept-based terminology consisting of more than 110,000 concepts with linkages to more than 180,000 terms with unique computer-readable codes

System maintenance and evaluation: The final phase of the systems development life cycle

System planning and analysis: The first phase of the systems development life cycle

Systems development life cycle (SDLC): A model used to represent the ongoing process of developing (or purchasing) information systems

Systems thinking: An objective way of looking at work-related ideas and processes with the goal of allowing people to uncover ineffective patterns of behavior and thinking and then finding ways to make lasting improvements

System testing(s): A type of testing performed by an independent organization to identify problems in information systems

Table: An organized arrangement of data, usually in columns and rows

Tactical decision making: A type of decision making that usually affects departments or business units (and sometimes policies and procedures) and includes short- and medium-range plans, schedules, and budgets

Tax Equity and Fiscal Responsibility Act of 1982 (TEFRA): The federal legislation that modified Medicare's retrospective reimbursement system for inpatient hospital stays by requiring implementation of diagnosis-related groups and the acute care prospective payment system

Technical component (TC): The portion of radiological and other procedures that is facility based or nonphysician based (for example, radiology films, equipment, overhead, endoscopic suites, and so on)

Technical safeguard provisions: Five broad categories of controls that can be implemented from a technical standpoint using computer software: access controls, audit controls, data integrity, person or entity authentication, and transmission security

Telecommunications: Voice and data communications

Temporary Assistance for Needy Families (TANF): A federal program that provides states with grants to be spent on time-limited cash assistance for low-income families, generally limiting a family's lifetime cash welfare benefits to a maximum of five years and permitting states to impose other requirements

Terminal-digit filing system: A system of health record identification and filing in which the last digit or group of digits (terminal digits) in the health record number determines file placement

Textual: A term referring to the narrative nature of much of clinical documentation to date

Third-party payers: An insurance company (for example, Blue Cross/Blue Shield) or healthcare program (for example, Medicare) that reimburses healthcare providers (second party) and/or patients (first party) for the delivery of medical services

Tort: An action brought when one party believes that another party caused harm through wrongful conduct and seeks compensation for that harm

Total length of stay (discharge days): The sum of the days of stay of any group of inpatients discharged during a specific period of time

Tracer methodology: An evaluation that follows (traces) the hospital experiences of specific patients to assess the quality of patient care; part of the new Joint Commission on Accreditation of Healthcare Organizations survey process

Traditional fee-for-service reimbursement: A reimbursement method involving third-party payers who compensate providers after the healthcare services have been delivered; payment is based on specific services provided to subscribers

Transaction-processing system: A computer-based information system that keeps track of an organization's business transactions through inputs (for example, transaction data such as admissions, discharges, and transfers in a hospital) and outputs (for example, census reports and bills)

Transaction standards: Standards that support the uniform format and sequence of data during transmission from one healthcare entity to another

Transcriptionists: A specially trained typist who understands medical terminology and translates physicians' verbal dictation into written reports

Transfer record: A review of the patient's acute stay along with current status, discharge and transfer orders, and any additional instructions that accompanies the patient when he or she is transferred to another facility; also called a **referral form**

Traumatic injury: A wound or injury included in a trauma registry

Treatment, payment, and operations (TPO): Term used in the HIPAA Privacy Rule pertaining to broad activities under normal treatment, payment, and operations activities, important because of the rule's many exceptions to the release and disclosure of personal health information

Trial court: The lowest tier of state court, usually divided into two courts: the court of limited jurisdiction, which hears cases pertaining to a particular subject matter or involving crimes of lesser severity or civil matters of lower dollar amounts; and the court of general jurisdiction, which hears more serious criminal cases or civil cases that involve large amounts of money

TRICARE: The federal healthcare program that provides coverage for the dependents of armed forces personnel and for retirees receiving care outside military treatment facilities in which the federal government pays a percentage of the cost; formerly known as Civilian Health and Medical Program of the Uniformed Services

TRICARE Extra: A cost-effective preferred provider network TRICARE option in which costs for healthcare are lower than for the standard TRICARE program because a physician or medical specialist is selected from a network of civilian healthcare professionals who participate in TRICARE Extra

TRICARE Prime: A TRICARE program that provides the most comprehensive healthcare benefits at the lowest cost of the three TRICARE options, in which military treatment facilities serve as the principal source of healthcare and a primary care manager is assigned to each enrollee

TRICARE Prime Remote: A program that provides active-duty service members in the United States with a specialized version of TRICARE Prime while they are assigned to duty stations in areas not served by the traditional military healthcare system

TRICARE Senior Prime: A program that provides active-duty service members in the United States with a specialized version of TRICARE Prime while they are assigned to duty stations in areas not served by the traditional military healthcare system

TRICARE Standard: A TRICARE program that allows eligible beneficiaries to choose any physician or healthcare provider, which permits the most flexibility but may be the most expensive

Turnkey system: A computer application that may be purchased from a vendor and installed without modification or further development by the user organization

UB-92 (CMS-1450): A Medicare form used for standardized uniform billing

Unbundling: The practice of using multiple codes to bill for the various individual steps in a single procedure rather than using a single code that includes all of the steps of the comprehensive procedure

Unified Medical Language System (UMLS): A program initiated by the National Library of Medicine to build an intelligent, automated system that can understand biomedical concepts, words, and expressions and their interrelationships

Unified messaging: The ability for an individual to receive and/or retrieve various forms of messaging at a single access point, including voice, e-mail, fax, and video mail

Unified modeling language (UML): A common data-modeling notation used in conjunction with object-oriented database design

Uniform Ambulatory Care Data Set (UACDS): A data set developed by the National Committee on Vital and Health Statistics consisting of a minimum set of patient/client-specific data elements to be collected in ambulatory care settings

Uniform Hospital Discharge Data Set (UHDDS): A core set of data elements adopted by the US Department of Health, Education, and Welfare in 1974 that are collected by hospitals on all discharges and all discharge abstract systems

Unique identification number: A combination of numbers or alphanumeric characters assigned to a particular patient

Unique physician identification number (UPIN): A unique numerical identifier created by the Centers for Medicare and Medicaid Services for use by physicians who bill for services provided to Medicare patients

Unit numbering system: A health record identification system in which the patient receives a unique medical record number at the time of the first encounter that is used for all subsequent encounters

Unit testing: The testing step in EHR implementation that ensures that each data element is captured, recorded, and processed appropriately within a given application

Universal precautions: A set of procedures designed specifically to minimize or eliminate the spread of infectious disease agents from one individual to another during the provision of healthcare services

Unstructured decision: A decision that is made without following a prescribed method, formula, or pattern

Upcoding: The practice of assigning diagnostic or procedural codes that represent higher payment rates than the codes that actually reflect the services provided to patients

Use case diagram: A systems analysis technique used to document a software project from a user's perspective

Use, disclosures, and requests: Three types of situations in which personal health information is handled: use, which is internal to a covered entity or its business associate; disclosure, which is the dissemination of PHI from a covered entity or its business associate; and requests for PHI made by a covered entity or its business associate

User groups: Groups composed of users of a particular computer system

Uses and disclosures: Referring to the use and disclosure of a patient's personal health information

Usual, customary, and reasonable (UCR) charges: Method of evaluating providers' fees in which the third party payer pays for fees that are "usual" in that provider's practice; "customary" in the community; and "reasonable" for the situation

Utility program: A software program that supports, enhances, or expands existing programs in a computer system, such as virus checking, data recovery, backup, and data compression

Utilization management (UM): 1. The planned, systematic review of the patients in a healthcare facility against care criteria for admission, continued stay, and discharge 2. A collection of systems and processes to ensure that facilities and resources, both human and nonhuman, are used maximally and are consistent with patient care needs

Utilization management organization: An organization that reviews the appropriateness of the care setting and resources used to treat a patient

Utilization review (UR): The process of determining whether the medical care provided to a specific patient is necessary according to preestablished objective screening criteria at time frames specified in the organization's utilization management plan

Utilization Review Act: The federal legislation that requires hospitals to conduct continued-stay reviews for Medicare and Medicaid patients

Values statement: A short description that communicates an organization's social and cultural belief system

Variable costs: Resources expended that vary with the activity of the organization, for example, medication expenses vary with patient volume

Variance: A measure of variability that gives the average of the squared deviations from the mean; in financial management, the difference between the budgeted amount and the actual amount of a line item; in project management, the difference between the original project plan and current estimates

V codes: A set of ICD-9-CM codes used to classify occasions when circumstances other than disease or injury are recorded as the reason for the patient's encounter with health-care providers

Vendor system: A computer system developed by a commercial company not affiliated with the healthcare organization

Videoconferencing: A communications service that allows a group of people to exchange information over a network by using a combination of video and computer technology

Vision statement: A short description of an organization's ideal future state

Vital Statistics: Data related to births, deaths, marriages, and fetal deaths

Vocabulary standards: A common definition for medical terms to encourage consistent descriptions of an individual's condition in the health record

Voir dire: The process of jury selection

Voluntary Disclosure Program: A program unveiled in 1998 by the OIG that encourages healthcare providers to voluntarily report fraudulent conduct affecting Medicare, Medicaid, and other federal healthcare programs

Web appliance: A computer without secondary storage capability that is designed to connect to a network

Web services architecture (WSA): An emerging architecture that utilizes Web-based tools to permit communication among different software applications

Wide area network (WAN): A computer network that connects devices across a large geographical area

Wireless local area network (WLAN): A data transmission network that uses an unguided medium such as radio waves or microwaves

Workers' compensation: The medical and income insurance coverage for certain employees in unusually hazardous jobs

Workflow: Any work process that must be handled by more than one person

Workstation: A computer designed to accept data from multiple sources in order to assist in managing information for daily activities and to provide a convenient means of entering data as desired by the user at the point of care

World Health Organization (WHO): The United Nations specialized agency for health, established on April 7, 1948, with the objective, as set out in its constitution, of the attainment by all peoples of the highest possible levels of health; responsible for *The International Statistical Classification of Diseases & Related Health Problems* **(ICD-10)**

Index

Capitation reimbursement methodology, 271
Care plans, 56
Career planning, 901–2
Case fatality rate, 476
Case management, 523
Case-mix group, relative weights of, 278, 288
Case-mixed index, 278
Cause-and-effect diagram in root-cause analysis, 575, 577
Cause-specific death rate, 475, 476
Census data, inpatient, 453–55
Centers for Disease Control and Prevention
    as healthcare data source, 170, 481–82
    National Immunization Program of, 409, 410
    standards for disease prevention maintained by, 518
Centers for Medicare and Medicaid Services
    administration of Medicare and Medicaid by, 241
    IRVEN provided to IRFs by, 288
    long-term care feedback from, 83
    medical service reporting requirements for Medicare by, 210
    as policy-making body, 35
    public reporting in hospitals introduced by, 128
    quality improvement organizations overseen by, 512–14, 524–25
    RBRVS system implemented by, 279
Central tendency, measures of, 434–36
Certification Commission on Health Information Technology, 128, 180
Certification for Medicare participation, 629
CHAMPVA healthcare program, 260
Change management, 566–67
    barriers to change in, 773
    in quality improvement model, 916
Chargemaster
    common elements in, 312
    in fee-for-service reimbursement, 268–69, 270
    maintenance of, 312, 314–15
    management of, 309, 311
    sample section of, 309
Chart conversion for EHR system, 147–48
Charts to display data, 444, 446–48
Checksheets as data collection tool, 578
Chief executive officer, hospital, 619, 818, 819
Chief financial officer, hospital, 620, 797
Chief information officer, 620
    roles of, 808, 818
Chief information security officer, role of, 818–19
Chief medical informatics officer, role of, 819
Chief nursing officer, 621
Chief operating officer, hospital, 620

Chief privacy officer, role of, 820
Chief security officer, functions of, 860, 861
Claims management, 529–32
Classification systems, 194
Clinical coding as HIM department function, 357–59, 374
Clinical data in health records, 51–52
Clinical data repository, 121
Clinical decision support for EHRs, 117, 118, 138–39
Clinical decision support systems, 121–22, 803, 837
Clinical forms committee, 371
Clinical information systems, inpatient, 119, 801–3
Clinical observations in hospital acute care records, 54, 56, 58, 59
Clinical practice guidelines and protocols, 504–8
    examples of, 505–7
Clinical privileges of medical staff, 620
Clinical problem solving, health record information used in, 41–42
Clinical quality assessment, 499, 502–19
    planning and implementing, 514–17
    sample summary report for, 516–17
    standards applied to, 504–14
Clinical quality management, 497–549
    processes included in, 499
    real-world case for, 546
    recent initiatives in, 544–46
Clinical quality standards, 503
Clinical representation standards, 184
Clinical trials, 416–17
Clinical vocabularies, 194
    HIPAA official, 196
    history and importance of, 195
    real-world case in, 230
    research in, 228–29
    users of, 195–96
CMS-1450 form. See UB-92 form
CMS-1500 form, 294, 297–300
    form locators for, 299
    sample, 298
Coding audits, 220–21, 323–24
Coding policies and procedures, 220
Coding practice
    ethical considerations in, 654–55
    relationship of corporate compliance and, 320–25
Coding process, 218–21
    quality assessment for, 220–21
    steps in, 220
Coding quality
    elements of, 218–19
    management of, 316–17
Coding sets, HIPAA official medical, 196

Ensure Career Success with an AHIMA Certification

Registered Health Information Technician (RHIT)

AHIMA's Registered Health Information Technician (RHIT) credential helps you stand out from the crowd, showing employers a higher competency level and a commitment to working in HIM.

RHITs ensure the quality of medical records by verifying their completeness, accuracy, reliability, and security. They also analyze patient data to improve patient care and manage costs.

RHITs enjoy job placements in a variety of settings, including hospitals, physician practices, nursing homes, home health agencies, and public agencies. RHITs are key team members and leaders in the delivery of successful health information management content and delivery.

"My current job as coding quality analyst is where my credentials have paid off— it was a requirement for the job. This job pays more and I really enjoy what I do"

Cathy M. Straub, RHIT, CCS
Mercy Hospital of Pittsburgh
Pittsburgh, PA

Make the right move…pair your degree and experience with AHIMA certification to maximize your career possibilities.

AHIMA is the premier organization for HIM professionals, with more than 50,000 members. AHIMA certification carries a strong reputation for quality and for mastering rigorous certification requirements.

For more information on AHIMA credentials, you can:
Visit our Web site at **www.ahima.org/certification**
E-mail AHIMA at **info@ahima.org**
Call **(800) 335-5535**

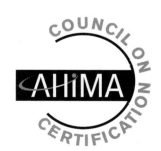

Look for These **Quality AHIMA Publications** at **Bookstores, Libraries,** and **Online**

- *Applying Inpatient Coding Skills under Prospective Payment*
- *Basic CPT/HCPCS Coding*
- *Basic ICD-9-CM Coding*
- *The Best of In Confidence*
- *Calculating and Reporting Healthcare Statistics*
- *Clinical Coding Workout: Practice Exercises for Skill Development*
- *Coding and Reimbursement for Hospital Inpatient Services*
- *Coding and Reimbursement for Hospital Outpatient Services*
- *CPT/HCPCS Coding and Reimbursement for Physician Services*
- *Documentation for Acute Care* (Book and CD)
- *Documentation for Ambulatory Care*
- *Documentation and Reimbursement for Behavioral Healthcare Services*
- *Documentation and Reimbursement for Long-Term Care* (Book and CD)
- *Documentation and Reimbursement for Home Care and Hospice Programs*

- *Effective Management of Coding Services*
- *Electronic Health Record*
- *Essentials of Healthcare Finance* (Workbook)
- *Healthcare Code Sets, Clinical Terminologies, and Classification Systems*
- *Health Information Management*
- *Health Information Management Technology*
- *Health Information Management Compliance* (Book and CD)
- *HIPAA in Practice*
- *ICD-9-CM Diagnostic Coding and Reimbursement for Physician Services*
- *ICD-9-CM Diagnostic Coding for Long-Term Care and Home Care*
- *ICD-10-CM and ICD-10-PCS Preview* (Book and CD)
- *Pocket Glossary of Health Information Management and Technology*
- *Principles of Healthcare Reimbursement*
- *Quality and Performance Improvement in Healthcare*
- *Statistical Applications for Health Information Management*

More Information

For details and easy ordering, visit **www.ahima.org/store.**

For textbook content questions, contact **publications@ahima.org** or **(800) 335-5535.**

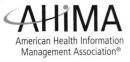

AHIMA
American Health Information
Management Association®

Play a Key Role in the Migration to an Electronic Health Record

AHIMA Helps You Take Center Stage in Advancing Healthcare

AHIMA Offers These Free Practice Standards

- Core Data Sets
- Delving into Computer-assisted Coding
- The Complete Medical Record in a Hybrid EHR Environment
- The Strategic Importance of Electronic Health Records Management
- Implementing e-Signatures
- E-mail as Provider-Patient Electronic Communication Medium and Its Impact on the EHR
- Electronic Document Management as a Component of the EHR
- Core Data Sets for the Physician Practice EHR
- Speech Recognition in the EHR

- HIM Practice Transformation
- The Role of the Personal Health Record in the EHR
- The Legal Process and EHR
- Guidelines for Defining the Legal Health Record
- Update: Maintaining a Legally Sound Health Record—Paper and Electronic
- Surveying the RHIO Landscape
- Guidelines for Developing a Data Dictionary
- Interpretation of Emerging Federal Guidelines for EHR as Legal Evidence and the Impact on Providers
- Standards for Minimum Content for the Legal EHR

And much more.
Go to www.ahima.org and click on "HIM Resources."

The e-HIM® work groups are supported in part by grants to the Foundation of Research and Education (FORE) from Dictaphone Corporation, McKesson, MedQuist, Meta Health Technology Inc., 3M Healthcare Services, Initiate Systems, Inc, and Precyse Solutions, Inc.

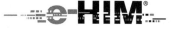

AHIMA provides its industry-leading e-HIM® education and advocacy programs to support the effective use of information technology to manage patient information and healthcare data.

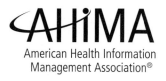

American Health Information Management Association®

AHIMA is the premier association of health information management (HIM) professionals. AHIMA's 50,000 members are dedicated to the effective management of personal health information needed to deliver quality healthcare to the public. Founded in 1928 to improve the quality of medical records, AHIMA is committed to advancing the HIM profession in an increasingly electronic and global environment through leadership in advocacy, education, certification, and lifelong learning. For information about the Association, go to www.ahima.org.

MDC major diagnostic category
MCO managed care organization
MIS management information system
MSO management service organization
MPI master patient index
MGMA Medical Group Management Association
MEDLINE Medical Literature, Analysis, and Retrieval System Online
MFS Medicare fee schedule
MMA Medicare Modernization Act of 2003
MSN Medicare Summary Notice
MDS Minimum Data Set for Long-Term Care
MDS 2.0 Minimum Data Set Version 2.0
NAHIT National Alliance for Health Information Technology
NCHS National Centers for Health Statistics
NCQA National Committee for Quality Assurance
NCVHS National Committee on Vital and Health Statistics
CF national conversion factor
NCCI National Correct Coding Initiative
NCPDP National Council for Prescription Drug Programs
NDC National Drug Codes
NGC National Guideline Clearinghouse
NHII national health information infrastructure
NHIN national health information network
NII-HIN National Information Infrastructure–Health Information Network Program
NIH National Institutes of Health
NLM National Library of Medicine
NPSGs national patient safety goals
NPDB National Practitioner Data Bank
NPI national provider identifier
NUCC National Uniform Claim Committee
NVAC National Vaccine Advisory Committee
NLP natural language processing
NAACCR North American Association of Central Cancer Registries
OODB object-oriented database

OSHA Occupational Safety and Health Act of 1970
ONC Office of the National Coordinator of Health Information Technology
OBRA Omnibus Budget Reconciliation Act
OSS operation support systems
OASIS Outcomes and Assessment Information Set
OCE outpatient code editor
OPPS outpatient prospective payment system
PAI patient assessment instrument
PSDA Patient Self-Determination Act
P4P pay for performance
P4Q pay for quality
PSI payment status indicator
PRO peer review organization
PMPM per member per month
PPPM per patient per month
PDA personal digital assistant
PHD personal health dimension
PHR personal health record
PBM pharmacy benefits manager
PHO physician-hospital organization
PACS picture archiving and communications system
PDSA plan-do-study-act cycle
POC point of care
POS point-of-service plan
PMS practice management system
PPO preferred provider organization
PCM primary care manager
PCP primary care physician
PBX private branch exchange
PC professional component
PSRO professional standards review organization
PACE Program of All-Inclusive Care for the Elderly
PMR proportionate mortality rate
PHI protected health information
QIO quality improvement organization
RLS record locator service
RAID redundant arrays of independent (or inexpensive) disks